Essentials for
PG Pediatric Exam

OSCE · Spotters · Viva · Procedures

For DNB, MD, Diploma, MRCPCH Exams

Essentials for PG Pediatric Exam

OSCE · Spotters · Viva · Procedures

For DNB, MD, Diploma, MRCPCH Exams

Baldev Prajapati
MD DPed FIAP MNAMS
Professor Emeritus and Director
Medical Education and Research
Bhagyoday Medical College and Multispecialty Hospital
Kadi, Gujarat, India

Forewords

Piyush Gupta
S Balasubramanian

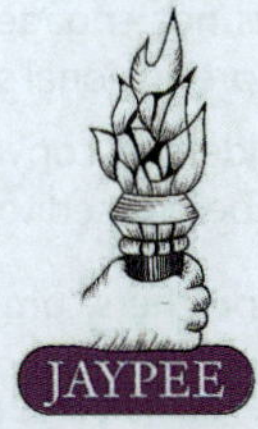

JAYPEE BROTHERS MEDICAL PUBLISHERS
The Health Sciences Publisher
New Delhi | London

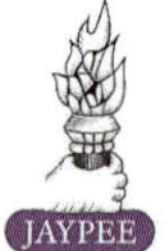

Jaypee Brothers Medical Publishers (P) Ltd

Headquarters
EMCA House, 23/23-B
Ansari Road, Daryaganj
New Delhi 110 002, India
Landline: +91-11-23272143, +91-11-23272703
+91-11-23282021, +91-11-23245672
e-mail: jaypee@jaypeebrothers.com

Corporate Office
4838/24, Ansari Road, Daryaganj
New Delhi 110 002, India
Phone: +91-11-43574357
Fax: +91-11-43574314
e-mail: jaypee@jaypeebrothers.com

Overseas Office
JP Medical Ltd.
83, Victoria Street, London
SW1H 0HW (UK)
Phone: +44-20 3170 8910
e-mail: info@jpmedpub.com

EU GPSR Authorised Representative
Logos Europe, 9 rue Nicolas Poussin
17000, La Rochelle, France
Phone: +33 (0) 6 67 93 73 78
e-mail: contact@logoseurope.eu

Website: www.jaypeebrothers.com
Website: www.jaypeedigital.com

Inquiries for bulk sales may be solicited at: jaypee@jaypeebrothers.com

Essentials for PG Pediatric Exam: OSCE · Spotters · Viva · Procedures *(For DNB, MD, Diploma, MRCPCH Exams)*

First Edition: **2026**

ISBN: 978-93-7545-456-4

Printed at: Samrat Offset Pvt. Ltd.

Dedicated to

My lovely granddaughter Mishika and my students who motivated and inspired me to leave a legacy for them

Foreword

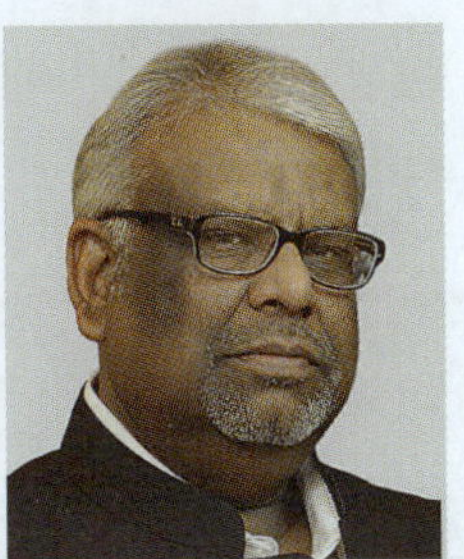

Postgraduate pediatric examinations today demand not only sound theoretical knowledge but also the ability to apply that knowledge with clarity, confidence, and clinical precision. The shift toward competency-based assessments—through OSCEs, structured viva formats, spotters, and skill-based evaluations—has made it essential for trainees to prepare with resources that are comprehensive, practical, and aligned with current examination standards. *Essentials for PG Pediatric Exam (OSCE, Spotters, Viva and Procedures)* by Dr Baldev Prajapati, an eminent Pediatrician and distinguished Medical Educator, fulfils this need with remarkable thoroughness.

Dr Prajapati brings to this work decades of academic leadership, clinical excellence, and a deep commitment to nurturing the next generation of pediatricians. His experience as Professor Emeritus and Director of Medical Education and Research at Bhagyoday Medical College and Multispecialty Hospital, Kadi, Gujarat, and his long-standing contributions at GCS Medical College, Ahmedabad, Gujarat, are reflected in the clarity, structure, and pedagogic strength of this book.

The text is thoughtfully organized into four sections:

Section 1, devoted to OSCEs, spans the full breadth of pediatrics—from history taking, physical examination, growth and development, nutrition, fluids, and ABG to system-wise stations covering neonatology, genetics, immunology, infections, cardiology, neurology, nephrology, endocrinology, and more. The inclusion of radiology, statistics, drugs, instruments, counseling, and preventive pediatrics makes this section exceptionally holistic.

Section 2 presents high-yield spotters on common genetic, metabolic, neuromuscular, and congenital conditions, enabling rapid recognition—an essential skill in both examinations and clinical practice.

Section 3 covers frequently tested viva topics such as nutrition, anemia, development, neonatal resuscitation, tuberculosis, nephrotic syndrome, vaccines, and ECG interpretation, offering trainees a concise yet concept-oriented revision tool.

Section 4 focuses on common pediatric procedures, reinforcing the practical competencies expected of every postgraduate trainee.

This book stands out for its exam-oriented approach, clarity of presentation, and its ability to distil complex subjects into accessible, structured learning points. It will undoubtedly serve as a valuable companion for DNB, MD, Diploma, and MRCPCH aspirants, as well as for practicing pediatricians seeking quick revision.

I congratulate Dr Baldev Prajapati for creating a resource that will strengthen pediatric training and support learners in achieving excellence. I am confident that this book will become an essential part of every postgraduate student's preparation.

Piyush Gupta
MD FAMS FRCPCH
ICMR—AS Paintal Distinguished Scientist
Chair
Former National President
Indian Academy of Pediatrics (IAP)
Former Principal and Professor
Department of Pediatrics
University College of Medical Sciences
New Delhi, India

Foreword

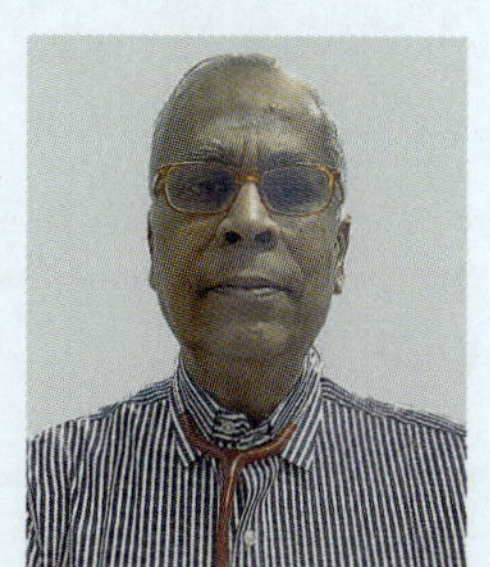

It is a privilege to write the foreword for Dr Baldev Prajapati's book intended for postgraduate students of pediatrics.

Dr Baldev Prajapati is among the most experienced and respected teachers in the field of pediatrics. With over four decades of dedicated involvement in postgraduate training across India, he has made a significant contribution to pediatric medical education. His teaching is highly regarded for its systematic and disciplined approach to the evaluation of complex clinical problems, as well as for his exceptional ability to convey core concepts of clinical pediatrics in a clear and practical manner.

Drawing upon his extensive experience, Dr Prajapati has developed this book in a structured and comprehensive format tailored to the needs of postgraduate students. The text addresses all major components relevant to MD, DNB, DCH, and MRCPCH clinical examinations, including OSCEs, spotters, viva, and procedures.

The book is enriched with high-quality illustrations sourced from Dr Prajapati's personal archives, which significantly enhance its practical utility. This publication will undoubtedly serve as a valuable and reliable reference for postgraduate students preparing for their clinical and practical examinations.

On a personal note, I sincerely commend Dr Baldev Prajapati for his dedication, perseverance, and commitment in producing this excellent academic resource.

S Balasubramanian
Senior Consultant Pediatrician
Former Medical Director
Kanchi Kamakoti CHILDS Trust Hospital
Chennai, Tamil Nadu, India

Preface

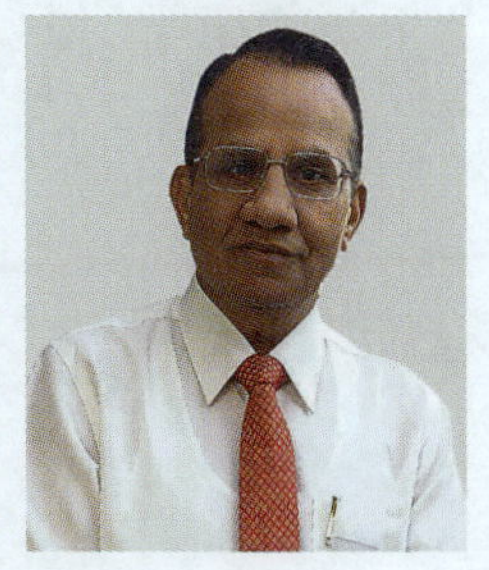

The case presentation in postgraduate examinations is conventional. The direction that discussion takes place during case presentation and the level of interrogation depend both upon the examinee's and examiner's approach. This leads to subjective assessment. Certain aspects of clinical pediatrics like interpretation of laboratory and radio-imaging pictures, clinical analysis of a given case scenario, counseling and communication skills, and statistics are most of the time overlooked in traditional examinations.

The Objective Structured Clinical Examination (OSCE) attempts to overcome these lacunae by providing a broad-based format to assess the candidate on several aspects of the subject. This objective pattern brings an element of uniformity. There is focus assessment because of a structured method of forming the questions. The variety of topics in childhood illnesses provides a wider source to the examiner to draw upon the OSCE questions. But OSCE is a nightmare for the candidate. Now, OSCE has become an integral part of every postgraduate practical examination. This book covers more than 600 OSCEs on almost all common topics. It is an attempt to sensitize and introduce the students to the OSCE format so that students can prepare accordingly. The student can assess himself by deciding the answer of each question and verifying it with the answer sheet given at the end of each chapter. This exercise will boost one's confidence and also guide for preparations accordingly.

"A picture is worth a thousand words and a video is worth a thousand pictures. I cannot define an elephant unless I have seen it." A glimpse of a clinical condition is sufficient for repercussion to your brain later, when you have come across a similar condition in the future. This is called spotter in clinical medicine. And spotter also is a part of postgraduate practical examinations. This book includes several common spotters. The students will find almost all conditions commonly asked in their practical examinations.

Many voluminous textbooks on pediatrics are available, and they need more concentration, time, and energy to read. Still, answers to many viva questions in the examination are not available in the textbooks. The students are always struggling to get answers of many viva questions. This book encompasses most common topics for viva questions, asked in postgraduate practical examinations. The answers provided are accurate, brief, and clear.

Common ward procedures asked in the examination are included in this book to complete all sections of practical examination.

The author had been an examiner for DNB, Diploma, MD, and other examinations for more than 40 years at different universities across the country. This book has taken present shape from his collective teaching experience, knowledge, experience of conducting practical examinations, and wisdom of more than four decades.

I hope that this book *Essentials for PG Pediatric Exam (OSCE, Spotters, Viva and Procedures)* would be useful to the students for their DNB, Diploma, MD, MRCPCH, and other examinations.

The readers are requested to send their suggestions regarding addition of specific topics, clarification in any of the questions included in this edition, modification in format, etc., at *baldevprajapati55@gmail.com*. Your feedback and suggestions will be invaluable for improving the next edition.

I am deeply indebted to two learned, eminent, and most popular academicians and teachers, Dr Piyush Gupta and Dr S Balasubramanium, for writing the foreword for this book.

This book is affectionately dedicated to my lovely granddaughter, Mishika. No amount of words can express my gratitude to my wife, Dr (Mrs) Rajal Prajapati; my daughters, Dr Aakanksha and Dr Aalapi; and my sons-in-law, Dr Mukund and Mr Sumit, who allowed me ample time for preparing this book.

Baldev Prajapati

Acknowledgments

I would like to profusely thank Nisarg Shah, who is sincere, dedicated, and meticulous in his work, for typesetting and composing.

My special thanks go to the staff of Aakanksha Children Clinic, Ahmedabad, Gujarat, India, for their help in preparing this book.

I extend my sincere gratitude to Shri Jitendra P Vij (Group Chairman), Mr Ankit Vij (Managing Director), Mr MS Mani (Group President), Mr Sabyasachi Hazra (Director—PG and PNR Content), Nikita Chauhan (Publishing Manager), and the staff of M/s Jaypee Brothers Medical Publishers (P) Ltd, New Delhi, India, for their generous help in all possible ways to bring out this book.

Baldev Prajapati

Contents

SECTION 1: OSCE

SECTION 2: Spotters Diagnosis

SECTION 3: Viva

SECTION 4: Common Procedures

SECTION

1

OSCE

1. History
2. Physical Examination
3. Growth
4. Development and Psychiatry
5. Nutrition
6. Fluid, Electrolytes and ABG
7. Neonatology
8. Genetics and Syndromes
9. Metabolic Disorders
10. Immunology
11. Rheumatology
12. Infections
13. Gastroenterology
14. Pulmonology
15. Cardiology
16. Neurology
17. Nephrology
18. Hematology–Oncology
19. Endocrinology
20. Ophthalmology
21. Dermatology
22. Radiology
23. Statistics
24. Drugs and Instruments
25. Counseling
26. Preventive and Social Medicine

CHAPTER 1

History

QUESTIONS

Q-1. What diagnosis is suggested by following pointers in history?

A. Changing handwriting
B. Micrognathia—small handwriting
C. Change or no perception of smell and taste
D. History of precipitation of skin rashes by amoxicillin
E. ACE inhibitor drugs are known to aggravate the symptom
F. Precipitation of an episode of abdominal pain by phenobarbitone in a case of recurrent abdominal pain

Q-2. Answer the following statements—True or False:

A. Mother is the most reliable informant.
B. Children above the age of 7 years often provide good information.
C. History should not be started with open-ended questions.
D. There is no place to close-ended questions in pediatric history taking.

Q-3. Answer the following questions pertaining to pediatric history taking:

A. Five illustrations of disease in pediatrics common at certain age groups
B. Examples of X-linked disorders
C. Examples of diseases known to have geographical distributions
D. Examples of disease known to have ethnic, caste or community distributions

Q-4. Answer the following questions on cough:

A. Most common causes of cough in neonates
B. Qualify a symptom of cough for presumptive tuberculosis
C. What are causes of cough with whoop?
D. A healthy 18-months-old child was playing with toys. He developed sudden choking and cough. What is most probable cause?
E. Qualify a symptom of cough for bronchial asthma
F. Which drugs are known to aggravate the cough?

Q-5. Define history of tuberculous contact as per NTEP.

Q-6. What are common causes of bad obstetric history with abortions, sill births or neonatal deaths?

Q-7. Define delayed passage meconium. What are common causes for delayed passage of meconium?

Q-8. Define delayed fall of umbilical cord. Name the conditions associated with delayed fall of umbilical cord.

Q-9. Define consanguinity. What are degrees of consanguinity? What disorders are common with consanguinity?

Q-10. What is modified Kuppuswamy scale?

Q-11. A 10-months-old boy presents from Lohana family with severe pallor and hepatosplenomegaly. What are important points to derive in the history?

Q-12. A 3-months-old infants presents with persistent jaundice, hepatomegaly and seizures due to hypoglycemia. No fever. Baby was delivered at full term with birth weight 2.6 kg with uneventful antenatal and postnatal periods. Mother noted bilateral cataract 15 days back, she was sure regarding absence of cataract before 15 days. What are important points to derive in the history?

Q-13. Match the following based on day of appearance of rash in a febrile child and probable diagnosis:

A. Day 1	Dengue fever
B. Day 2	Typhus fever
C. Day 3	Typhoid fever
D. Day 4	Varicella
E. Day 5	Scarlet fever
F. Day 6	Measles
G. Day 7	Smallpox

Q-14. Match the following as named first to sixth disease, presenting as fever with rash:

A. First	Human herpes virus 6 and 7 (HHV6 and 7)
B. Second	Erythema infectiosum (slapped Cheek syndrome)
C. Third	Filatov–Duke disease
D. Fourth	Rubeola (measles)
E. Fifth	Scarlet fever
F. Sixth	Rubella

Q-15. Answer the following questions pertaining to pica.

A. Definition of pica
B. Common types of pica
C. Complications of pica

ANSWERS

A-1. A. Rheumatic chorea, Wilson's disease
B. Parkinson's disease
C. COVID-19
D. Epstein–Barr virus infection
E. Cough
F. Porphyria

A-2. A. True
B. True
C. False
D. False

A-3. A. Common age for certain childhood diseases.

Disease	*Age*
Febrile seizures	6 months to 5 years
Kawasaki disease	<5 years
Rheumatic fever	5–15 years
Rheumatic chorea	10–13 years
Infantile tremor syndrome	6 months to 2 years
Breath-holding spells	6 months to 2 years
Cyanotic spell in TOF	2 months to 2 years
Systemic lupus erythematosus (SLE)	Adolescents
Wilson's disease	>5 years

B. *X-linked disorders:*
- Hemophilia A
- Duchenne muscular dystrophy
- Color blindness
- G-6-P-D deficiency
- Fragile X-syndrome
- Rett syndrome
- X-linked agammaglobulinemia

C. *Diseases with geographical distributions:*
- *Leishmaniasis (Kala-azar):* Bihar
- *Yellow fever:* Africa, South America
- *Japanese encephalitis:* Assam, Uttar Pradesh, Bihar, Odisha
- *Thyroid goiter:* Himalayan and Sub-Himalayan regions in India

D. *Examples of disease having ethnic or community:*
- *Thalassemia:* Lohana, Jain, Bhanushali
- *Sickle-cell disease:* Scheduled tribes

A-4. A. *Causes of cough in neonates:*
- Aspiration syndrome
- Pertussis (Whooping cough)
- Chlamydial infection

B. Persistent, non-remittent cough for more than two weeks

C. *Causes of cough with whoop:*
- Pertussis
- Parapertussis
- Adenovirus
- Chlamydial infection

D. Foreign body aspiration in airway

E. Dry, paroxysmal, nocturnal cough, may follow post-tussive vomiting suggests bronchial asthma

F. *Drugs aggravating cough:*
- ACE inhibitors
- Beta-blockers
- Calcium-channel blockers
- NSAIDs
- Opioid analgesics
- Glaucoma eyedrops

A-5. A contact is defined as a child who lives in a household with an adult taking anti-tuberculous therapy or having taken such therapy in past 2 years due to any form of active tuberculosis.

A-6.
- Genetic causes
- Maternal diabetes mellitus, thyroid dysfunctions
- Anatomical conditions with uterus or the cervix-like incompetent OS
- Infections like congenital syphilis and TORCH infections
- Pre-eclampsia
- Thrombophilia
- Rh-incompatibility

A-7.
- Passage of meconium after 48 hours is defined as delayed passage of meconium.
- Common causes for delayed passage of meconium are Hirschsprung disease, intestinal pseudo-obstruction, cystic fibrosis and hypothyroidism

A-8.
- Fall of umbilical cord after 3 weeks is defined as delayed fall of umbilical cord.
- Leukocyte adhesion defect (LAD) and factor XIII deficiency are associated with it.

A-9.
- Consanguinity is defined as marriage between blood relatives who have at least one common ancestor, no more remote than a great great grandparents.
- *Degree of consanguinity:*
  - *First degree:* Relationship between sibling and sibling, parent and child
  - *Second degree:* Relationship between uncle and niece, aunt and nephew, stepbrother and stepsister, grandparents and grandchildren
  - *Third degree:* First cousins
- Autosomal recessive and genetic diseases are more common with consanguinity.

A-10.

Educations of head of family	***Score***
Profession or honors	7
Graduate or postgraduate	6
Intermediate or post high-school diploma	5
High school certificate	4
Middle school certificate	3
Primary school certificate	2
Literate	1
Occupation of head of family	
Profession	10
Semi-profession	6
Clerical, shop-owner	5
Skilled owner	4
Semi-skilled worker	3
Unskilled worker	2
Unemployed	1
Monthly income of family (2017)	
>41,430	12
20,715–41,429	10
15,536–20,714	6
10,357–15,535	4
6,214–10,356	3
2,092–6,213	2
<2091	1

Socioeconomic status		***Total score***
I	Upper	26–29
II	Upper middle	16–25
III	Lower middle	11–15
IV	Upper lower	5–10
V	Lower	<5

A-11.
- *Birth history:* Preterm/low birthweight, NICU admission
- Age of development of pallor (acute/chronic)
- Progressive/Static
- *Feeding history:* Breastfeeding, complementary feeds, top milk (goatmilk/amount per day)
- History of neonatal jaundice
- History of iron therapy
- History of blood transfusion to the child and in family

A-12.
- Blood groups of mother and baby (for any blood group incompatibility)
- History of MMR vaccine to mother to rule out rubella infection to mother
- Any observation to suspect hearing impairment
- Day of appearance of jaundice
- History of fever and skin rash to mother during antenatal period on first trimester (TORCH infection—?Rubella)
- Cardiac examination for any congenital heart disease (congenital rubella syndrome)

A-13.

A. Day 1	Varicella
B. Day 2	Scarlet fever
C. Day 3	Smallpox
D. Day 4	Measles
E. Day 5	Typhus fever
F. Day 6	Dengue fever
G. Day 7	Typhoid

A-14.

A. First	Rubeola (measles)
B. Second	Scarlet fever
C. Third	Rubella
D. Fourth	Filatov–Dukes disease
E. Fifth	Erythema infectiosum (slapped cheek syndrome)
F. Sixth	Human herpes virus 6 and 7 (HHV 6 and 7)

A-15. A. Pica is defined as persistent or compulsive perversion of appetite with ingestion of inedible or nonnutritive substances over a period of at least 1 month

B. *Common types of pica:*
- Geophagia (eating earth, soil, clay, chalk, etc.)
- Pagophagia (consumption of ice)
- Amylophagia (consumption of starch)
- Trichophagia (consumption of hairs and wool)
- Xylophagia (consumption of wood)
- Coprophagia (consumption of excrement)
- Hyalophagia (consumption of glass)

C. *Complications of pica:*
- Iron deficiency anemia
- Worms infestations
- Lead poisoning
- Intestinal obstruction
- Constipation
- Trichobezoar
- Intestinal ulceration and perforation

CHAPTER 2

Physical Examination

QUESTIONS

Q-1. Demonstrate palpation of liver.

Q-2. Demonstrate palpation of spleen.

Q-3. Examination for signs of ascites.

Q-4. Examination for direction of blood flow in superficial abdominal wall veins.

Q-5. Examination for tracheal position by palpatory method.

Q-6. Clinical examination for jugular venous pressure.

Q-7. Examination for hepatojugular reflux.

Q-8. Demonstration of apex beat.

Q-9. An 8-year-old boy presented with history of fever, headache and vomiting with Glasgow Coma Scale (GCS) 10. He was found in following posture:

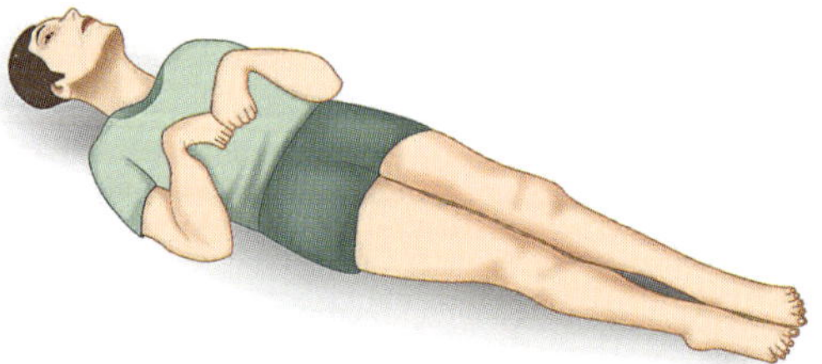

A. Identify the posture.
B. Describe the characteristics of this posture.
C. What is the anatomical site of lesion?
D. What prognosis is predicted?

Q-10. A 10-year-old boy had fever of 6 weeks duration, headache and vomiting 10 days, seizures for 4 days. It was diagnosed as tuberculous meningitis. His posture was as follows:

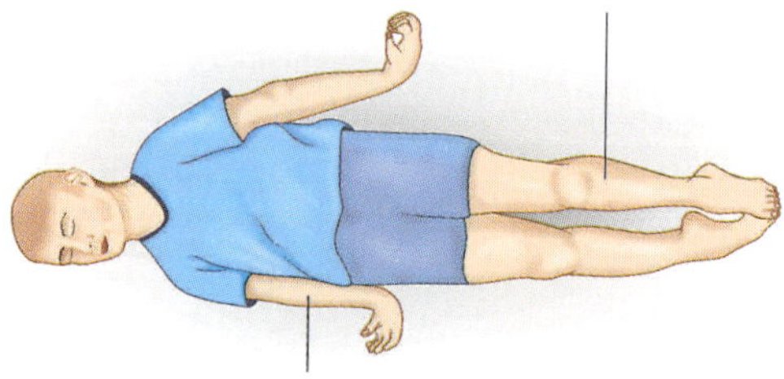

A. Identify the posture.
B. What are the characteristics of this posture?
C. What is the anatomical site of lesion?
D. What prognosis is predicted?

Q-11. Examination for elicitation of planter reflex.

Q-12.

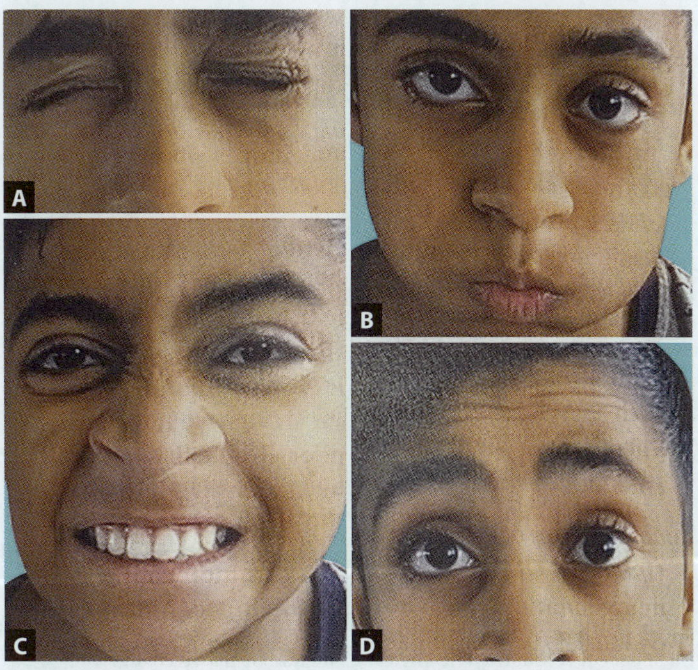

A. What clinical examination performance is shown in the above picture?
B. What are the signs of upper motor neuron lesion in this testing?
C. What are the signs of lower motor neuron lesion in this testing?
D. Give an example for each type, upper motor and lower motor neuron lesions of this structure.

Q-13. Clinical examination for signs of meningeal irritation.

Q-14.

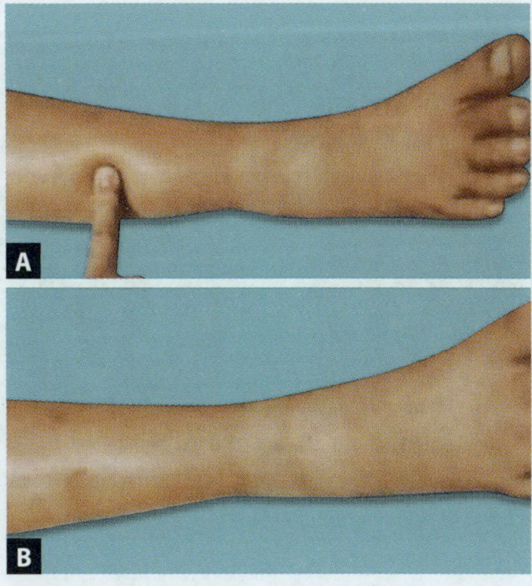

A. What does it show?
B. For what time is to be pressed to demonstrate this sign?

C. What are common sites to demonstrate this sign?
D. Two years female presents with bilateral present this sign over feet and mid upper arm (MUA) circumference <11.5 cm. What is the diagnosis?

Q-15.

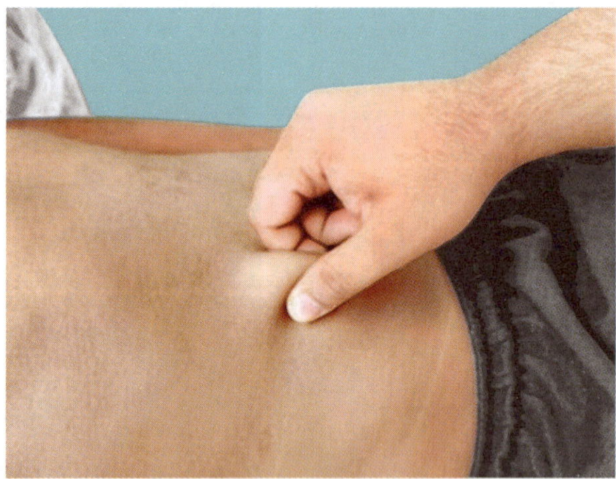

A. The examiner demonstrates this sign over abdominal wall in a case of nephrotic syndrome. What does he want to check for?
B. For what time one should pinch the skin over abdomen to check for this sign?
C. What would be seen on releasing the pinch in a case of positive sign?

Q-16. Answer the following questions pertaining to capillary refill time (CRT).

A. What are the sites to be examined for CRT?
B. For how much time, the tissue should be blanched?
C. What is normal CRT?
D. In which type of shock CRT may be normal?
E. What are the pre-requisites for proper interpretation of CRT?

Q-17.

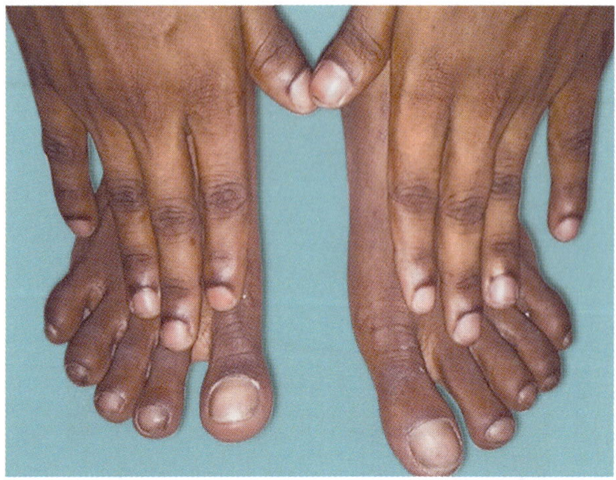

A. Identify the clinical sign.
B. What are the different grades of this clinical sign?
C. What are the common causes of this clinical sign in children?

Q-18. Answer the following questions related to 'observation'.

A. It is emphasized in clinical medicine for observation—general appearance before initiating examination proper. What are the important points to be noted on observation?

B. What are the Red Flag signs on general appearance?

Q-19. Define the following clinical signs.

A. Single breath count

B. Ashworth scale of muscle tone

Q-20. Ascites with following condition is an important clues for the probable diagnosis. Name the disease.

A. Splenomegaly

B. Cor pulmonale

C. Pericardial rub

D. Diffuse abdominal pain

E. Abdominal pain radiating to back

F. Lymphedema

Q-21. Explain the importance of following clinical signs in cardiovascular system.

A. Loud P_2

B. Wide fixed splitting of S_2

C. Precordial bulging

D. Epigastric and subxiphoid pulsations

E. Pulsations in right second intercostal space

F. Pulsations in left second or third intercostal spaces

ANSWERS

A-1. *Palpation of liver:*

- Introduce yourself
- Explain the parents and the child regarding examination
- Take their consent
- Warm your hands before examination
- Child should be in supine position with flexed knees to keep abdomen relaxed

Define the lower border of liver:

- Place the right hand over right iliac fossa such that your fingers are parallel to the ribs.
- Ask the child to take deep breaths
- Wait for the liver edge to come down and strike the lateral border of the index finger with inspiration. The fingers should be placed gently over the abdomen and not to dug deep which may lead to missing soft liver.
- Measure the size of liver below the right costal margin at midclavicular line in centimeters.

Define the upper border of liver:

- Locate the sternal angle. The intercostal space at the level of sternal angle is second intercostal space.
- Start the percussion from right second intercostal space to downward. It will be resonant till the upper border of liver is reached, then it will become dull note.

Span of liver:

- The upper border of liver is defined by percussion and lower border by palpation.
- The distance between these two borders at midclavicular line is span of liver.

Liver span in normal children:

- *Infants:* 5–6.5 cm
- *1–5 years:* 6–7 cm
- *5–10 years:* 7–9 cm
- *10–15 years:* 8–10 cm

Surface:

- Gently rolling the fingers over surface of liver
- Smooth (normal), nodular (cirrhosis of liver)

Consistency:

- Soft (viral hepatitis, congestive heart failure)
- Firm (chronic conditions like tuberculosis, malaria)
- Hard (Malignancy)

Margin:

- Round (normal)
- Sharp and leafy (cirrhosis)

Tenderness:

- Viral hepatitis
- Congested liver (Dengue fever, congestive heart failure)
- Liver abscess

A-2. *Palpation of spleen:*

- Introduce yourself
- Explain the parents and child regarding examination
- Take the consent
- Warm your hands before examination

Classical method:

- Palpation of spleen should begin from right iliac fossa, not to miss a massively enlarged spleen.
- Palpate the spleen with the right hand over abdomen with fingers pointing toward the left hypochondrium and slowly press the fingers a little into abdomen with each breath.
- Try and feel for the lower end of the spleen as it comes and strikes your fingers at the peak of inspiration.
- The spleen moves with respiration and has a palpable notch and one cannot get above it. These are confirmatory findings for spleen.

Bimanual method:

- If the spleen is not palpable by classical method, not to miss a small palpable spleen, one should examine with bimanual method, before it is declared that spleen is not palpable.
- The child should be turned on his right side.
- Try to insinuate the fingers of your right hand beneath the thoracic cage in left hypochondrium.
- Try to push the spleen forward and downward by putting your left hand over his left thoracic cage.
- Ask the child to take the deep breath.
- By insinuating fingers beneath the thoracic cage in left hypochondrium, pushing spleen forward and downward from back and asking the child to take deep breath, spleen may become palpable, if it is enlarged.

Dipping method:

- This method is used to palpate the spleen with massive ascites.
- Palpate the spleen by exerting sudden thrust by the palpating fingers which will displace the fluid and spleen may become palpable, if it is there.

Hooking method:

- This method is crude method and not recommended in routine examination. It may cause injury to soft spleen.
- One should stand on left side of the patient and try to palpable the spleen by making hook of the fingers of your right hand and insinuating it on the left hypochondrium in the thoracic cage.

A-3. *Signs of Ascites:*

- Introduce yourself
- Established rapport with parents and patients
- Take the permission for examination
- Warm your hands before examination

Shifting dullness:

- Child should be in supine position. Expose the abdomen and stand on the right side of the patient.
- Start the percussion from umbilicus, it is tympanic in a normal child. With mild ascites, you may get tympanic note at umbilicus.
- Start percussion from umbilicus laterally toward right or left flank. If it remains tympanic throughout up to flank, it indicates absence of free fluid in the peritoneal cavity.
- A dull not in the dependent flank suggests presence of fluid
- If the flank is dull, turn the patient to the opposite side without displacing your pleximeter finger. Wait for some time and let the fluid shift toward opposite flank because of gravity
- Again, percuss over the same area. A dull note has now changed to tympanic which confirms that fluid has shifted to dependent opposite side and intestine has floated up.
- The shifting can be confirmed by making the child supine again, waiting for some time and percussing over the same point which becomes dull again.

Horseshoe shape dull note:

- In moderate ascites, the whole peritoneal cavity is filled up with fluid, except some area between and around xiphisternum and umbilicus.
- Start the percussion from epigastric region, which would be tympanic to umbilicus till you get the dull note. Mark the point.
- From epigastrium to this point, percuss laterally and define dull not at various points both the sides.
- If you join these points, it will give the shape of horseshoe shape.

Fluid thrill:

- In case of massive, huge ascites, it is not possible to elicit shifting dullness because shift of the fluid by gravity is not possible. The whole peritoneal cavity is filled up with fluid, therefore, hoarseness space is also not available.
- Ask an assistant or a nurse to keep her hand longitudinally in the middle of the abdomen in such a way that ulnar border of her hand presses the abdomen firmly.
- Keep your left palm over the right flank and with right hand give a flick over the left flank. You will feel a thrill that gets transmitted through the fluid under left hand.
- To prevent transmission of tapping impulse to travel through the abdominal wall, an assistant or nurse is asked to keep her hand firmly over the middle of the abdomen.

A-4. *Examination for direction of blood flow in superficial abdominal veins:*

- Introduction
- Explanation to parents and child
- Take their permission
- Warm your hands before examination
- Small superficial veins may be visible normally over abdomen. If the veins are distended, prominent and tortuous, they are abnormal and check the direction of blood flow into them.
- The normal flow of blood into superficial veins of the abdomen is from umbilicus upward to the thorax and from the umbilicus downward to groin.
- Empty the vein of blood by placing two fingers side by side over the vein.
- Move one finger away while keeping the other fixed.
- Now, release the finger one-by-one to see the direction through which the blood fills the vein.
- Direction of flow of flood is away from umbilicus in portal hypertension. There are periumbilical engorged veins with exaggerated flow. It is also called caput medusae.
- In inferior vena cava obstruction, the engorged veins are at the flanks with flow of blood from below upward.
- In superior vena cava obstruction, the engorged veins are above the umbilicus with flow of blood from above downward.

A-5. *Examination for tracheal position by palpation:*

- Introduce yourself
- Explain the parents and the child regarding examination
- Take the permission
- It is examined in supine position of the child or sitting with slight flexion of neck.

There are two methods:

- *First method:* Place the index finger into the suprasternal notch and gently pushed backward. The finger would touch the trachea in the midline in the normal child. If the trachea is deviated, the finger will slide into the trachea sternomastoid space.
- *Second method:* Place the ring and index fingers on the two sternal attachments of the sternocleidomastoid muscles. Gently, pass the middle finger over the trachea to assess its relationship to the fixed two landmarks, whether trachea is central or on either side.

A-6. *Clinical examination for jugular venous pressure (JVP):*

- Introduce yourself
- Explain the parents and the child regarding examination
- Take the permission
- The child should be in supine, a reclining posture on the bed
- Elevate the head and shoulder at an angle of 45° with the help of backrest.
- Keep the neck slightly extended and to the left making sure that the neck muscles are not contracted.
- The sternal angle is located. Identifying internal jugular venous pulsations seen in between two heads of the sternocleidomastoid muscles.
- Measure the vertical height in centimeters by keeping a scale horizontally projected from the top most point of JVP to a measuring centimeter ruler or scale kept vertically at the level of sternal angle.

A-7. *Examination of hepatojugular reflux:*

- Introduce yourself.
- Explain regarding the examination and take permission.
- The child should be in supine position with flexed knees.
- Warm your hands before examination.
- The liver (right hypochondrial area) should be pressed for 30 seconds simultaneously looked for JVP.
- There may be transient rise in JVP up to 3 cm normally.
- If the rise is >3 cm or if the rise is for >15 seconds, the hepatojugular reflux is said to be positive.
- It is seen in right heart failure and tricuspid regurgitation.

A-8. *Clinical examination for palpation of apex beat:*

- Introduce yourself.
- Explain the parents and the child regarding examination.
- Take the consent.
- Put the palm over the precordium and try to locate the position of heart and cardiac impulse.
- Putting the finger in intercostal spaces with cardiac impulse, try to locate the intercostal space with maximum intensity of cardiac impulse.
- Put the tip of the finger perpendicularly at the point with maximum thrust. It is the apex beat.
- Count the intercostal space from second intercostal space (corresponding to sternal angle) to downward and decide intercostal space in which apex beat is located.
- Apex beat is described in relationship to midclavicular line or anterior and midaxillary line in case of cardiomegaly.
- If the apex beat is not found in supine position, it should be sought with left lateral position of the child or in sitting posture.

A-9. A. Decorticate rigidity

B.

- Abnormal flexor response
- Consisting of rigid extension of the lower limbs and flexion and supination of the arms with fisting of hands

C. It is cortical lesion. There is lack of cerebral and diencephalic control of brainstem.

D. Favorable prognosis is predicted.

A-10. A. Decerebrate rigidity

B.

- Abnormal extensor response
- Consisting of rigid extension of legs, arms, trunk and head with hyper-pronation of arms

C. Anatomical site of lesion is midbrain or pons.

D. Prognosis is not favorable.

A-11. *Elicitation of Plantar reflex:*

- Your introduction
- Explain the parents and patient regarding examination
- Take permission
- The child should be in supine position.
- The object used for elicitation of reflex should be blunt like a key and not sharp. Sharp objects may cause injury to the patient and there will be withdrawal of foot and not exact elicitation of reflex.
- Start stroking the lateral aspect of the sole from heel to little toe, and then medially from the base of the toes to a great toe.
- Plantar flexion of the great toe, along with flexion and abduction of other toes indicate flexion plantar response
- Extension (dorsiflexion) of the great toe with fanning of the other toes is called as extensor planter response.
- Extensor planter response is also called as Babinski response. It may be present normally in infants.
- Plantar extensor response indicates pyramidal tract lesion. It is an important sign.

A-12. A. Testing facial nerve motor function

B. In upper motor neuron lesion of facial nerve

- Upper part of face is spared as it is bilaterally innervated
- Wrinkling over forehead, eye closing and blinking are not affected.
- Only lower half of face on the opposite side is involved.

C. In lower motor neuron lesion of facial nerve

- Half of the whole face, both upper and lower halves are involved on the same side of lesion.

D.

- Upper motor facial nerve palsy is seen in involvement of anterior horn at genu of the internal capsule. It is common with involvement of middle cerebral artery. It manifests with hemiplegia on same side of lesion and upper motor neuron facial palsy on the opposite side.
- Bell's palsy is common condition with lower motor neuron type of facial palsy. It develops following lesion from facial nerve nucleus in the brainstem to anywhere along its pathway.

A-13. *Clinical examination of signs of meningeal irritation:*

- Your introduction
- Explain the parents regarding examination
- Take the permission for examination

Neck rigidity (nuchal rigidity, neck stiffness):
- Child should be in supine position.
- One hand is placed behind the head of the child and the neck is gently flexed. If there is resistance to flexion of neck, the sign is considered positive.

Kernig Sign
- The patient should be in supine position.
- His hip and knee joints are flexed to 90° and then knee is slowly extended by the examiner.
- The appearance of resistance or pain during extension of patient's knee beyond 135° constitute a positive Kernig sign.

Brudzinski Sign
- The child should be in supine position.
- The examiner keeps one hand behind patient's head and other hand on the chest to prevent the patient rising with passive flexion of patient's hips and knees in a positive Brudzinski sign.
- *Brudzinski leg sign:* When one leg is passively flexed, there is reflexed flexion of the opposite leg.

A-14. A. Pitting edema
B. 30 seconds
C.
- Shin of tibia
- Malleolus

D. Severe acute malnutrition

A-15. A. Abdominal wall edema
B. 10 seconds
C. Indentation or pits over abdominal wall

A-16. A. Sternum or forehead
B. 3 seconds
C. <2 seconds
D. Warm septic shock
E. Neutral thermal environment, extremity should be raised above the level of heart

A-17. A. Digital clubbing
B. *Grades of clubbing:*
- *Grade I:* Fluctuation and softening of the nailbed
- *Grade II:* Loss of normal angle between the nailbed and the fold
- *Grade III:* Increased convexity of the nails, parrot-beak appearance
- *Grade IV:* Drumstick sign, due to the thickening of the whole distal finger resembling the drumstick
- *Grade V:* Hypertrophic pulmonary osteoarthropathy

C. *Causes of clubbing:*
- *Respiratory causes:*
  - Bronchiectasis (tuberculosis, cystic fibrosis, ciliary dyskinesia)
  - Suppurative lung diseases (lung abscess, empyema)
  - Interstitial lung disease
  - Pleural malignancy (rare)
- *Cardiac causes:*
  - Cyanotic congenital heart diseases (Fallot's tetralogy)
  - Bacterial endocarditis

- *Gastrointestinal causes:*
  - Celiac disease
  - Crohn's disease
  - Ulcerative colitis
  - Cirrhosis of liver
- *Miscellaneous causes:*
  - Familial
  - Local trauma of digit
  - Scleroderma
  - Arteriovenous fistula

A-18. A. *Points on observation:*
- Look of face—sick/ill-looking or well-looking
- Dysmorphic facial features
- Posture and attitude
- Nutrition and built
- Breathing
- Perfusion
- Nature of cry
- Mental status
- Abnormal movements

B. *Red flags on general appearance:*
- Ill look/sick look
- Altered sensorium (drowsiness, irritability)
- Lethargic/generalized weakness (poor perfusion, hypoxia)
- Abnormal posture (dyskinesia, dystonia, opisthotonus, decerebrate or decorticate rigidity)
- Increased work of breathing (tachypnea, indrawing, sounds)
- Petechial/purpura skin lesions (dengue fever, sepsis, meningococcemia)
- Faucial membrane (diphtheria)

A-19. A. Ask the patient to count out loud after maximal inspiration. Ability to reach 50 indicates normal function of respiratory muscles. Single breath count <15 typically correlates with low-forced vital capacity and respiratory muscle weakness in a conditions like GBS.

B. *Ashworth scale of muscle tone:*
1. No increase in muscle tone
2. Slight increase 'catch' when limb is moved.
3. Marked increase muscle tone passive movements are difficult.
4. Affected part is rigid in flexion or extension

A-20. A. Portal hypertension
B. Congestive heart failure
C. Constrictive pericarditis
D. Peritonitis
E. Pancreatitis
F. Lymphangiectasia

A-21. A. Pulmonary hypertension
B. Atrial septal defect
C. Precordial bulging indicates chronic cardiac condition, right ventricular hypertrophy or dilatation
D. If pulsations are felt at tip of thumb, it is due to enlarged right ventricle and at the pulp, it indicates aortic pulsations.
E. Ascending aorta or aortic aneurysm
F. Dilated pulmonary artery

CHAPTER 3

Growth

QUESTIONS

Q-1.

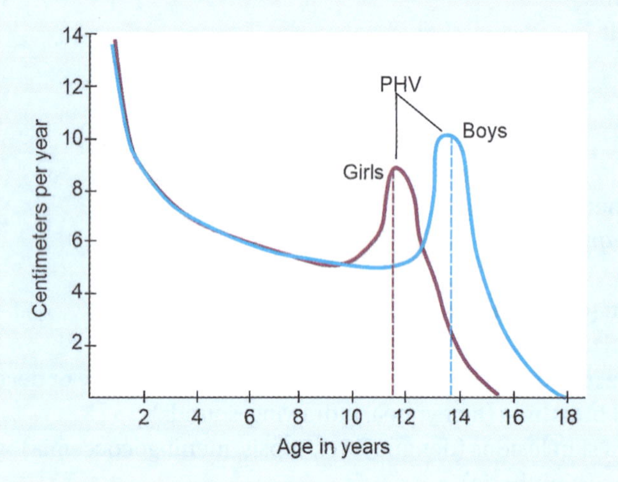

A. What do you call this graph?
B. What is the rate of increase in height at different ages?
C. What is growth velocity in boys during puberty?

Q-2.

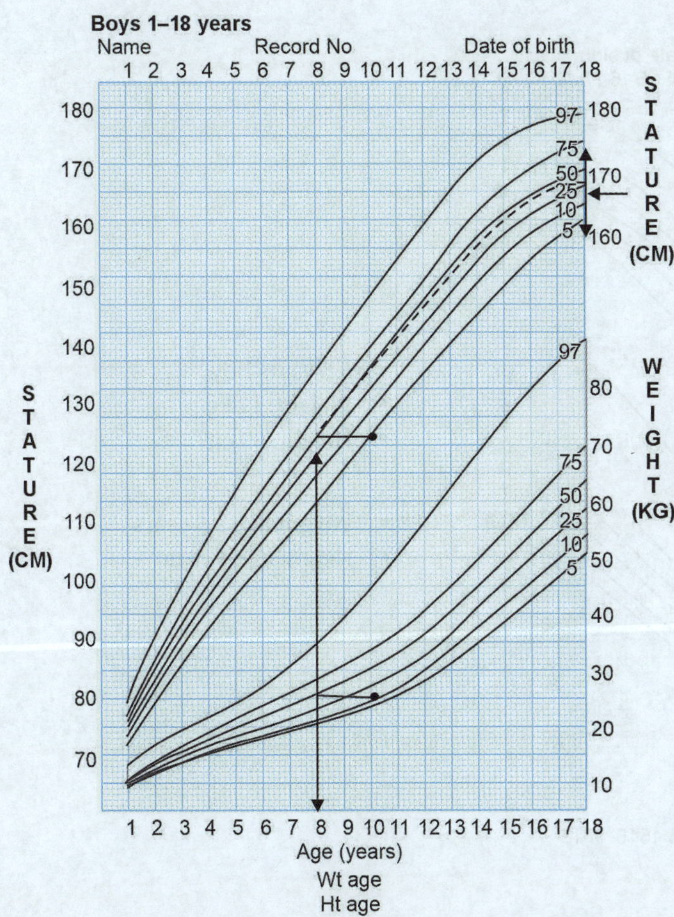

- 10 years Boy
- Weight: 23 kg
- Height: 123 cm

- MPH 168 cm (162–174 cm)
- Weight age 8 years
- Height age 8 years
- BA 8 years

A. Arrange weight age, height age, bone age and chronological age in ascending order.
B. What problem does it suggest?
C. What point in the history may be favoring the condition?
D. What investigations are suggested?
E. What is the treatment of this condition?

Q-3.

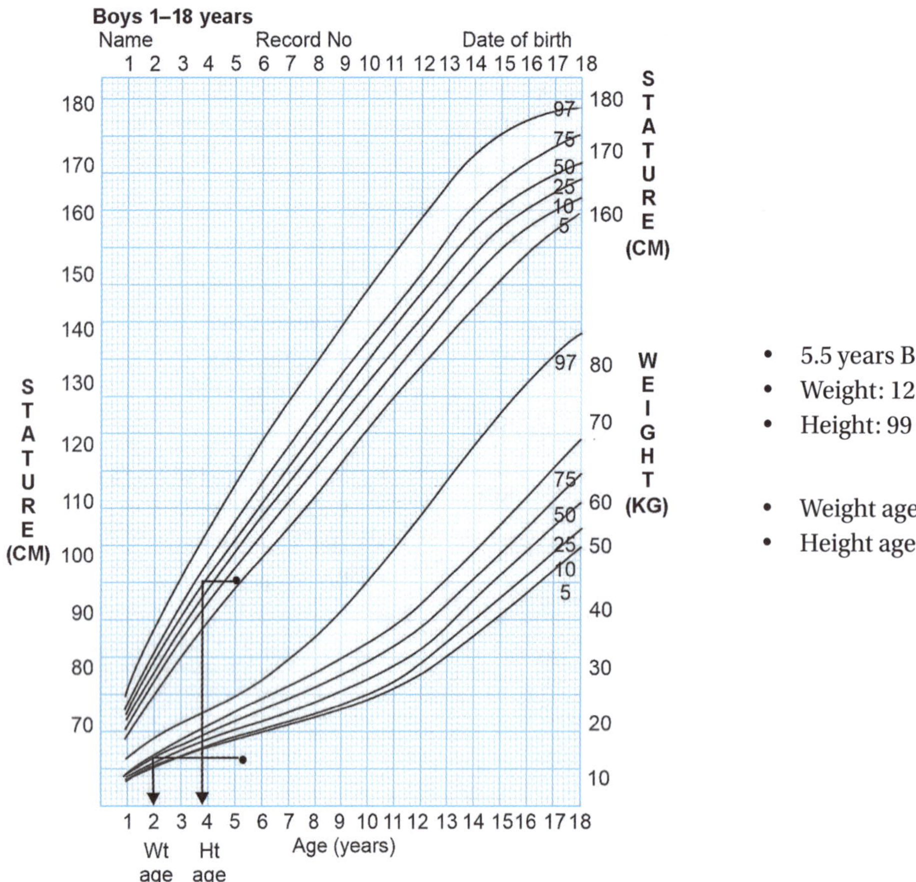

- 5.5 years Boy
- Weight: 12 kg
- Height: 99 cm

- Weight age 2.5 years
- Height age 4 years

A. Arrange chronological age, height age, and weight age in descending order.

B. What type of disorder does it indicate?

Q-4.

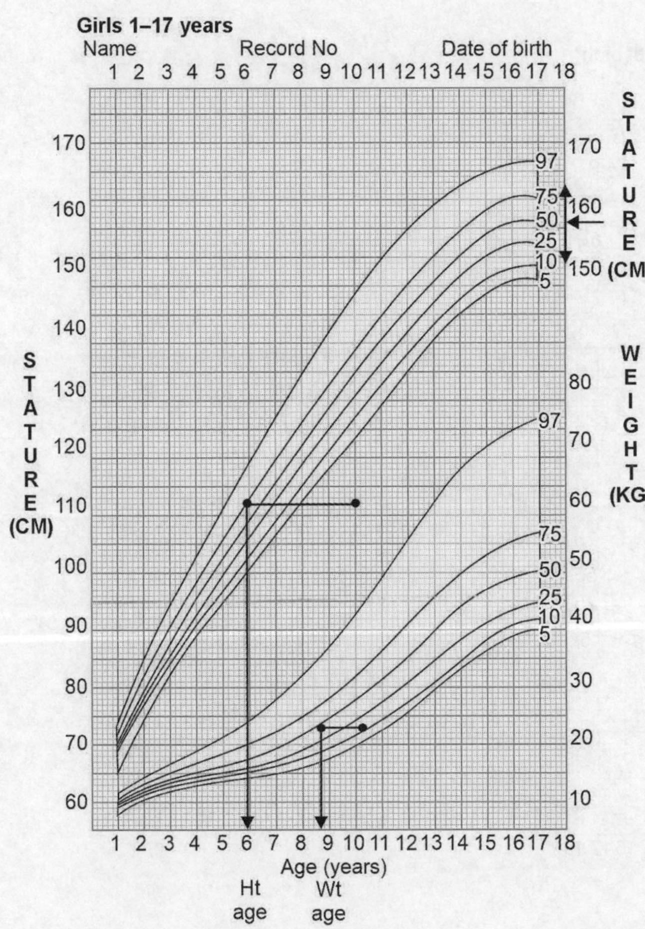

- 10 years Female
- Weight: 22 kg
- Height: 110 cm

- MPH 157 cm (151–163 cm)
- Weight age 8.5 years
- Height age 5.75 years
- Bone age 5.5 years

A. Arrange chronological age, height age, bone age and weight age in ascending order.
B. What does it suggest?

Q-5.

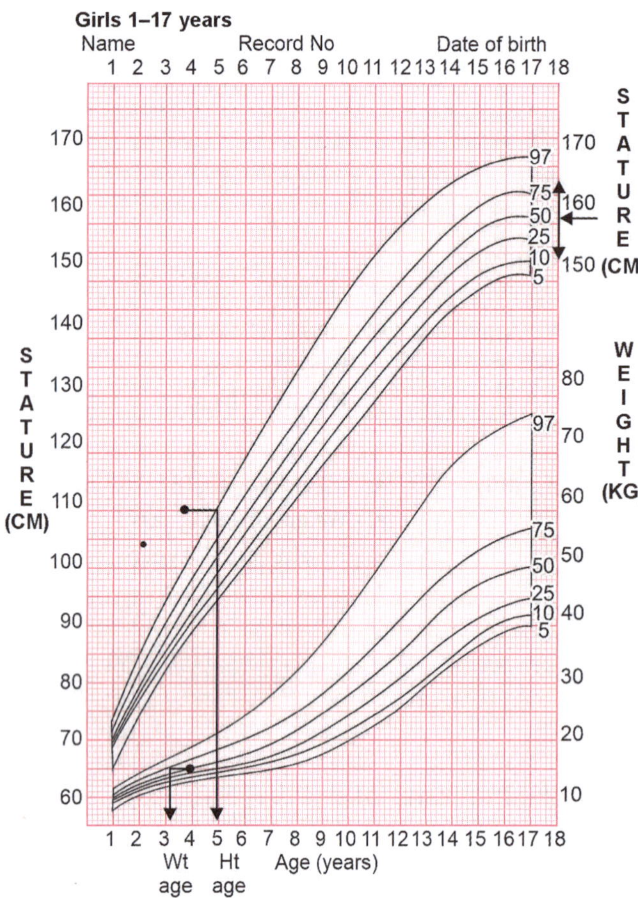

- 4.5 years Female
- Weight: 15 kg (10–25th)
- Height: 110 cm (75–97th)

- Weight age: 3.75 years
- Height age: 5.5 years
- Bone age: 6.5 years

A. Arrange bone age, height age, weight age and chronological age in descending order.

B. What type of disorder does it show?

Q-6.

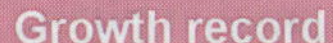

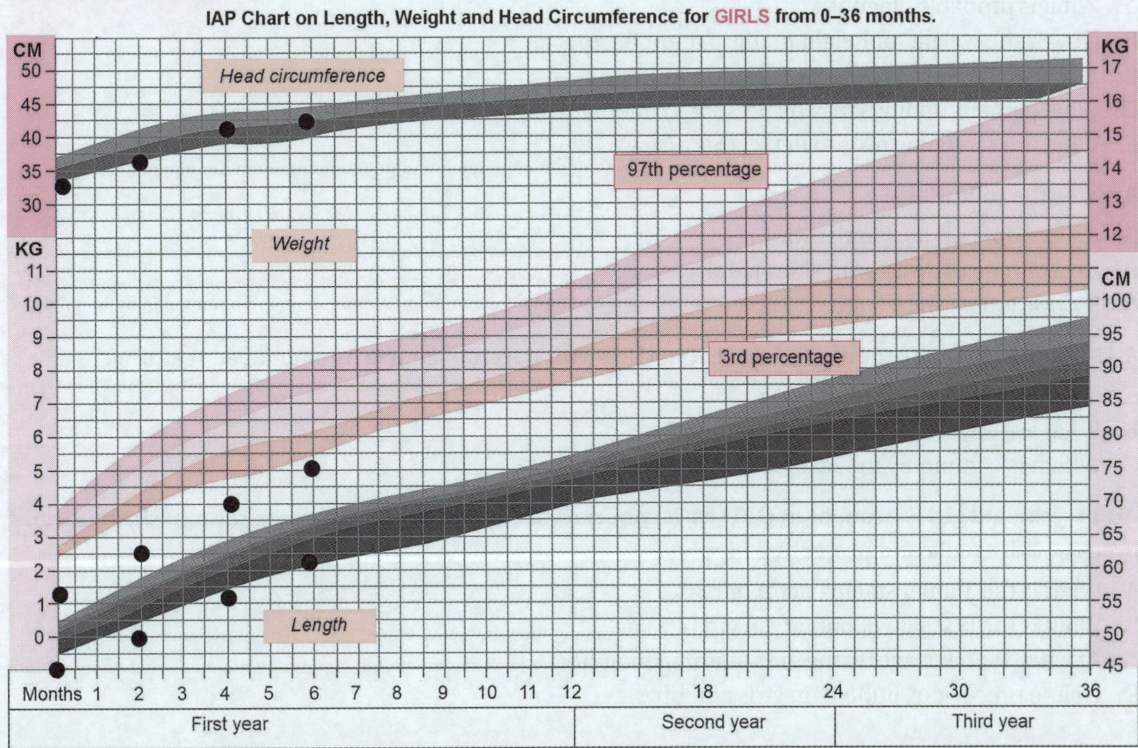

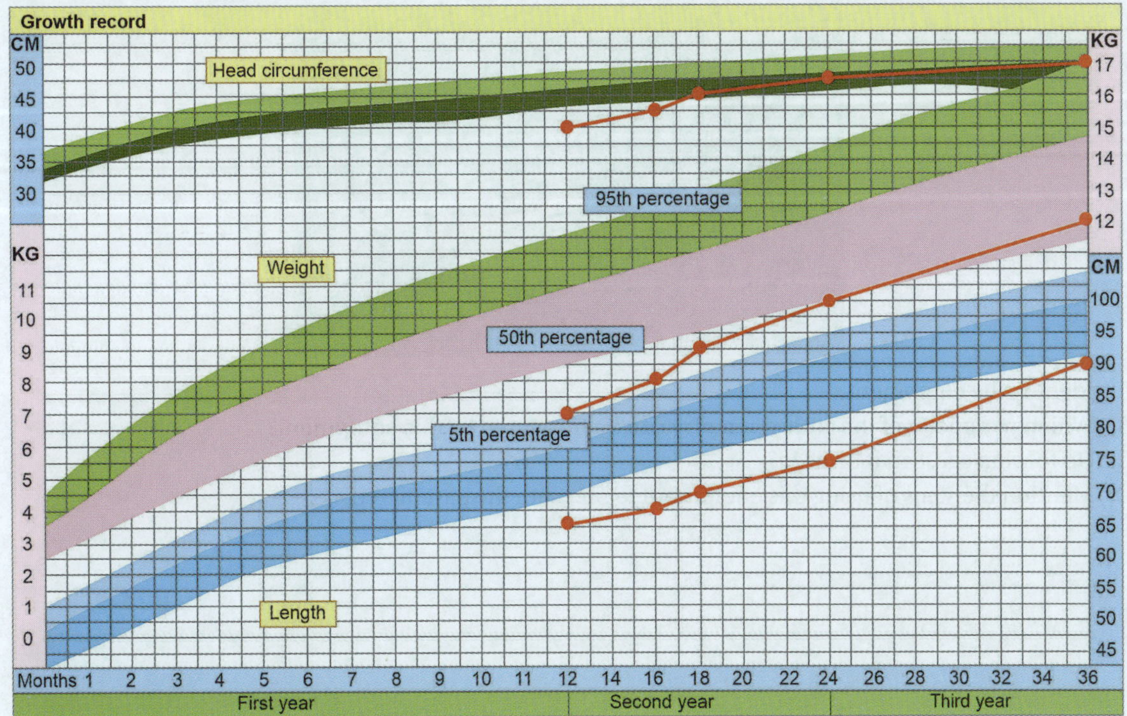

A. Interpret these two growth charts.

B. What is pattern of catch-up growth in all parameters?

Q-7. An 11-year-old boy presented in the OPD with height less than 1st percentile. He was hospitalized in NICU during neonatal period for hypoglycemia and prolonged jaundice. He was apparently looking chubby with round face. He is short but body proportions are normal. His anthropometry was normal at birth.

A. What is probable diagnosis?
B. How is the weight for height in this patient is expected?
C. Any specific voice is expected in this condition?
D. What genitals findings may be present in neonatal period in this disorder?
E. What are screening tests to detect this disease?

Q-8. Answer the followings:

A. An example of short limb dwarf
B. An example of dwarf with short trunk
C. Proportionate short stature

Q-9. A 15-month-old male toddler is brought in OPD with parental concerns of delayed teething:

A. What is delayed teething?
B. What are the causes of delayed teething?
C. Which is commonly the first tooth to appear?

Q-10. An 11-year-old girl is brought in OPD with concerns of early puberty. On examination, she has well-formed breasts with areola and projecting nipples.

A. What is the Tanner staging of this girl?
B. What is the first sign of puberty in girls?
C. At what Tanner stage do the girls attain menarche?
D. Define precocious puberty in girls and boys.

Q-11.

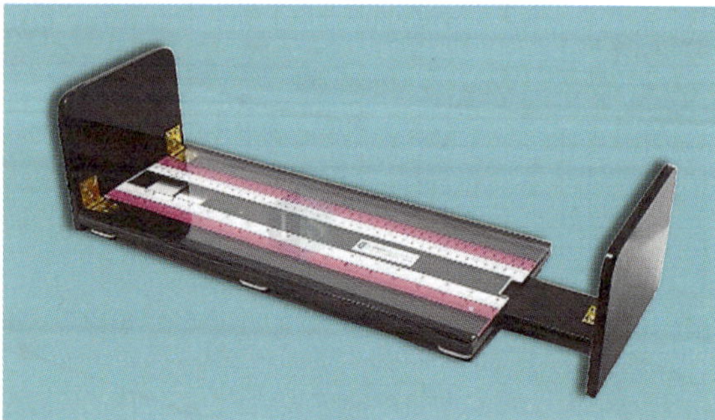

A. Identify the equipment.
B. Which parameter of the anthropometry can be measured by this equipment?
C. Up to what age, can it be used?
D. Mention the steps of using this equipment to measure the parameter.

Q-12.

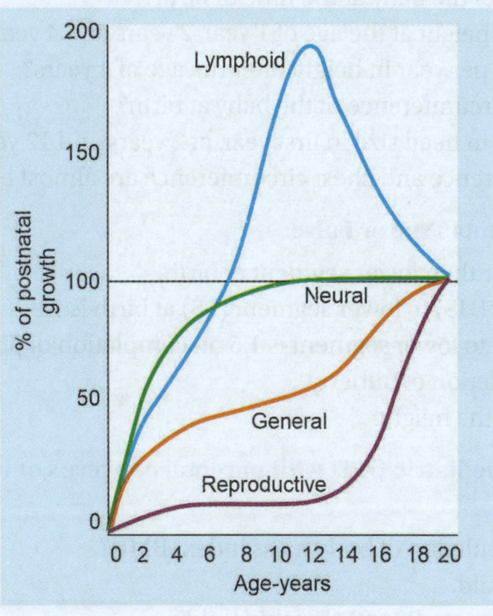

A. Name the growth curves.
B. Describe the growth pattern of different tissues and organs.
C. What is the critical phase of brain development?
D. At what age enlarged tonsils and lymph nodes may be physiological?

Q-13. Answer the following questions pertaining to estimation of bone age.

A. Assessment of bone age postnatally based on which observations?
B. Commonly bone age is assessed on radiograph of which part of body?
C. What are the other methods used for assessment of bone age?
D. Which epiphyses are present at the time of birth?

Q-14. Answer the following question on growth hormone (GH).

A. FDA approved indications for growth hormone use in pediatric practice.
B. What is the dose of GH in mg/kg/week and µg/kg/day?
C. What is the route of administration of GH?
D. What is the biomarker of adherence to GH?
E. Up to what age, GH can cause growth augmentation in males?
F. Up to what age, GH can cause growth augmentation in females?
G. Which year of therapy has maximum auxological response?
H. What are the side effects of GH?

Q-15. Answer the followings in true or false response, pertaining to Tanner stage.

A. Growth acceleration is observed during Tanner stage 2 in boys.
B. Thickening of scrotum is a sign of puberty in boys.
C. Menarche in girls usually occurs 2–2.5 years after the onset of thelarche.
D. Pubarche appears 6–12 months after the onset of thelarche.
E. Pubarche precedes the growth of penis in boys.
F. Axillary hairs appear during late puberty in boys.

Q-16. Answer the following questions pertaining to anthropometry.

A. What is the average length of the baby at the time of birth?
B. What is the average length/height at the age of 1 year, 2 years and 4 years?
C. What is the rate of increase per year in height after the age of 4 years?
D. What is the average head circumference of the baby at birth?
E. What is the rate of increase in head size in first year, at 2 years and 12 years of age?
F. At what age, head circumference and chest circumference are almost equal?

Q-17. Answer the following statements True or False:

A. The trunk is relatively larger than lower segment at birth.
B. The ratio of upper segment (US) to lower segment (LS) at birth is 1.9.
C. The ratio of upper segment to lower segment is 1.5 on completion of puberty.
D. LS >US by 5 cm after completion of puberty.
E. Arm span is within 5 cm of the height.

Q-18. A 10-year-old boy is seen in pediatric OPD with parental concerns of being underweight. He has weight of 40 kg and height of 140 cm.

A. What is the formula for calculation of body mass index (BMI)?
B. Calculate the BMI of this child.
C. What is your interpretation regarding BMI of this child?

Q-19. What are effects of constitutional growth delay on following parameters?

A. Birth weight and length
B. Skeletal maturation
C. Timing of puberty
D. Growth velocity
E. Treatment

ANSWERS

A-1. A. Growth velocity curve

B.

- 25 cm in first year
- 12 cm in second year
- 6 cm in third year
- 5 cm/year till puberty

C.

- 9.5 cm/year in boys
- 8.3 cm/year in girls
- Boys have 2 years longer duration of pubertal growth than girls.

A-2. A. WA = HA = BA < CA

B. Constitutional delay

C. History of delayed puberty in either parent

D. No investigations

E.

- Assurance to parents
- Follow-up for growth velocity

A-3. A. CA > HA > WA
B. Acute on chronic malnutrition

A-4. A. BA = HA < WA < CA
B. Endocrinal disorder

A-5. A. BA > HA > CA > WA
B. Precocious puberty

A-6. A.
- At birth, weight, length and head by all were low (preterm/LBW).
- Head is growing faster than weight and length is still slower.
- Second growth chart shows catch up growth of head, weight and height.

B.
- Head by 18 months
- Weight by 24 months
- Height by 40 months

A-7. A. Hypopituitarism
B. Normal, proportionate weight to his height
C. High-pitched voice in hypopituitarism
D. Micro-penis and/or undescended testis
E. IGF-1 and IGFBP-3 (insulin-like growth factor binding protein 3)

A-8. A. *Short limb dwarfs:* Achondroplasia, hypochondroplasia
B. *Short trunk dwarfs:* Mucopolysaccharidosis
C. *Proportionate short stature:* Growth hormone deficiency

A-9. A. The appearance of first tooth may be delayed until after first year in some children. It is considered delayed, if there is no tooth by 13 months of age.
B. *Causes of delayed teething:*
- Familial
- Rickets
- Hypothyroidism
- Osteogenesis imperfecta
- Idiopathic

C. Central incisors are first to appear

A-10. A. Stage 5
B. Appearance of breast buds
C. Stage 3–4
D. Pubertal onset before the age of 8 years in girls and 9.5 years in boys is suggestive of precocious puberty.

A-11. A. Infantometer
B. Length of a child
C. It is used up to the age of 2 years of the child.
D. *Steps of using infantometer to measure the length of the child:*
- Head is placed in Frankfort plane, with crown of head touching the headboard (fixed board).
- Shoulders and buttocks should be touching the backboard.
- Long axis of the body should be in line with center line of backboard.
- Heels should be against foot board (moving end).
- See the upper end of moving board indicating length of the baby.

A-12. A. Scammon growth curves

B.

- *Brain growth:* At birth, head size is 60–70% of expected head size in adults. It reaches 90% of adult head size in first 2 years of life.
- *Somatic growth:* It is sigmoid curve. During early childhood and adolescence, there is phase of rapid growth. There is slower growth in between these rapid phases. A period of stasis with little or no growth as the individual reaches adulthood.
- *Growth of gonads:* Gonadal growth is dormant during childhood and becomes conspicuous during puberty.
- *Lymphoid growth:* The growth of lymphoid tissue is most notable during mild childhood. During this period, the lymphoid tissue is overgrown and its mass may appear larger than that of a fully mature adult.

C. The fetal period and first two years are a critical phase for brain development.

D. Between 4 and 8 years

A-13. A.

- Number, shape and size of epiphyseal centers
- Size, shape and density of ends of bones

B. Left hand and wrist

C.

- Bone age atlases like Gruelich and Pyle or Tanner and Whitehouse
- Software such as BoneXpert

D.

- Distal femoral epiphysis
- Proximal tibial epiphysis
- Calcaneus, cuboid, capitate and hamate
- Head of humerus

A-14. A. FDA approved indications of GH:

- GH deficiency
- Turner syndrome
- Chronic renal failure
- Prader–Willi syndrome
- Noonan syndrome
- Small for gestational age with short stature
- Idiopathic short stature

B.

- 0.16–0.24 mg/kg/week
- 22–35 μg/kg/day

C. Subcutaneous

D. IGF-1

E. 16 years

F. 14 years

G. First year

H. *Side effects of GH:*

- Type II diabetes mellitus
- Gynecomastia
- Scoliosis
- Slipped capital femoral epiphyses
- Pseudotumor cerebri

A-15. A. False (growth acceleration is observed during Tanner stage 4 in boys)
B. False (thinning of scrotum is a sign of puberty in boys)
C. True
D. True
E. False (pubarche usually follows the growth of penis in boys)
F. False (axillary hairs appears during mid-puberty in boys)

A-16. A. 50 cm
B. *1 year:* 75 cm, *2 years:* 87.5 cm, *4 years:* 100 cm
C. 6 cm per year
D. 34 cm
E.
- *First 3 months:* 2 cm per month
- *3–6 months:* 1 cm per month
- *6–12 months:* 0.5 cm per month
- *2 years*: 48 cm
- *12 years*: 52 cm

F. 1 year

A-17. A. True
B. False (It is 1.7)
C. False (It is 1–1.1)
D. True
E. True

A-18. A. $\text{BMI} = \dfrac{\text{Weight in kg}}{(\text{Height in meter})^2}$
B. BMI of this child $\dfrac{40}{(1.4 \times 1.4)} = 40/1.96 = 20.4\ \text{kg/m}^2$
C. Normal BMI for this child

A-19. A. Normal
B. Delayed
C. Delayed
D. Delayed
E. Normal
F. Only assurance

CHAPTER 4

Development and Psychiatry

QUESTIONS

Q-1.

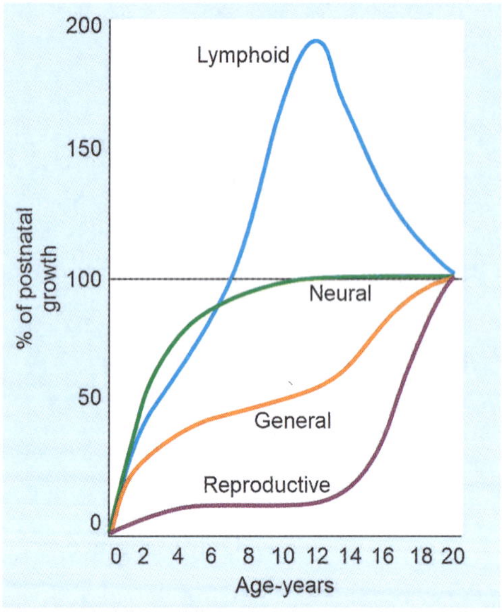

A. What does it show?

B. What is its name?

C. Describe its interpretation.

Q-2.

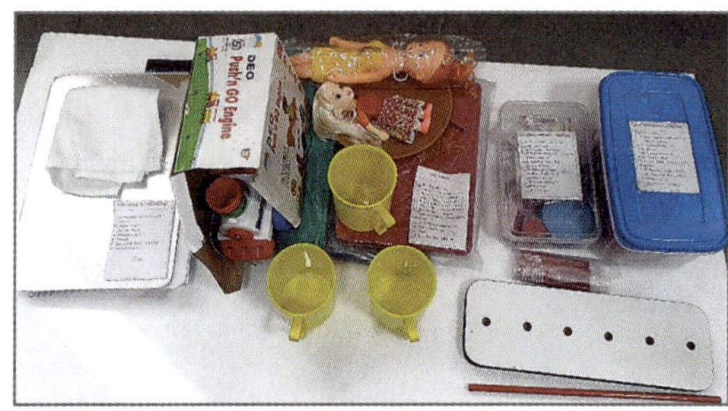

A. What is the name of this kit used in child development clinic?

B. What is the utility of this kit?

C. What age is recommended to use this kit?

D. What are the key features of this kit?

E. Who developed this kit?

Q-3.

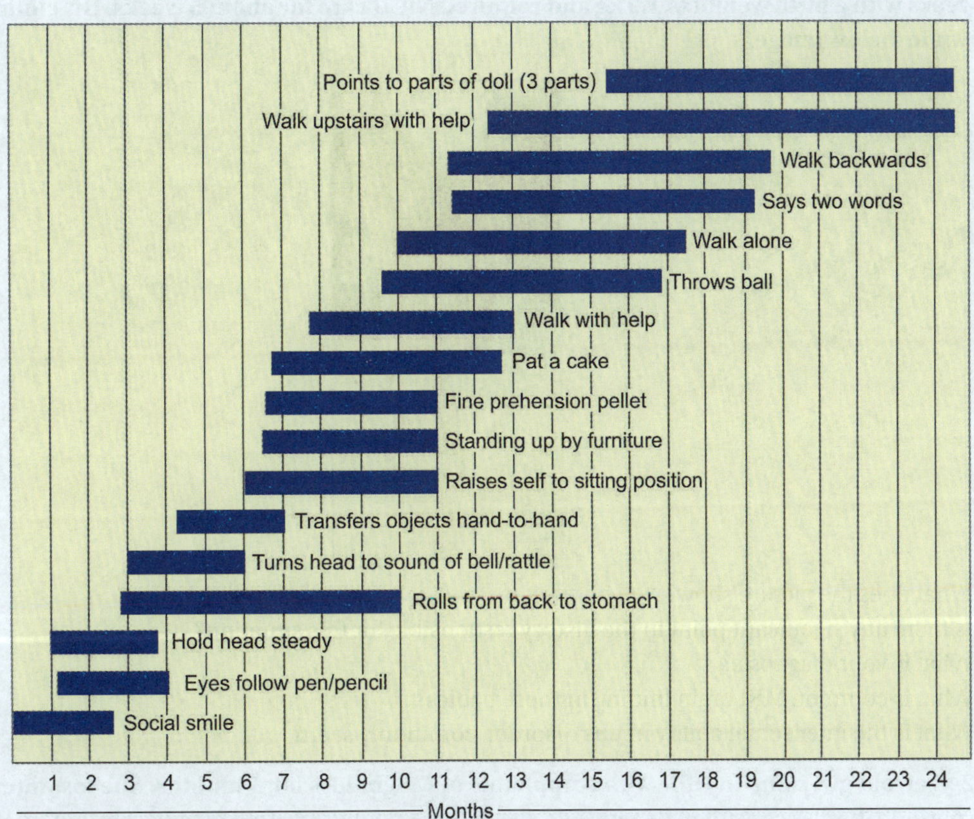

A. What is the name of this development screening tool?
B. At what age, this development screening tool can be used?
C. What is the utility of this screening tool?
D. How one should interpret this screening tool?
E. What are the other developmental screening tools that can be used?

Q-4.

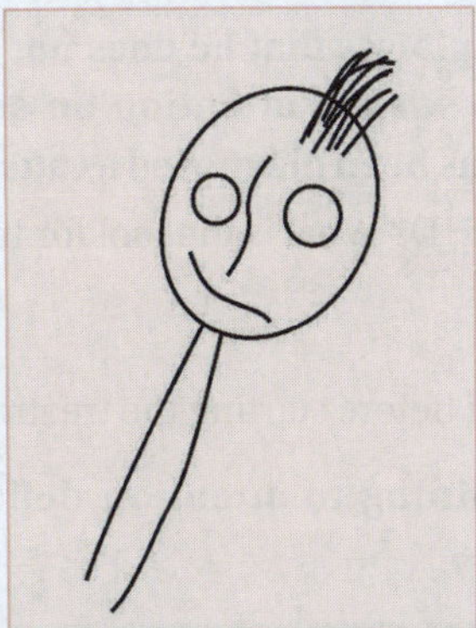

A. What is this simple bedside test for assessing the cognition of a child called?
B. Beyond what age can this test be used?
C. What is the mental age of the child who has drawn this image? How will you calculate?

Q-5. A 2-year-old child is brought with concerns of notable to walk without support. He was delivered as a 32 weeks with a birth weight of 1.2 kg and required NICU care for about 5 weeks. His clinical observations is shown in below image.

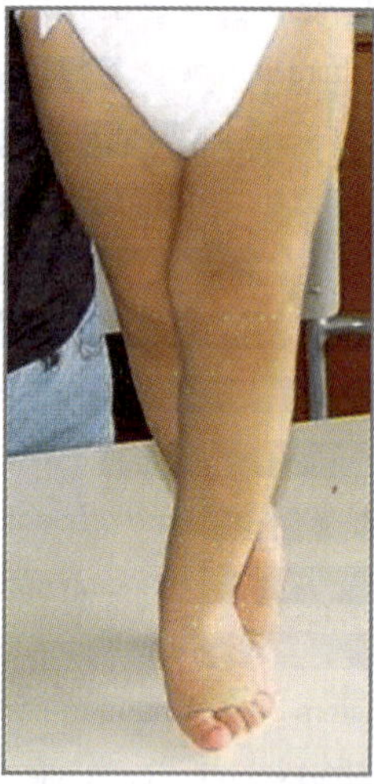

A. What does the picture show?
B. Is there any significant point in the history responsible for this situation?
C. What is your diagnosis?
D. What is common MRI brain finding in these babies?
E. What is the intellectual ability in this disorder, commonly seen?

Q-6. A 12-year-old girl came in OPD with complaints of weight loss for 6 months. She lost more than 10 kg over this period. She was consulted by multiple specialists and investigated extensively, but no medical cause was found. Parents informed avoidance of food, prefers vegetables and salad and following vigorous physical exercise. On psychological, she denied any cognition related to abnormal body image and fear of weight gain.

A. What is probable diagnosis?
B. What are the types of this disorders?
C. What are differential diagnosis?
D. What are the complications of this disorder?
E. What symptoms and signs required hospitalization of this patient?

Q-7. A 5-year-old boy is brought with complaints that he does not sit in class room or at home, keeps running around, talks too much, not able to sustain attention on any work given, often easily distracted and forgetfulness for past 10 months. He has been diagnosed as attention deficit hyperactivity disorder (ADHD).

A. What are the diagnostic tools for ADHD? What is the tool for Indian children?
B. What are the differential diagnosis?
C. What are the treatment modalities?
D. What conditions should be excluded before starting the treatment?

Q-8. The following statements are pertaining to attention deficit hyperactivity disorder (ADHD), Write True/False.

A. Impulsive behavior is a feature.
B. Is associated with high rate of teenage pregnancy.
C. Is associated with high rate of tic disorders.
D. Is associated with higher rate of expulsion from school.
E. May respond to treatment with stimulants such as amphetamines.

Q-9. A 2.5-year-old child was brought in OPD by parents with complaints of impaired verbal response, plays alone, stereotype and restrictive behavioral problems.

A. What is probable diagnosis?
B. Which diseases are associated with this disorder?
C. What is the triad of symptoms required to label this disorder?
D. What is the pharmacotherapy for this condition?

Q-10. A 9-month-old girl was brought as an emergency case with complaints that following crying, she suddenly stops breathing and lips become bluish followed by a seizure-like movement for few seconds and then becomes normal.

A. What is probable diagnosis?
B. What are the types of this disorder?
C. What are the differential diagnosis?
D. What is the management of this condition?

Q-11. A 20-month-old boy is brought in the OPD with classical features of autistic spectrum disorder (ASD). Answer the following questions pertaining to the condition.

A. What are differential diagnosis?
B. What key features should be checked in his clinical examination?
C. What are the indications of radio-imaging of brain in ASD?
D. What are the principles of the treatment?

Q-12. A 2-year-old boy was brought in OPD by parents with complaints of not responding to oral commands, not making eye contacts, not playing with other children, remains alone and repeats similar actions. It is observed since last 6 months.

A. What is probable diagnosis?
B. What is most consistent findings on his clinical examination in this disorder?
C. What drugs are approved for this disease?

Q-13. A 6-year-old boy is brought with complaints of sudden and recurrent movements of eye blinking, jerking of neck and repeating his words often. This occurs several times in a day and has been present for 14 months. His development is normal and no fever or altered sensorium. There is no history of any drug intake.

A. What is most probable diagnosis?
B. What are the associated disorders with this condition?
C. What are differential diagnosis?
D. What are the treatment modalities?

Q-14. A 14-year-old adolescent girl is brought by her mother with complaints of repetitive paroxysmal episodes for last 1 year. The events are variable but she develops sudden loss of consciousness and fall every time. The episode is classical with jerking movements of head, tight closing of eyes, open mouth and deep breathing. Her development is normal. There is no history of seizures in family. She has taken multiple antiepileptic drugs without any benefit. Clinical examination, including CNS is essentially normal. On deep probing, mother revealed the information regarding her separation from her husband.

A. What is most probable diagnosis?
B. What are the risk factors for this disorder?
C. How to manage her?

Q-15. A 10-year-old boy is presented with complaints of difficulty in reading and writing for 2 years. He is not able to keep up with his classmates academically despite of special efforts by his teachers and tuition classes. His development, hearing and vision are normal. His family is stable.

A. What is the diagnosis?
B. What are possible comorbid conditions with this disorder?
C. What interventions should be done?

Q-16. Answer the following question pertaining to specific learning disability.

A. Define specific learning disability.

B. What is the most common specific learning disability?

C. What is the etiology of this disorder?

D. What are the features suggestive of specific learning disability?

Q-17. Define following developmental and behavioral disorders in children.

A. Juvenile delinquency

B. Munchausen by proxy

C. Pica

D. Temper tantrum

E. Thumb-sucking

F. Stuttering

G. Enuresis

H. Encopresis

Q-18. What is the age of development of motor milestones shown in images A, B, and C?

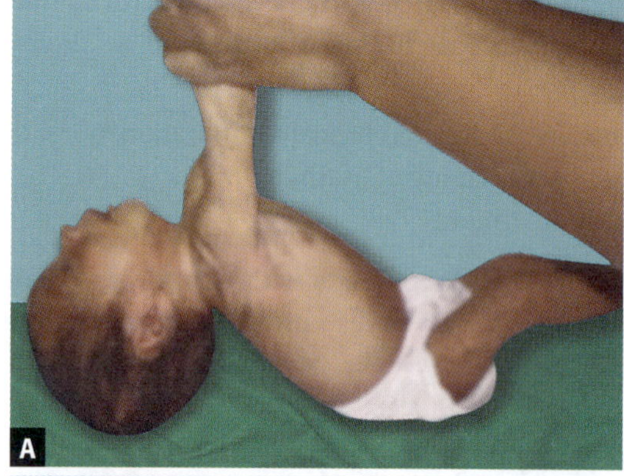

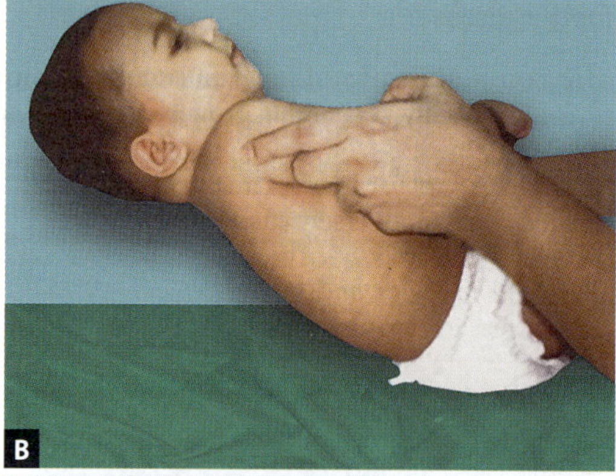

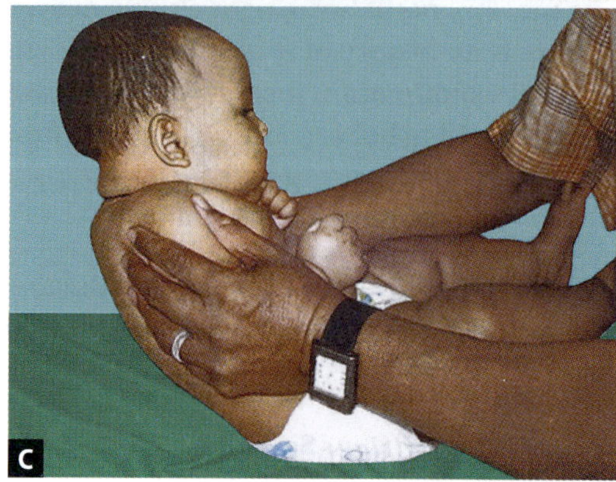

Q-19. What is the age of development of motor milestones as shown in images A, B, and C?

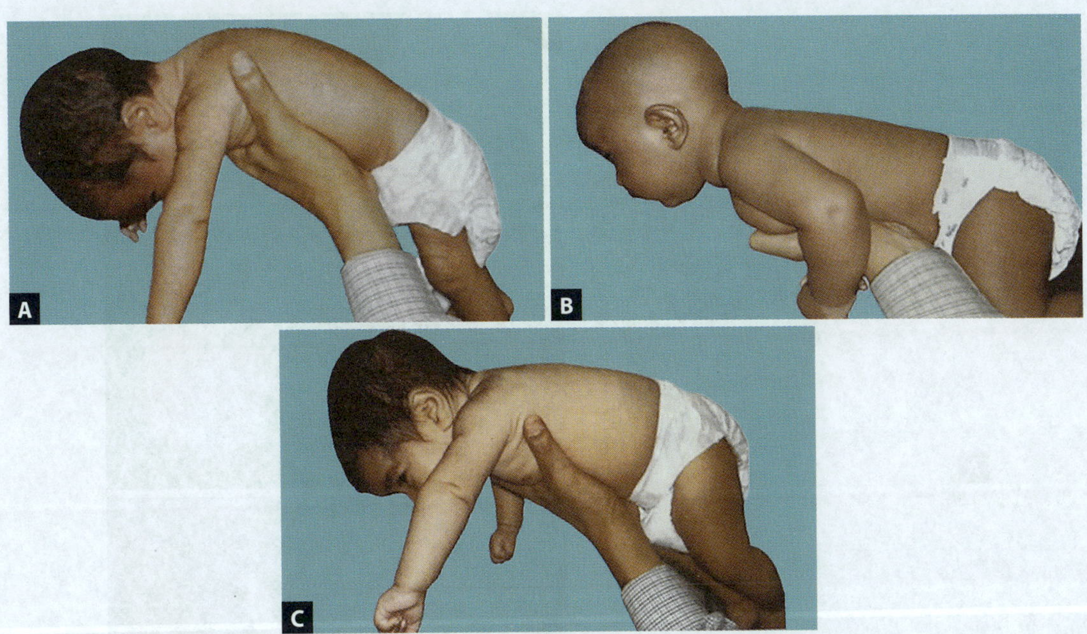

Q-20. What is the age of development of the child as shown in images A, B, C, D, and E?

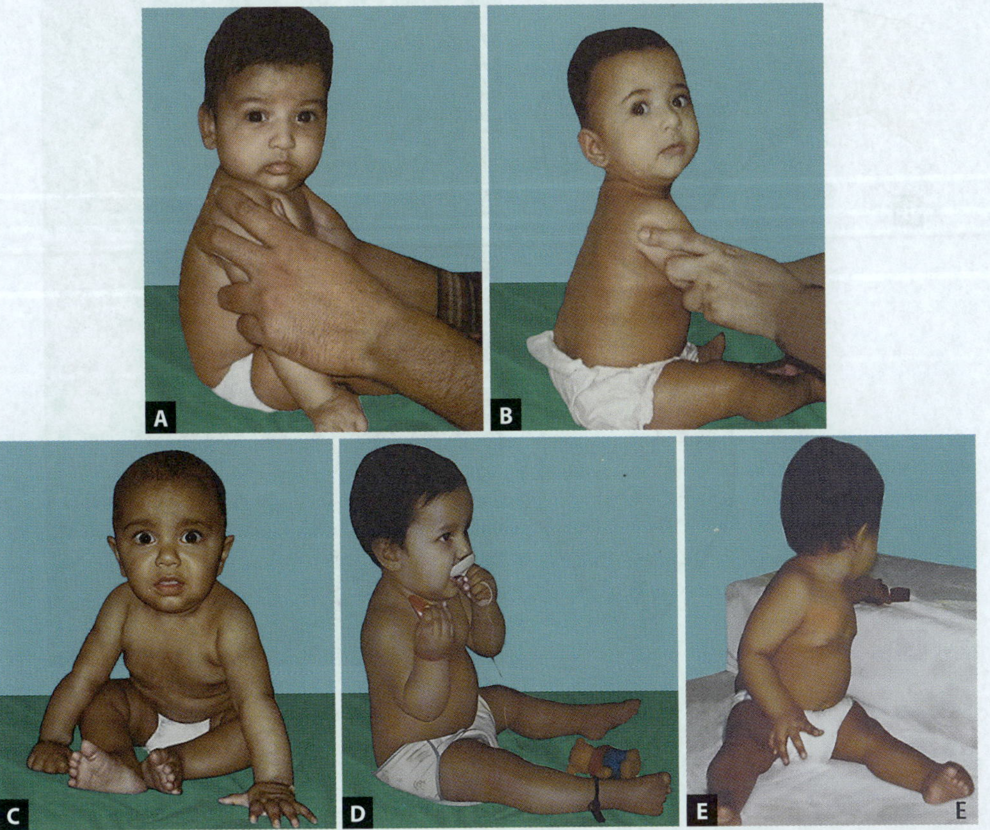

Q-21. What is the age of development of different stages of grasp as shown in images A, B and C?

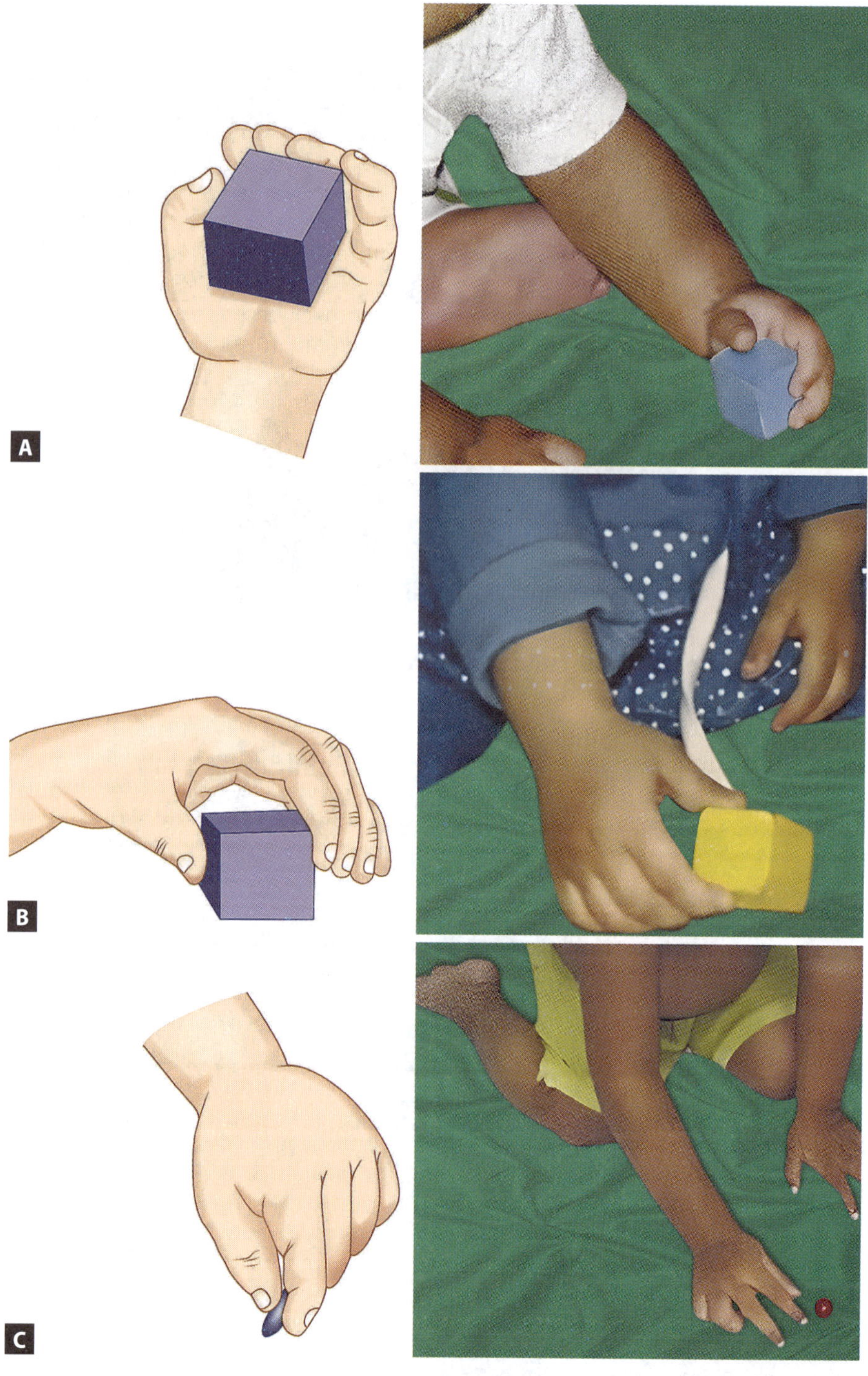

Q-22.

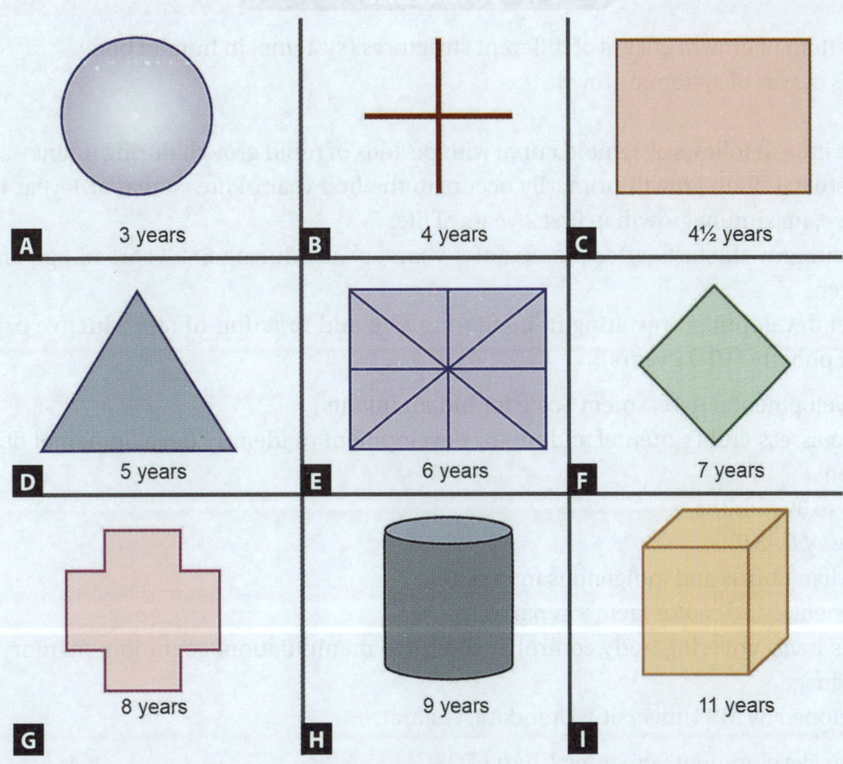

At what age different drawing skills develop as shown in images A, B, C, D, E, F, G, H, and I?

Q-23.

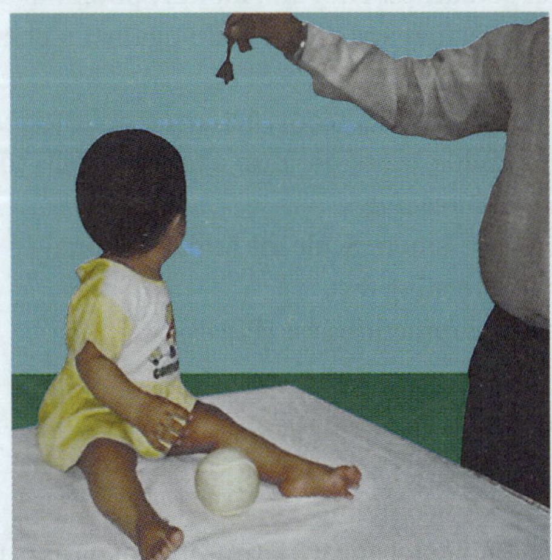

A. What the examiner is trying to assess in this picture?

B. At what age of the child do you expect this response?

ANSWERS

A-1. A. It shows pattern of growth curves of different structures (systems) in human body.

B. Scammon's curves of systemic growth

C.

- Somatic growth follows a sigmoid curve with periods of rapid growth during infancy and puberty.
- The postnatal brain growth primarily occurs in the first year of life so that at 1-year infant has 90% adult brain size, maximum growth in first 2 years of life.
- Lymphoid growth starts after the age of 5 years, peaks during 6–9 years of age and declines steadily thereafter.
- Gonadal development resulting in increasing size and function of reproductive organs starts after the onset of puberty (10–14 years).

A-2. A. DASII (Developmental Assessment Scale for Indian Infants)

B. It is used to assess child's mental and motor development to identify developmental delays and to monitor interventions.

C. From birth to 30 months

D. *Key features of DASII:*

- Uses Indian norms and indigenous material
- Scores mental and motor factors separately
- Includes items covering body control, locomotive manipulation, cognition, memory, social interactions and language

E. It was developed by MS University, Vadodara, Gujarat.

A-3. A. Trivandrum Development Screening Chart (TDSC)

B. 0–6 years

C. The primary utility of TDSC is easy for community health workers to administer, without requiring specialized training in developmental pediatrics. They can identify potential delays in cognitive and motor function.

D. The test giver compares the actual age of the child against a chart that plots the typical ages for achieving specific milestones.

- A 'pass' is recorded if the child has already, achieved milestones to the left of their age line.
- A 'delay' is assumed if a child cannot perform a task that falls to the left of their age line.

E. *Other tests for developmental screening:*

- DASII (Developmental Assessment Scale for Indian Infants)
- Denver Developmental Screening test
- Parent's evaluation of development status (PEDS)
- Age and stage questionnaire

A-4. A. Good enough draw a Man Test

B. Beyond 3 years of age

C.

- Formula for calculation of mental age = 3 + (number of parts/4)
- Mental age of this child = 3 +(6/4) 4.5 years

A-5. A. Scissoring of legs

B. Significant points in the history are prematurity, low birth weight and prolonged NICU admission

C. Spastic diplegia (spastic bilateral cerebral palsy)

D. Periventricular leukomalacia with dilated ventricles is commonly seen in MRI of brain in these babies.

E. Intellectual ability may be normal or minimal affected in spastic diplegic cerebral palsy

A-6. A. Anorexia nervosa

B. Binge eating and restricting types

C. Obsessive compulsive disorder (OCD), hyperthyroidism, malignancy, inflammatory bowel disease (IBD), etc. are differential diagnosis.

D. *Complications of anorexia nervosa:*
- Cardiac complications like hypotension, bradycardia, refeeding syndrome, tachyarrhythmias
- Hypothalamic dysfunction
- Decreased bone and mineral density
- Endocrinal problems

E. *Indications for hospitalization:*
- Heart rate <50/min
- Arrhythmias
- Hypotension and postural hypotension
- Hypokalemia
- Hypoglycemia
- Dehydration
- Suicidal intent

A-7. A. *Diagnostic tools for ADHD:*
- Child behavior checklist
- Conners abbreviated rating scale
- Vanderbilt ADHD diagnostic rating scale

INCLEN diagnostic tool for ADHD is validated for Indian Children

B. *Differential diagnosis of ADHD:*
- Thyroid disorders
- Neurodegenerative diseases
- Hearing and vision impairment
- Fragile X syndrome
- Heavy metal poisoning

C. Multidisciplinary treatment including behavioral, interventions, educational interventions, psychostimulant drugs like methylphenidate, amphetamine, parents counseling.

D. History of cardiomyopathy, arrythmia, syncope, etc.

A-8. All are true.

A-9. A. Autism spectrum disorder (ASD)

B. Diseases associated with ASD (in 10% cases)
- Fragile X syndrome
- Tuberous sclerosis
- Angelman syndrome
- Phenylketonuria
- Hypothyroidism

C. Triad of impaired communication, defect in social interactions and stereotypic and restrictive behavioral patterns is required to label ASD.

D. *Pharmacotherapy in ASD:*

Medication	*Indication*
Antipsychotics (risperidone, olanzapine)	Anxiety, aggression, repetitive behavior
Methylphenidate	Inattention, hyperactivity, impulsivity
Clonidine, atomoxetine	Hyperactivity
Melatonin	Sleep-related problems
Iron supplementation	Iron deficiency

A-10. A. Breath-holding spell

B. Cyanotic spell, Pallid spell or mixed

C. *Differential diagnosis:*

- Seizures
- Dystonia
- Cardiac arrhythmia

D. Counseling to parents regarding self-resolving condition and to ignore it. They should not be panic. Iron supplementation may reduce the episodes.

A-11. A. *Differential diagnosis of ASD:*

- Language disorders
- Intellectual disability
- Developmental delay
- Hearing impairment

B. *Physical examination points in ASD:*

- Head circumference (may be macrocephaly)
- Dysmorphic features
- Muscle tone and DTR

C. Macrocephaly or microcephaly, developmental regression or focal findings on CNS examination are indications for radioimaging of brain

D. *Treatment of ASD:*

- Applied behavioral analysis methods such as joint attention, shared enjoyment and reciprocal communication and educational approaches
- Speech and language therapy
- Augmentative communication
- Parent-mediated early intervention
- Social skills program

A-12. A. Autism

B. 20% of children with autism have macrocephaly

C. Risperidone and Aripiprazole are FDA approved drugs for autism

A-13. A. Tourette syndrome

B. Obsessive compulsive disorder (OCD), learning disabilities, autism spectrum disorders, anxiety, depression and ADHD are associated disorders.

C. *Differential diagnosis of Tourette syndrome:*

- Stereotypies
- Movement disorders
- Torticollis
- Sandifer syndrome
- Shuddering attacks

D. *Treatment modalities:*

- Psychoeducation
- Habit reversal therapy (HRT)
- Drugs like haloperidol, clonidine, aripiprazole, etc.

A-14. A. Conversion disorder (functional neurological disorder)

B. *Risk factors for conversion disorder:*

- Genetic factor
- Childhood trauma
- External environmental stress in school or family

- Sensitive or insecure temperament
- Psychiatric comorbid conditions
- Preexisting other illnesses

C. *Management:*

- Multidisciplinary
- Modification of parental responses
- Treatment of psychiatric and other associated illnesses

A-15. A. Specific-learning disorder

B. ADHD, autism, communication disorders and developmental coordination disorders may be associated comorbid conditions

C.

- Changes in teaching assessment
- Modifications like lowering level of teaching
- Remediation methods for critical and numeracy skills

A-16. A. Specific learning disability is defined as persistent impairment in reading (dyslexia), writing (dysgraphia) and/or arithmetic (dyscalculia) skills in an individual with preserved cognition, vision, hearing and adequate opportunities

B. Dyslexia is the most common specific learning disability (almost 80%)

C. Possible etiology is functionally disrupted networks in the cerebral cortex with intact anatomy

D. *Features suggesting specific learning disability:*

- Reading slowly and incorrectly
- Skipping lines while reading aloud
- Making repeated spelling mistakes
- Untidy or illegible handwriting
- Poor sequencing and inability to perform even simple mathematics

A-17. A. *Juvenile delinquency:* Children who show oppositional defiant behavior or conduct disorders and come into conflict with the juvenile system are called juvenile delinquents.

The term refers to a person under 18 years of age who is brought to the attention of juvenile justice system for committing a criminal act or displaying other illegal behaviors like the use of alcohol or illicit drugs.

B. *Munchausen by proxy:* Munchausen syndrome by proxy is a disorder in which a caregiver, usually mother deliberately makes up a history of illness in her child and/or harms the child to create illness. In this condition, the abusing caregiver gains attention from the relationship formed with healthcare providers, her family and as a result of problem created.

C. *Pica:* Pica is the persistent ingestion of non-nutritive substances such as plaster, charcoal, paint and soil for at least one month, inappropriate to the child's developmental level and cultural practice. It is common in children less than 5 years of age.

D. *Temper tantrums:* It is a child's response to physical or emotional challenges by attention seeking tactics like crying, kicking, pushing, throwing objects, hitting, head banging, etc. Tantrums typically begin at 18–36 months of age and gradually subsides by the age of 3–6 years.

E. *Thumb-sucking:* It is normal in infants and toddlers. It peaks by 18–21 months of age and usually disappears by the age of 4 years. If it persists, can lead to malalignment of teeth.

F. *Stuttering:* It is a defect in speech characterized by hesitation or spasmodic repetition of syllabuses with pauses. There is difficulty in pronouncing the initial consonants caused by spasm of lingual and palatal muscles. It can affect up to 5% of children between 2 and 5 years of age.

G. *Enuresis:* It is defined as passage of urine in the clothes beyond an age when bladder control should be established, usually 5 years. Both psychological stress and physiological dysfunction can be seen in affected children. Enuresis may be primary or secondary (after an initial control for 6 months or more). Primary monosymptomatic nocturnal enuresis is the commonest variety. Before labeling as primary enuresis, UTI, diabetes and bowel bladder dysfunction should be ruled out.

H. *Encopresis:* It is defined as passage of stools in clothes beyond an age when bowel control should have been achieved, usually 4 years. It may be retentive (associated with constipation) or non-retentive, primary (never achieved bowel control) or secondary (loss of control after an initial phase of control for at least 6 months). Primary encopresis is usually associated with constipation, while secondary is associated with significant psychological stressors.

A-18. A. Newborn
B. 4 months
C. 5 months

A-19. A. 4 weeks
B. 8–10 weeks
C. 12 weeks

A-20. A. 8 weeks
B. 4 months
C. 6 months
D. 8 months
E. 11 months

A-21. A. At birth
B. 5–6 months
C. 9–12 months

A-22. A. 3 years
B. 4 years
C. 4.5 years
D. 5 years
E. 6 years
F. 7 years
G. 8 years
H. 9 years
I. 11 years

A-23. A. Hearing assessment. Make a sound of a bell kept at 1.5 feet away and out of the field of vision of the child.
B. 10 months

CHAPTER 5

Nutrition

QUESTIONS

Q-1. A 2-year-old child presented with edema, hair changes and these skin lesions.

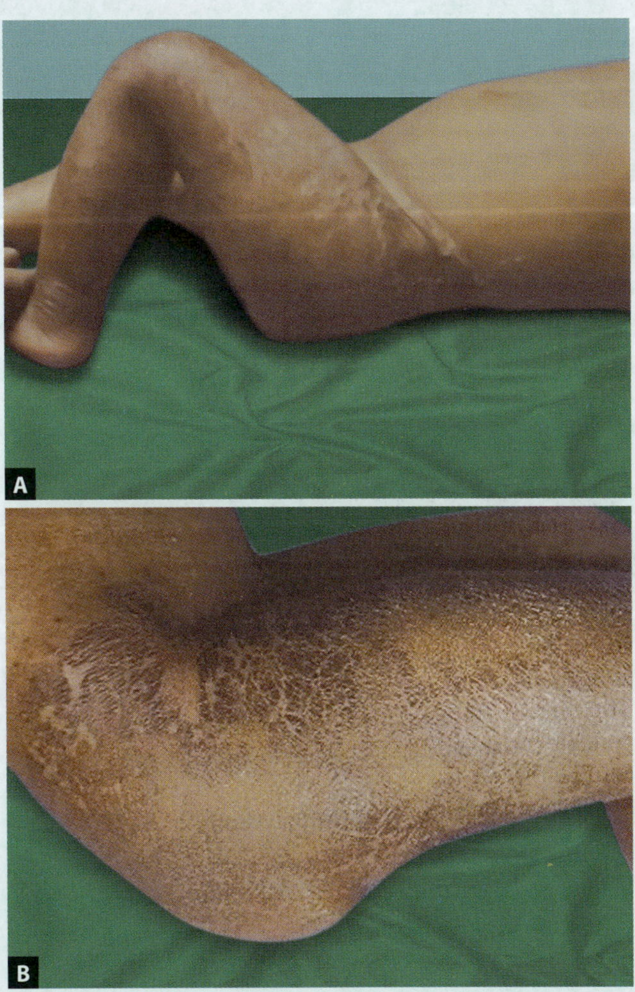

A. What is your diagnosis?
B. What are essential (cardinal) features of this disorder?
C. What are characteristics of skin lesions in this condition?
D. What deficiencies cause these skin changes?
E. What are common sites of these skin lesions?

Q-2.

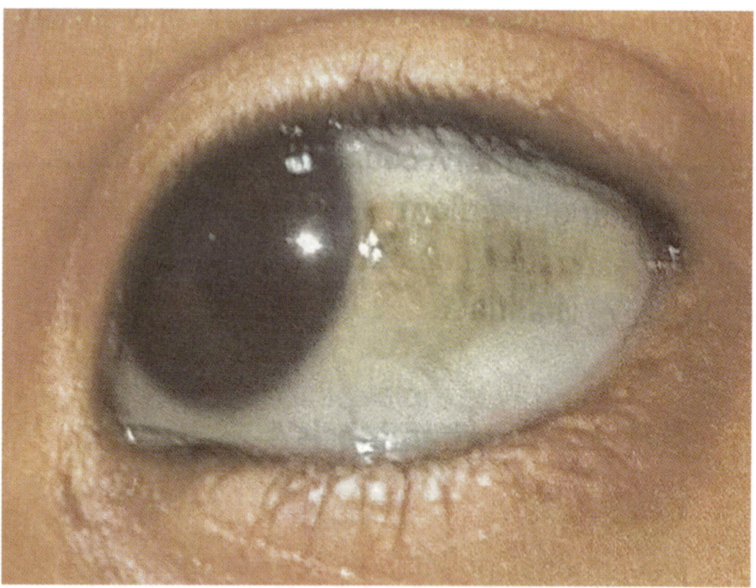

A. What does it show? Diagnosis?
B. What is the treatment of this condition?
C. What is the prophylaxis program against this nutritional disorder?
D. What is the dose and schedule of this nutrient for a child presenting with measles or SAM?

Q-3. An infant presented with severe anemia, regression of motor milestones, irritability and vacant look.

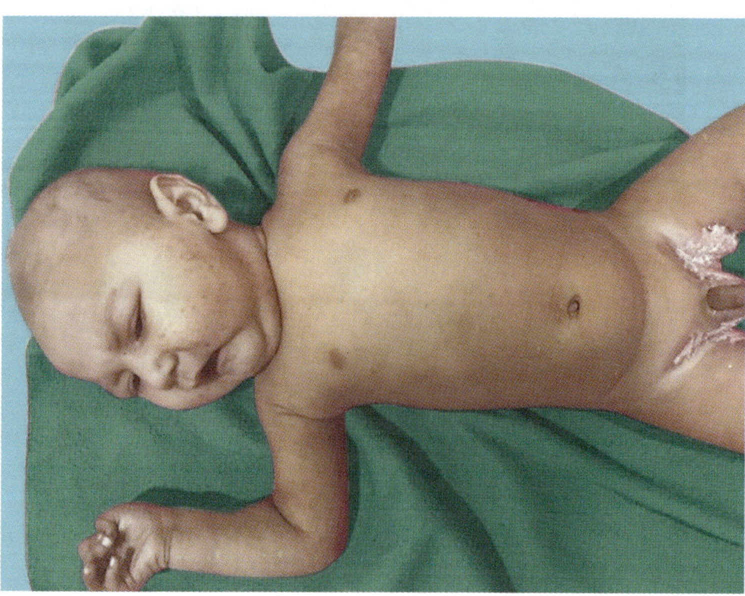

A. What is your diagnosis?
B. What deficiencies cause anemia in this disorder?
C. What are treatment components of this condition?

Q-4. All the three children from one family presented with diarrhea and this clinical picture. All of them responded well to therapy.

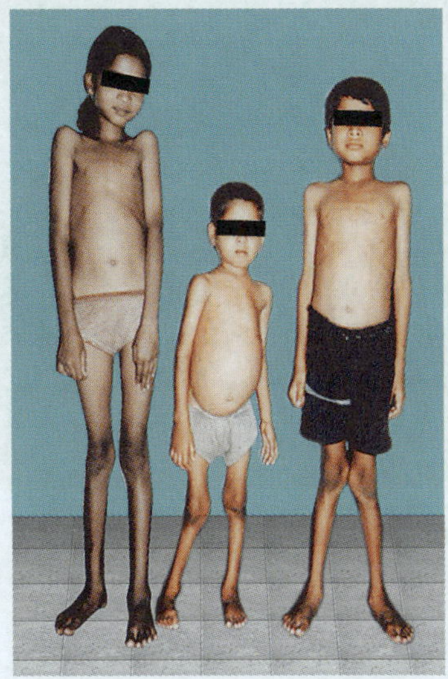

A. Name the condition.
B. Which amino acid deficiency results in this condition?
C. Which metabolic disorder can manifest with these features?

Q-5. A 3-year-old boy presented with hair loss of scalp and eye brows, non-healing ulcers over legs and perineum and edema both legs. He had history of diarrhea on and off, treated with various antibiotics without any benefit. These are the pictures of pre- and post-treatment.

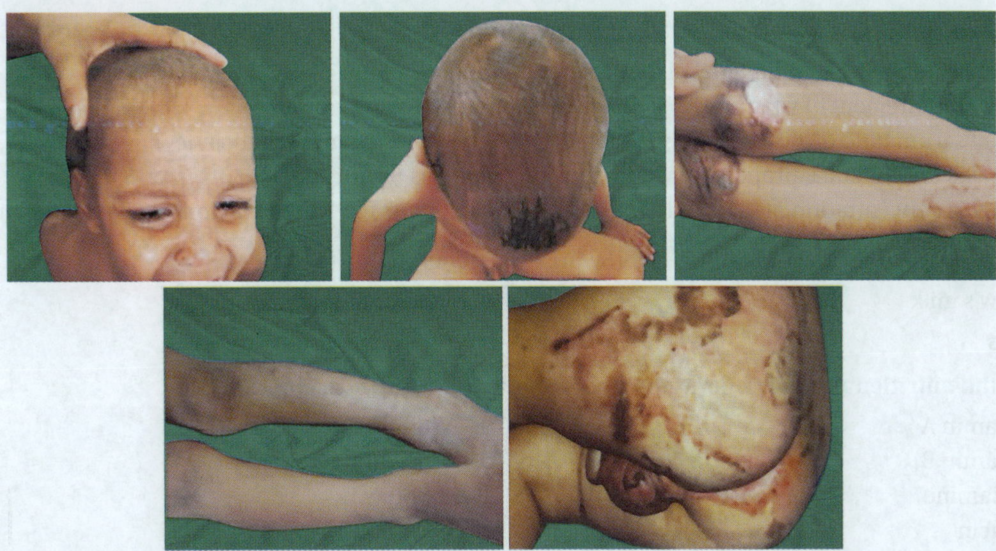

A. What is your diagnosis?
B. What is the treatment?
C. What are the manifestations of deficiency of this element?
D. What is the dose of this element in acute diarrhea disease?

Q-6.

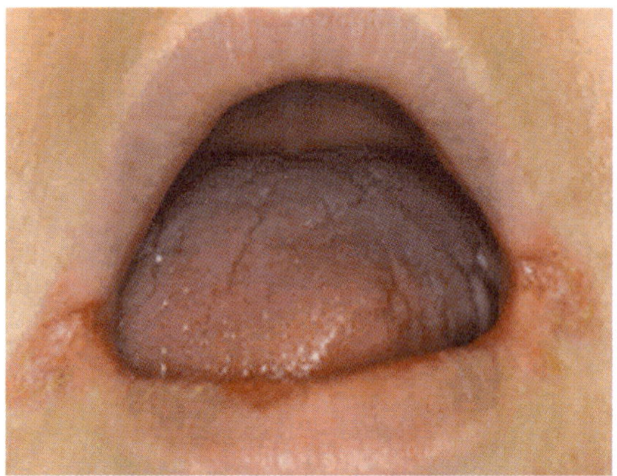

A. Identify the condition shown in image.
B. What is the underlying cause of this condition?
C. What are other features of this disease?
D. What is the treatment?

Q-7. Answer the following questions based on mid-day meal program,

A. What are the principles?
B. Write a model menu.

Q-8. A 5-year-old boy was brought with a history of abdominal pain, refractory anemia and sensory neuropathy. His father is working in chemical factory and family is staying in the campus of factory.

A. What is probable diagnosis?
B. What urine investigation suggests the possibility of condition?
C. What investigation would guide for indication for treatment in this disease?
D. What are the treatment options?

Q-9. Answer the following questions pertaining to vitamin E.

A. Manifestations of vitamin E deficiency in preterm babies
B. Daily requirement of vitamin E in preterm babies
C. What serum ratio of alpha-tocopherol: lipid is diagnosed as vitamin E deficiency?
D. What is the chemical property of vitamin E, considered as useful effect?
E. What is concentration of α-tocopherol in international unites in 1 mL of 'Evion' available preparation?

Q-10. What is the ideal age for introducing following food items?

A. Cow's milk
B. Peanut and seafood
C. Egg
D. Meat

Q-11. Write the nutritional requirements for a child of the following nutrients.

A. Vitamin A
B. Vitamin D
C. Vitamin B_{12}
D. Vitamin E
E. Thiamine
F. Riboflavin
G. Niacin
H. Vitamin C

Q-12. Answer the nutritional deficiencies commonly associate with followings:

A. Prolonged exclusive breastfeeding
B. Goat's milk
C. Cow's milk

Q-13. What are ingredients and kcal/100 g and protein /100 g of the following food preparations?

A. Hyderabad mix
B. Shakti ahar

Q-14. What are the calories contents of the following food items (100 g)?

A. Rice
B. Bengal gram
C. Fish
D. Egg
E. Groundnut
F. Dates
G. Almond
H. Apple

Q-15. Match the following:

A. Ujjawala
B. ASHA
C. Vademataram Scheme
D. Kishori Shakti Yojana
E. The Sharda Act

1. NRHM
2. Child trafficking
3. Adolescent girl health
4. Sage motherhood services
5. Child marriage prevention

Q-16. What is the nutritional values-calories and protein of the following cooked food items?

A. One chapati
B. One biscuit
C. One egg
D. One TSF cooked dal
E. One TSF mashed potato
F. One slice of bread

Q-17. Write content of the following human milk fortifier.

A. Protein
B. Fat
C. Vitamin D
D. Vitamin B_{12}
E. Zinc
F. Sodium
G. Calcium
H. Thiamine

Q-18. Match the followings—Trace element and its deficiency.

A. Manganese
B. Copper
C. Selenium
D. Molybdenum
E. Chromium

1. Central scotoma
2. Hyperglycemia
3. Refractory anemia
4. Red hair
5. Cardiomyopathy

Q-19. A one-year-old child has a weight of 6 kg and length 68 cm, there is no edema. What is the nutritional status as per following classification?

A. Gomez classification
B. Welcome classification
C. Water low classification
D. IAP classification

ANSWERS

A-1. A. Kwashiorkor

B.

- Bilateral pedal edema
- Growth failure
- Apathetic
- Muscle wasting

C.

- Flaky paint
- Crazy pavement
- Ulcers
- Petechiae, ecchymosis

D.
- Tyrosine
- Niacin
- Zinc
- Vitamins

E. Buttocks, perineum, thigh

A-2. A.
- Bitot spot
- Vitamin A deficiency

B.

Age	Dose in IU
<6 months	50,000
6–12 months	1 lakh
>1 year	2 lakhs

3 doses:
- First day
- Next day
- 4 weeks later

C.
- 6–59 months
- Vitamin A 1,00,000 units at 9 months with measles vaccine
- 2,00,000 units at 15–18 months with DPT booster
- Then 6 monthly till the age of 5 years (total 9 doses)

D.
- *<1 year:* 1,00,000 units
- *Older children:* 2,00,000 units
- Consecutive 2 days

A-3. A.
- Infantile tremor syndrome
- Anemia tremor syndrome

B.
- Iron
- Vitamin B_{12}
- Folic acid

C.
- Iron
- Vitamin B_{12}
- Folic acid
- Magnesium
- Zinc
- Calcium

A-4. A. Pellagra (Niacin deficiency)
B. Tryptophan
C. Hartnup disease

A-5. A. Acrodermatitis enteropathica
B. Oral zinc

C. A
- Malnutrition
- Dermatitis
- Growth retardation
- Hypogonadism
- Thymic atrophy
- Alopecia
- Diarrhea
- Acrodermatitis enteropathica
- Reduced taste sensation

D.
- <6 months 10 mg/day for 14 days
- >6 months 20 mg/day for 14 days

A-6. A. Angular cheilitis and glossitis
B. Riboflavin deficiency
C. Other features of riboflavin deficiency are keratitis, seborrheic dermatitis, photophobia and lacrimation.
D. Riboflavin 3–10 mg/day orally

A-7. A. *Principle of mid-day meal:*
- It is a supplement, not a substitute to home diet
- Should supply 1/3 of total energy, ½ of protein
- Low cost
- Can be cooked easily in school
- Use locally available food
- Frequent change of menu

B. *Model menu of mid-day meal:*
- *Cereals and millets:* 75 g
- *Pulses:* 30
- *Oil and fat:* 8
- *Leafy vegetables:* 30
- *Non-leafy:* 30

A-8. A. Lead poisoning
B. Urine protoporphyrin which is increased in lead poisoning.
C. Blood level of lead. Treatment is indicated, if lead level is >45 µg%
D. BAL and $CaNa_2$ (calcium versenate) are treatment options for lead poisoning.

A-9. A. Hemolytic anemia, thrombocytosis and edema are manifestations of vitamin E deficiency in preterm babies.
B. 5–25 IU/day
C. 0.8 mg/gm
D. Antioxidant
E. 50 IU

A-10. A. 1 year
B. 3 years
C. 18 months
D. 1 year

A-11. A. 500 µg
B. 400 IU
C. 0.5–1 µg
D. 5–15 IU
E. 0.5–1.5 mg
F. 0.5–1.5 mg
G. 5–15 mg
H. 40–50 mg

A-12. A. Iron deficiency anemia
B. Folate deficiency
C. Iron deficiency anemia

A-13. A. Hyderabad Mix 330 kcal and 11.3 g protein/86 g
- *Whole wheat:* 40 g
- *Bengal gram:* 16 g
- *Groundnut:* 10 g
- *Jaggery:* 20 g

B. *Shakti Ahar:* 390 kcal and 11.4 g protein/100 g
- *Roasted wheat:* 40 g
- *Roasted gram:* 20 g
- *Roasted peanut:* 10 g
- *Jaggery:* 30 g

A-14. A. 350 kcal B. 360 kcal
C. 80 kcal D. 80 kcal
E. 560 kcal F. 317 kcal
G. 655 kcal H. 59 kcal

A-15. A. 2 B. 1
C. 4 D. 3
E. 5

A-16. A. 70 kcal and 2 g protein B. 20 kcal and 0.5 g protein
C. 80 kcal and 6 g protein D. 10 kcal and 0.5 g protein
E. 40 kcal and no protein F. 80 kcal and 2.5 g protein

A-17. A. 0.2 G B. 0.1 G
C. 250 IU D. 0.05 μg
E. 0.18 mg F. 1.5 mg
G. 50 mg H. 12 μg

A-18. A. 4 B. 3
C. 5 D. 1
E. 2

A-19. A. Grade II malnutrition B. Undernutrition
C. Normal D. Grade II PEM

CHAPTER 6

Fluid, Electrolytes and ABG

QUESTIONS

Q-1.

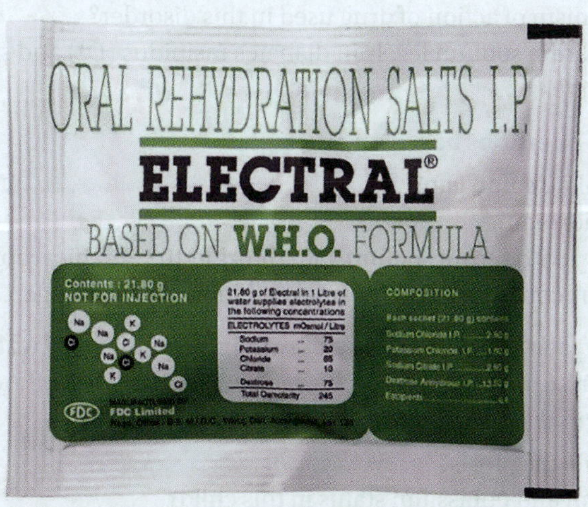

A. What is the osmolarity of low osmolar ORS?

B. Which day is celebrated as ORS day?

C. Bicarbonate in ORS is replaced by citrate. What are the advantages of citrate?

D. When was ORS introduced by WHO?

E. Name the condition in which standard WHO-ORS is appropriate.

Q-2 A 1.5-year-old child presented with failure to thrive, muscle weakness, constipation and polyuria. His arterial blood gas was as below:

***pH:* 7.57**

***pCO_2:* 36**

***pO_2:* 78**

***HCO_3:* 38**

***Oxygen saturation:* 98%**

A. What is your interpretation of the ABG?

B. Mention 4 clinical conditions in which this type of ABG finding can be seen.

C. On further investigations, he was noted to have hypokalemia. What is your diagnosis?

D. What is the line of treatment of this disorder?

Q-3. Answer the following questions:

A. Na^+ content of 0.9% NaCl
B. Na^+ content of 3% NaCl
C. Concentration of K^+ in Ringer's lactate
D. Elemental calcium in 1 mL 10% of calcium gluconate

Q-4. A 3-year-old girl was referred with complaints of high-grade fever for 5 days, vomiting, irritability followed by altered sensorium and generalized tonic-clonic seizures. It was diagnosed clinically as acute bacterial meningitis and admitted in PICU. Besides, necessary investigations for CNS infection, other investigations were performed for intractable seizures. Her serum sodium was 120 mEq/L, potassium 4 mEq/L, Chloride 100 mEq/L, bicarbonate 22 mEq/L, serum osmolarity 260 mOsm/kg, urine sodium 58 mEq/L, urine osmolarity 310 moSm/kg and urine output 1.5 mL/kg/hour.

A. What is the most probable diagnosis?
B. What happens if treating person rapidly corrects sodium in this patient?
C. What is the mechanism of action of drug used in this disorder?
D. What happens to serum sodium levels in diabetes insipidus (DI) and syndrome of inappropriate antidiuretic hormone (SIADH)?

Q-5. Answer the following questions based on anion gap.

A. How will you calculate anion gap?
B. What is normal anion gap?
C. Calculate anion gap with serum sodium 136, chloride 102 and bicarbonate 10.
D. Mention the various conditions with normal and increased anion gap.

Q-6. A 2.5-year-old girl presented with history of multiple episodes of watery stools. Her weight was 8 kg and height 90 cm and mid upper arm circumference 10.5 cm with bilateral pedal edema. She had signs of dehydration with normal sensorium.

A. What is the probable diagnosis?
B. What will be sodium and potassium status in this child?
C. What is the preferred route for correction of dehydration in this patient?
D. What are the clinical signs of shock in this child?
E. Mention the composition of rehydration solution for the children with this type nutritional status.
F. How will you prepare ReSoMal using low osmolar ORS?

Q-7. A 7-year-old boy with nephrotic syndrome is hospitalized with complaints of edema, lethargy and altered sensorium for a day only. The patient had no any sign of shock. The fundus examination revealed papilledema. His blood investigations showed serum sodium 125 mEq/L, potassium 3.8 mEq/L, chloride 100 mEq/L and bicarbonate 22 mEq/L.

A. What type of hyponatremia in this patient?
B. What CNS complications is expected in this type of hyponatremia?
C. How one should correct hyponatremia in this child?

Q-8. A 18-month-old girl was brought for regular booster doses of vaccination. On physical examination, wide open anterior fontanelle, rachitic rosary and widening of wrists were noted. Laboratory investigations showed serum calcium 7.3 mg/dL, phosphorus 1.3 mg/dL, alkaline phosphatase 1400 IU/L, parathyroid hormone (PTH) 360 pg/mL, 25-hydroxy vitamin D_3 35 ng/mL and serum magnesium 2 mg/dL.

A. What is the probable diagnosis?
B. When does this condition develop in this disorder?
C. What are other conditions predisposing to this disorder?
D. What happens to urine calcium and phosphorus in this disease?

Q-9. A 8-year-old girl, diagnosed to have minimal change nephrotic syndrome, on steroids has no edema and is in remission phase. On follow-up, laboratory investigations were performed and reported as serum albumin 4.5 g/dL, serum cholesterol 320 mg/dL, serum sodium 128 mEq/L, potassium 4 mEq/L, chloride 105 mEq/L and bicarbonate 22 mEq/L.

A. What is the cause of hyponatremia in this patient?
B. Mention other conditions, known to present like this situation.
C. What changes in serum osmolarity is seen in true and pseudohyponatremia?
D. How to diagnose pseudohyponatremia?

Q-10. A 9-year-old boy was admitted in PICU following traumatic brain injury. He developed polyuria and dehydration on second day. Investigations showed serum sodium 130 mEq/L, potassium 4 mEq/L, chloride 104 mEq/L, bicarbonate 22 mEq/L, serum osmolarity 210 mOsm/kg, urine sodium 180 mEq/L with urine osmolarity 310 mOsm/kg.

A. What is probable diagnosis in this patient?
B. What is the pathophysiology of this condition?
C. What should be treatment of this child?
D. What is the concentration of sodium in mEq/L in 1 mL of 3% saline?

Q-11. A 6-year-old boy was referred for polyuria and polydipsia. His vitals were within normal limits. His blood glucose was 80 mg/dL, urine routine and renal function tests normal. Blood and urine ketones were negative.

A. What are two common differential diagnosis?
B. Name conditions, known to present with above-mentioned clinical picture.
C. Which test can confirm central diabetes insipidus?
D. What is triple response?

Q-12. A 3-year-old girl presented with acute diarrheal disease with reduced oral intake, lethargy and oliguria. The clinical examination was suggesting compensated shock. CBC showed Hb 13 g/dL, TLC 18,500 with 70% Polymorphs and 30% lymphocytes. Platelets were 7,50,000. Her blood glucose was 70 mg/dL, serum sodium 170 mEq/L, potassium 3.8 mEq/L, chloride 108 mEq/L, bicarbonate and serum creatinine 0.6 mg/dL.

A. What is the type of hypernatremia in this patient?
B. What are other causes of seizures in a child with hyponatremia in such a case apart from sodium disturbance?
C. What is the line of treatment in this child?
D. What are indications of renal replacement therapy in a child with hypernatremia?
E. What is the maximum correction of sodium allowed in this patient?

Q-13. A 2.5-year-old girl was brought for delayed motor development. Antenatal, natal and post-natal periods were uneventful. The child had no history of seizures. Clinical examination showed generalized hypotonia, wide- open anterior fontanelle, wide wrists and double malleoli. Laboratory investigations showed serum calcium 5.8 mg/dL, phosphorus 1.6 mg/dL, Alkaline phosphatase 1850 IU/L, parathyroid hormone 650 pg/mL, 25 hydroxy vitamin D_3 20 ng/mL and 1,25, dihydroxy vitamin D_3 very low.

A. What is the probable diagnosis?
B. What is the confirmatory test of this condition?
C. What is the treatment of this child?
D. If this disorder is associated with alopecia and similar problem in another sibling, then what is your diagnosis?

ANSWERS

A-1. A. 245 mmol/L

B. 29th July

C. Increased self-life of ORS. Better taste
Unsoiled packets

D. 1971

E. Cholera

A-2. A. Uncompensated metabolic alkalosis

B.
- Gastric losses (persistent vomiting or nasogastric suction)
- Diuretics
- Gitelman syndrome
- Bartter syndrome

C. Bartter syndrome

D. Potassium supplementation and indomethacin

A-3. A. 154 mEq/L

B. 500 mEq/L

C. 5 mEq/L

D. 8.9 mg (0.45 mEq/L)

A-4. A. SIADH (Syndrome of Inappropriate Antidiuretic Hormone)
The patient with CNS infection, likely bacterial meningitis, has hyponatremia with normal urine output, suggesting euvolemia. Her serum osmolarity is low hence it is true hyponatremia, urine osmolarity is more than serum osmolarity and urine sodium is 58 mEq/L which suggests natriuresis despite low serum osmolarity. It is classical presentation of SIADH, which is known complication in a case of CNS infection.

B. This child is symptomatic for more than 72 hours, means chronic hyponatremia. The chronic hyponatremia should be corrected slowly, 6–8 mEq/day because rapid correction can result in osmotic demyelination.

C. Vasopressin receptor antagonism is the mechanism of action of drug used in SIADH.

D. Hypernatremia in DI and hyponatremia in SIADH.

A-5. A. Anion gap = (Serum sodium) – (Serum chloride + Serum bicarbonate)

B. Normal anion gap is 8 to 12.

C. (136) – (102 + 10) = 24

D. *Conditions with normal anion gap:*
- Acute diarrheal disease (ADD)
- Renal tubular acidosis (RTA)

Conditions with increased anion gap:
- Diabetic ketoacidosis (DKA)
- Lactic acidosis
- Acute renal failure (ARF)
- Inborn error of metabolism (IEM)
- Septic shock
- Salicylate poisoning

A-6. A. Severe acute malnutrition (SAM) with acute diarrheal disease (ADD) with some dehydration

B. In a child with SAM, there will be an increase in cellular sodium and depletion of serum potassium levels. Hence, in children with SAM, diet should be supplemented with low sodium with supplemented potassium. Magnesium should also be supplemented.

C. Oral or nasogastric tube-feeding with ReSoMal is preferred for correction of dehydration in this situation. IV fluid is indicated in such children only when a child is in shock, altered sensorium or not able to take orally. IV fluid of choice is 0.45% NS with 5% glucose.

D. *Clinical sign of shock in children with SAM:*
- Lethargy
- Thirst
- Cold clammy skin
- Weak or absent pulses
- Oliguria

E. *Composition of ReSoMal:*
- *Glucose:* 125 mmol/L
- *Sodium:* 45 mmol/L
- *Potassium:* 40 mmol/L
- *Chloride:* 70 mmol/L
- *Magnesium:* 3 mmol/L
- *Zinc:* 0.3 mmol/L
- *Copper:* 0.045 mmol/L
- *Lactate:* 7 mmol/L
- *Osmolarity:* 300 mmol/L

F. *Preparation of ReSoMal using low osmolar ORS:*
- Take one sachet of WHO-ORS and mix in two liters of water
- Add 50 g of glucose
- 20 mL of Potklor
- 40 mL of electrolyte and mineral solution (containing zinc, magnesium and copper)

A-7. A. Acute hyponatremia, hypervolemic hyponatremia due to low intravascular volume

B. Cerebral edema is known complication of acute hyponatremia.

C. *Correction of acute hyponatremia:*
- 3–5 mL/kg of 3% saline in euvolemic and hypervolemic hyponatremia
- In hypovolemic hyponatremia 20 mL/kg of NS over 30–60 minutes by IV route
- The goal is to increase the sodium up to 5 mEq/L from baseline values which is sufficient to correct symptoms. It is done in addition to stabilization of the patient and control of seizures.

A-8. A. This patient has clinical and biochemical findings of rickets with a normal 25-hydroxy vitamin D_3 level, suggesting calcium deficiency. With normal 25-hydroxy vitamin D_3 level, if the child has rickets, there are two possibilities, VDDR type I and II and dietary calcium deficiency.

B. When dietary intake of calcium is less than 200 mg/day, rickets is likely to develop.

C. *Other conditions predisposing to dietary calcium deficiency leading to rickets are:*
- Celiac disease
- Abetalipoproteinemia
- Small bowel resection

D. In this disease, there is low urine calcium and high urine phosphorus due to secondary hyperparathyroidism.

A-9. A. It is pseudohyponatremia in this case due to hypercholesterolemia.

B. *Conditions presenting as pseudohyponatremia:*
- Hyperglycemia
- Hyperproteinemia
- Improper sampling
- Osmolar agents like mannitol

In this conditions, there is increased plasma volume, hence sodium is erroneously measured as low due to dilution, actually total serum sodium is normal.

C. Serum osmolarity is low in true hyponatremia while it is high or normal in pseudohyponatremia

D. Ion-selective electrode (ISE) method measures the sodium in total serum, therefore true hyponatremia and pseudohyponatremia becomes obvious with this method.

A-10. A. Cerebral salt wasting. Polyuria with hypovolemia, hyponatremia, low serum osmolarity and high urinary sodium excretion are classical features of cerebral salt wasting.

B. Increased atrial natriuretic peptide (ANP) which inhibits arginine vasopressin (AVP) and aldosterone causing natriuresis.

C. Sodium and water replacement using isotonic saline and fludrocortisone is the line of treatment.

D. 1 mL of 3% saline = 513 mEq/L sodium

A-11. A. Diabetes insipidus and psychogenic polydipsia are common differential diagnosis with this type of presentation.

B. *Conditions known to present with this clinical picture:*

- Craniopharyngioma
- Sarcoidosis
- Pituitary trauma
- Congenital malformation
- Familial central diabetes insipidus
- Langerhans cell histiocytosis
- Idiopathic

C. Water deprivation test can confirm central diabetes insipidus.

D. Triple response is following pituitary stalk injury from traumatic brain injury or in a neurosurgical procedure.

In Triple response, initially there is a central diabetes insipidus followed by SIADH and finally established central diabetes insipidus. The initial phase of central diabetes insipidus is due to stunning of arginine vasopressin neurons and serving to downstream nerve terminals in the posterior pituitary followed by SIADH due to unregulated release of vasopressin from the remaining degenerating neurons followed by an established diabetes insipidus as the damaged neurons can no longer produce arginine vasopressin.

A-12. A. The presence of dehydration and hypernatremia suggest hypovolemic hypernatremia in this patient.

B. *Causes of seizures in such patients:*

- Intracranial bleeding
- Venous sinus thrombosis
- Hypocalcemia

C. *Line of treatment in this patient:*

- Establish airway breathing and circulation
- Oxygen
- The child is in compensated shock, hence give bolus with NS at 20 mL/kg over 30–60 minutes and further boluses, if needed to be decided as per clinical status.
- Followed by boluses, fluid therapy consisting of deficit correction plus ongoing loss replacement plus daily maintenance. Choice of fluid should be ½ NS

D. *Indications of renal replacement therapy:*

- Serum sodium >180 mEq/L
- Multiple electrolyte abnormalities
- Acute kidney injury

E. Maximum correction of sodium allowed in this patient is 8–10 mEq/day. The fall of serum sodium should not exceed beyond 0.5 mEq/hour.

A-13. A. This child has clinical features of rickets with low serum calcium and phosphorus, elevated alkaline phosphatase, raised parathyroid hormone, normal 25-hydroxy vitamin D_3 and very low 1, 25-dihydroxy vitamin D_3 suggesting the diagnosis of vitamin D dependent rickets type I (VDDR type I)

B. Molecular testing is the confirmatory investigation.

C. 1,25-dihydroxy vitamin D_3 (calcitriol) in the dose of 0.25 μg/day along with calcium and phosphorus.

D. Vitamin D dependent rickets type II (VDDR type II)

CHAPTER 7

Neonatology

QUESTIONS

Q-1. Mother noticed a swelling over scalp in two-day-old Infant as shown below:

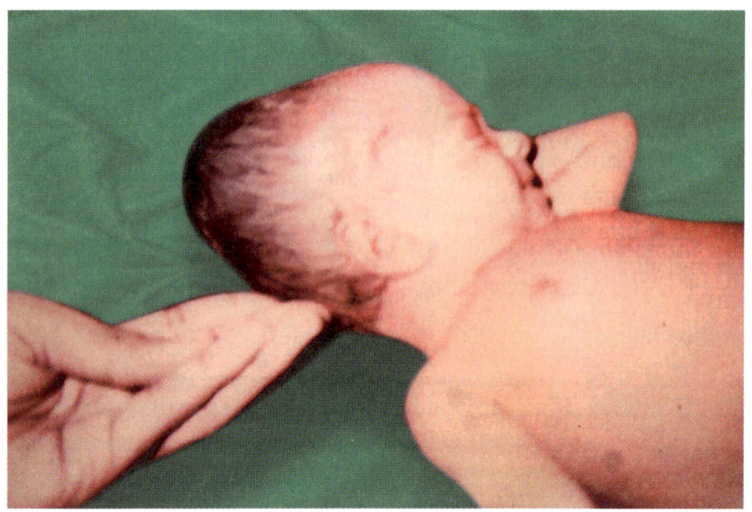

A. What is your diagnosis?
B. What is cause of it?
C. What are its clinical characteristics?
D. What is its usual course?
E. What is the treatment?
F. What are its known complications?

Q-2. Antenatal corticosteroids in preterm labor:

A. Indication
B. Optimal timing
C. Dosage
D. Which preparation is preferred? Why?

Q-3. The findings on ophthalmoscopic of newborn are shown below:

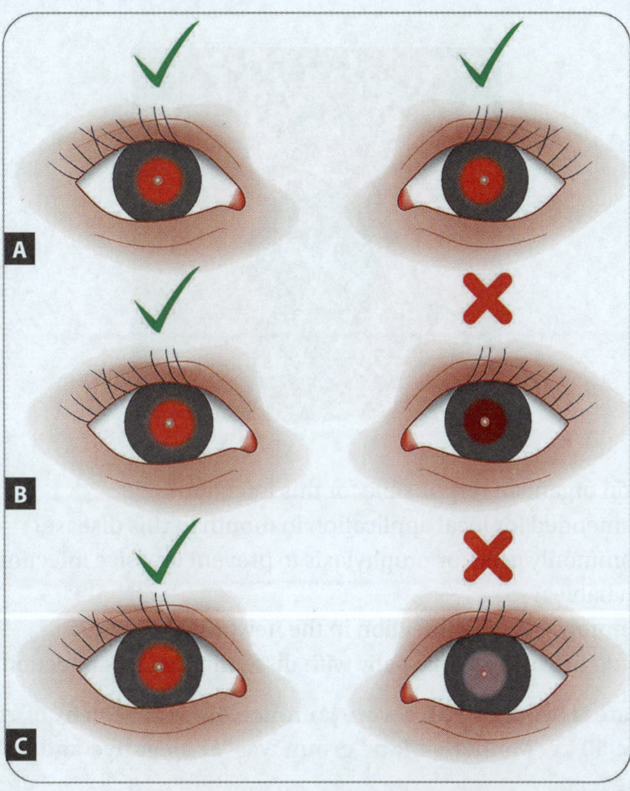

A. Name the test.

B. What are the findings in **Figures A, B and C**.

Q-4. A mother was worried for the whitish spots over nose and face of her baby as shown in below:

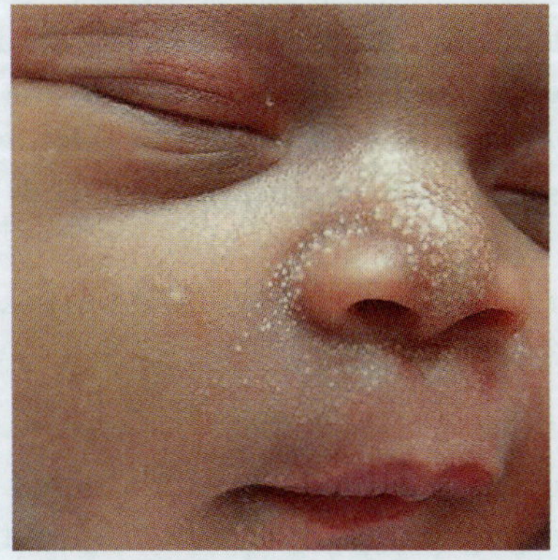

A. What is this condition?
B. Which structure of skin is involved in this disorder?
C. What treatment will you suggest?
D. What are these retention cysts called when present in midline palate?

Q-5. A neonate, exclusively breastfed was brought with complaints of not taking breastfeeding adequately and these oral lesions.

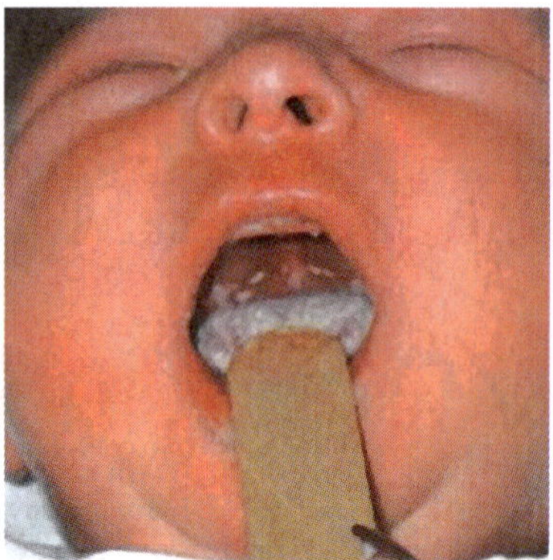

A. Name the condition.
B. What is most common organism responsible for this infection?
C. Which drug is recommended for local application in mouth in this disease?
D. Which are the two commonly used for prophylaxis to prevent invasive infection due to this organism in NICU in extremely preterm babies?
E. What is the most common source of infection in the newborns?
F. Which infection should be rules out in a baby with disseminated this infection?

Q-6. A 6-day-old term neonate is brought with severe jaundice. He was born by normal vaginal delivery at home. His birth weight was 2.950 kg. Mother's blood group was 'O' negative and baby 'B' positive. The baby was lethargic and not taking feed.

A. What is your diagnosis?
B. What are the sign of this disease?
C. Which part of brain are specific predilection for this condition in neonates?

Q-7. A 72 hours old term baby presented with severe jaundice. The serum bilirubin was 32 mg/dL. He was born by a normal vaginal route to a primigravida mother, cried soon after birth, birth weight was 2.9 kg. Mother's blood group was 'O" positive. There was some problem in establishing breast feeding. On admission, his weight was 2.5 kg. He was irritable and not accepting the oral feeds now.

A. What is the diagnosis?
B. What are the risk factors for severe neonatal jaundice in a term baby?
C. How will you manage this baby?

Q-8.

A. What are two disease preventive measures routinely administered to all newborns?
B. Name three early disease detection measures which should be routinely done in all newborns before hospital discharge.

Q-9. A neonate was brought with complaints of swelling of left eye and pus discharge as shown in image below:

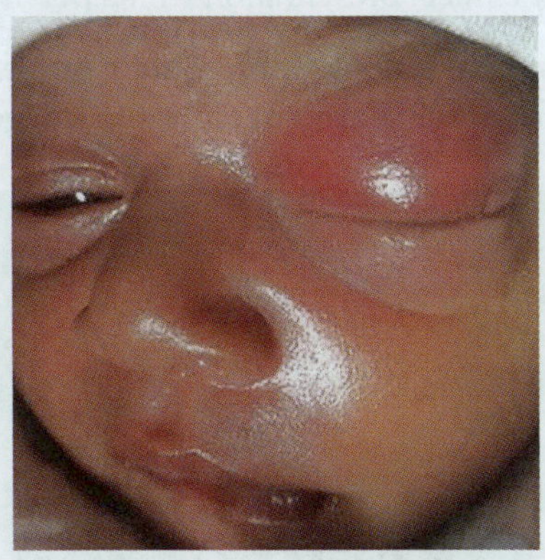

A. What is the probable diagnosis?
B. What are common predisposing factors?
C. What are common organisms responsible for this condition?
D. What is the treatment?
E. What complications are known following this problem?

Q-10. A newborn presented with a painless lesion on the forearm as shown in image below:

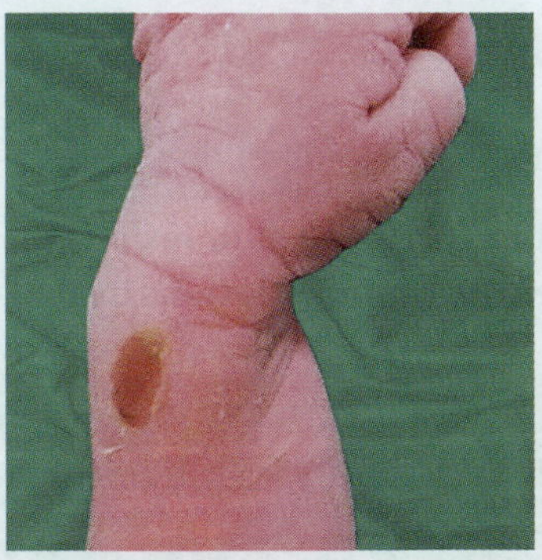

A. What is likely condition?
B. What are other sites where similar lesions may be found?
C. What is the line of treatment?

Q-11. A neonate developed reticular mottling of the skin of extremities on day 4 of life as shown in image. The baby was otherwise asymptomatic, taking feeds well and vitals within normal limits. He skin lesions disappear and reappear within few hours.

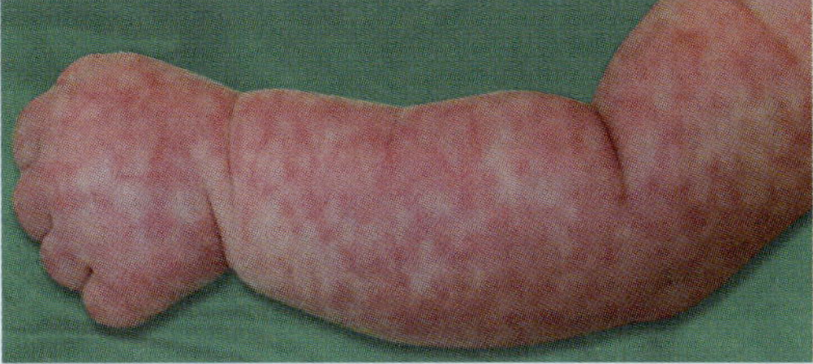

A. What is the probable condition?
B. What causes these skin changes?

C. How these lesions get resolved?
D. Name the condition with similar clinical presentation which persists in spite of a remedial measure?

Q-12. A 10-day-old neonate was brought with tender, hard, mobile and erythematous violaceous nodules lateral aspect of right arm and back in the winter season as shown in image. Serum calcium level was 7 mg/dL.

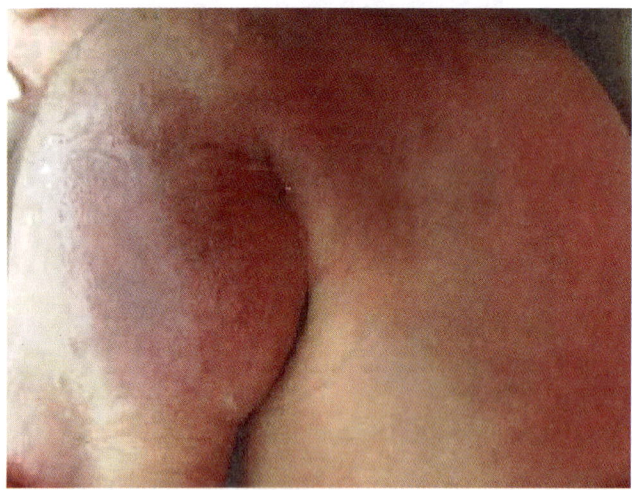

A. What is likely condition?
B. What is the risk factor for this disorder?
C. What is known complication in this disease?
D. What is the course and prognosis of this condition?

Q-13. A 3-day-old baby was brought in OPD with skin lesions as shown in following image. The blisters were flaccid with erythematous base. The ruptured lesions healed with yellowish crusting.

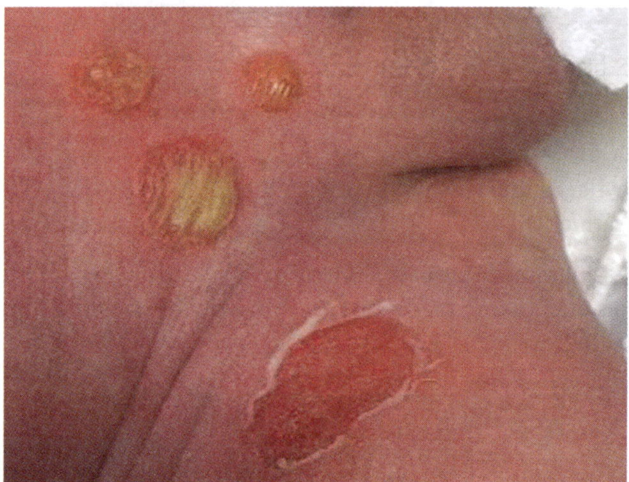

A. What is probable diagnosis?
B. What is the most common organisms causing this condition?
C. What are choice of drugs to treat the disease?

Q-14. A 8-day-old neonate was brought in pediatric OPD with complaints of multiple pustular skin lesions over the trunk and limbs. The skin swab examination showed gram positive cocci in cluster.

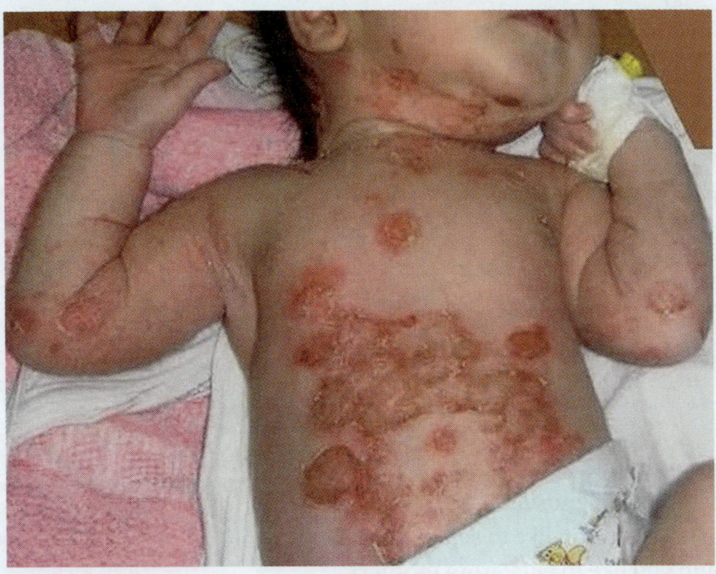

A. What is most probable diagnosis?
B. Which are common organisms responsible for this condition?
C. What is the treatment?

Q-15. A full-term neonate presented on day 4 with following rashes all over body, maximum over face and trunk, sparing palms and soles.

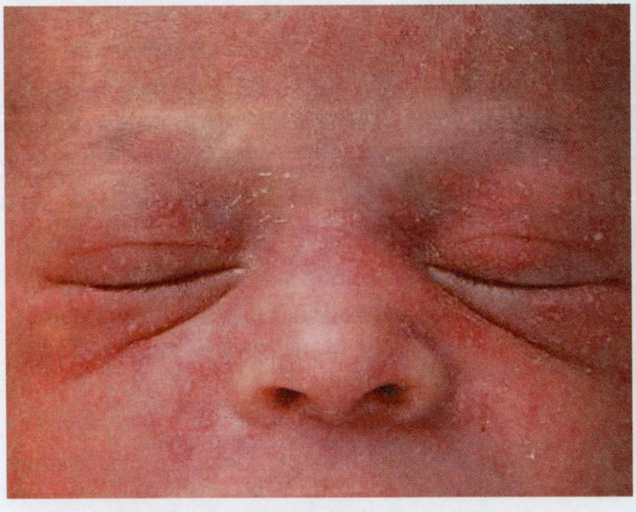

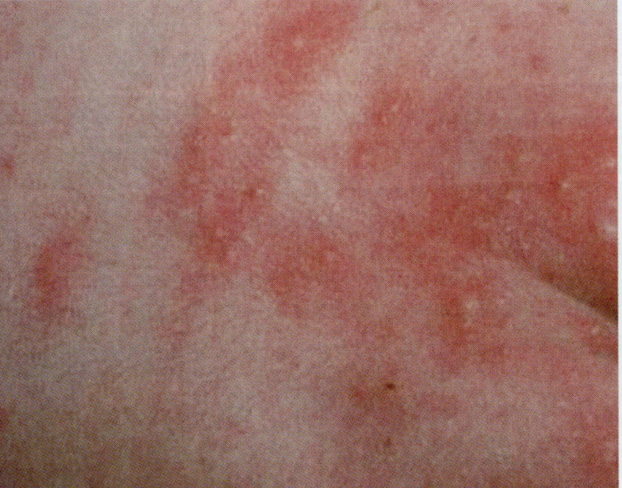

A. What is probable diagnosis?
B. What are the two vanities of this condition?
C. What cells from WBC series will be seen in smear from these lesions?
D. What is the treatment?

Q-16. A neonate presented with maculopapular rashes all over body, more on face as shown in image. On examination, he also had blueberry muffin rashes and hepatomegaly.

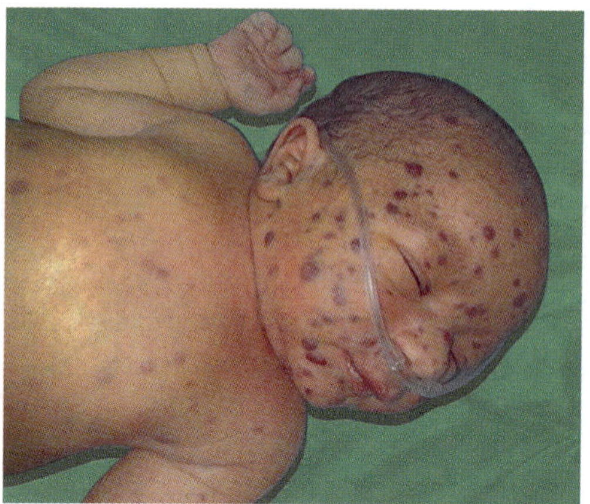

A. What is probable condition?
B. What are the differential diagnosis?
C. What other features would you like to see in the patient?
D. What history would you like to elicit from mother?
E. What investigations would you like to perform?

Q-17. A 1.5-month-old infant was brought with following scalp lesions:

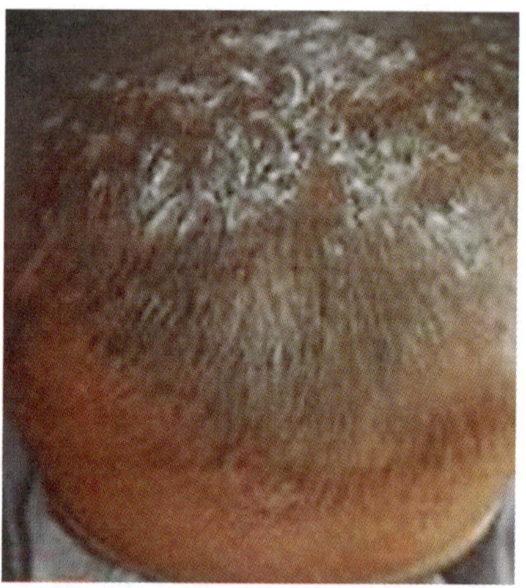

A. What is probable diagnosis?
B. Which structure of skin is involved in this disease?
C. What is the morphological description of these lesions?
D. Name the associated causative organisms.
E. What drugs are used as the treatment?
F. Which disease in infants and toddlers is known to present with these scalp lesions, hepatosplenomegaly and lymphadenopathy?

Q-18. Answer the following questions on neonatal jaundice:

A. What is breastfeeding jaundice?
B. What is breast milk jaundice?

C. *True/False for following statements pertaining to neonatal jaundice:*
   a. Physical examination is not a reliable measure for serum bilirubin level.
   b. When clinically jaundice is evident in a newborn, serum bilirubin is more than 5 mg/dL.
   c. Jaundice in first 24 hours is always physiological.
   d. Breastfeeding is contraindicated in breast milk jaundice.
   e. ABO group incompatibility occurs when mother is 'A' or 'B' group and baby 'O'.

Q-19. Name the probable clinical diagnosis in a given scenario in newborns.

A. Dextroposition of heart, respiratory distress and scaphoid abdomen
B. Bilious vomiting and scaphoid abdomen
C. Bilious vomiting, blood in stool and scaphoid abdomen
D. Frothing from mouth and scaphoid abdomen

Q-20. What is warm chain in neonatology?

ANSWERS

A-1. A. Right-sided parietal cephalohematoma
B. It is due to subperiosteal hemorrhage.
C. Swelling appears after few hours to days as subperiosteal bleeding is a slow process, It does not cross the suture line.
D. Most cephalohematomas are reabsorbed within 2 weeks to 3 months
E. No treatment is required.
F. Hyperbilirubinemia, may require phototherapy. It may get infected, if aspiration is tried.

A-2. A. *Indication:* Risk of preterm delivery between 24 and 34 weeks of gestation
B. *Optimal timing:*
- Beneficial, if delivery occurs after 24–48 hours.
- Effect lasts for 7 days

C. *Dosage:*
- Injection betamethasone 12 mg IM every 24 hours for 2 doses
- Injection dexamethasone 6 mg IM every 12 hours for 2 doses

D. Dexamethasone is preferred.

A-3. A. Red reflex test
B. Findings are as follows:
A: Symmetric red reflex
B: Normal red reflex in one eye but diminished in another eye (refractive error, retinoblastoma)

A-4. A. Milia neonatorum
B. Sebaceous glands
C. No treatment is required. Counsel the mother that it is benign condition and lesions will resolve spontaneously in 2–3 weeks
D. Epstein pearls

A-5. A. Oral thrush (oral candidiasis)
B. Candida albicans
C. Clotrimazole mouth paint
D. Fluconazole and amphotericin B
E. Maternal candida vaginal infection
F. HIV

A-6. A. Acute bilirubin encephalopathy
B. Kernicterus is the conditions with chronic sequelae following bilirubin encephalopathy in a neonate. It is irreversible damage to brain.

Sequelae of kernicterus:
- Cerebral palsy
- Choreoathetosis type of cerebral palsy
- Sensorineural deafness
- Upward gaze paresis
- Dental enamel dysplasia

C. *The most common affected parts of brains are:*
- Basal ganglia, particularly Globus pallidus and subthalamic nuclei
- Hippocampus
- Substantia nigra
- Oculomotor, vestibular, cochlear and facial nerves nuclei
- Reticular formation of pons
- Inferior olivary nucleus
- Anterior horn cell of spinal cord

A-7. A. Bilirubin encephalopathy

B. *Risk factors for severe jaundice in a term baby:*
- Jaundice in first 24 hours of life
- Rh-incompatibility
- ABO incompatibility
- G-6-P-D deficiency
- History of severe neonatal jaundice in sibling
- Feeding problem
- Neonatal infections
- Cephalohematoma

C. *Management of this baby:*
- Double volume blood exchange transfusion at the earliest
- Intensive phototherapy
- IV fluid
- Intravenous immunoglobulin for iso-immune hemolytic anemia

A-8. A.
- Vitamin K
- *Birth vaccines:* BCG, Hepatitis B and OPV

B.
- Transcutaneous bilirubinometer
- SpO_2
- Metabolic disorders blood screen
- OAE screen
- TSH
- Pulse oximetry screen

A-9. A. Orbital cellulitis

B. Eyelid infection, dental abscess, hematogenous spread can lead to orbital cellulitis.

C. Common organisms are *Staphylococcus aureus, Streptococcus*, and *Klebsiella pneumoniae.*

D.
- *Antibiotics:* Cloxacillin, amoxicillin-clavulanic acid combination, vancomycin
- Surgical intervention

E. *Complications:*
- Intracranial abscess

- Bacterial meningitis
- Cavernous sinus thrombosis
- Loss of vision
- Sepsis

A-10. A. Sucking blister
B. Hands, forearm, and lips are common sites for sucking blisters.
C. No treatment is required. It is self-limiting condition.

A-11. A. Neonatal cutis Marmorata
B. It is due to vascular response to cold, variable vascular constriction and dilatation.
C. Making the limb warm, the lesion get resolved.
D. Cutis marmorata telangiectasia congenita

A-12. A. Subcutaneous fat necrosis of newborn
B. Hypothermia is the risk factor. Brown fat of neonate has increased ratio of saturated palmitic acid to unsaturated oleic acid. Palmitic acid has a higher melting point than oleic acid making it more susceptible to solidification and crystallization in response to cold.
C. Hypercalcemia
D. Self-limiting disease with favorable prognosis

A-13. A. Bullous impetigo
B. *Staphylococcus aureus*
C. *Choice of antibiotics:*
- Cloxacillin
- Cefazolin
- Vancomycin
- Mupirocin or Fusidic acid for local application

A-14. A. Impetigo
B. *Common organisms:*
- *Staphylococcus aureus* (bullous impetigo)
- Streptococcal infection

C.
- Oral or IV cloxacillin
- *Local antibiotics:* Mupirocin or Fusidic acid

A-15.
A. Erythema toxicum neonatorum
B. *Types of disorder:*
- Erythematous
- Pustular variety

C. Eosinophils
D. It is begin condition, will resolve by his own in few days. Only reassurance to mother is the treatment.

A-16. A. Congenital infection
B. Congenital toxoplasmosis, rubella, CMV infections
C. Other features
- Icterus
- Pallor
- Cardiac anomaly
- Eye examination for cataract, chorioretinitis, etc.
- Hydrocephalus, microcephaly

D.
- History fever and skin rashes during pregnancy in first trimester
- History of vaccines received by mother like MMR
- History of pets in family

E. *Investigations:*
- CBC for anemia, thrombocytopenia
- Liver function tests
- Serological tests (IgM and IgG) in baby and mother
- *Radio-imaging*: MRI brain of baby for intracranial calcifications, hydrocephalus, congenital anomalies

A-17. A. Seborrheic dermatitis of scalp (cradle cap)

B. Sebaceous glands

C. These lesions are erythematous and greasy scales.

D. Malassezia furfur

E. *Drugs used in treatment:*
- Petrolatum
- Ketoconazole shampoo
- Tar containing shampoo
- 1% hydrocortisone

F. Langerhans cell histiocytosis (LCH)

A-18. A. *Breastfeeding jaundice:* Due to inadequate feeding, there is weight loss of the baby and increased enterohepatic circulation which results in hyperbilirubinemia.

B. A metabolite substance 3α-20β pregnanediol, lipase and free fatty acids interfere with conjugation of bilirubin results in persistent and prolonged physiological jaundice in an otherwise healthy term baby, beyond 14 days.

C.
  a. True
  b. True
  c. False
  d. False
  e. False

A-19. A. Congenital diaphragmatic hernia on left side

B. Duodenal atresia

C. Volvulus of intestine

D. Esophageal atresia

A-20. *Components of warm chain:*
- Warm delivery room
- Warm resuscitation
- Immediate drying the baby
- Skin-to-skin contact
- Breastfeeding
- Bathing postponed
- Appropriate clothing-coving head
- Mother and baby together
- Professional alertness
- Warm transportation

CHAPTER 8

Genetics and Syndromes

QUESTIONS

Q-1. An infant girl was brought with swelling on the dorsum of both hands and feet. She also had non pitting edema over legs. The clinical photographs are given below:

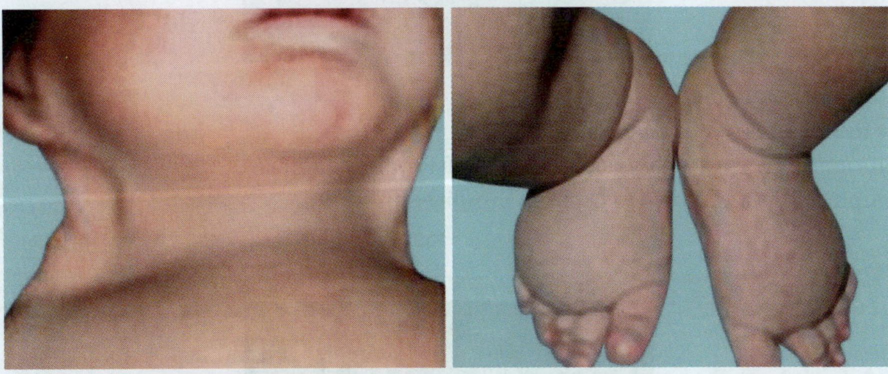

A. What is the probable diagnosis?
B. Name two characteristic cardiac anomalies seen in this condition.
C. Name two common endocrinal problems in this disorder.
D. Which gastrointestinal disorders are known to occur in this disease?
E. What is the most common renal anomaly seen in this disease?

Q-2.

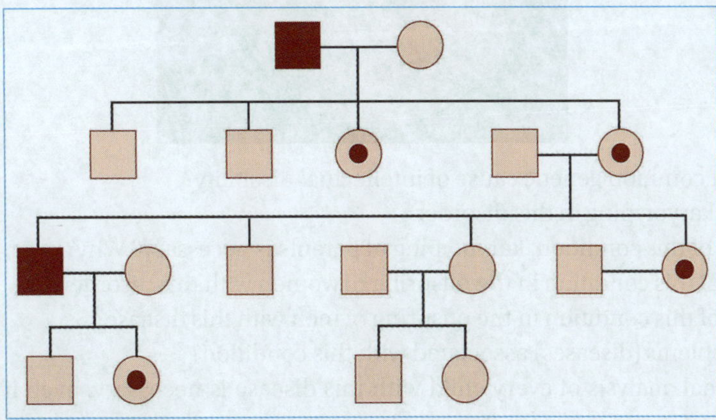

A. Identify the pattern of inheritance.
B. Name other conditions with similar inheritance.
C. What is the risk of getting affected in each pregnancy?

Q-3. A 10-month-old male child was brought with a large tongue. Birth weight was 4.2 kg and no perinatal complications.

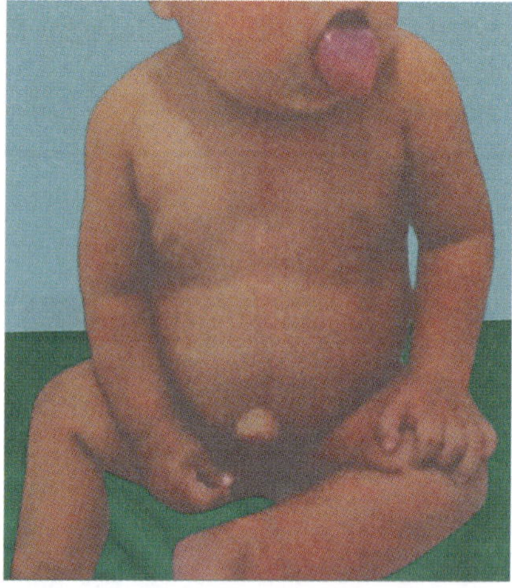

A. What is the most probable diagnosis?
B. What are the features of this condition?
C. Which chromosome carries this gene responsible for the disorder?
D. What complications are known to occur in this disease?

Q-4.

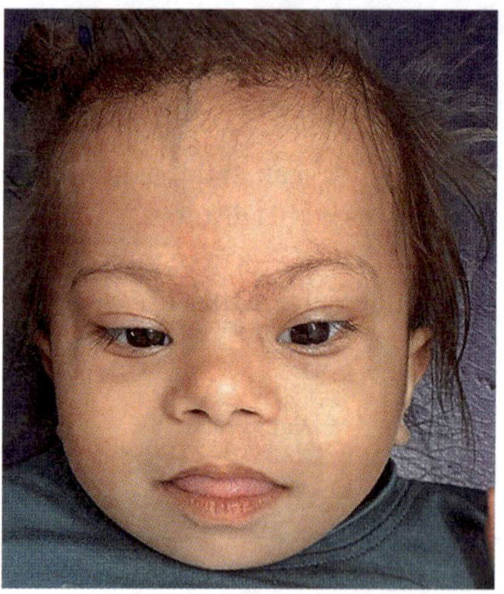

A. What is the most common genetic cause of intellectual disability?
B. Various types of karyotyping in this disorder.
C. In which variety of this condition, karyotyping of parents is necessary? Why?
D. What is the risk of this condition in the offspring of women with this disorder?
E. What is the risk of this condition in the offspring of men with this disease?
F. What are the problems (diseases) associated with this condition?
G. Why chromosomal analysis of every child with this disease is necessary, even if the diagnosis is clinically obvious?
H. What points to be checked or assessed during follow-up of a child with this disorder?

Q-5. A 32-year-old pregnant lady is at 20 weeks of gestation. She is referred for Triple test.

A. What are the components of Triple test? What constitutes an abnormal test and which disease do they screen for?
B. Name three radiological findings that suggest the presence of the disease
C. How can a definitive diagnosis can be offered at this stage?

Q-6. A long faced mentally retarded boy presents with prominent ears and large testes.

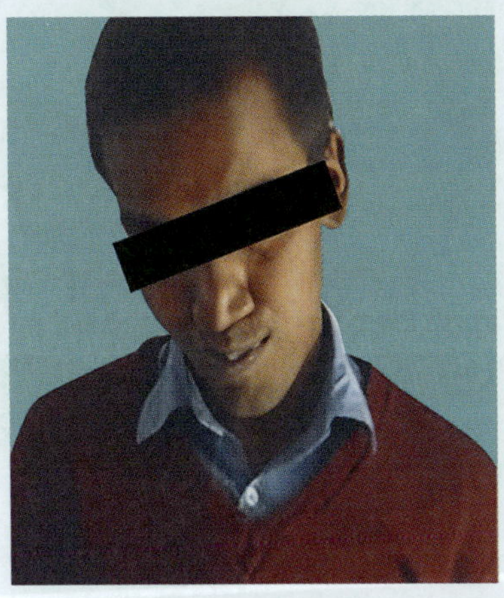

A. Name the condition
B. What causes feminization of these boys?
C. Name other two conditions associated with testicular enlargement.

Q-7. A 7-year-old boy presented with massive lymphedema, webbing of neck and short stature as shown in following picture.

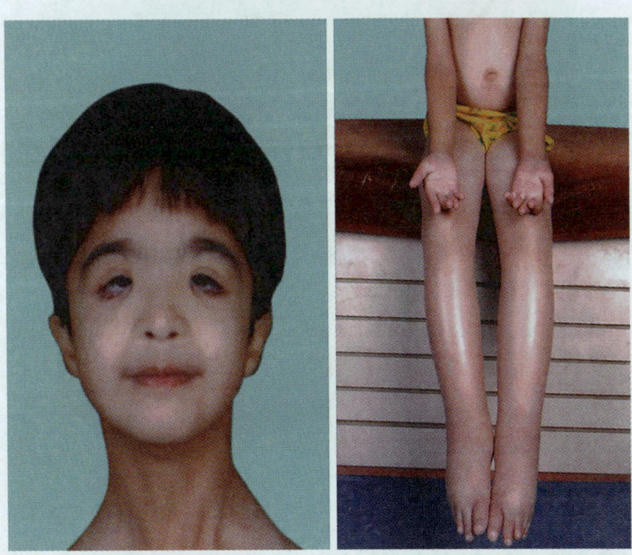

A. Name the condition.
B. What is it's another name?
C. What is the most common cardiac anomaly?
D. What anomalies of external genitals are common in this disorder?

Q-8. This neonate has undescended tests and urinary tract abnormality.

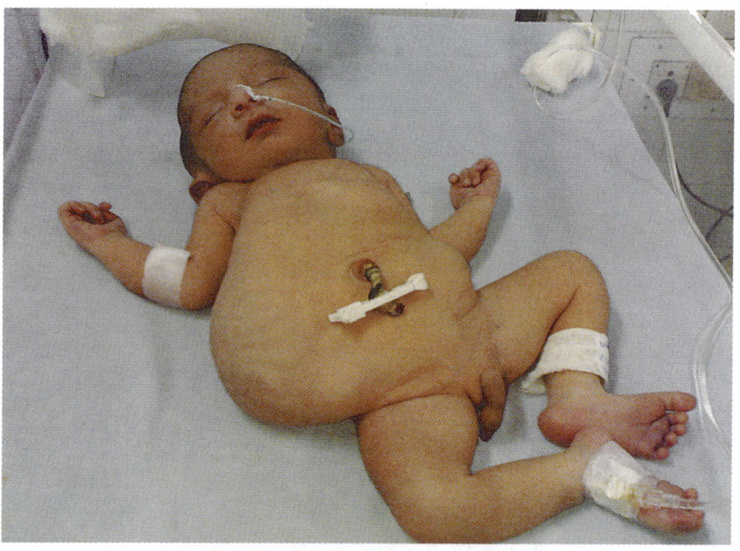

A. What is the diagnosis?
B. What are the common associated urinary tract abnormalities with this condition?
C. What is the known pulmonary complication associated with this condition?

Q-9. This child also had holoprosencephaly, hemangioma, ventricular septal defect and other anomalies.

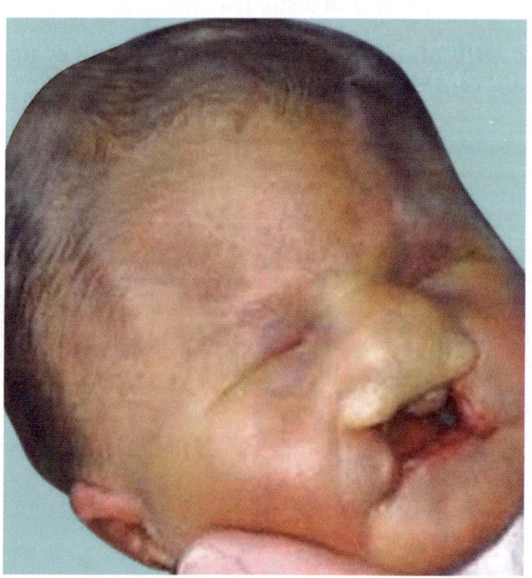

A. What is probable diagnosis?
B. What is most common cause of death?
C. What skeletal anomalies are common in this condition?

Q-10.

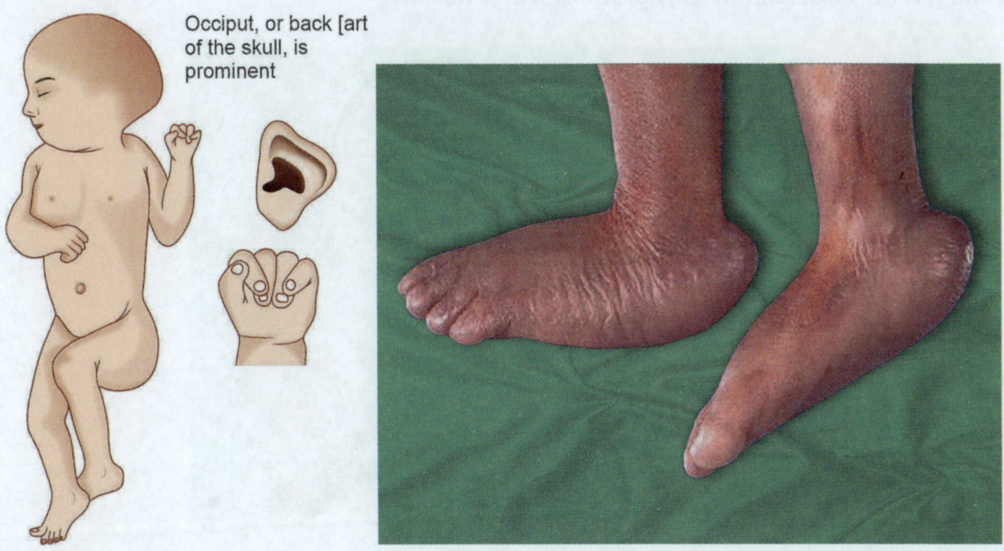

A. Describe the features shown in pictures?
B. What is probable diagnosis?
C. What is most common cardiac defect in this condition?
D. What is the most common cause of death in this disorder?

Q-11. A child presented with obesity, intellectual disability and polyuria and polydipsia with other features shown in picture.

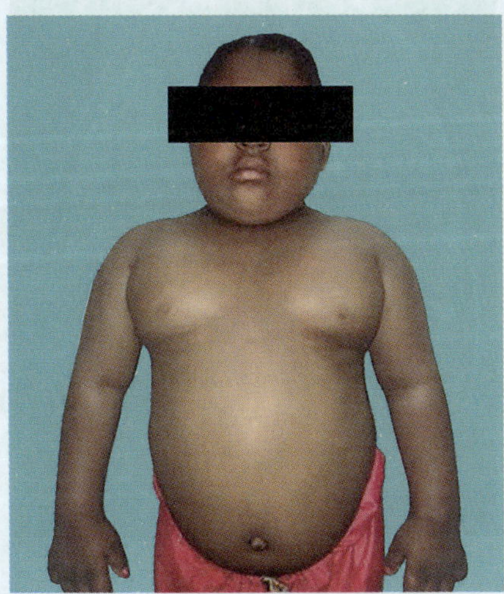

A. What is the probable diagnosis?
B. What is the most common gastrointestinal disorder associated with it?
C. What is the cause of polyuria and polydipsia?
D. What is the mode of inheritance?
E. What are common eye problems with this disorder?

Q-12. Absent sense of satiation, obsession with eating, micropenis and cryptorchidism are other features of this condition. It is the most common syndromic form of obesity.

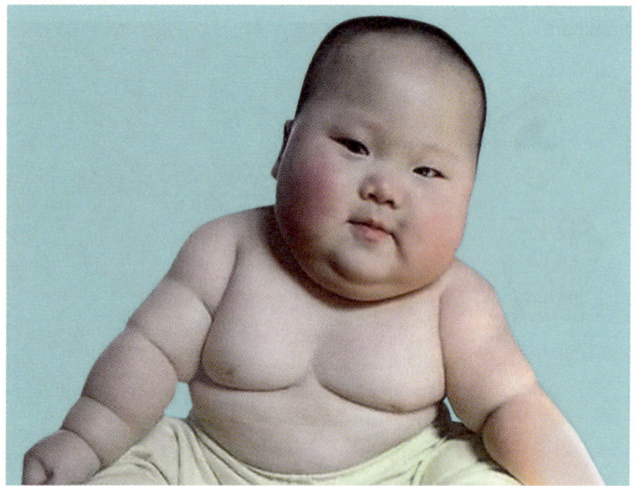

A. What is probable diagnosis?
B. What eyes abnormalities are characteristics of this condition?
C. Which medication is FDA approved to be used in this disorder?
D. Why they develop short stature, central obesity and hypogonadism?

Q-13. This baby was large for date, excessive growth in first year of life, large hand and feet and premature tooth eruption. The CT brain finding was characteristic as shown in the picture.

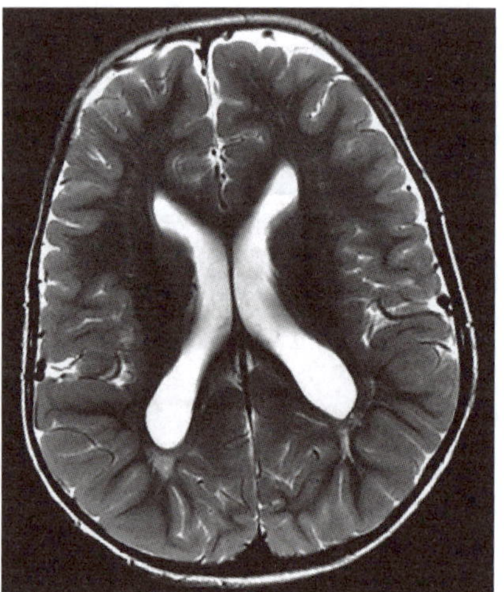

A. What is probable diagnosis?
B. What is the mode of inheritance?
C. Which malignancies are at increased risk with this condition?
D. What radiological findings are common with CT scan of brain?

Q-14. Ataxia and jerky arm movements, inappropriate bouts of laughter and seizures are other features of this disorder.

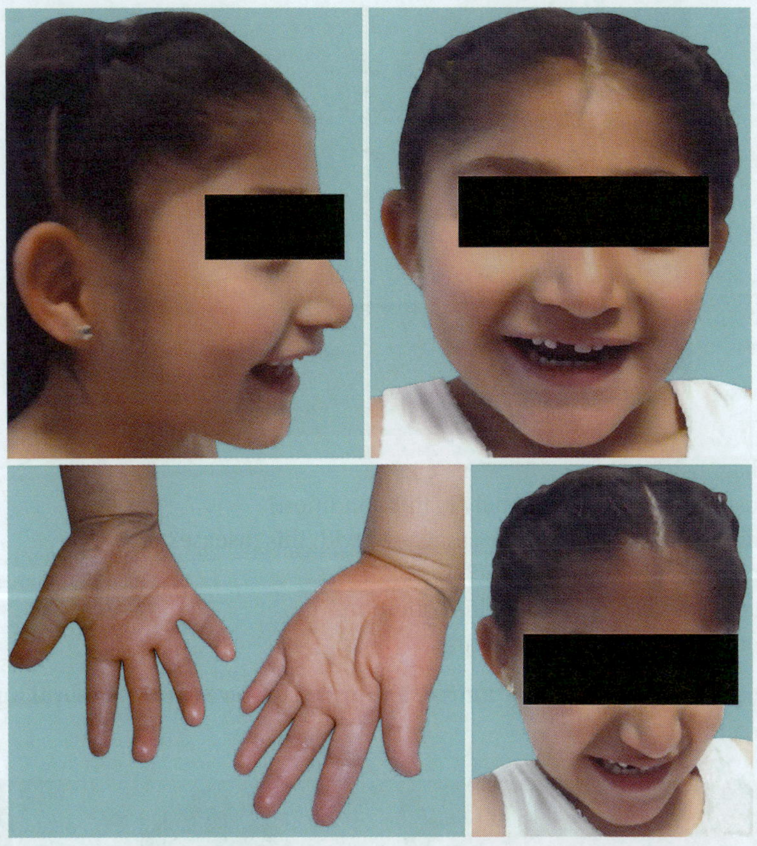

A. Name the condition.
B. What is another name of this condition?
C. Which higher function of brain is severely affected?
D. Which medication should be avoided in seizure treatment in this disorder?

Q-15. This condition also presents with growth and mental retardation.

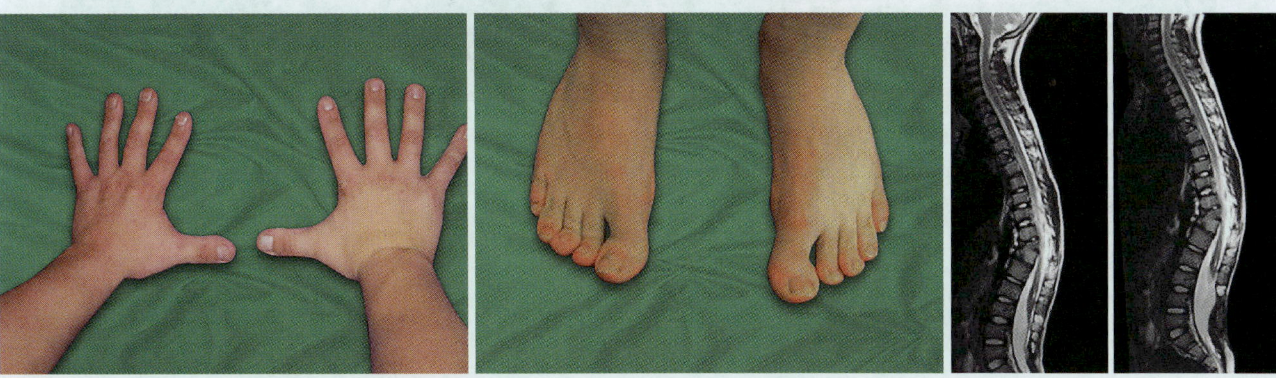

A. What is probable diagnosis?
B. What is the mode of inheritance of this condition?
C. What is the most common cardiac defect associated with this disorder?
D. What are common skeletal anomalies associated with this disorder?

Q-16. This female was brought for short stature, and abnormal features as shown in picture. She had swollen hands and feet at birth.

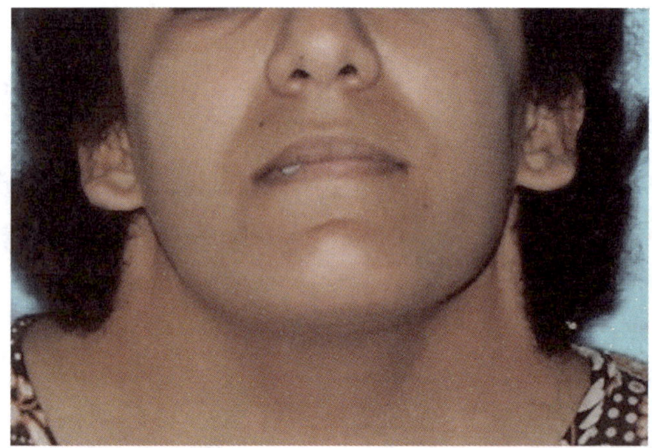

A. What is your diagnosis?
B. What is the most common renal anomaly in this condition?
C. What cardiac anomalies are commonly associated with this disease?
D. What risks are increased in this disorder?
E. Which malignancy risk is increased in this condition?
F. Which treatment may help to some extents?

Q-17. This child presented with persistent jaundice, abnormal features and vertebral anomaly as shown in the pictures.

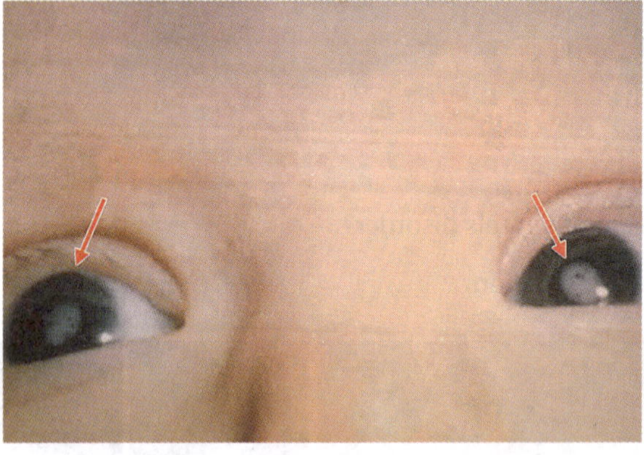
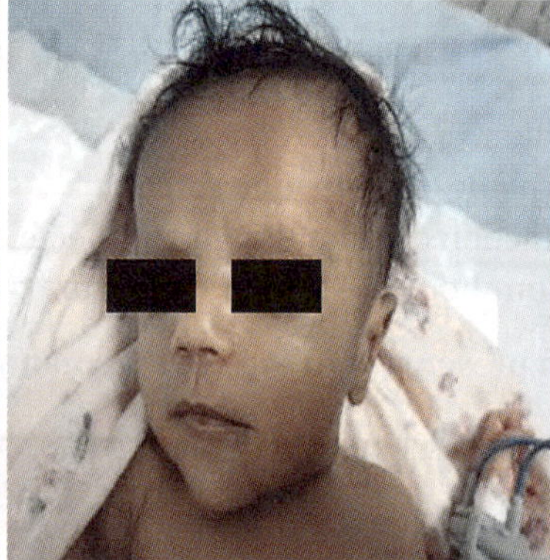
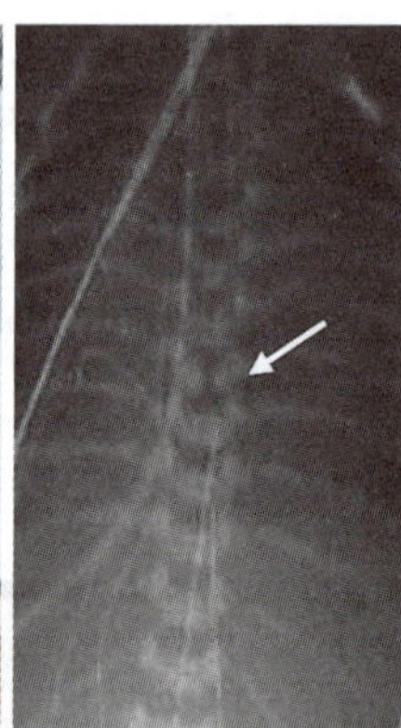

A. Describe the features shown in pictures.
B. What is common hepatic disorder associated with it?
C. Name the condition.

D. What is most common cardiac defect in this disease?
E. What is the hallmark of diagnosis on liver biopsy?
F. What treatment options are available?

Q-18. This child had high-pitched (cat's like) cry.

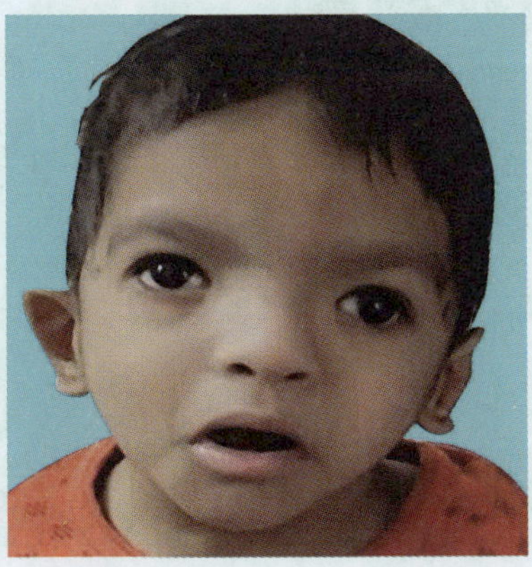

A. What is probable diagnosis?
B. What is the mode of inheritance of this disorder?
C. What cardiac defects are known associated with this condition?

Q-19. A child presented with seizures. The investigations reveled hypocalcemia as a cause of seizures. He also had ear anomaly as shown in the picture, also noted craniofacial anomalies. Chest X-rays (AP and lateral views) showed important clues for a condition. Further work-up confirmed aortic arch anomaly.

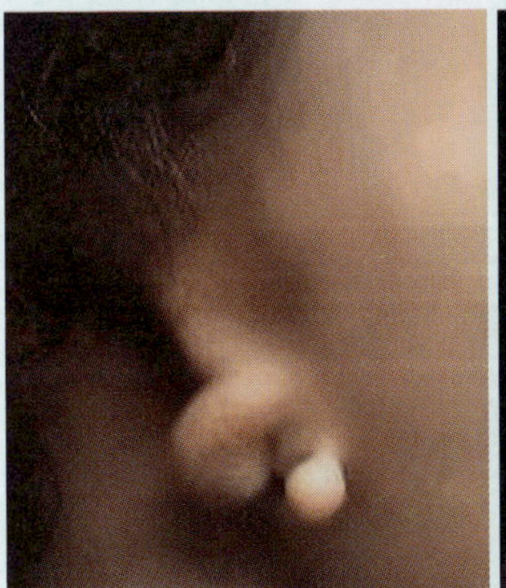

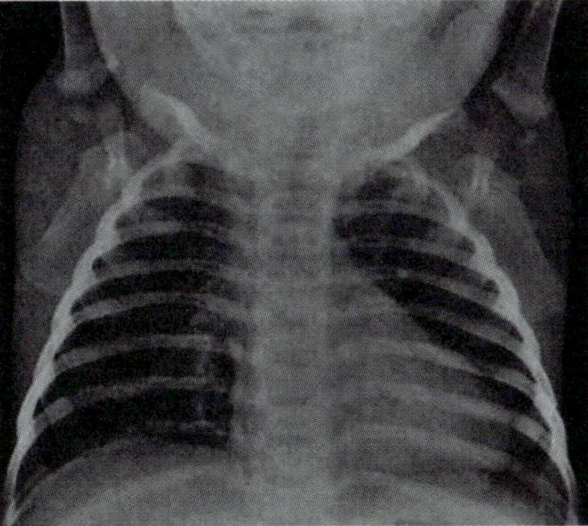

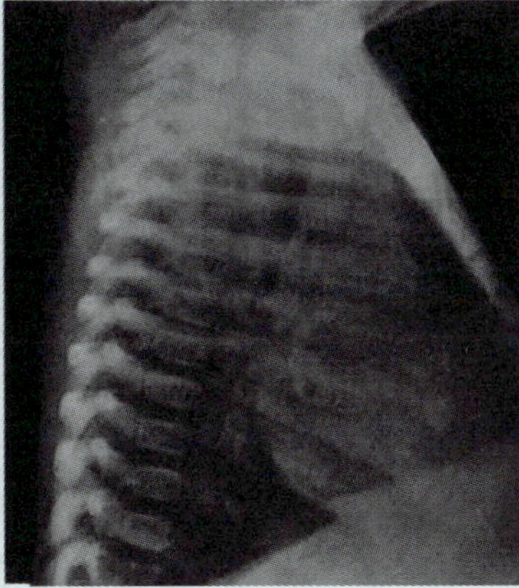

A. What is important clue on X-rays?
B. What is your diagnosis?
C. What is the cause of hypocalcemia?
D. What are common cardiac defects in this disorder?

Q-20. A 4-month-old boy presented with fever of 3 weeks duration and extreme irritability. His activity and weight gain were normal. Clinical examination revealed swelling of left jaw and left leg as shown in pictures. CBC showed mild anemia, leukocytosis and thrombocytosis. His X-ray skull and leg were taken.

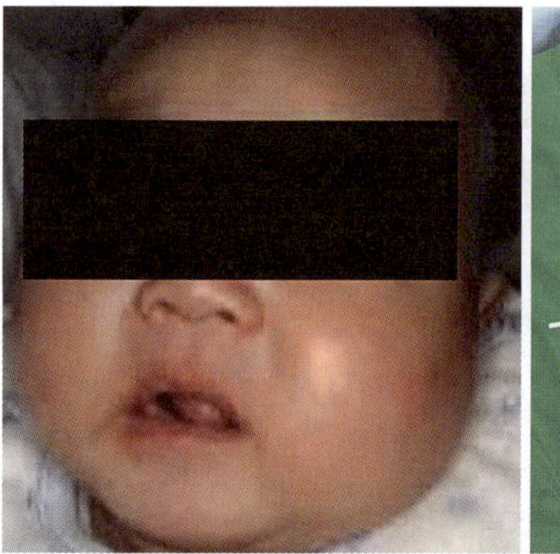

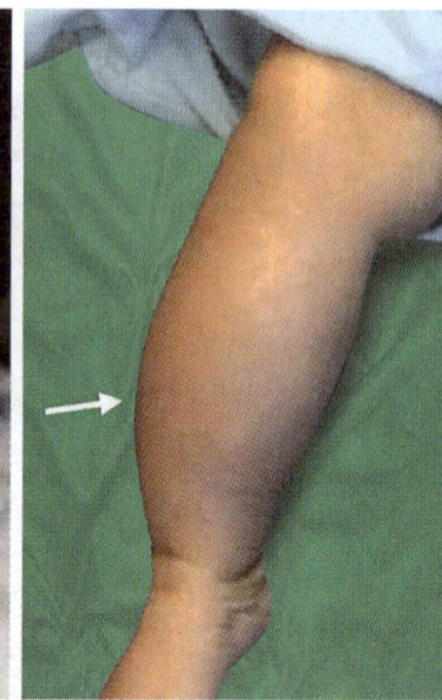

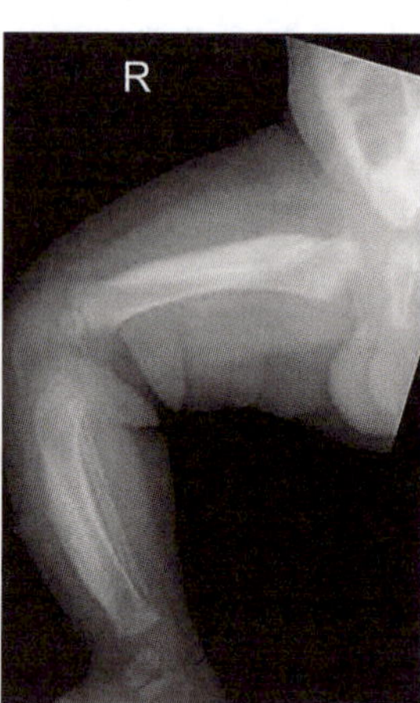

A. What is probable diagnosis?
B. What are differential diagnosis?
C. Which bone is most commonly affected?
D. What are diagnostic laboratory tests?
E. What is the mode of inheritance?

Q-21. This tall person also had characteristic eye and cardiac findings favoring a clinical diagnosis.

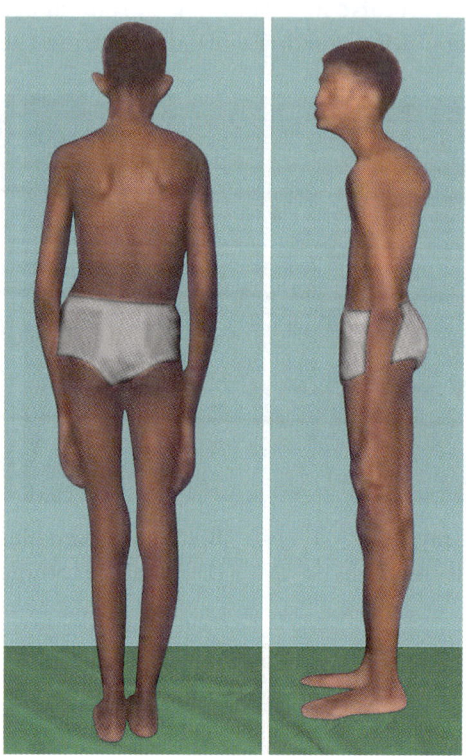

A. What is probable diagnosis?
B. What eye and cardiac features are common in this condition?
C. What annual monitoring is recommended?
D. What is most common cause of death?

Q-22. The parents noted unusual skin and joint extensibility. The skin was found fragile with increased bruising.

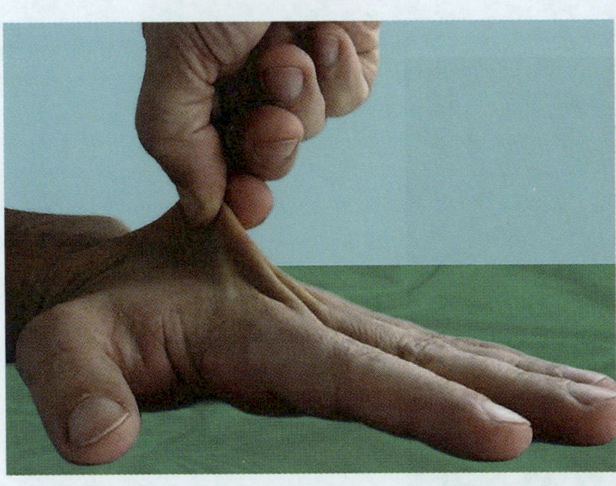
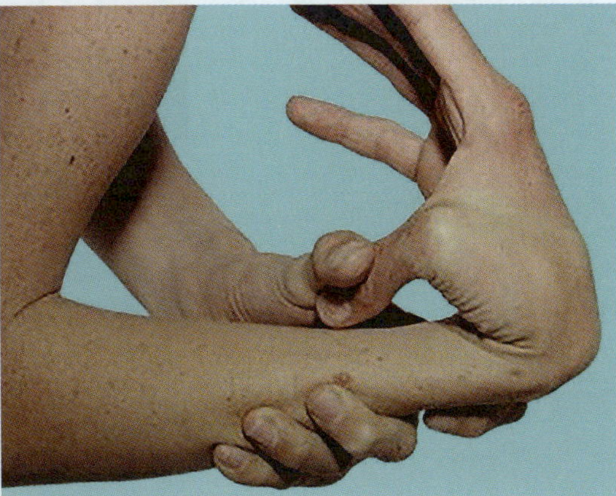

A. What is probable diagnosis?
B. What is the characteristic of wound healing in this condition?
C. What is most common cardiac defect?
D. What coagulation test is abnormal in this condition?

Q-23. Cleft lip and/or cleft palate and conductive hearing loss are other features of this condition.

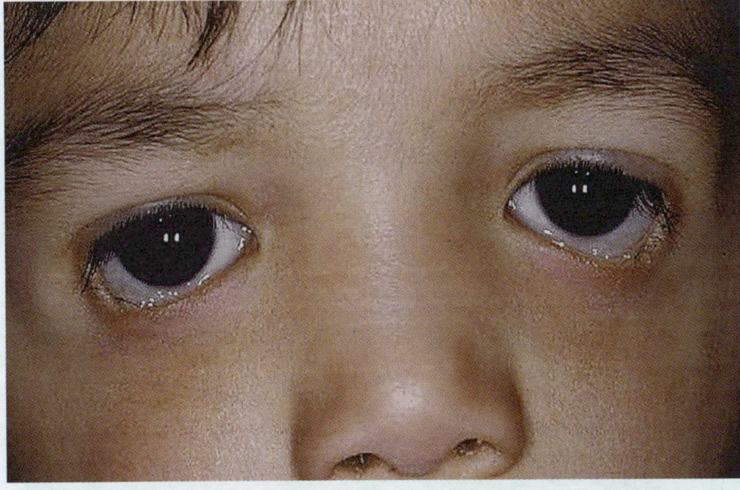
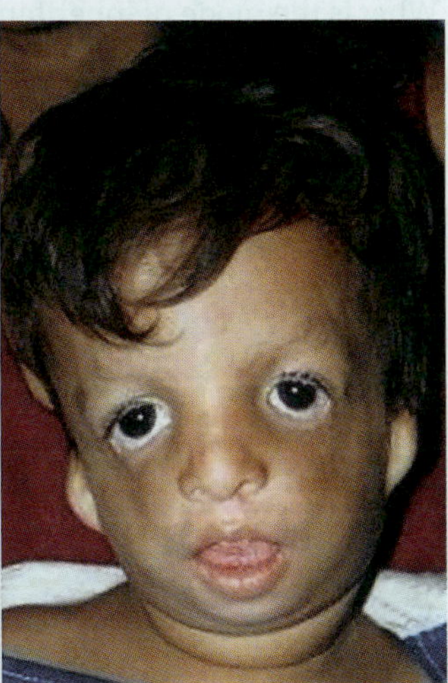

A. What is probable diagnosis?
B. What is most common neonatal problem with this disorder?
C. What is the level of intelligence?
D. What issues are common on follow-up?

Q-24. A 16 days full-term baby was brought with complaints of breathing and feeding difficulties. Mother notes less difficulty in breathing in prone position.

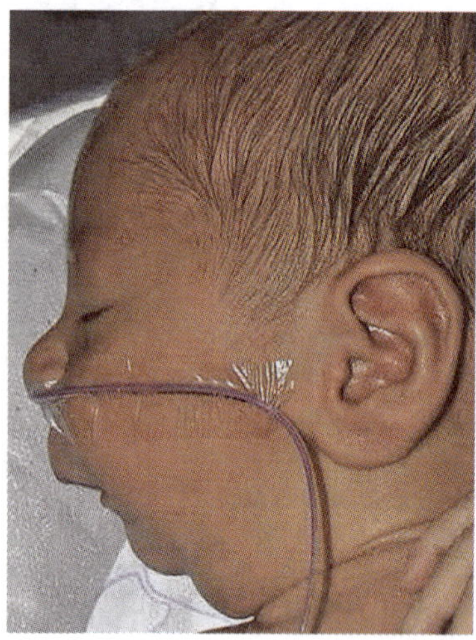

A. What is probable diagnosis?
B. What causes difficulty in breathing in this condition?
C. What is the most common cause of death?
D. What is the mode of inheritance?

Q-25. This patient also had hearing problem and constipation.

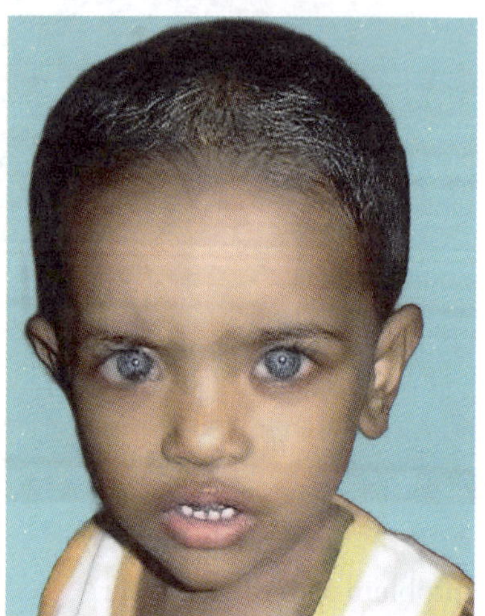

A. What is probable diagnosis?
B. What is the cause of constipation in this condition?
C. What is the mode of inheritance of this disorder?
D. What other skin conditions may be associated with this disease?

Q-26. This child presented with cerebellar ataxia and recurrent pulmonary infections.

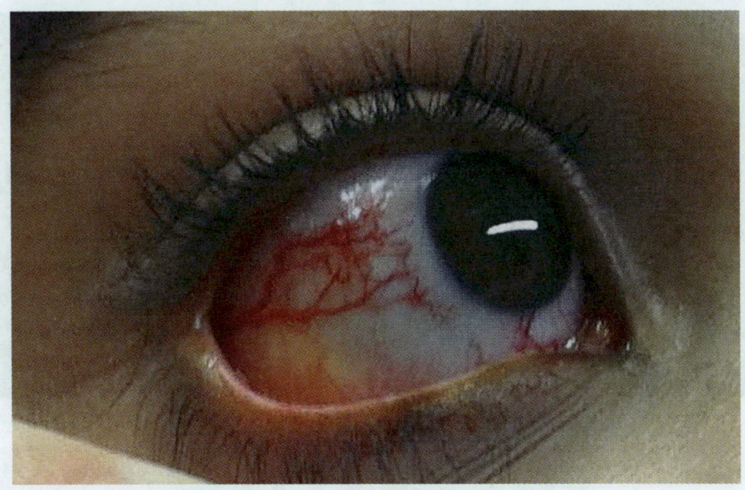

A. What is the diagnosis?
B. What is the cause of recurrent infections in this condition?
C. What is the most consistent laboratory abnormality?
D. What malignancies are at increased risk in this disorder?

Q-27. This child developed seizures first at the age of 14 months and then refractory epilepsy.

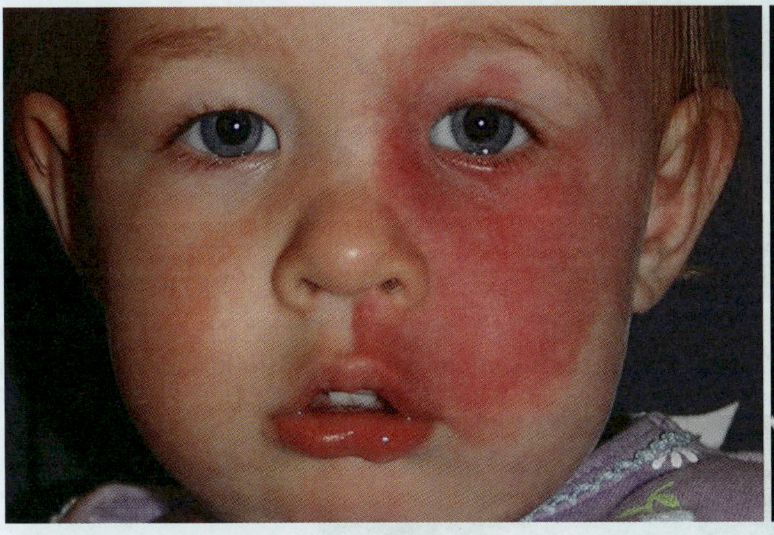

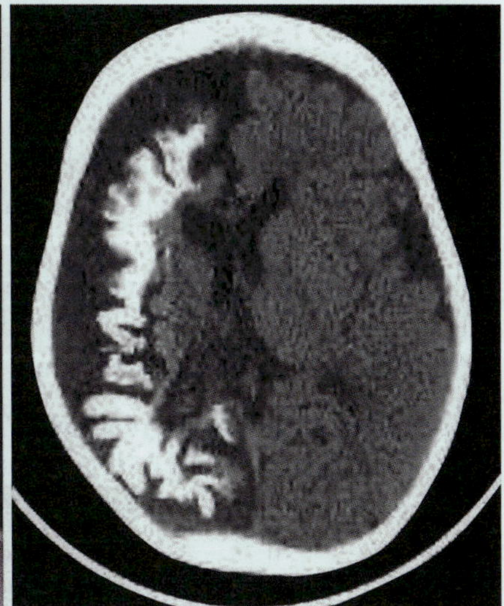

A. What is the diagnosis?
B. What are MRI brain findings in this condition?
C. What CNS manifestations are known in this disease?
D. What is the mode of inheritance?

Q-28. This patient also is suffering from epilepsy and autism spectrum disorders.

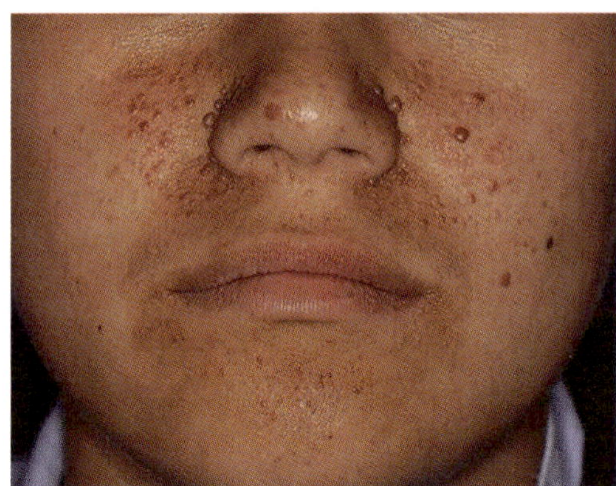

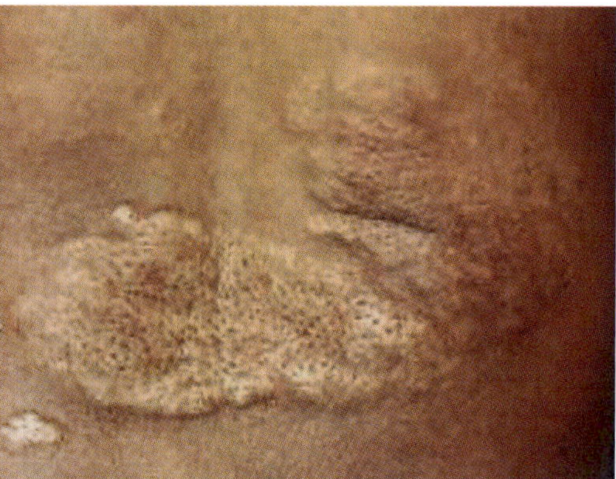

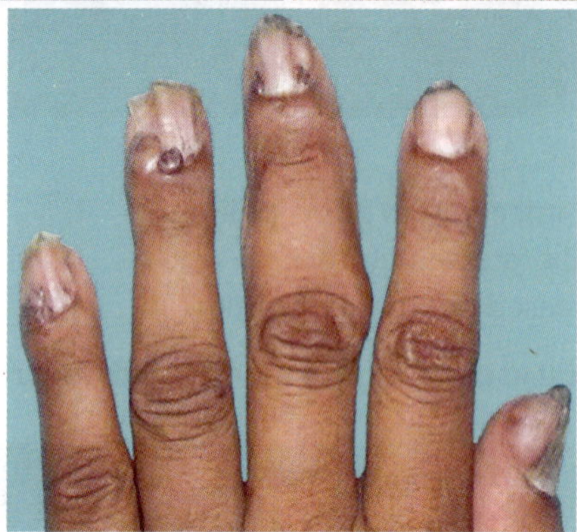

A. What is probable diagnosis?
B. What are CNS lesions known to occur in this disorder?
C. What are common neurological manifestations?
D. What skin lesions are common in this condition?
E. What is most common cardiac defect?
F. What is most common renal manifestation?
G. What is the mode of inheritance?

Q-29. This child presented with Failure to Thrive, delayed closure of anterior fontanel and history of hypoglycemia.

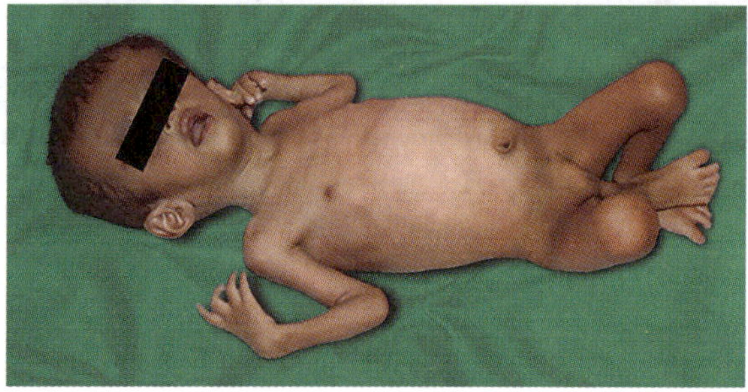

A. What is probable diagnosis?
B. What skeletal defects are common with this disease?
C. What abnormality of skull is characteristic of this condition?

Q-30. This condition was found associated with absence of one chest muscles.

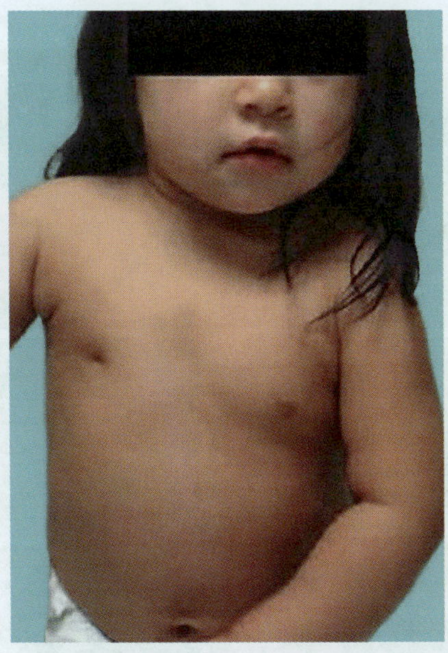

A. What is probable diagnosis?
B. Which maternal disease increases the risk of this disorder?
C. What is the mode of inheritance?

Q-31. This child was normal at the time of birth. Then, developed dystonia, spasticity and delayed development. The pictures show self-injury which started at the age of 18 months.

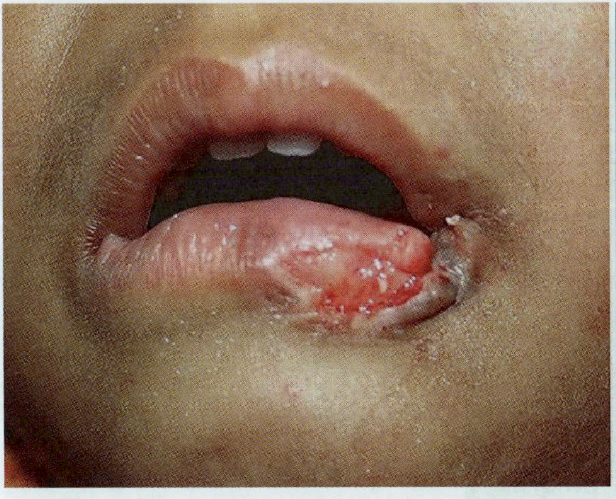
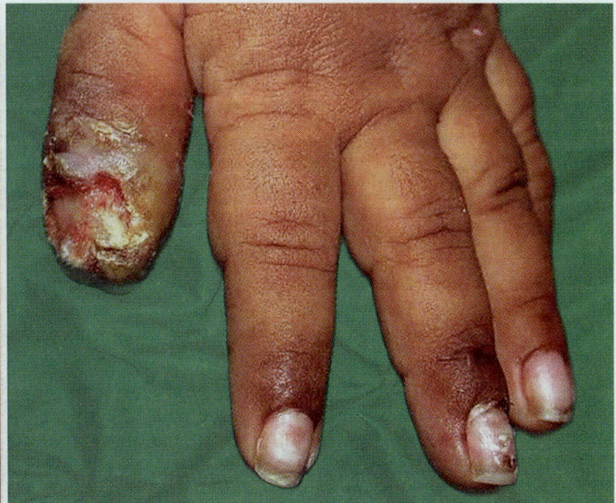

A. What is probable diagnosis?
B. What is basic defect in this disorder?
C. What is characteristic laboratory finding for this condition?
D. What complications are known to occur in this disease?
E. What is the most common cause of death?
F. What treatment can be offered?

Q-32. This patient was brought for recurrent epistaxis, especially during night and USG abdomen revealed liver vascular malformation.

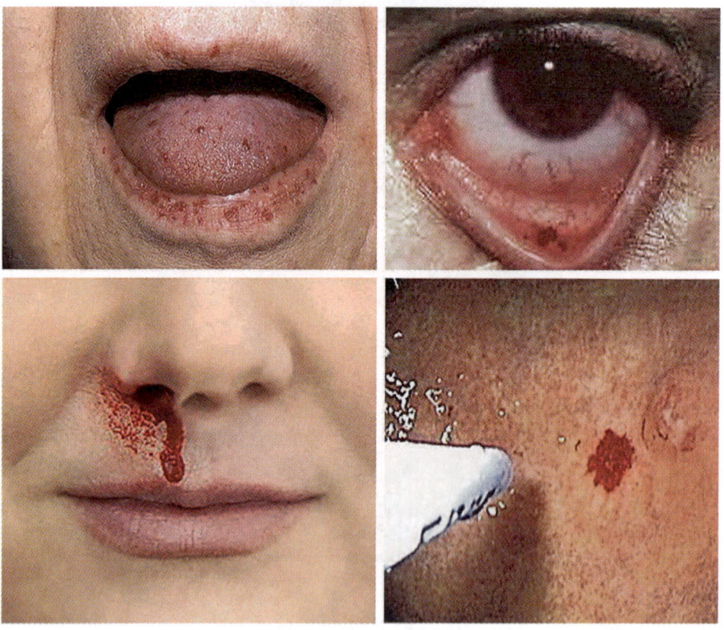

A. What is probable diagnosis?
B. What complications are known to occur in this disorder?
C. What is the mode of inheritance?

Q-33. As shown in the picture, this disorder has mainly skeletal and cardiac defects.

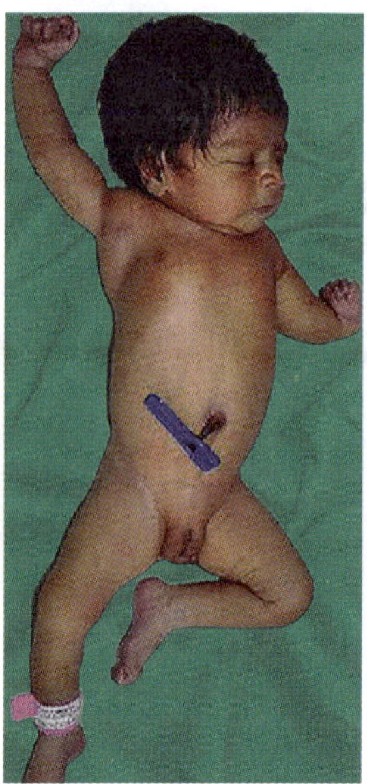

A. What is probable diagnosis?
B. What skeletal defects are common in this disorder?
C. What cardiac defect is the most common?
D. What is mode of inheritance?

Q-34. An adolescent boy presented with tall stature and features as shown in pictures.

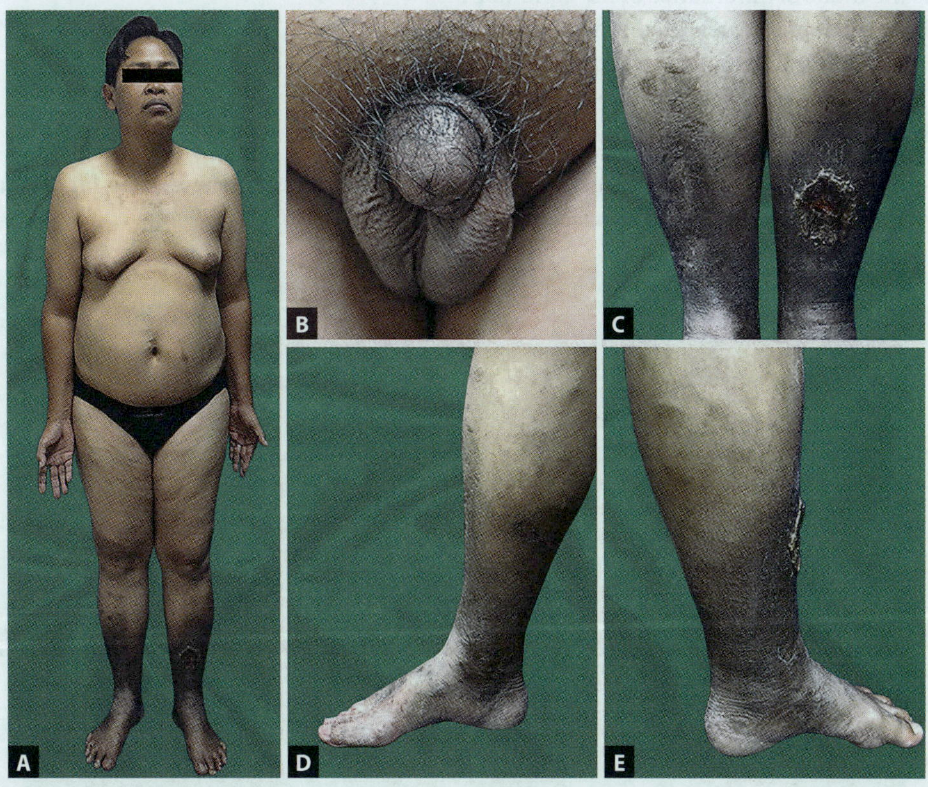

A. Identify the features shown in pictures.
B. What is the probable diagnosis?
C. What is the karyotyping in most cases?
D. What are the abnormalities in hormonal levels?
E. What malignancies are at increased risk in this disease?
F. What is the effective treatment?

Q-35. Intellectual disability, autism and loose joints are common manifestations of this condition.

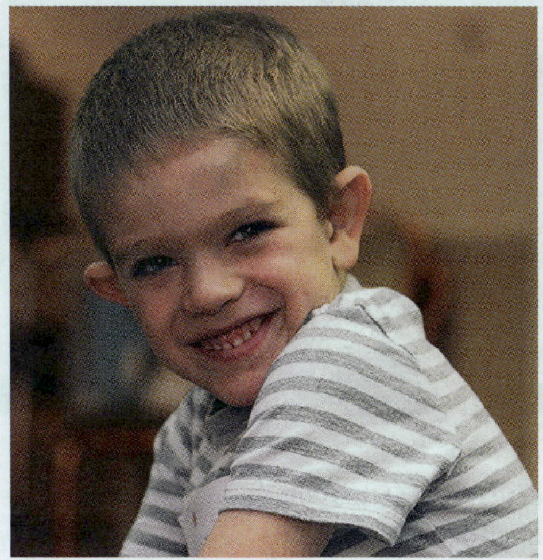

A. What is probable diagnosis?
B. What is the mode of inheritance of the condition?
C. What behavioral problems are common with this disease?
D. What is the confirmatory test for this condition?
E. Can a female have this disorder?
F. What is the most common cardiac defect?

Q-36. A 6-year-old boy presented with intellectual disability and the characteristic facial features. Routine laboratory investigations revealed hypercalcemia.

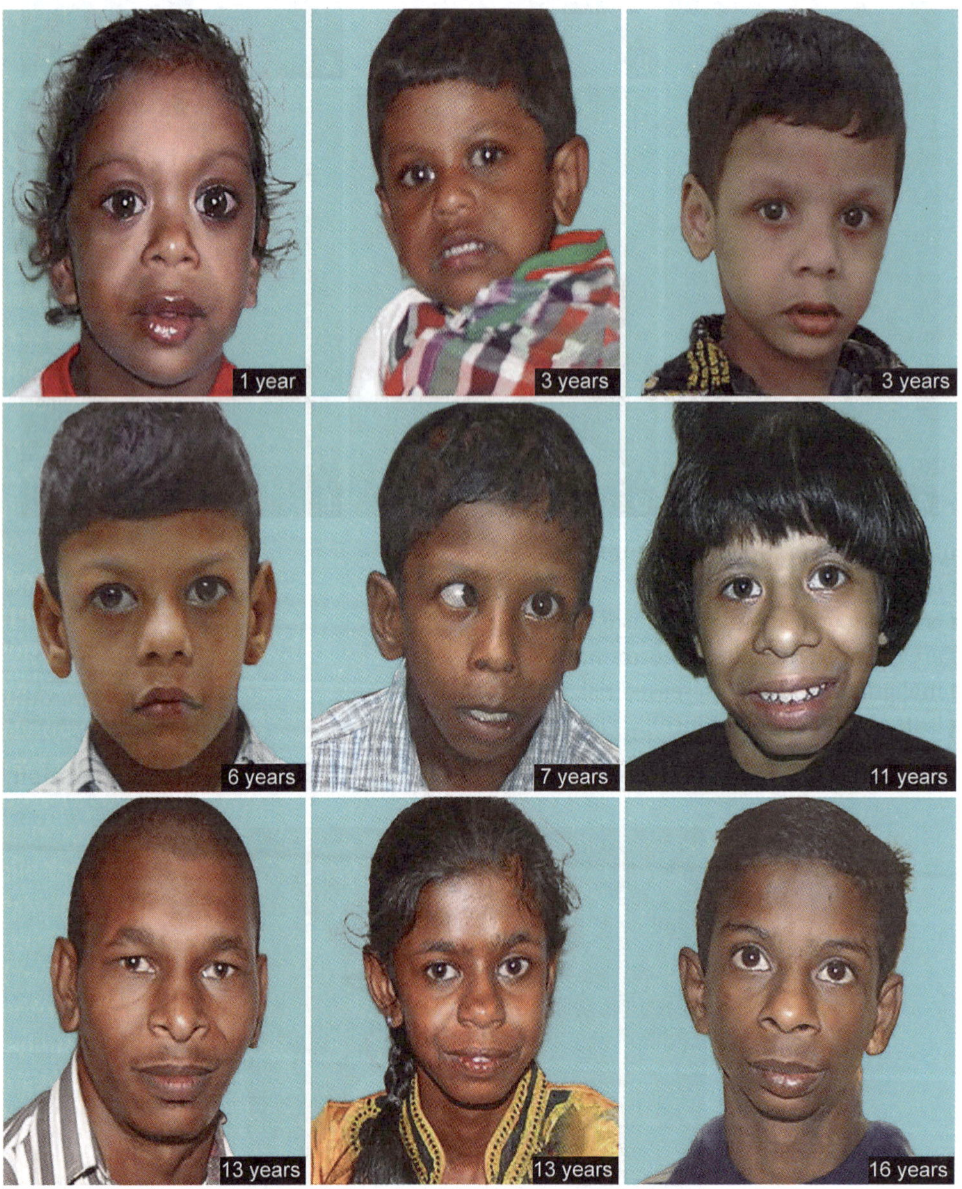

A. What is probable diagnosis?
B. What are characteristic facial features of this condition? Name the facies.
C. What is the mode of inheritance of this condition?
D. What is most common cardiac defect?

Q-37. A 2-year-old boy was brought with complaints of sitting at one year of age and still not walking, rest milestones are normal. His head circumference was 52 cm, length 76 cm and weight 11.7 kg. He had hypotonia.

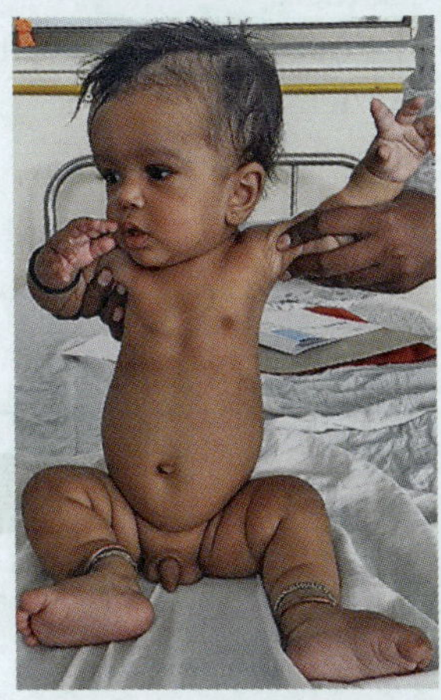

A. What is your diagnosis?
B. What type of disorder is it?
C. What are life-threatening complications?
D. What hormonal therapy may be useful?
E. What are skeletal characteristic?

Q-38.

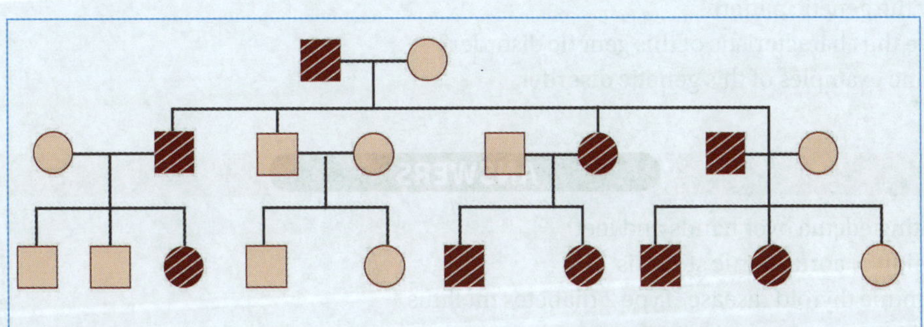

A. Identify the genetic pattern.
B. What are the characteristics of this genetic disorder?
C. What is the risk of recurrence in this disorder?
D. Give some examples of this genetic disorder.

Q-39.

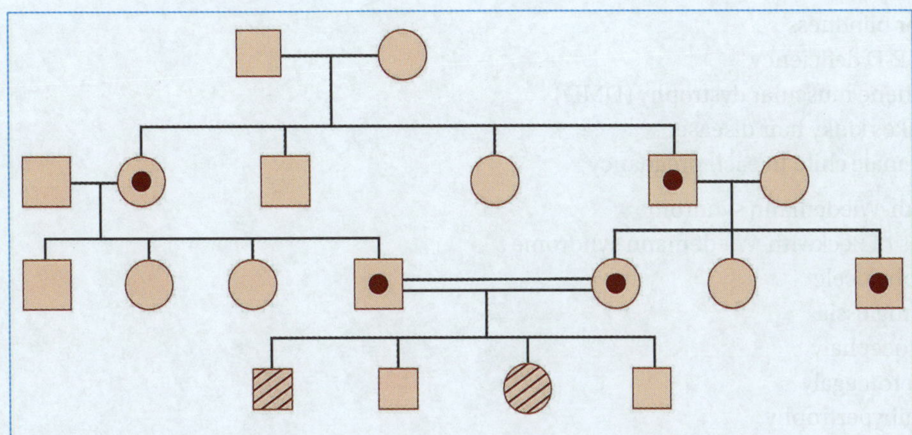

A. Identify genetic pattern.
B. What are the characteristics of this genetic disorder?
C. What is the risk of recurrence in this disorder?
D. Which factor among a couple may play a role in inheritance in this genetic disorder?
E. Give some examples of this genetic disorder.

Q-40.

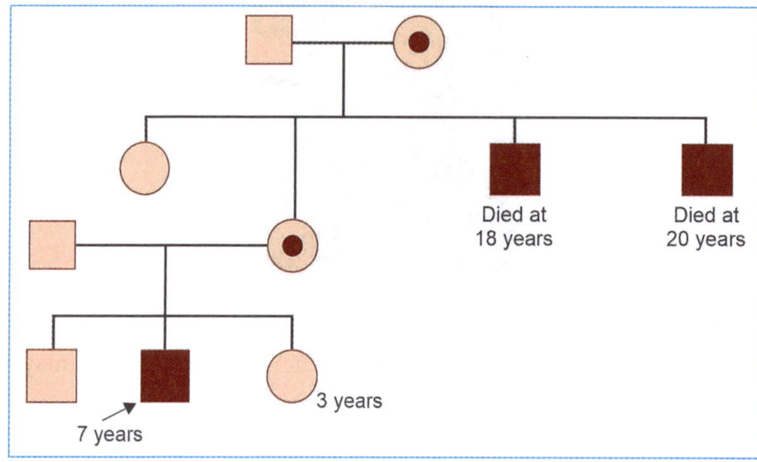

A. Identify the genetic pattern.
B. What are the characteristic of this genetic disorder?
C. Give some examples of this genetic disorder.

ANSWERS

A-1. A. Non-pitting edema over hands and feet
B. Coarctation of aorta, aortic stenosis
C. Autoimmune thyroid disease, Type 2 diabetes mellitus
D. Celiac disease
E. Most common renal anomaly: Horseshoe shape kidney

A-2. A. X-linked recessive
B.
- Hemophilia
- Color blindness
- G-6-P-D deficiency
- Duchene muscular dystrophy (DMD)
- Menkes kinky hair disease

C. 50% for male child in each pregnancy

A-3. A. Beckwith-Wiedemann syndrome
B. Features of Beckwith-Wiedemann syndrome
- Omphalocele
- Macroglossia
- Microcephaly
- Visceromegaly
- Hemihypertrophy

C. 11

D. Complications in Beckwith-Wiedemann syndrome
- Wilmar's tumor
- Hepatoblastoma
- Gonadoblastoma
- Adrenal carcinoma
- Rhabdomyosarcoma

A-4. A. Down syndrome (20–30% cases with intellectual disability)

B. *Trisomy 21:*
- *>90% non-disjunction:* Extra chromosome from mother due to failure of separation of chromosome during meiosis (more common with advanced maternal age)
- *4% translocation:* Translocation of chromosome 21 to any of D group chromosome, 13, 14, 15 or G group chromosome, 21, 22.
- *1% mosaics:* One cell line with 47 chromosome and normal cell line with 46 chromosomes.

C. Down syndrome caused due to translocation, one of the parents may be a carrier of a balanced translocation (risk of Down syndrome in the offspring of a translocation carrier mother 10–15% and carrier father 1–5%)

D. 30%

E. Males with trisomy 21 are usually infertile.

F.
- Hypothyroidism
- Deafness
- Leukemia
- Atlantoaxial instability
- Epilepsy

G.

Age of mother	*Risk of having a child with down syndrome*
20	1:1925
25	1:1205
30	1:885
35	1:365
40	1:110
45	1:32

H. Depending upon the type of chromosomal abnormality and carrier status of the parents, the risk of recurrence may vary from 1 to 100

I. *Assessment of growth and development:*
- Eye examination (especially for cataract)
- Hearing assessment
- Yearly evaluation for thyroid functions
- Assessment for atlantoaxial instability
- Peripheral smear examination for leukemia

A-5. A.
- Maternal serum alpha-fetoprotein (low)
- Unconjugated estradiol (high)
- Free beta-hCG (high)

Triple test is used to screen for fetal trisomy chromosomal anomalies.

B. *Second trimester USG findings:*
- Increased nuchal fold thickness
- Short femur and humerus
- Duodenal atresia

First trimester USG findings:
- Nuchal fold thickness,
- Nasal bone evaluation

C. Fetal karyotyping by amniocentesis

A-6. A. Fragile X syndrome
B. Excessive production of aromatase
C. Henoch-Schönlein purpura, lymphangiectsia

A-7. A. Noonan syndrome
B. Male Turner syndrome
C. Pulmonary valve stenosis
D. Small penis and cryptorchidism

A-8. A. Prune-belly syndrome (Eagle-Barrett syndrome)
B. Megaureter, megalourethra, large, bladder, posterior urethral valve, vesicoureteric reflux
C. Pulmonary hypoplasia

A-9. A. Patau syndrome (Trisomy 13)
B. Central apnea
C.
- Postaxial polydactyly
- Hypoplastic or absent ribs

Trisomy 13 (Patau Syndrome)

- Third most common autosomal trisomy
- *Clinical features:*
  - Midline defects
  - Aplasia cutis congenita
  - Micro ophthalmia
  - Post-axial polydactyly
  - Hypotonia
  - Holoprosencephaly
  - Hypoplastic/absent ribs
  - Abdominal wall defect
  - Deafness
  - Colobomas
  - Capillary hemangioma
  - Genital anomalies
  - Clenched fist
  - Common cardiac defects
- *Most common cardiac defects:*
  - Ventricular septal defect (VSD)
  - Atrial septal defect (ASD)
  - Patent ductus arteriosus (PDA)

A-10. A.

- Prominent occiput
- Micrognathia
- Low set ears
- Short sternum
- Rocker bottom feet
- Overlapping fingers
- Hypoplastic nails

B. Trisomy 18 (Edward syndrome)

C.

- Ventricular septal defect (VSD)
- Others are ASD and PDA.

D. Central apnea

Trisomy 18 (Edward Syndrome)

- Second most common autosomal trisomy
- *Clinical features:*
  - Rocker bottom feet
  - Overlapping fingers
  - Clenched fist
  - Small and premature appearance
  - Tight palpebral fissures
  - Narrow nose
  - Hypoplastic nasal alae
  - Narrow bifrontal diameter
  - Prominent occiput
  - Micrognathia
  - Cleft lip or palate
  - Microcephaly
  - Short sternum
  - Hypoplastic nails
  - Hypertonia
- Most common cardiac defects
  - VSD
  - ASD
  - PDA
- Most common cause of death
  Central apnea

A-11. A. Laurence–Moon–Biedl syndrome (Bardet–Biedl Syndrome)

B. Hirschsprung disease

C. Nephrogenic diabetes insipidus

D. Autosomal recessive

E.

- Retinitis pigmentosa
- Rods and cones dystrophy

A-12. A. Prader–Willi syndrome
B.
- Almond-shaped appearance of palpebral fissures
- Upward slanting

C. Growth hormone therapy
D. Secondary to hypothalamic and pituitary dysfunction

A-13. A. Soto syndrome (Cerebral gigantism)
B. Autosomal dominant
C.
- Wilms tumor
- Hepatic carcinoma

D.
- Ventriculomegaly
- Partial agenesis or hypoplasia of septum pellucidum

A-14. A. Angelman syndrome
B. Happy puppet syndrome
C. Speech
D.
- Carbamazepine
- Vigabatrin

A-15. A. Rubinstein-Taybi syndrome
B. Autosomal dominant
Microdeletion 16q
C. Ventricular septal defect
D.
- Scoliosis
- Spina bifida occulta
- Cervical hyper kyphosis
- Small, flared iliac wings

A-16.
A. Turner Syndrome
B.
- Horseshoe kidney
- Double-collecting system

C.
- Bicuspid aortic valve
- Coarctation of aorta

D.
- Hypothyroidism
- Hashimoto disease
- Celiac disease
- Inflammatory bowel disease

E. Gonadal blastoma
F.
- Growth hormone
- Estrogen therapy

A-17. A.

- Triangular face with pointed chin
- Long nose
- Hypertelorism
- Deeply set eyes
- Butterfly vertebrae in X-ray spine
- Posterior embryotoxon on eye examination

B. Cholestatic jaundice

C. Alagille syndrome

D. Peripheral pulmonary artery stenosis/Pulmonary valve stenosis.

E. Paucity of bile duct

F.

- Ursodeoxycholic acid (UDCA) for pruritus
- Supplementation of fat soluble vitamins including vitamin K
- Liver transplantation

A-18. A. Cri-du-chat syndrome

B. De novo mutation
5p deletion

C. VSD, ASD, PDA and TOF

A-19. A. Absence of thymic shadow

B. DiGeorge syndrome

C. Hypocalcemia is due to parathyroid hypoplasia or aplasia

D.

- Interrupted aortic arch
- Truncus arteriosus
- Tetralogy of Fallot
- VSD

A-20. A. Caffey Disease—infantile cortical hyperostosis

B.

- Osteomyelitis
- Hypervitaminosis A
- Leukemia
- Child abuse
- Scurvy

C. Mandible

D.

- Raised serum alkaline phosphatase
- Hypercalciuria

E. Autosomal dominant
COLIAI gene

A-21. A. Marfan syndrome

B.

- Ectopia lentis (Subluxation of eye lens)
- Aortic dilatation or dissection

C. Echocardiogram

D. Rupture aortic root dilatation

A-22. A. Ehlers–Danlos syndrome

B. There is poor wound healing leaving parchment thin scar. It is also called as cigarette paper scar.

C.
- Mitral valve prolapse
- Aortic arch dilatation

D. Capillary fragility test

A-23. A. Treacher Collins syndrome (Mandibulofacial dysostosis)

B. Airway difficulties

C. Normal

D.
- Airway difficulties
- Feeding difficulties
- Hearing impairment
- Speech disorders
- Vision assessment

A-24. A. Pierre Robin syndrome

B. It is due to glossoptosis backward displacement of the tongue, causing obstruction. The tongue is of normal size but mouth is foreshortened due to micrognathia.

C. Upper airway obstruction

D. De novo mutation
SOXq gene

A-25. A. Waardenburg syndrome

B. Hirschsprung disease

C. Autosomal dominant

D.
- Vitiligo
- Hypomelanosis of IgA

A-26. A. Ataxia Telangiectasia

B.
- Humoral immunologic abnormality
- Selective absence of IgA

C. High serum alfa-fetoprotein

D.
- Lymphoreticular type
- Adenocarcinomas

A-27. A. Sturge–Weber syndrome

B.
- Ipsilateral cortical atrophy
- Tram track calcifications
- Leptomeningeal angioma

C.
- Seizures
- Hemiparesis
- Stroke like episodes
- Headache
- Developmental delay

D. Not inherited, due to somatic mutation

A-28. A. Tuberous sclerosis

B.

- Cortical tuber
- Subependymal nodules causing candle-dripping appearance
- Subependymal giant cell astrocytoma

C.

- Epilepsy
- Cognitive impairment
- Autistic spectrum disorders
- Infantile spasms and hypsarrhythmia EEG changes in infancy
- Myoclonic epilepsy

D.

- Ash-leaf macules
- Facial angiofibromas
- Shagreen patch
- Ungal and periungal fibromas

E. Rhabdomyoma

F. Angiomyolipomas

G. Autosomal dominant

A-29. A. Russel Silver Syndrome

B.

- 5th finger clinodactyly
- Syndactyly
- Asymmetry of limbs

C. False hydrocephalus

A-30. A. Poland syndrome

B. Maternal diabetes

C. Not inherited

A-31. A. Lesch–Nyhan disease

B.

- It is purine metabolism disorder
- Hypoxanthine-guanine phosphoribosyl Transferase (HPRT) deficiency is the basic defect.

C. X-linked recessive

D. Hyperuricemia

E.

- Gouty arthritis
- Renal and bladder stones
- Renal failure

F. Renal failure

G.

- Allopurinol
- High-fluid intake
- Behavioral therapy

A-32. A. Osler-Weber-Rendu syndrome (Hereditary hemorrhagic telangiectasia)

B.
- Pulmonary hemorrhage
- Intracranial hemorrhage
- GI bleeding

C. Autosomal dominant

A-33.

A. Holt-Oram syndrome

B.
- Thumb—aplasia, hypoplasia, triphalangeal, bifid
- Radial hypoplasia
- Clavicle hypoplasia

C. Atrial Septal Defect (ASD)

D.
- Autosomal dominant
- Cardiac arrhythmia (First degree block)

A-34. A.
- Gynecomastia
- Micropenis
- Small testes
- Varicose veins and leg ulcers

B. Klinefelter syndrome

C. 47, XXY (80% cases)

D.
- Low testosterone
- High FSH and LH

E.
- Breast cancer
- Testicular cancer

F. Testosterone replacement

A-35. A. Fragile X Syndrome

B.
- X-linked dominant
- >200 CGG repeats in *FMR1* gene

C.
- Autism
- Attention deficit hyperactivity disorder (ADHD)

D. Molecular genetic test for CGG allele repeat size

E.
- Yes, but milder symptoms
- Premature ovarian failure

F. Mitral valve prolapse

A-36. A. Williams syndrome

B.
- Triangular face
- Long philtrum

- Short nose with bulbous nasal tip
- Small chin
- Broad mouth

It is Elfin face.

C.

- Autosomal dominant
- Microdeletion 79

D.

- Supravalvular aortic stenosis (80%)
- Peripheral pulmonary stenosis
- Pulmonary valvular stenosis

A-37. A. Achondroplasia

B. It is short limb dwarf. The limb shortening is greatest in the proximal segment (Rhizomelia). The trunk is long and narrow. Head is larger and may have hydrocephalus.

C.

- Quadriparesis
- Central and obstructive apnea
- Sudden death

D. Growth hormone

E.

- Calvarial bones are large, whereas cranial base and facial bones are small.
- The vertebrae pedicles are short.
- The iliac bones are short and round and the acetabular roofs are flat.
- The tubular bones are short.
- The fibula is disproportionately large compared to tibia.

A-38. A. Autosomal dominant (AD)

B. *Characteristics of AD disorder:*

- Successive or multiple generations are affected.
- The change of the progeny being affected by an autosomal dominant disorder is independent of the sex, both males and females are affected in equal proportions.
- Both males and females can transmit the disease to their offspring or either sex.

C. The risk of transmission of the disease from an affected parent to his or her children is 50%.

D. *Examples of AD disorder:*

- Marfan syndrome
- Achondroplasia
- Neurofibromatosis
- Familial hypercholesterolemia
- Polycystic kidney disease
- Von Willebrand disease
- Acute intermittent porphyria
- Huntington disease

A-39. A. Autosomal recessive (AR)

B. *Characteristics of AR:*

- Both males and females are affected.
- The disorder normally occurs in only one generation, usually within a single sibship.
- The parents can be consanguineous, especially if the disorder is rare.

However, consanguinity is not essential.

C. The risk of their second child being affected with the disorder is 25%.
D. Consanguinity
E. *Examples of AR disorder:*
- Cystic fibrosis
- Wilson's disease
- Thalassemia major
- Sickle cell anemia
- Tay-Sachs disease
- Bartter syndrome
- Gaucher's disease
- Galactosemia
- Spinal muscular atrophy

A-40. A. X-linked inheritance
B. *Characteristics of X-linked disorders:*
- Disease is caused by mutation in gene on X-chromosome
- No male-to-male transmission

X-linked Recessive
- Mostly males are affected, females are usually normal or only mildly affected.
- Affected males in a family are always related to each other through female carriers.
- For a carrier mother, risk of male offspring being affected is 50% and chance of female off springs being carrier is 50%.
- For an affected father, the risk of male offspring being affected is zero and chance of female offspring being carrier is 100%.

X-linked Dominant
- Both males and females are affected, but males usually have a more severe phenotype.
- Some disorders are perinatally lethal in males and compatible with survival only in females, disease phenotypes seen only in females.
- For an affected mother, risk of male offspring being affected is 50% and the risk of female offspring being affected is 50%

C. *X-linked disorders:*
- Fragile X syndrome
- Duchenne muscular dystrophy (DMD)
- G-6-P-D deficiency
- Hemophilia
- Color blindness
- Ornithine transcarbamylase deficiency (Urea Cycle disorder)
- Adrenoleukodystrophy
- Alport syndrome

CHAPTER 9

Metabolic Disorders

QUESTIONS

Q-1. A 6-year-old child presents with muscle cramps on exercise with urine test positive for myoglobinuria. His CPK is raised and has been found more raised after exercise.

A. Name the condition.

B. Name the enzyme deficiency.

C. Name the type of this disorder presenting with hypertrophic cardiomyopathy in infancy.

Q-2. A 6-year-old girl born of consanguineous parents presented with swollen, painful joints. It was not rheumatoid arthritis. The biopsy of nodule confirmed the diagnosis.

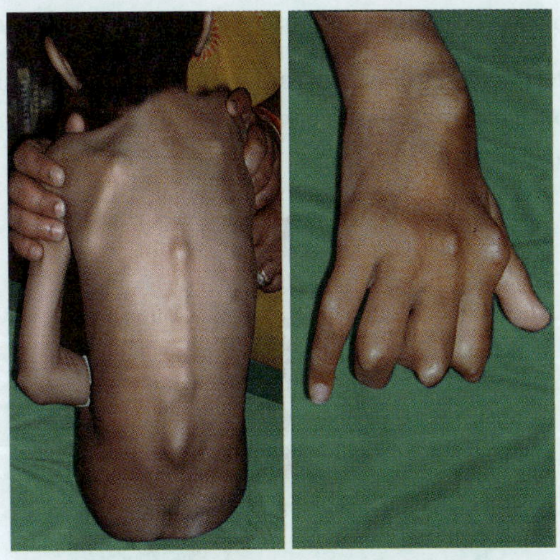

A. What is the disorder?

B. Name the enzyme deficiency.

C. What causes hoarseness of voice and breathing difficulties in this disease?

D. What causes death in this disease?

Q-3. A 2-year-old girl presented with failure to thrive, severe anemia and splenohepatomegaly. The bone marrow picture given below confirmed the diagnosis.

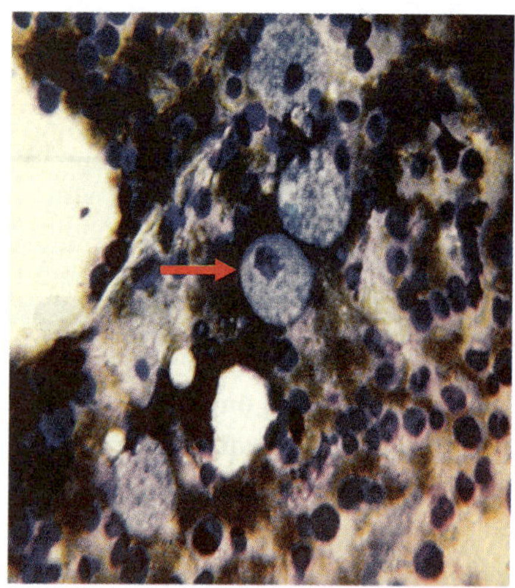

A. Name the condition.
B. What enzyme deficiency causes this disorder?
C. Describe the cell.
D. What are the treatment options available for management of this disease?

Q-4. A 10-month-old boy presented with regression of milestones, dysmorphism, macrocephaly and blue sclera. He also had hypotonia and brisk deep tendon reflexes. High concentration of some metabolite substance in urine and blood confirmed the diagnosis.

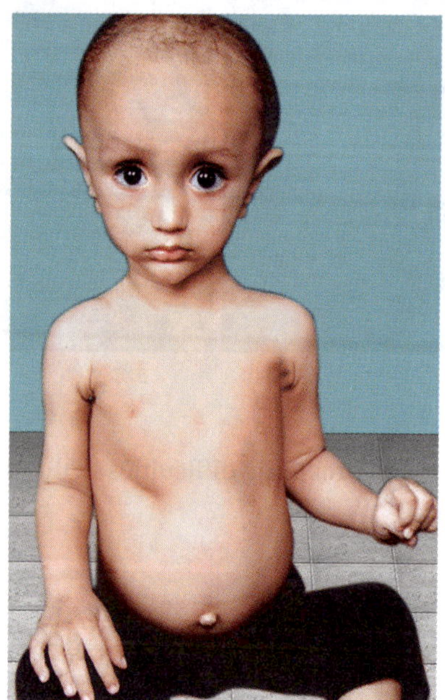

A. What is your diagnosis?
B. What metabolite substance is likely found in high concentration in urine and blood?
C. Name the group of inborn error of metabolism (IEM) in which this disorder is classified.
D. What deficiency is cause of this disorder?

Q-5. A 5-month-old boy presented with regression of milestones and seizures. One sibling died at the age of 3 years due to same illness. His fundus examination picture was as below.

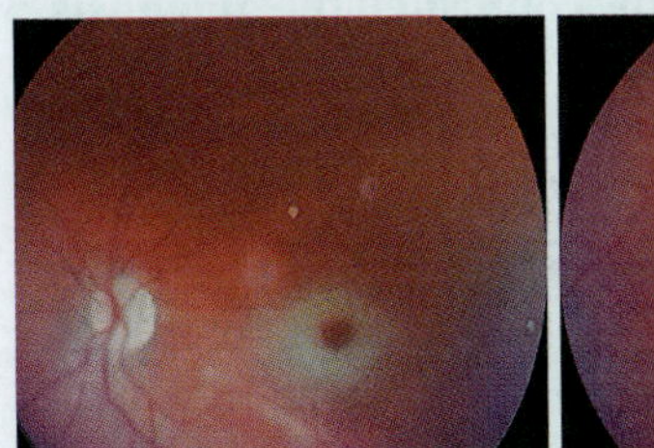
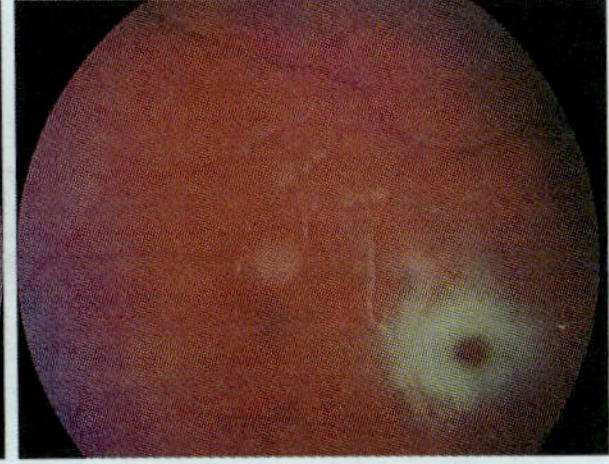

A. What does the fundus examination of eye show?
B. Name the conditions with this ophthalmic finding.

Q-6. A 6-year-old boy presented with difficulty in walking due to knee pain both sides. Mother also complained of darkish staining of the toilet commode following voiding. The urine when kept in a sterile container for a few hours turned black.

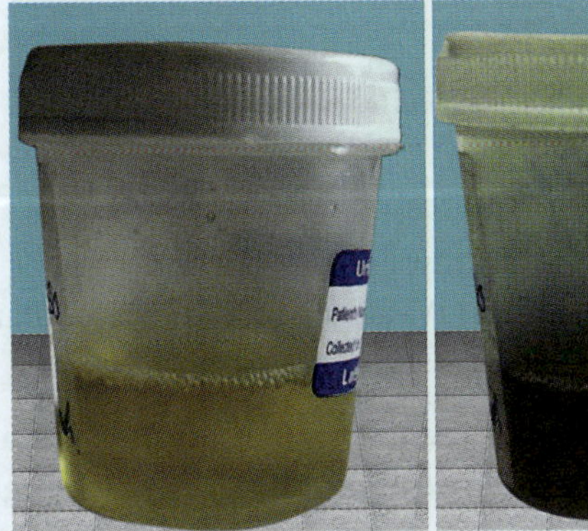

A. What is your diagnosis?
B. Which substance present in the urine turns it black on standing at the room temperature for few hours?
C. What are the other features of the disease?
D. What is treatment of this disease?

Q-7. A 10-year-old boy presented with vomiting. He had photosensitivity on face. Parents noted change in color of urine on standing at room temperature for some time as shown in figure.

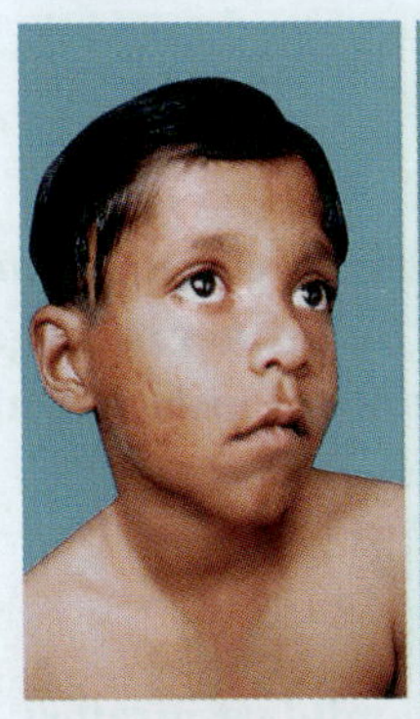
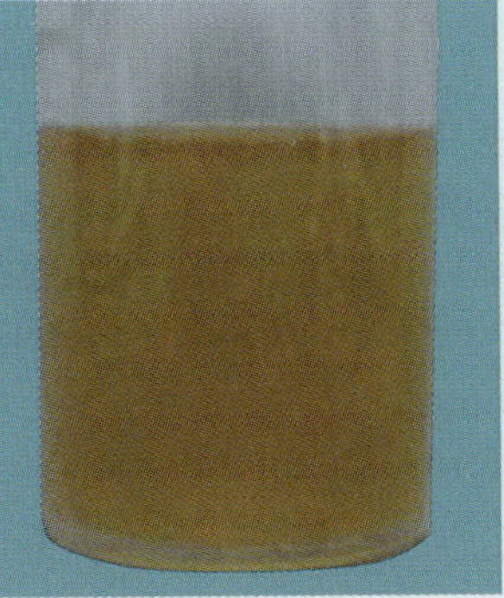
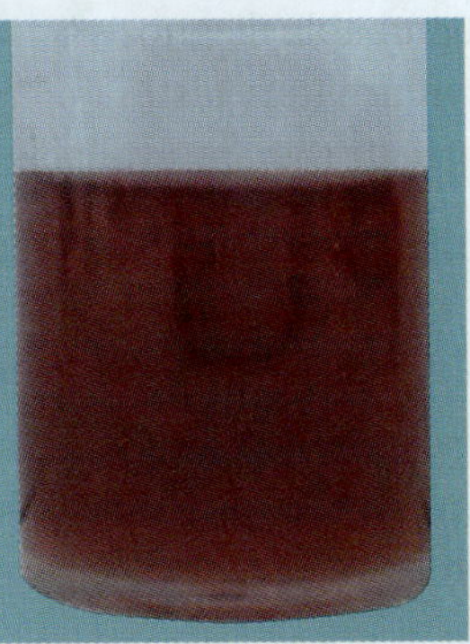

A. What is your diagnosis?
B. What metabolite is responsible for change in color?
C. What is the diagnostic test?

Q-8. A 18-month-old male child presented with huge splenomegaly, hepatomegaly and cachexia. There was no fever, no lymphadenopathy. CBC revealed, Hb 4.5 g/dL, TLC 4200/cumm with polymorphs 36% and lymphocytes 60%, platelets 22,000. Bone marrow confirmed the diagnosis.

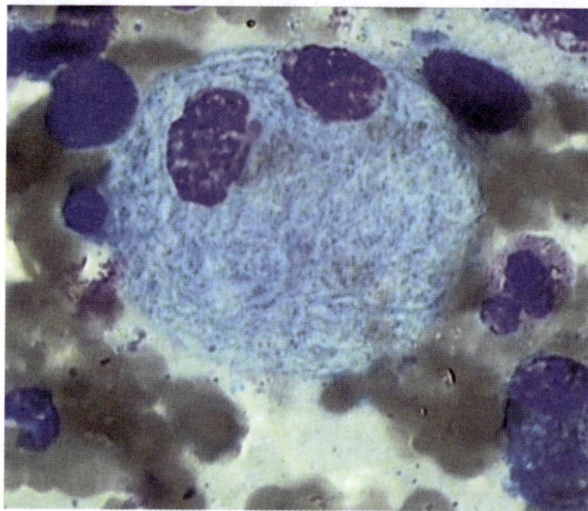

A. What is probable diagnosis?
B. What is its pattern of inheritance?
C. What is the hallmark of diagnosis on bone marrow examination?
D. What is the enzyme deficiency in this disorder? What substance is accumulated in organs?
E. What treatment options are available?

Q-9. A 2-month-old boy presented with vomiting, feeding problems and lethargic for 3 weeks. He also had erythematous rash and partial alopecia. The investigations showed hypoglycemia, ketosis, acidosis and raised ammonia.

A. What is most probable diagnosis?
B. What is genetic inheritance of this disease?
C. What is the treatment?

Q-10. A 5-year-old boy was referred for progressively increasing spleen and pancytopenia. All investigations for infections conditions and malignancy has been ruled out with appropriate investigations. The ophthalmologist detected supranuclear gaze palsy.

A. What is most probable diagnosis?
B. What is the confirmatory test?
C. What is the specific therapy available for this disease?

Q-11. A 4-month-old infant presented in emergency with poor feeding, lethargy, vomiting and respiratory distress. She was treated as bronchiolitis but deteriorating and was referred for further management. Investigations suggested low blood glucose, raised acetone, ketonuria and metabolic acidosis with high anion gap.

A. What investigation is essential at this point?
B. What other investigation should be performed in this infant?
C. What is the probable diagnosis?

Q-12. A 7-month-old boy referred for dystonia and dyskinesia following mild respiratory infection. Antenatal, natal and postnatal periods were uneventful. He was born at full term by vaginal route in the hospital.

Development was normal. Anthropometry showed weight and length normal for age, but head large (>90th centile). He has 4 years old brother who is normal. Family history for dystonia was negative. On further evaluation, CT scan of brain revealed bilateral subdural effusion.

A. What is possible diagnosis?
B. What tests will help for diagnosis?
C. What is the line of treatment?
D. Why is there subdural effusion in this condition?

Q-13. A term male baby born to non-consanguineous parents presented on day 3 with poor feeding, lethargy and irregular respiration. On admission, the baby was encephalopathic, developed seizures and apnea. Sepsis screen was negative. The cousin of the baby died in neonatal period following similar illness. IEM was suspected. ABG showed pH 7.6, HCO_3 decreased marginally and $PaCO_2$ decreased. Plasma ammonia was 1900 µmol/L.

A. What is the interpretation of ABG?
B. Common causes of hyperammonemia in IEM?
C. What is probable diagnosis?
D. What tests should be performed to establish the diagnosis?
E. What urgent lifesaving procedure is indicated in this patient?
F. What are principles of management of such type of disorders?

Q-14. A term baby delivered uneventfully was discharged from hospital on day 3. He was again admitted on day 5 with complaints of poor feeding, lethargy, cyclical movements and hypertonia of limbs followed by progressive encephalopathy. Baby had a typical odor of urine with clinical possibility of inborn errors of metabolism (IEM), basic investigations were performed. Blood glucose, ammonia and lactate wee normal. Metabolic acidosis, ketosis and ketonuria were noted. MRI brain was as below.

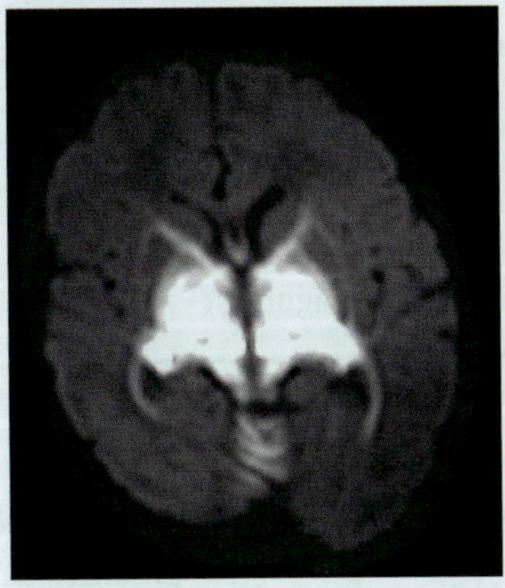

A. What is the characteristic findings in MRI brain?
B. What is probable diagnosis?
C. What tests would be diagnostic?
D. What is the treatment? Is it effective in neonates?

Q-15. A 13-year-old boy had episodes of severe acute abdominal pain not responding to medicines. All the investigations for abdominal pain were normal. On examination, he had hypertension and features of peripheral neuropathy and photosensitivity.

A. What is probable diagnosis?
B. What biochemical test would clinch the diagnosis?
C. What is the definitive treatment?

Q-16. A 6-month-old male infant presented with gray brittle hairs since 3 months of age, reduced activity since 4 months of age and left-sided turning of head and facial twitching lasting for 8–10 minutes since 4 months of age. His serum biotinidase level was normal.

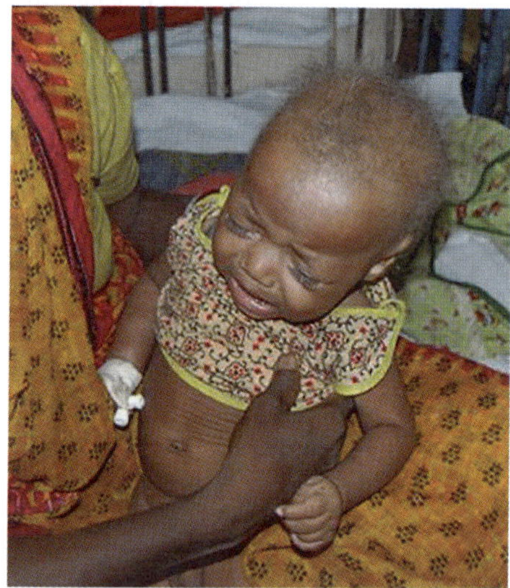

A. What is probable diagnosis?
B. What biochemical test will help for diagnosis?
C. Which specific investigations and its findings will confirm the diagnosis?
D. What is the treatment of this disease?

Q-17. A 4-month-old child presented with seizures hypotonia, loss of scalp hairs and delayed development with clinical diagnosis of IEM, TMS and urine GCMS were performed. TMS showed raised C5OH and urine GCMS was normal.

A. What is probable diagnosis?
B. What are differential diagnosis?
C. What biochemical test would confirm the diagnosis?
D. What is treatment of this condition?
E. What is the prognosis of this disease?
F. What are preventive steps of this disorder?

Q-18. Match the following antenatal ultrasound findings with IEM disorder:

A. Nonimmune hydrops	1. Glutaric aciduria type 2
B. Corpus callosal agenesis	2. Mitochondrial respiratory chain defects
C. Antenatal ventriculomegaly	3. Zell Verger syndrome
D. Renal cyst	4. Pyridoxine-dependent seizures
E. VACTERI association	5. Mucopolysaccharidosis type VII
F. Epiphyseal stippling and binder phenotype	6. Chondrodysplasia punctata

Q-19. A 7-day-old baby presented with encephalopathy. Her perinatal period was normal. Baby was managed with supportive therapy before that blood samples and urine samples were sent for TMS and urine GSMS. Molecular analysis revealed the diagnosis of carbonic anhydrase VA deficiency.

A. What biochemical abnormalities can present in this patient?
B. What diagnosis was labeled in the past in such patients before the availability of molecular diagnosis?
C. If these patients are managed well with metabolic crisis, they generally do well. How it happens so?

Q-20. A 7-year-old boy was admitted for stroke. On evaluation, he had marfanoid features. Ophthalmic examination revealed subluxation of lens and myopia.

A. What is probable diagnosis?
B. Which enzyme deficiency is there in this disorder?
C. What tests should be performed to confirm the diagnosis?
D. What drug therapy may help in this condition?

Q-21. A 14-day-old neonate was brought for poor feeding, lethargy, FTT and respiratory distress. She was born as second child out of third degree consanguineous marriage. First child died in immediate neonatal period due to unknown cause. She had a typical sweaty feet odor. Her basic investigations revealed severe metabolic acidosis, ketosis and hyperammonemia. TMS showed elevated C5 carnitine levels.

A. What is most probable diagnosis?
B. Why sodium benzoate should not be used to treat hyperammonemia in this condition?
C. What chelating agents can be used to remove toxic metabolism in this condition?

Q-22. A 10-day-old infant referred for refractory seizures, not responding to multiple anticonvulsants. EEG showed burst suppression pattern.

A. Name the treatable condition presenting as refractory seizures.
B. How would you treat this patient?
C. What is an important clue in the history to be elicited from mother?
D. Which biochemical tests will confirm the diagnosis?
E. What are differential diagnosis for treatable refractory neonatal seizures?

Q-23. A 4-week-old girl is admitted with complaints of poor feeding, vomiting and fever. On physical examination, body temperature is 102°F, she has jaundice, 4 cm hepatomegaly and hypotonia with normal tendon reflexes. Blood culture shows no growth after 72 hours. CSF microscopy showed coliform organisms. She had direct type hyperbilirubinemia and not responding to antibiotics.

A. What is the probable diagnosis?
B. What is the confirmatory test?
C. What clinical findings helps in the diagnosis?
D. What is the treatment of this patient?

Q-24. A 2-week-old infant is brought in OPD for routine follow-up. The mother showed his newborn metabolic screening test report. It shows high levels of phenylalanine.

A. What will be your approach for this baby?
B. How will you confirm the diagnosis?
C. Which conditions can have high phenylalanine levels?
D. What is the treatment of this disease?

Q-25. A 9-month-old child was referred for failure to thrive, rickets and features suggesting liver failure. Antenatal and natal history was uneventful. As a part of routine new born screening was performed and it showed raise tyrosine.

A. What is probable diagnosis?
B. What biochemical tests should be performed to confirm the diagnosis?
C. Why is there rickets in this disorder?
D. What is the specific drug used in this condition?
E. What is permanent solution to this disease?

Q-26. A 4-year-old girl, born to third degree consanguineous parents presented with encephalopathy seizures following mild viral URTI. She had history of hypoglycemia during neonatal period, medical record of evaluation is not available. On examination, she had continuous seizures, tonic posturing with Glasgow

coma scale 5. Investigations showed hypoketotic hypoglycemia, hyperammonemia, raised hepatic enzymes and metabolic acidosis. CSF was normal.

A. What is probable diagnosis?
B. What biochemical test would help to confirm the diagnosis?
C. What preventive advice should be given to the patient on discharge?

Q-27. A 10-month-old infant was referred for hypoglycemic seizures with generalized hypotonia and protuberant abdomen. Clinical examination showed hepatomegaly.

A. What is probable diagnosis?
B. What biochemical tests are specific for the disorder?
C. What are long-term complications of this disease?
D. What diet is advised in this condition? What is specific diet for this disease?

Q-28. A 4-year-old girl was admitted in PICU with severe metabolic acidosis, hypoglycemia, ketosis and lactic acidosis. She required dialysis. She had similar episodes in the past 3 times since neonatal period. Her weight was less than 3rd centile, although height and development were within normal range. She was well in between the episodes. TMS showed high alanine and urine GCMS elevated glycerol.

A. What is probable diagnosis?
B. What is the confirmatory test for the condition?
C. What other IEM can present with elevated urine glycerol?
D. What precautious should be taken in collecting the urine sample in such patients
E. What is the long-term outcome in this disease?

Q-29. Match the following with disorders responding to specific vitamin supplementation:

A. Homocystinuria	1. Biotin
B. Methylmalonic acidemia	2. Riboflavin
C. Propionic acidemia	3. Vitamin B_{12}
D. Maple syrup urine disease	4. Pyridoxine
E. Glutaric aciduria type I	5. Thiamine

Q-30. A 3-year-old child was brought in OPD with complaints of joint pain and change of color of urine to black on exposure to atmosphere. Parents also noted some dark-colored areas over skin.

A. What is probable diagnosis?
B. What biochemical test would confirm the diagnosis?
C. What is the basic defect in this disorder?
D. What is the treatment?

ANSWERS

A-1. A. McArdle disease (Type V glycogen storage disease)
B. Muscle phosphorylase deficiency
C. Pompe disease (Type II glycogen storage disease)

A-2. A. Farber disease
B. Lysosomal enzyme ceramidase
C. Nodule or granulomatous formation on the vocal cords
D. Recurrent pneumonias

A-3. A. Gaucher disease
B. Lysosomal hydrolase, acid beta-glucosidase
C. 20–100 μm in diameter, wrinkled paper appearance
D. Enzyme replacement and bone marrow transplantation

A-4. A. Glutaric aciduria type 1
B. Glutaric acid
C. Organic aciduria
D. Glutaryl-CoA dehydrogenase

A-5. A. Cherry-red spot
B. Tay-Sachs disease, Sandhoff disease, Generalized gangliosidosis

A-6. A. Alkaptonuria
B. Homogentisic acid
C.
- Ochronosis (dark spots on ear cartilage and sclera)
- Changes of osteoarthritis with X-rays of knee, hips and spine

D.
- Nitisinone
- Phenylalanine and tyrosine restricted diet

A-7. A. Acute intermittent porphyria
B. Porphobilin
C.
- Increased urinary porphobilinogen
- Erythrocyte PBGD

A-8. A. Gaucher disease
B. Autosomal recessive
C. *Gaucher cell:* This is a large uninucleate or multinucleate cell measuring 20–100 μm in diameter. The nucleus is small, round or oval and eccentric and the cytoplasm is abundant. It has wrinkled tissue paper appearance
D.
- Glucocerebrosidase enzyme deficiency
- Glycosphingolipids is collected in organs.

E. *Treatment options:*
- Enzyme replacement therapy
- Substrate reduction therapy
- Enzyme enhancement therapy
- Bone marrow transplantation
- Hematopoietic stem cell transplantation (HSCT)

A-9. A. Multiple carboxylase deficiency
B. Autosomal recessive
C. Biotin 10 mg/day, orally

A-10. A. Gaucher disease
B. Beta-glucosidase enzyme activity is reduced.
C. Enzyme replacement therapy and substrate reduction—miglustat are definitive therapy for Gaucher disease

A-11. A. Plasma ammonia
B. TMS and urine GCMS are important investigations for further evaluation
C. Organic acidemia

A-12. A. Glutaric aciduria type 1
B. TMS and urine GMS. TMS will show elevated glutarylcarnitine and glutaric aciduria.
C. Low protein diet and special formula devoid of offending amino acid.
D. A hallmark of glutaric aciduria type 1 is cerebral atrophy and enlarged CSF spaces particularly in frontotemporal regions, which leads to wide, expanded CSF spaces. These enlarged CSF spaces cause stretching of delicate cortical veins bridging the dura and brain. It causes rupture of vessels and results in subdural effusion.

A-13. A. Respiratory alkalosis

B. *Common causes of hyperammonemia in IEM:*
- Ornithine transcarbamylase (OTC) deficiency
- Citrullinemia type II
- Organic acidemias
- Carnitine deficiency

C. Ornithine transcarbamylase deficiency (OTC), type of urea cycle disorders

D. Plasma amino acids, plasma acylcarnitine profile and organic acids and orotic acid

E. Extracorporeal toxin removal—hemodialysis or peritoneal dialysis

F. *Principles of management:*
- *Substrate reduction:*
  - Stop feeding
  - IVF with dextrose and intralipid
- *Provision of deficient metabolites:* Pyridoxine in pyridoxine dependent epilepsy
- *Removal of toxic metabolites:* Sodium benzoate for hyperammonemia, hemodialysis
- Increase in enzyme activity
- Liver transplantation

A-14. D. MRI brain shows cytotoxic edema of myelinated white matter involving brainstem and cerebellum producing characteristic double swan appearance.

E. Maple syrup urine disease (MSUD)

F. *Investigations:*
- Plasma amino acid profile by high performance liquid chromatography (HPLC) will show marked elevation in leucine, isoleucine and valine.
- *Tandem mass spectrophotometry (TMS):* Marked elevation in leucine, isoleucine and valine
- *Urine gas chromatography mass spectrometry:* Elevation of multiple alpha-keto acids.

G. Thiamine supplementation can be given, but in neonatal onset MSUD, it is not effective.

A-15.

A. Acute intermittent porphyria

B. Urinary porphobilinogen will be raised.

C. Liver transplantation

A-16. A. Menkes kinky hair disease

B. Serum copper and ceruloplasmin levels

C.
- Microscopy of hair which shows pili torti hair
- MRI of brain shows intracranial arterial tortuosity

D. Parenteral copper histidine therapy

A-17. A. Biotinidase deficiency

B. Holocarboxylase deficiency is nearby differential diagnosis. Urine GCMS usually shows elevated organic acids in holocarboxylase deficiency.

C. Serum biotinidase level

D. Oral biotin supplementation

E. Earlier treatment is started, better is the prognosis. If treatment is started beyond neonatal period, hearing and visual impairment and affected intellectual ability may develop.

F. Neonatal screening and early biotin supplementation are most effective preventive measures.

A-18. A. 5 B. 4

C. 3 D. 1

E. 2 F. 6

A-19. A. Hyperammonemia, metabolic acidosis, lactic acidosis and normal ketones are common metabolic derangement in these patients.
B. Transient hyperammonemia of neonate (THAN)
C. Activation of carbonic anhydrase B-enzyme

A-20. A. Homocystinuria
B. Cystathionine beta-synthetase
C. Plasma total homocysteine levels. Confirmatory tests by mutational analysis of the *CBS* gene.
D. Pyridoxine

A-21. A. Isovaleric acidemia
B. Sodium benzoate acts by combining glycine and can deplete the glycine levels, whereas glycine acts as a chelating agents in isovaleric acidemia.
C. Carnitine and glycine

A-22. A. Pyridoxine-dependent seizures
B. Intravenous pyridoxine 100 mg under EEG monitoring
C. Increased fetal movements (Fetal seizures)
D. CSF and plasma α-aminoadipic semialdehyde and pipecolic acid
E.
- Pyridoxine-5-phosphate oxidase deficiency treatable with pyridoxine phosphate
- Cerebral folate deficiency, treatable with folinic acid

A-23. A. Galactosemia
B. Estimation of an enzyme, galactose-1-phosphate uridyl transferase.
C. Red reflex examination of eye will detect cataract.
D. Galactose free diet

A-24. A. Initial assessment includes thorough history including antenatal and natal periods. One should check for unusual odor, hypopigmentation, etc.
B. A positive screening test should be confirmed by quantitative amino acid analysis in plasma. Phenylalanine >120 µmol/L is considered as positive. Phenylalanine/Tyrosine ratio >3 is positive for phenylketonuria.
C. Classical phenylketonuria and protein defects can have high phenylalanine levels.
D. *Treatment of phenylketonuria:*
- Phenylalanine restricted diet
- Maintain blood phenylalanine levels 120–360 µmol/L. Care must be taken to avoid low levels of phenylalanine as it is also harmful because phenylalanine is required for brain development and its function.
- Breast milk contains low phenylalanine levels. Hence, breastfed infants are given phenylalanine free formula in measured quantity followed by breastfeeding.

A-25. A. Tyrosinemia
B. Urine succinyl acetone is specific test for tyrosinemia.
C. Rickets in tyrosinemia is secondary to renal tubular acidosis.
D. Nitisinone
E. Liver transplantation

A-26. A. Fatty acid oxidation defect
B. TMS will show elevated acyl carnitine profile.
C. Avoid fasting

A-27. A. Glycogen storage disease GSD lb
B. Hypoglycemia, hyperlactatemia, hypertriglyceridemia, hyperuricemia and hypokalemia are common biochemical findings.
C. Hepatic adenoma, pancreatitis, inflammatory bowel disease and polycystic ovaries in females are common long-term complications.

D. Complex carbohydrate with high-protein and low-fat diet is the treatment. Uncooked corn starch is specific diet for this disease.

A-28. A. Fructose 1-6 diphosphatase deficiency

B. Molecular testing/exome sequencing is the test for definite diagnosis

C. Glycerol kinase deficiency and essential fructosuria present with elevated urine glycerol

D. Do not use glycerol containing soap for cleaning the genitals before collection of urine sample for GCMS analysis.

E. Normal development and intellectual ability is not affected

A-29. A. 4

B. 3

C. 1

D. 5

E. 2

A-30. A. Alkaptonuria

B. Raised homogentisic acid in blood and urine

C. Homogentisate 1,2-dioxygenase enzyme deficiency

D. Vitamin C. It prevents binding of homogentisic acid to cartilage.

CHAPTER 10

Immunology

QUESTIONS

Q-1. A 8-year-old boy developed swelling of lips suddenly following eating chiki containing nuts. He developed severe swelling of eyelids, lips and neck and stridor within 2 hours of onset of symptoms. There is history of similar problem to sibling.

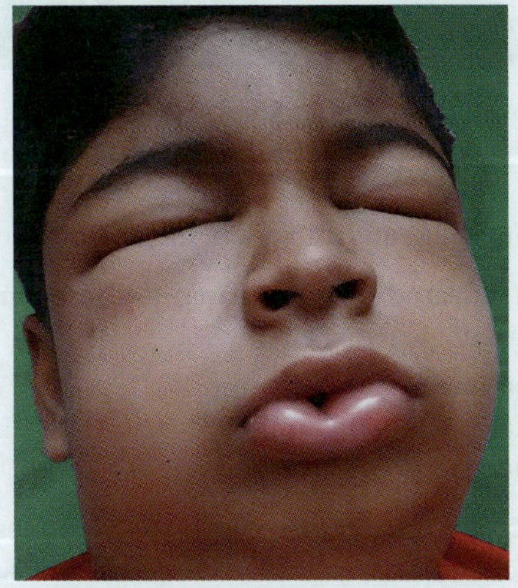

A. What is your diagnosis?
B. What type of immune reaction is it?
C. What is the investigation of choice for this disorder?
D. Which drugs are lifesaving?

Q-2. An infant presented with this swelling over left thigh following DTwP vaccination within few hours:

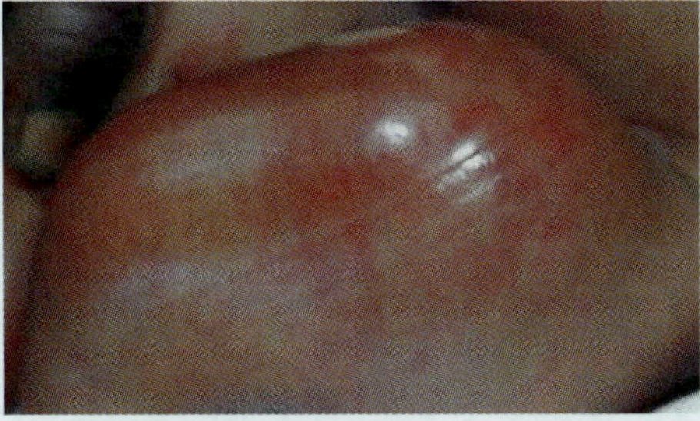

A. What type of reaction is it?
B. What are absolute contraindications of DPT vaccination?
C. What are considered as precautions, but not contraindications for DPT vaccination?

Q-3. Emergency management of anaphylaxis.

Q-4. This development is following BCG vaccination in an infant:

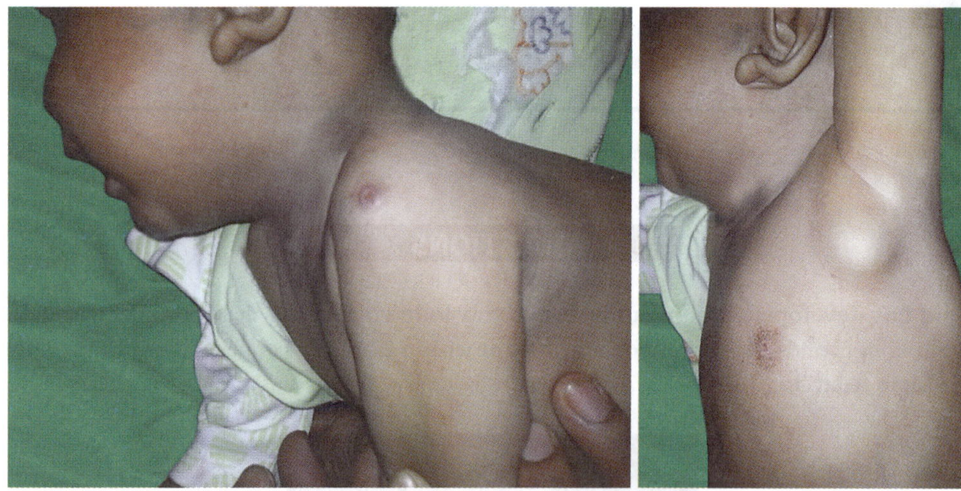

A. Is it normal or abnormal following BCG? When do you call it abnormal?
B. When this type of complication is common following BCG vaccination?
C. Line of treatment.
D. What is role of anti-tuberculous drugs and antibiotics in this situation?

Q-5. A 7-year-old child presents with repeated episodes of non-pitting edema and abdominal cramps. His parents are told that the child has immunological disorder.

A. What immunological disorder is likely?
B. What complication can be fatal in this condition?
C. Which other disorders have been reported in these patients?

Q-6. A 12-year-old boy presented with high-grade fever, cough and breathlessness. Chest X-ray showed necrotizing pneumonia. He had history of pneumonia four times in past, once with pneumatocele formation. He also had recurrent abscesses and once psoas abscess.

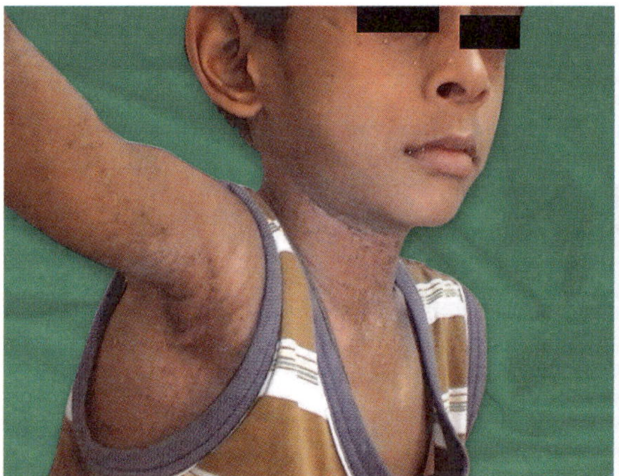

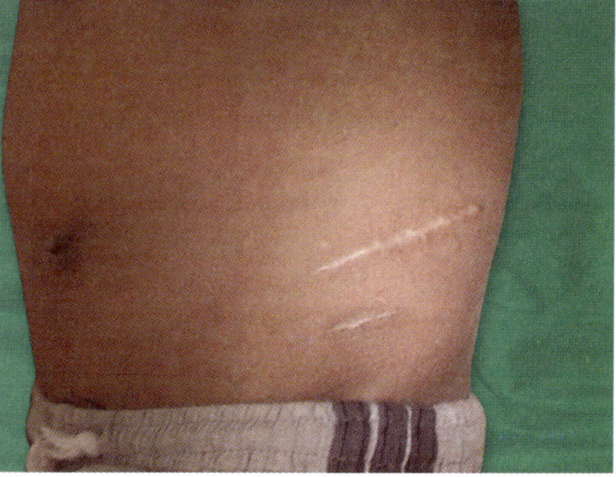

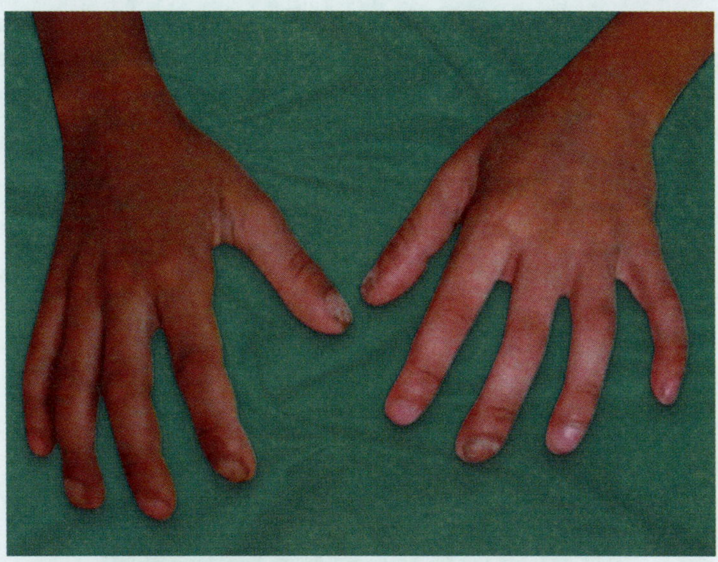

A. What is most probable diagnosis?
B. What are common features of this disorder?
C. What is considered as confirmed diagnosis?

Q-7. A 10-year-old boy had fever 102–103°F, pain in abdomen and vomiting for 5 days, followed by skin rashes as shown in the pictures. He had seizures one month back and pediatric neurologist started oxcarbamazepine and clobazam. On physical examination, he had 101.0°F fever, skin rashes, mild jaundice, lymphadenopathy and hepatomegaly. CBC showed WBC count 18,400/cumm with 15% eosinophils, raised direct type bilirubin and SGPT.

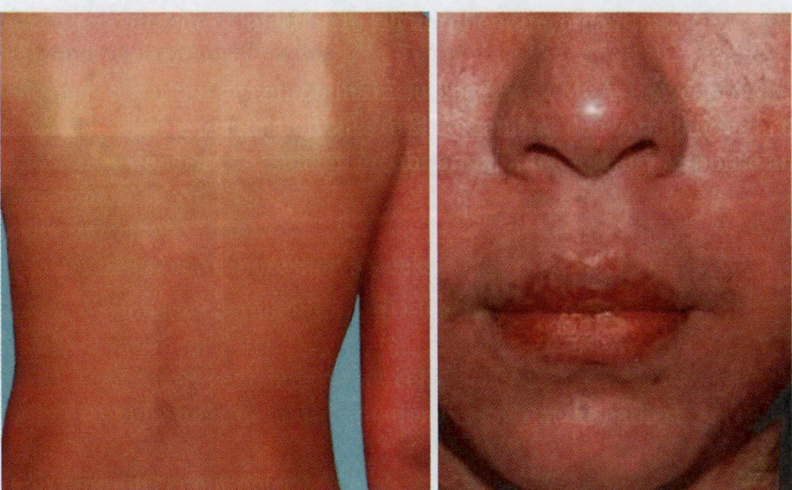

A. What is probable diagnosis?
B. What are differential diagnosis for skin rashes?
C. Which drugs are known to cause this disorder?
D. What is the new name for this condition?

Q-8. An 8-years boy presented with mild fever and cough of 6 weeks duration. His mother was diagnosed as pulmonary tuberculosis 3 months back and she is on anti-tuberculous treatment. The patient had also complaint of pain at legs and examination revealed lesions as shown in picture. These skin lesions were inflamed and tender. His Mantoux test was strongly positive.

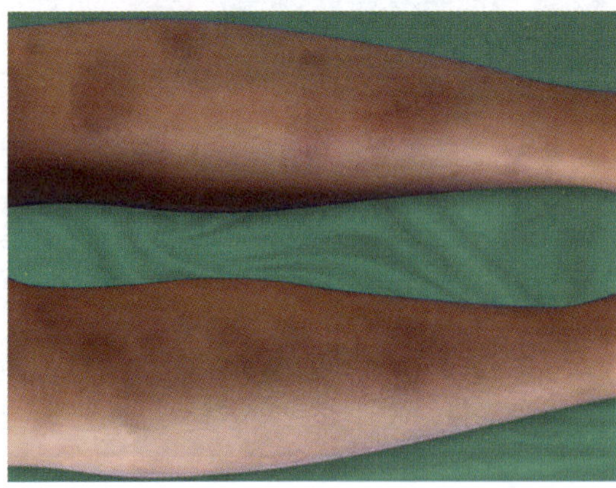

A. What are called this skin lesions?
B. What are common sites for these lesions? what is morphological description of lesions?
C. What type of immune reaction can cause this type of skins lesions?
D. What are other manifestations of this infection following same immune reaction?
E. What are other causes of these type of skin lesions?

Q-9. A 9 year-old girl was brought in emergency room with complaints of high-grade fever of 5 days duration, knees and elbows swollen and tender. She started to deteriorate leading to shock. She had an abrasion over left knee 15 days back while playing in school, got it infected. On physical examination, she had high-grade fever, tachycardia, tachypnea and narrow pulse pressure. Tongue was red. Skin lesions, and joint swelling and generalized edema are shown in the pictures. CBC showed leukocytosis and raised CRP. Blood culture showed growth of *Staphylococcus aureus*.

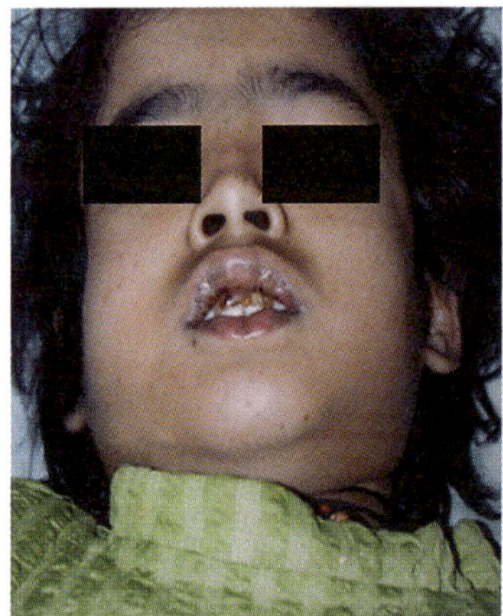
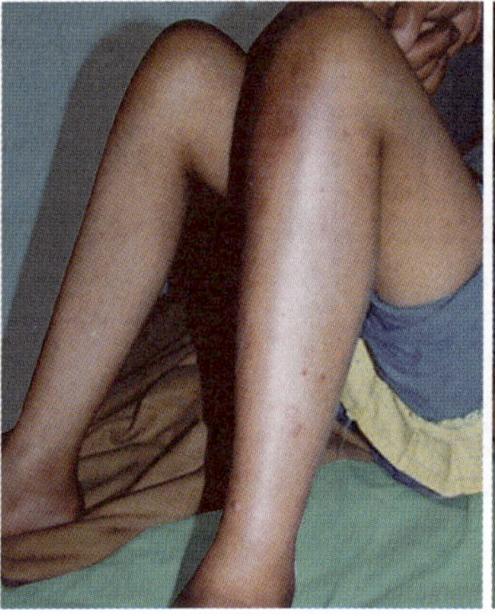
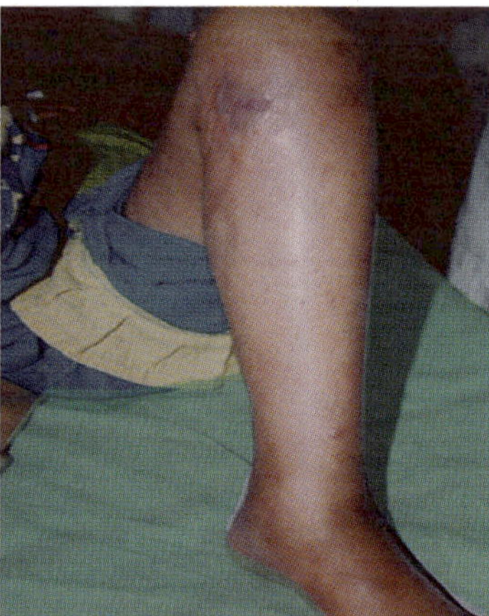

A. What is probable diagnosis?
B. What are differential diagnosis?
C. Which specific substance is responsible for the condition?
D. What should be antibiotics of choice?

Q-10. A 4-year-old boy presented with high-grade fever for 8 weeks. He also has complaint of skin rashes, erythematous, salmon-colored, like urticaria, non-pruritic, especially during fever, disappearing during afebrile period. He had pain at thighs and morning stiffness since 10 days. CBC showed mild anemia, leukocytosis, thrombocytosis, ESR and CRP more than 100. No response to antibiotics.

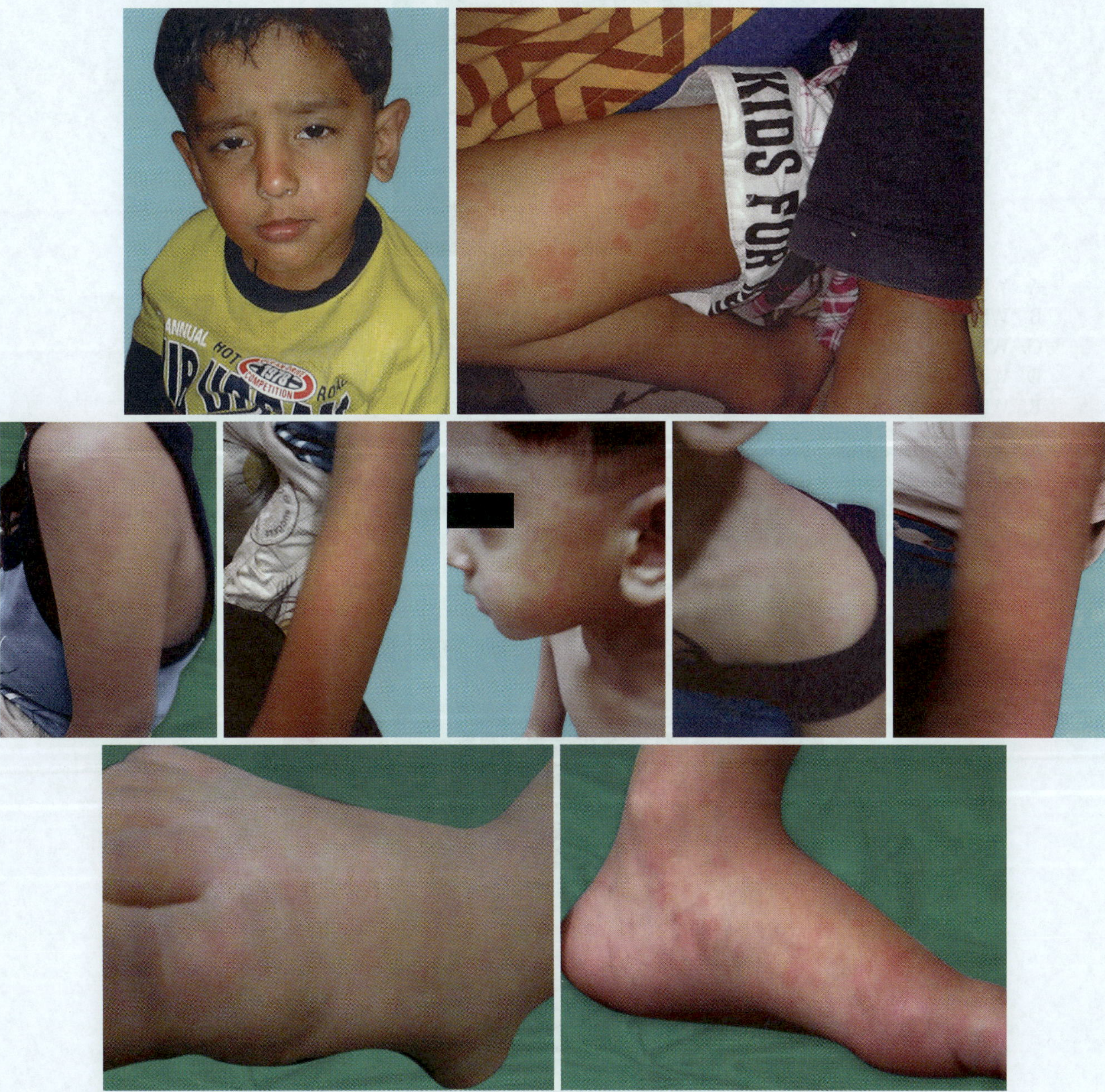

A. What is probable diagnosis?
B. What factors can evoke reappearance of skin rash?
C. What is specific name of skin rashes as described in this case?
D. What is the known complication associated with condition with development of pancytopenia and drop of ESR?

Q-11. A 12-year-old girl was brought with complaints of mild-to-moderate fever, decreased appetite, oral ulcers, fatigue, and skin rashes over face as shown in the picture.

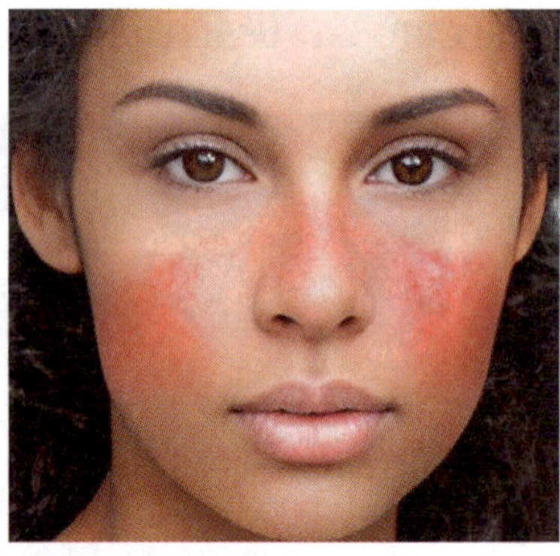

A. What is probable diagnosis?
B. What are neurological manifestations of this disease?
C. What are common CBC findings in this disorder?
D. What are confirmatory immunological investigations in this disease?
E. What complication may develop to the neonate of a mother suffering from this disease?

Q-12. A 3-year-old boy presented with high-grade fever of 10 days duration. He also had erythema over palms and soles, bilateral conjunctivitis without exudate and red tongue as shown in the pictures. After few days, he developed swelling over dorsum of hands and fingers. CBC showed leukocytosis, thrombocytosis and raised CRP and ESR. There was no response to antibiotics.

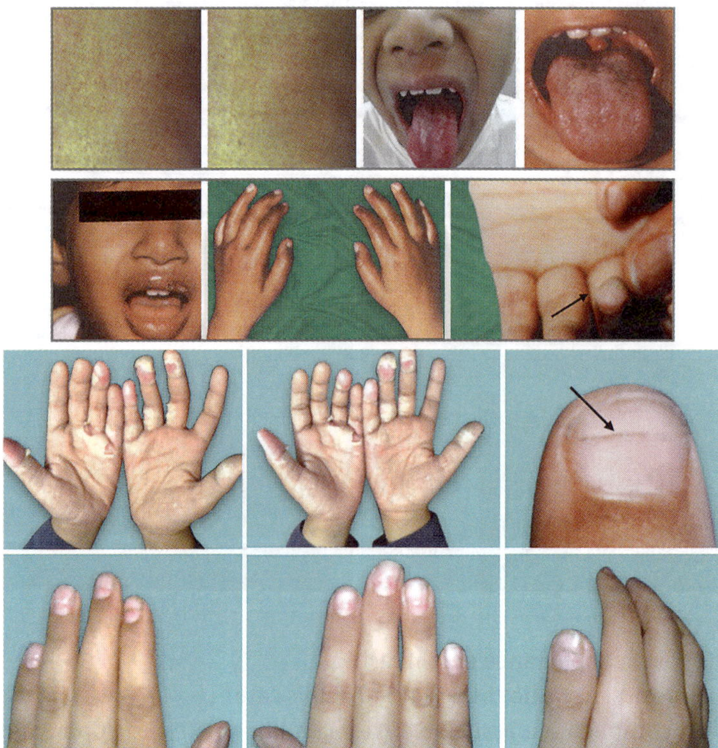

A. What is probable diagnosis?
B. What features are not suggesting this disorder and may suggest alternate diagnosis?
C. What are the variants of this condition, missed in the clinical practice?
D. What treatment modalities are recommended in this disease?

Q-13. A 9-year-old girl was brought with complaints of difficulty in getting up from sitting position, difficulty in opening the eyes and change of voice. She also had mild-to-moderate fever and joint pain. She had skin changes over eyelids, knuckles and elbows as shown in picture.

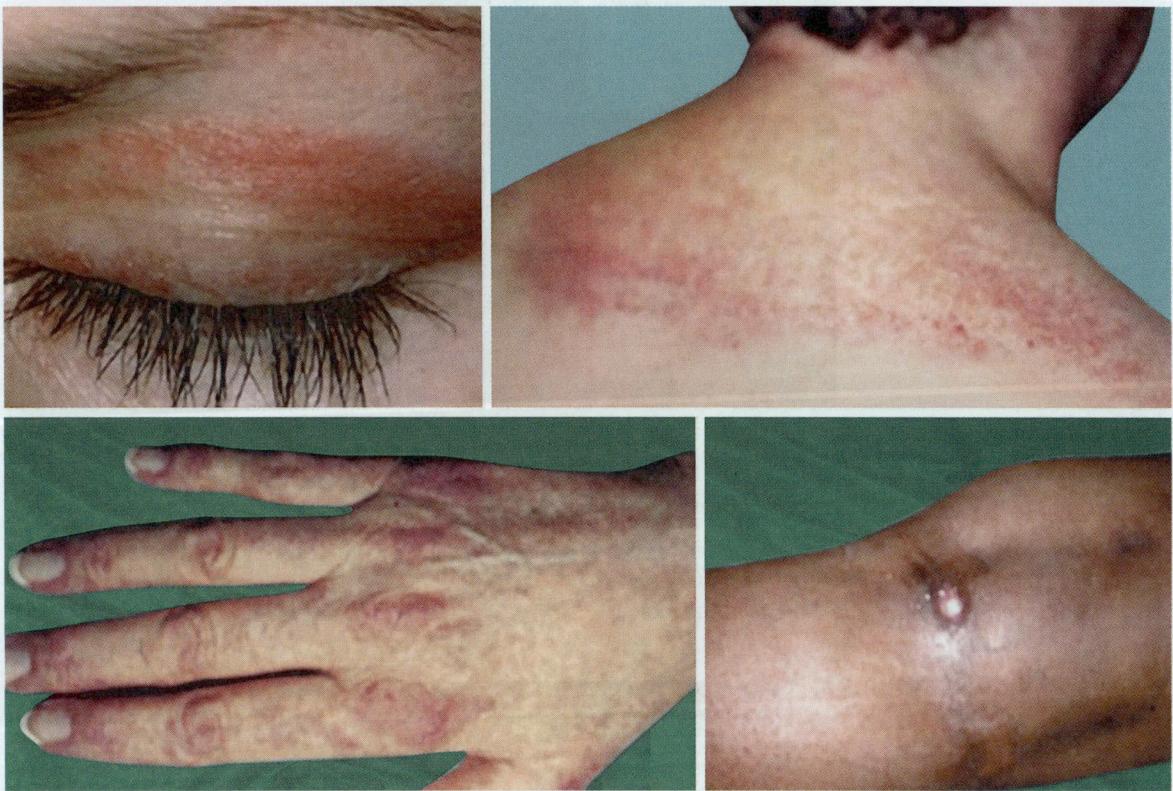

A. What is probable diagnosis?
B. Identify the lesions seen in the pictures.
C. What is the cause of difficulty in getting up from sitting position? Which investigation may support your reasoning?
D. What complications are known to be associated with this disease?

Q-14. Term baby born to third degree consanguineous parents with birth weight of 2.9 kg and normal transition is brought on Day 23 with history of loose stool 12–15 times a day for 7 days. Baby was exclusively breastfed. There was history of discharge from umbilicus from 7th day of life. On examination, there was severe erythema and induration around umbilicus and cellulitis at perianal region. Hb was 14 g/dL and total leukocyte count 60,500/cumm, platelets 3.5 lakhs.

A. What is probable diagnosis?
B. What is the basic defect in this disorder?
C. What are the immunologic features of this disease?
D. What is an important marker in neonatal history is associated with this condition?

Q-15. A neonate was admitted on 20 DOL for fever and respiratory distress for 6 days. Antenatal and birth history were uneventful. The baby had generalized extensive skin rash, hepatosplenomegaly and lymphadenopathy. Chest X-ray was reported as pneumonia and hypoplasia of thymus. CBC showed Hb 8, TLC 18,500, P_{56}, L_{20}, E_{18}. Absolut eosinophils were 3330, Platelets 3,50,000. bronchoalveolar lavage (BAL) showed *Pneumocystis jirovecii*. Immunoglobulin study revealed elevated IgE level. The clinical photograph was as below:

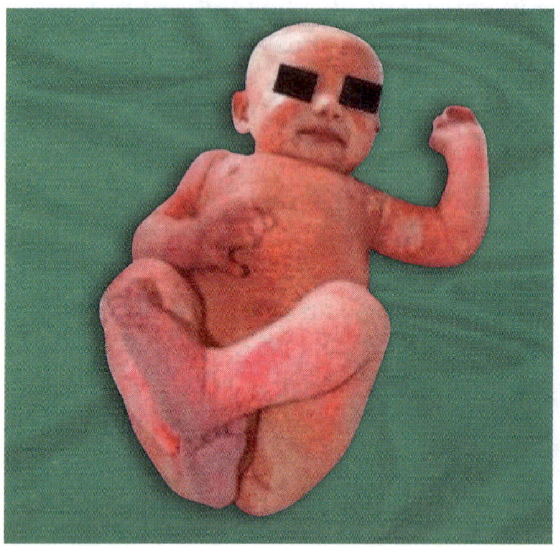

A. Identify the rash.
B. What is probable diagnosis?
C. What is expected on lymphocyte subset analysis?
D. What is treatment?
E. What is prognosis in untreated patient?
F. What are common genetic defects in this disease?

ANSWERS

A-1. A. Hereditary angioedema
B. Type I hypersensitivity
C.
- Serum C4 level (decreased)
- C1 esterase inhibitor

D.
- Epinephrine
- Antihistaminic
- Steroids

A-2. A. Type III (Immune Complex Hypersensitivity) (Arthus reaction)
B.
- Severe allergic reaction to vaccine component following prior dose
- Encephalopathy
- Anaphylaxis

C.
- Persistent inconsolable crying for >3 hours
- Hyperpyrexia (Fever >40.5°C)
- Hypotonic hyporesponsive episode (HHE) within 48 hours
- Febrile seizures

A-3.
- Administer epinephrine (1:1000 solution) 0.01 mL/kg/dose (maximum 0.5 ml) IM on anterolateral aspect of thigh
- Set-up IV access
- Lay patient flat and elevate legs if tolerated. Give high flow oxygen and airway or ventilation, if needed.
- If hypotensive also, set-up additional wide bore access and give normal saline 20 mL/kg over 1–2 minutes.
- IM adrenaline may be repeated after 5 minutes, if required
- Oral antihistaminic (No IV)
- Oral/injectable steroids has no definite role.

A-4. A. *Normal BCG reaction:* Wheal of 5 mm at injection site (successful ID–Peau d'orange) subsides within 30 minutes → No visible change for several days → Development of papule after 2–3 weeks → 4–8 mm size by 5–6 weeks → pustule formation → bursts open and gets sealed off (may be repeated 2–3 times) → Ulceration → scab formation → scab falls of → superficial, tiny scar of few mm size

B. Ipsilateral axillary or cervical enlarged lymph node (<1 cm size) may develop a few weeks or months after BCG vaccination → Lymph nodes regress spontaneously → Anti-tuberculous therapy (ATT) is not indicated.

C. Lymph node size >1 cm or signs of suppuration (abscess formation) → Needle aspiration, may require repeated aspirations or surgical excision. No ATT.

D. BCG adenitis is more common with subcutaneous BCG administration. No ATT, no antibiotics are indicated.

A-5. A. C1 inhibitor deficiency

B. Laryngeal edema

C. SLE and glomerulonephritis

A-6. A. Hyper IgE syndrome (Job syndrome)

B.
- Staphylococcal abscess
- Pneumatocele formation
- Unusual facial features
- *Candida albicans* is second most common pathogen
- Pruritic dermatitis
- Delay in shedding primary teeth, recurrent fractures and scoliosis

C. Serum IgE level >2000 Iu/mL

A-7. A. DRESS syndrome (Drug, Rash, Eosinophilia, Systemic Symptoms)

B.
- Erythema multiforme
- Stevens-Johnson syndrome
- Toxic epidermal necrolysis

C.
- Phenytoin, carbamazepine, phenobarbitone, primidone
- Antibiotics

D. Drug hypersensitivity syndrome

A-8. A. Erythema nodosum

B. The common sites for erythema nodosum are shin of tibia, forearms, thighs and trunk. These lesions are nodular, tender, look-like bruises and turned into violaceous color and fades to normal skin

C. Hypersensitivity reaction (Type III)

D. Phlyctenular conjunctivitis, pleural effusion, tuberculous lymphadenopathy

E. *Other causes of erythema nodosum:*
- *Infections:* Group A streptococcal pharyngitis, tuberculosis, histoplasmosis
- *Inflammatory conditions:* Sarcoidosis, inflammatory bowel disease
- *Drugs:* Sulfonamides, phenytoin

A-9. A. Staphylococcal toxic shock syndrome

B.
- Streptococcal toxic shock syndrome
- Septic shock

C. Toxic shock syndrome Toxin-1 (Superantigen)

D.
- Vancomycin + Clindamycin in a case of MRSA
- Cloxacillin + Clindamycin in a case of MSSA

A-10. A. Systemic-onset juvenile idiopathic arthritis (SOJIA)

B. Heat, warm bath can evoke the reappearance of skin rash

C. Evanescent (Vanishing)

D. Macrophage activation syndrome (MAS)

A-11. A. Systemic lupus erythematous (SLE)

B.
- Seizures
- Neuropsychiatric manifestations such as headache, psychosis, stroke, transverse myelitis
- Peripheral nervous system manifestations

C.
- Hemolytic anemia with reticulocytosis
- Leukopenia
- Lymphopenia
- Thrombocytopenia

D.
- ANA
- Anti Ds-DNA
- Anti-SM
- Antiphospholipid antibody
- Low C3 and C4
- Direct Coomb's test positive

E. Complete heart block

A-12. A. Kawasaki disease

B. *Features not suggesting Kawasaki disease:*
- Exudative conjunctivitis
- Exudative pharyngitis
- Generalized lymphadenopathy
- Discrete oral lesions
- Bullous/pustular/vesicular rashes
- Splenomegaly
- Lymphocytosis

C. *Variants of Kawasaki disease:*
- Incomplete Kawasaki disease
- Atypical Kawasaki disease
- Neonatal Kawasaki disease
- Refractory (Resistant) Kawasaki disease

D.
- Intravenous immunoglobulin
- Infliximab
- Pulse methyl prednisolone
- Cyclosporine
- Abciximab

A-13. A. Juvenile dermatomyositis

B.
- Heliotrope rash of eyelids
- Malar rash over face
- Photosensitive rash
- Calcinosis
- Acanthosis nigricans at back of neck
- Gottron's papules over joints

C.
- Myopathy
- CPK, SGOT, LDH

D.
- Muscle atrophy
- Cutaneous calcinosis
- Interstitial lung disease
- GI bleeding and perforation
- Lipodystrophy

A-14. A. Leucocyte adhesion defect (LAD)

B. LAD is an immune deficiency disorder involving both B- and T-cells and is characterized by an inability of leukocytes to migrate to the site of infection to kill the offending organisms.

C. *Immunologic features of LAD:*
- There is deficiency of various glycoproteins including LFA–1/MCA–1, glycoprotein 150/95.
- Leucocytes cannot migrate to infection sites to kill organisms due to mutations in the CD18 glycoprotein.
- Adhesion molecules deficiency results in an abnormal inflammatory response and eventually recurrent bacterial infections
- There is no pus formation.

D. Delayed falling of umbilical cord, more than 3 weeks.

A-15. A. Erythroderma rash—exfoliative dermatitis, GVHD-like rash

B. Omenn syndrome—a variant of SCID

C. *LSSA:* Oligoclonal T-cell, low B-cells, normal NK cells

D. Definitive treatment is bone marrow transplantation or HSCT at the earliest.

E. Fatal in infancy

F. RAG1, RAG2 are common genetic defects

CHAPTER 11

Rheumatology

QUESTIONS

Q-1. A 14-year-old girl has been brought with history of high-grade fever since 3 weeks and progressive breathlessness and swelling of feet. History of generalized seizures to day. She is drowsy, but arousable, has oral ulcers, arthritis both knees, pleural effusion. No jaundice, no neck stiffness. Liver 4 cm. 2D echo showed pericardial effusion.

A. What is most probable diagnosis?
B. What are confirmatory investigations for this disorder?
C. What hematological parameters are expected to be present?
D. Name two drugs that can lead to this condition.

Q-2. An 8-year-old girl presented with fever, joint pain, abdominal pain and skin rashes as shown in picture below.

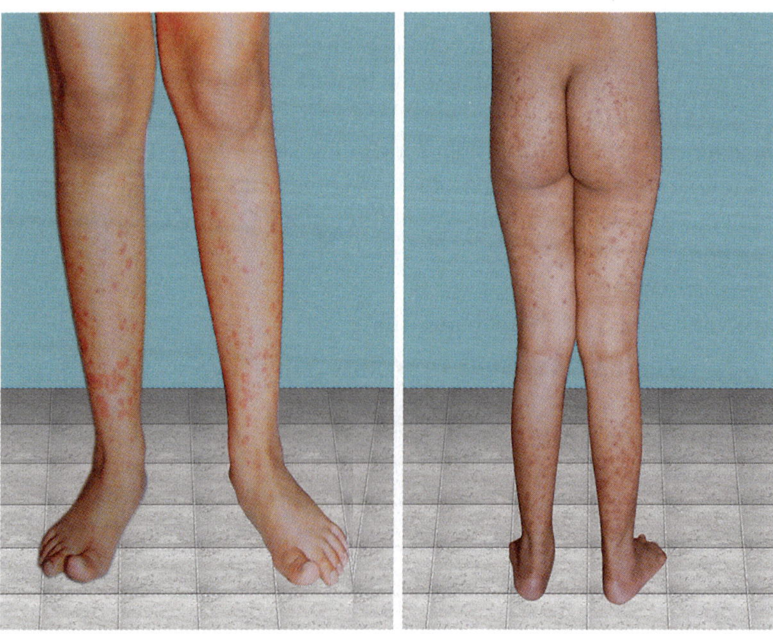

A. What is your diagnosis?
B. What is the cause of pain in abdomen in this disorder?
C. What emergency surgical complications are known to develop in this disease?
D. What is another major complication of this disorder deciding course of disease?
E. What is the new name of this condition?

Q-3. A 10-year-old boy presented with high-grade fever for 15 days, swelling and excruciating pain right ankle and then right knee, gradually involved elbows and wrists. Involvement of joints was by turn. Child had joint pain even on touch with clothes.

A. What is probable diagnosis?
B. What are latest modified criteria for diagnosis of this condition?
C. What clinical manifestations of this disease may not require to follow the diagnostic criteria?
D. What is choice of antibiotics to treat this disease? What is the role of antibiotics in treating this disease?
E. Outline the treatment plan of this disorder as an acute one.

Q-4. A 13-year-old girl presented with complaints of difficulty in getting up and not able to climb the stairs. She also had fever off and on and skin lesions over eyes, back, hands and elbows as shown in the pictures.

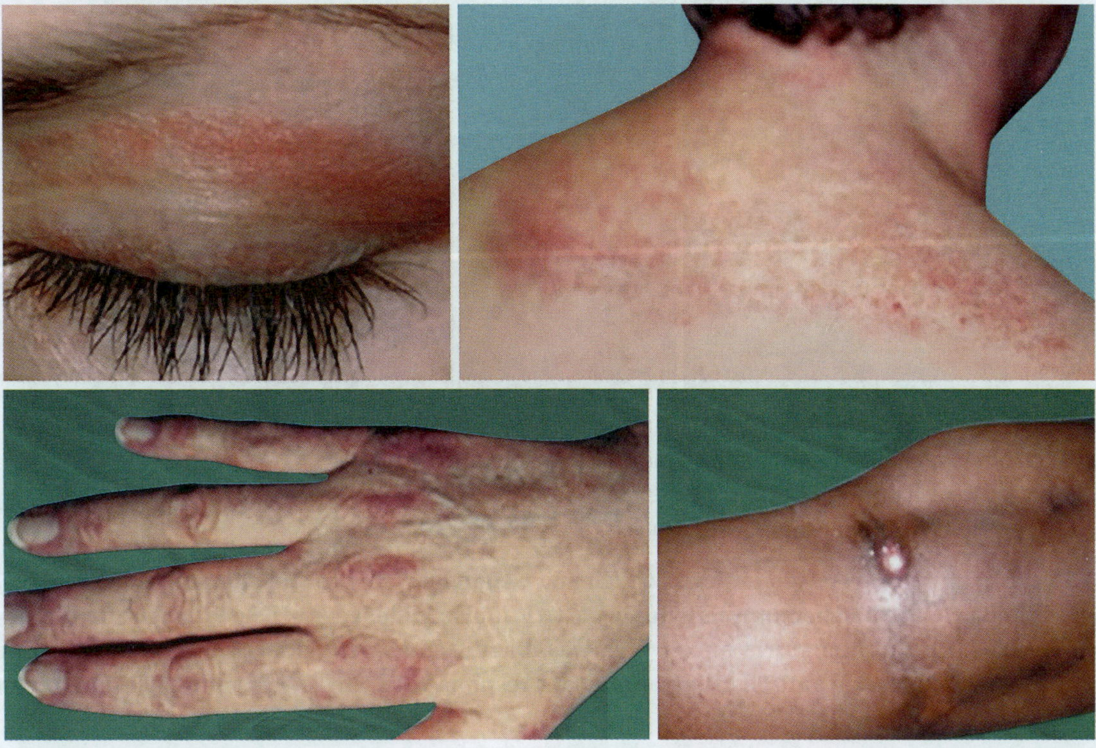

A. Name the lesions over eyelids, back, hands and elbows.
B. What is the probable diagnosis?
C. What specific clinical sign due to muscle weakness may be present in this patient?
D. What other systemic involvement is known in this disease?
E. What investigation may be useful in diagnosis of this disorder?
F. What are principles of management of this disease?

Q-5. A 9-year-old boy presented with high-grade fever, 2 spikes a day for 6 weeks, each spikes of fever associated with erythematous rashes over trunk and extremities. He was active and playful during inter febrile period. He was investigated for multiple times, showing leukocytosis with polymorphonuclear reaction, thrombocytosis and raised ESR and CRP. Initial chest X-ray, USG abdomen, blood culture were negative. Echo study of heart was normal. He was treated with multiple courses of antibiotics. The pattern of skin rashes was as shown in the picture.

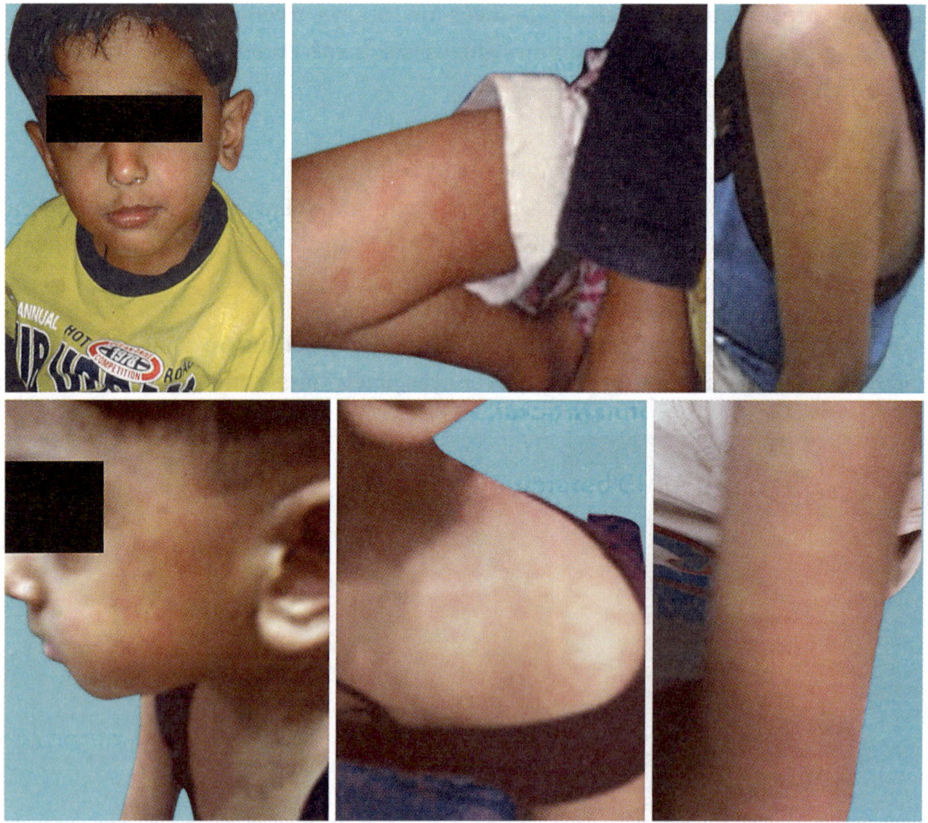

A. What is most probable diagnosis?
B. What other systemic clinical findings may develop later on?
C. What do we call this type of skin rashes?
D. Outline stepwise management with drugs.

Q-6. A 15-year-old boy was referred for fever, cough and weight loss. He has sinusitis since long, not responding to treatment. He also had hemoptysis twice in past. He is also under care of dermatologist for ulcers, papules and vesicles. He had hematuria once which was diagnosed as nephritis. He was treated with multiple courses of antibiotics and anti-TB drugs without any response. His chest x-ray and skin lesions pictures were as below:

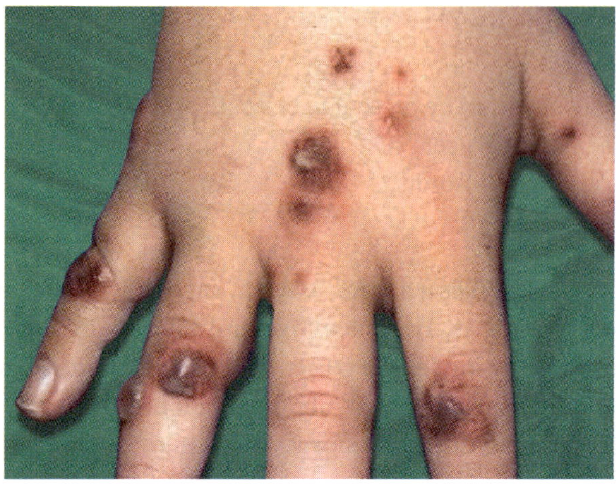

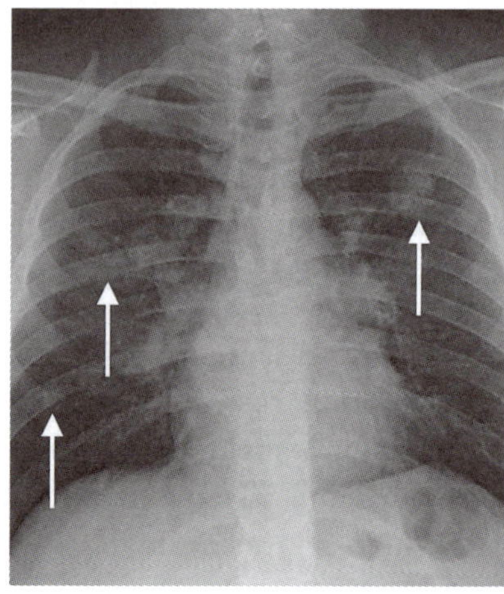

A. What is probable diagnosis?
B. What are diagnostic criteria of this disease?
C. What is the triad for this disorder?
D. What investigations should be performed in this condition?

Q-7. A 13-year-old boy was referred for painful oral ulcers, fever and diarrhea off and on for 3 years. He had significant weight loss. He also had violaceous, painful skin lesions over shin of tibia as shown in picture. His Hb was 7.6, TLC 4300, platelets 66,000. ANA profile and RA factor negative.

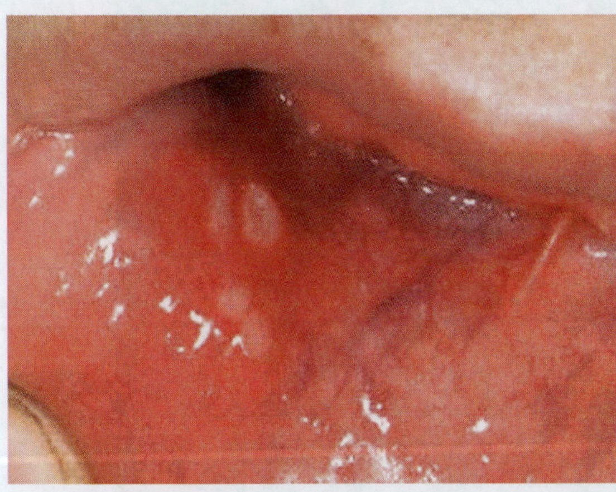

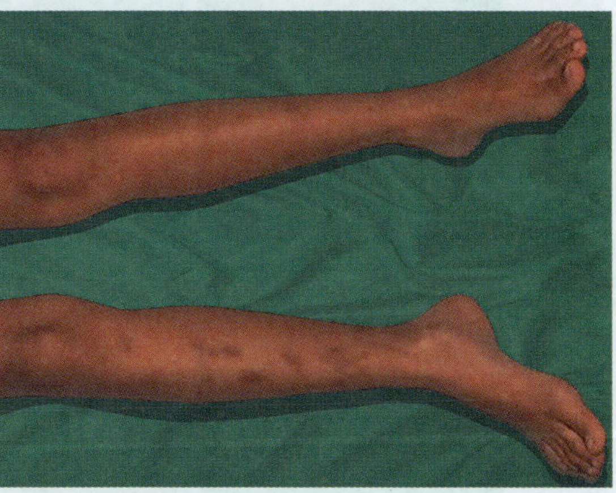

A. What is probable diagnosis?
B. What other clinical examination points are important for diagnosis of this condition?
C. What is the life-threatening complication of this disease?
D. What is the drug therapy for this disease?

Q-8. A 10-year-old boy was referred for right knee joint swelling for 3 weeks duration with limitation of movement and mild-to-moderate fever. He had frequency of stool with blood 3 weeks back and was treated with oral antibiotics with good recovery. His right knee was swollen and tender. Investigations showed leukocytosis with raised ESR and CRP.

A. What is probable diagnosis?
B. What is HLA associated with this condition? What percentage of patients are associated with this HLA?
C. What organisms are associated with this disease?
D. What is prognosis?

Q-9. Answer the following questions based on the antinuclear antibody (ANA) test in pediatrics: True/False

A. ANA can be positive in 5–18% of normal population.
B. Up to 50% Indian descent children can have a positive ANA.
C. ANA is also elevated in some viral infections and drug intake like INH.
D. ELISA is currently recommended for purpose of screening for ANA.
E. ANA testing by indirect immunofluorescence (IIF) is the gold standard method.
F. The titer cut-off points for ANA is 1:80 or 1:160.

Q-10. Answer the followings: True/False

A. ANA is good screening test for SLE because it is associated with 95% cases of SLE.
B. Hip joint is never involved in oligoarticular arthritis.
C. Congenital deficiency of C1q, C2 and C4 associated with SLE
D. High C3 level can be seen in many inflammatory conditions.
E. Low C3 and C4 levels are uncommon in SLE.

Q-11. An infant presented with high-grade fever of 10 days duration without any focus. She developed edema of hands and irritability. Physical examination revealed a 3 cm size solitary right anterior cervical lymph node. There was no response to IV antibiotics for 6 days. Investigations showed Hb 10.2 g/dL, TLC 16,500 with 80% neutrophils, platelets 5,60,000 and CRP 84 mg/dL. Blood culture was negative after 5 days. Chest X-ray was normal. USG neck confirmed solitary right cervical lymphadenopathy. BCG site was found erythematous and hands were swollen as shown below in the pictures:

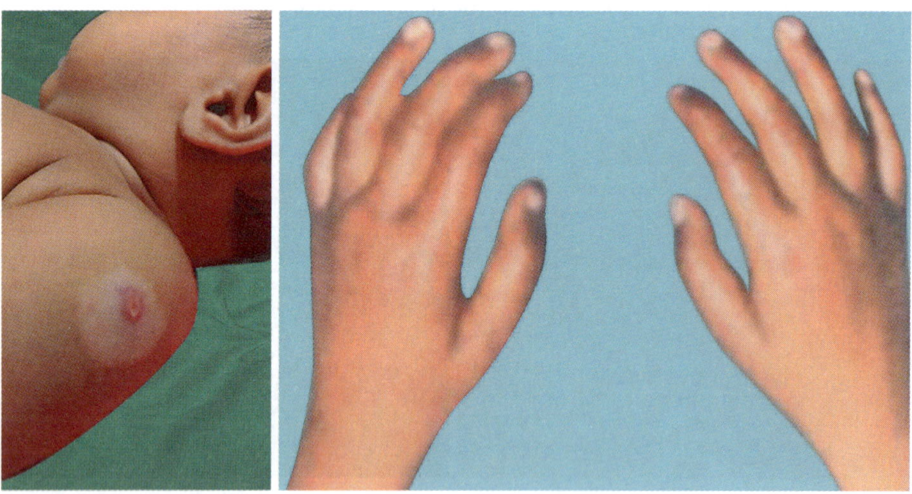

A. What is probable diagnosis?
B. What are the diagnostic criteria of this disease?
C. What is the next important investigation on suspecting this condition? Is it for confirmation?
D. What are different presentations of this disorder?
E. What is the treatment of this condition?

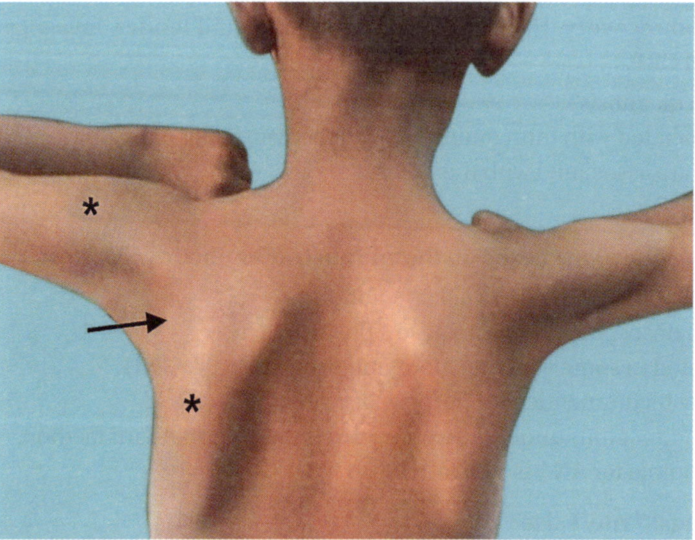

Q-12.

A. Identify the clinical sign.
B. How does this sign develop?
C. Name the condition in which this sign has high sensitivity and specificity.

ANSWERS

A-1. A. SLE

B. Anti ds-DNA
Anti-Smith antibody

C. Hemolytic anemia with raised reticulocyte count
Leucopenia, Lymphopenia and thrombocytopenia

D. Phenytoin, sulfonamides, hydralazine

A-2. A. Henoch-Schönlein purpura
IgA-mediated, small vessel leukocytoclastic vasculitis

B. Vasculitis and ischemia of intestine

C. Intussusception, bowel perforation, testicular torsion

D. Renal involvement (nephritis/nephrosis)

E. IgA-mediated small vessel leukocytoclastic vasculitis

A-3 A. Acute rheumatic fever with arthritis

B. Johns Criteria—Updated 2015

Major manifestations:

- Carditis
- Polyarthritis
- Erythema marginatum
- Subcutaneous nodules
- Chorea

Minor manifestations:

- *Clinical features:*
  - Arthralgia
  - Fever
- *Laboratory features:*
  - Elevated acute phase reactants, ESR and CRP
  - Prolonged P–R interval

Supporting evidence of antecedent Group A streptococcal infection (GAS):

- Positive throat culture or rapid streptococcal antigen test
- Elevated or increasing streptococcal antibody titer

Interpretations

- *Initial attack:* Two major manifestations or one major and two minor manifestations plus evidence of recent GAS infection.
- *Recurrent attack:* Two major or one major and two minor or three minor manifestations (the latter only in the moderate or high-risk population) plus evidence of recent GAS infection.
- *Recent modifications:*
  - *Low-risk population* is defined as ARF incidence <2 per 1,00,000 school-age children per year or all age RHD prevalence of <1 per 1000 population.
  - *Moderate-/high-risk population:* ARF incidence >2 per 1,00,000 school-age children per year or all age RHD prevalence of >1 per 1000 population
  - Carditis is now defined as clinical and/or subclinical (echocardiographic valvulitis)
  - Arthritis (major) refers only to polyarthritis in low-risk population but also to mono-arthritis or polyarthritis in moderate/high-risk population.

- Minor criteria for moderate-/high-risk population only include mono-arthralgia (polyarthralgia for low-risk population), fever of 38°C (>38.5°C for low-risk population), and ESR >30 mm/hour (>60 mm in low-risk population)

C.
- Rheumatic chorea
- Indolent carditis
- Recurrent of acute rheumatic fever in particularly high-risk population

These clinical manifestations do not require to fulfill the criteria for diagnosis of rheumatic fever.

D.
- Bedrest till inflammation is there, longer duration in patients with carditis.
- Once the diagnosis of acute RF has been established and regardless of the throat culture result, the patient should receive 10 days of orally administered penicillin or amoxicillin or a single dose of IM injection of benzathine penicillin to ensure eradication of GAS from the upper respiratory tract.
- If allergic to penicillin, 10 days of erythromycin, 5 days of azithromycin or 10 days of clindamycin is indicated.
- After the initial course of antibiotics therapy, long-term antibiotic prophylaxis for secondary prevention should be instituted.

E. *Treatment plan:*
- Antibiotics course penicillin or amoxicillin for 10 days. If allergic to penicillin, then 10 days of erythromycin or 5 days or azithromycin or 10 days of clindamycin, followed by long-term prophylaxis for secondary prevention.
- *Anti-inflammatory therapy:*
  - Aspirin 50–70 mg/kg/day in 4 divided doses orally for 3–5 days, followed by 50 mg/kg/day in 4 divided doses orally 2–3 weeks and half the dose for another 2–4 weeks
  - Patients with carditis and more than minimal cardiomegaly and/or CCF, prednisolone 2 mg/kg/day in 4 divided doses for 2–3 weeks, followed by half the dose for 2–3 weeks, and then tapering the dose by 5 mg/kg every 2–3 days.
  - When steroids is being tapered, aspirin should be started at 50 mg/kg/day in 4 divided doses for 6 weeks to prevent rebound inflammation.
- Supportive therapy includes digoxin, fluid and salt restriction, diuretics and oxygen.

A-4. A. *Identification of lesion:*
- Heliotrope rash over eyelids
- Shawl sign over back
- Gottron's papule over hands
- Calcinosis over elbows

B. Juvenile dermatomyositis

C. Gower's sign is often present.

D. *Systemic involvement:*
- *GI tract:* Ischemic pain and acute abdomen, hematemesis, melena and perforation
- *Cardiac involvement:* Cardiomegaly, murmurs
- *Respiratory:* Restrictive pulmonary disease

E. *Investigations:*
- *CBC:* Leukocytosis and thrombocytosis
- Raised ESR and CRP
- Raised CPK, SOGT, LDH
- Autoantibodies
- MRI
- EMG
- Muscle biopsy

F.
- Steroids
- Methotrexate
- IV immunoglobulins
- Cyclophosphamide, mycophenolate mofetil

A-5. A. Systemic onset juvenile idiopathic arthritis (SOJIA)

B. Other systemic findings may appear later are:
- Hepatosplenomegaly
- Lymphadenopathy
- Polyarthritis
- Serous cavity effusions

C. Evanescent (vanishing) maculopapular, skin rashes

D. *Drugs for SOJIA:*
- NSAIDs such as naproxen, ibuprofen, indomethacin, diclofenac, etc.
- Methotrexate
- Azathioprine
- Steroids
- Cyclosporine
- Biologic agents like anakinra, tocilizumab, etc.

A-6. A. Wegener's granulomatosis, now known as granulomatosis with polyangiitis (GPA)

B. *Diagnostic criteria (two of the following four criteria are present):*
1. Nasal or oral inflammation
2. Abnormal chest radiograph
3. Abnormal urinalysis
4. Granulomatous inflammation on biopsy

C. The triad of upper and lower respiratory tract inflammation and renal disease is the characteristic of Wegener's granulomatosis.

D. *Investigations findings:*
- Normocytic, normochromic, anemia, leukocytosis, thrombocytosis and raised CRP and ESR
- *Urinalysis:* Hematuria, proteinuria, RBC casts
- Elevated blood urea and serum creatinine
- Antinuclear antibody serology positive like rheumatoid factor (50%), antiphospholipid antibodies (22%) CANCA (85%), etc.

A-7. A. Behçet's disease

B. Genital ulceration, uveitis on slit-lamp examination of eyes and venous and arterial thrombosis are characteristics of Behçet's disease.

C. Large vessel thrombosis is life-threatening complication of this disease.

D. Colchicine and thalidomide are drugs used in Behçet's disease. Methotrexate and chlorambucil have also been used.

A-8. A. Postinfectious reactive arthritis

B. HLA B27 in 75% of patients

C. *Campylobacter*, *Shigella*, *Salmonella*, *Yersinia*, CMV, Herpes simplex, Rubella are common organisms causing reactive arthritis.

D. Usually, resolves without complications or sequelae.

A-9. A. True
B. False (15–20%)
C. True
D. False
E. True
F. True

A-10. A. False
B. True
C. Ture
D. True
E. False

A-11. A. Kawasaki disease (KD)

B. *Diagnostic criteria for Kawasaki disease:*
- Fever lasting for at least 5 days
- Presence of 4 of the following 5 conditions
  - Bilateral non-purulent conjunctival injection (without discharge)
  - Changes of mucosa of oropharynx (injected pharynx, lips, strawberry tongue)
  - Changes of peripheral extremities
    Acute stage: Edema, erythema of hands and feet
    Convalescent stage: Desquamation which usually begins periungual
  - Polymorphous rash (never bullous or vesicular)
  - Cervical lymphadenopathy (at least one node 1.5 cm, usually unilateral)
- Illness not explained by any other known disease process.

C. 2D echo study of heart to check of dilatation of coronary vessels. It is not for confirmation. On the contrary, normal echo in case of Kawasaki is the time to treat so that future cardiac complications can be prevented.

D. *Different presentations of KD:*
- Typical case fulfilling standard diagnostic criteria
- Incomplete KD refers to a patient with fulfill less than 4 criteria in the presence of fever and laboratory features suggestive of KD.
- Atypical KD refers to some unusual clinical manifestations of KD such as nephritis.
- Important clues to KD are sterile pyuria, hydrops of gallbladder, aseptic meningitis and BCG reactivation.

E. *Treatment of KD:*
- Intravenous immunoglobulins (IVIG) 2 g/kg over 10–12 ours
- Aspirin 30–50 mg/kg/day until child is afebrile, followed by 3–5 mg/kg/day for 4–6 weeks.
- 10–20% patients of KD remain refractory to this treatment, may require second dose of IVIG, infliximab or corticosteroids.
- Coronary artery abnormalities may develop in 3–5% of children with KD even after treatment.
- Left untreated 15–25% children with KD develop coronary artery abnormalities

A-12. A. Valley sign

B. Even though the deltoid and infraspinatus muscles are enlarged, parts of these muscles along with other muscles, which traverse through posterior axillary fold, are wasted. On the other hand, subtle enlargement of a muscle is best observed when the muscle in question is under mild contraction.

C. Duchenne muscular dystrophy (DMD)

CHAPTER 12

Infections

QUESTIONS

Q-1.

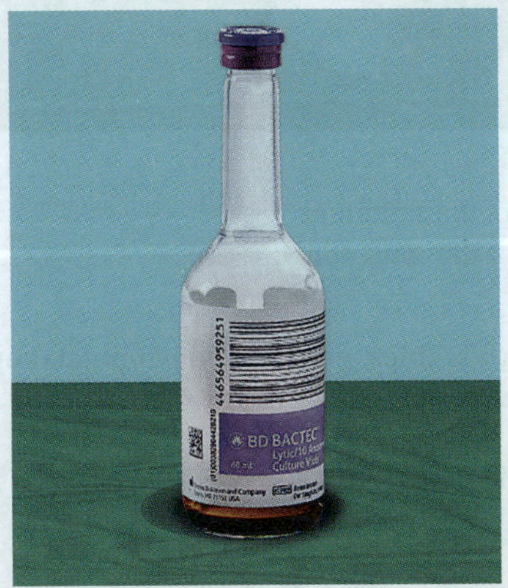

A. In which investigation, this container is used?
B. Skin antisepsis during collection of sample.
C. Volume of blood.
D. Preservation before sending to laboratory.

Q-2. A 20-day-old child presented with staccato cough and sticky eyes. There was no fever and child was non-toxic. Auscultation of chest revealed fine crackles.

A. What is your clinical diagnosis?
B. What findings are expected in chest X-ray of this patient?
C. What is the choice of antibiotic in this condition?

Q-3. An infant developed high-grade fever, irritability and generalized erythema. The child developed peeling of skin on touching, resulting in this type of picture.

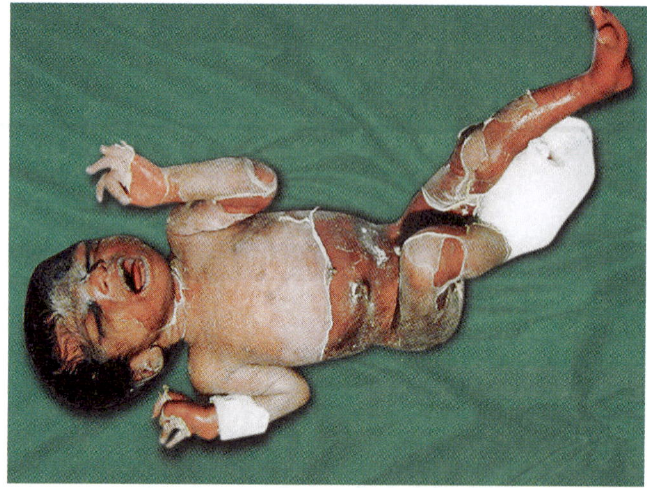

A. Name the condition.
B. Name the characteristic sign of the condition.
C. Name the toxin responsible for the condition.
D. Name the drugs to treat it.

Q-4. A 2-year-old boy presented with scabies, generalized lymphadenopathy and failure to thrive. A test for systemic infection confirmed the diagnosis.

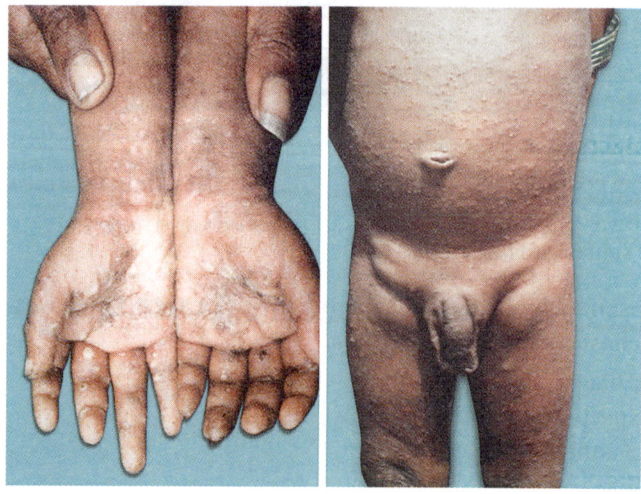

A. Name the systemic infection.
B. Which variant of human scabies is commonly associated with this disease?
C. Which drug is given orally for scabies in this situation?
D. Name mite causing scabies in human being.

Q-5. An 8-year-old boys presented with difficulty in chewing and swallowing. He had injury over leg while playing in school. He did not receive any vaccine. He had spasms on sound, touch or light.

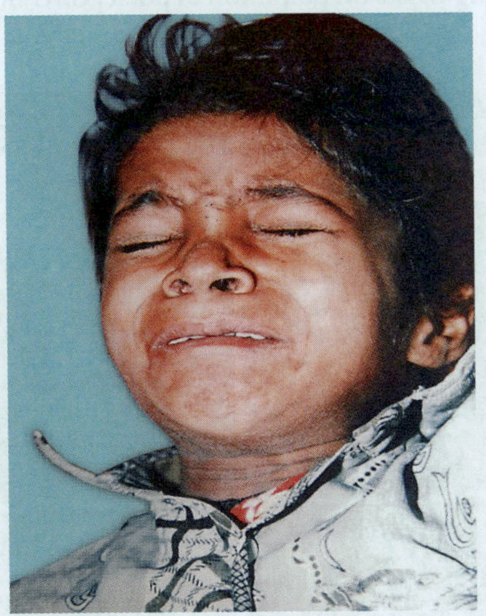

A. What is your diagnosis?
B. Name the sign.
C. What is the mechanism of this sign?
D. What is the cause of sudden death in this disease?
E. Name the antibiotics of choice in this condition.

Q-6. A child presented with fever and maculopapular, vesicular lesions over hands, feet and buttocks. He also had sore throat and ulcers in mouth.

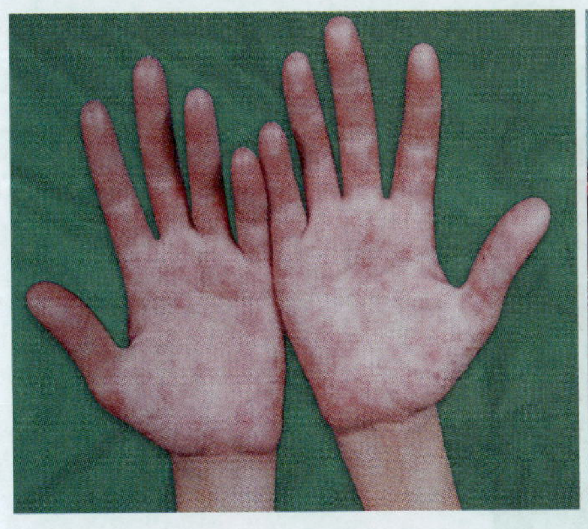

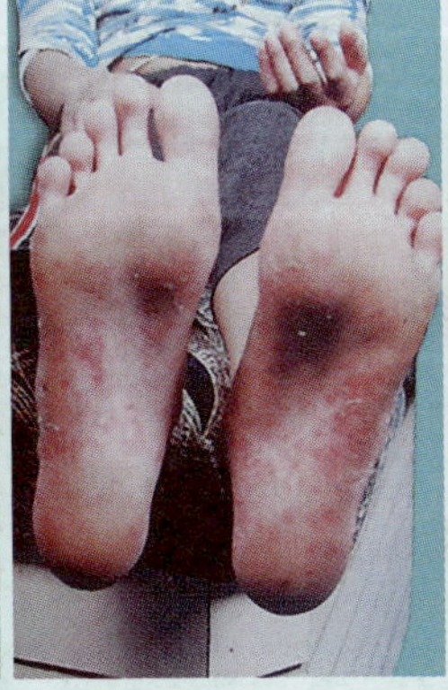

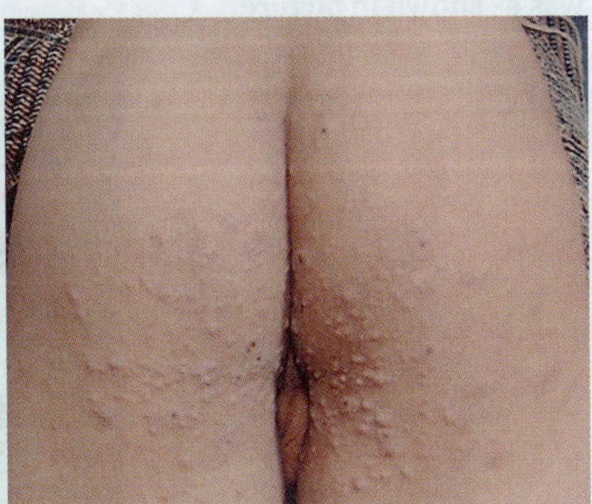

A. What is your clinical diagnosis?
B. Name most frequent causative agent.
C. What other organisms are known to cause it?
D. What are known serious complications of this disease?

Q-7. A 2-month-old baby was brought for fever, nasal discharge, irritability, persistent jaundice and not gaining weight. Physical examination revealed hepatosplenomegaly, lymphadenopathy and perianal excoriation. The baby was crying on touching wrists on palpation of pulse. CBC showed anemia and thrombocytopenia. X-ray wrists was performed.

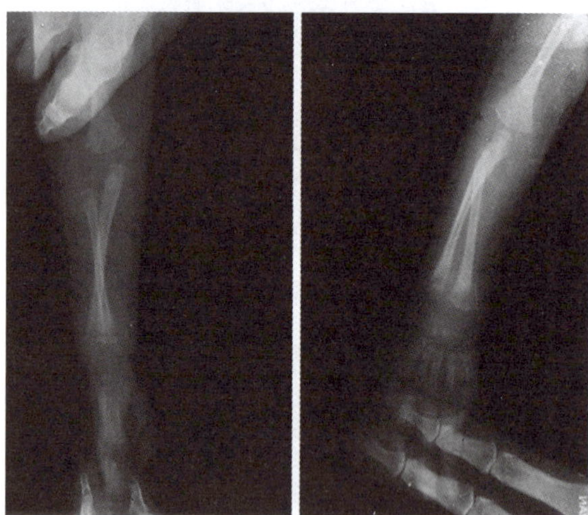

A. What does the X-ray wrists show?
B. What is your clinical diagnosis?
C. What serological tests should be performed to confirm the diagnosis?
D. What is the first choice of antibiotics to treat it?

Q-8. An 11-year-old boy presented with high-grade fever and chest pain on right side of 2 days duration. He developed difficulty in breathing on third day and no chest pain. His chest X-ray and USG study of thorax revealed right side pleural effusion. It was tapped and collected for examination. The appearance of fluid was as shown in picture.

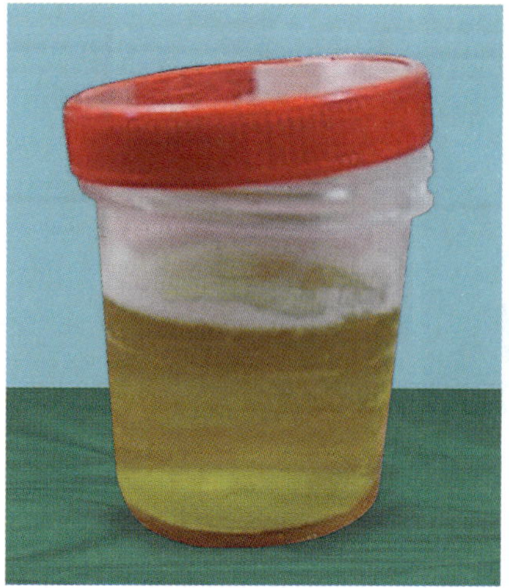

A. What is most probable etiological diagnosis?
B. What type of immune reaction causes this type of pleural effusion in said disease? What type of protein is considered responsible for this reaction?
C. What type of reaction is predicted to Mantoux test?

D. Give some other examples of manifestations of this disease based on the same immune reaction?
E. What is the sensitivity of GeneXpert in this case?

Q-9. A 3-year-old girl was brought with complaint of something coming out per rectum. She passed similar thing in vomitus 15 days back. She also complaint of pain in abdomen and cough off and on.

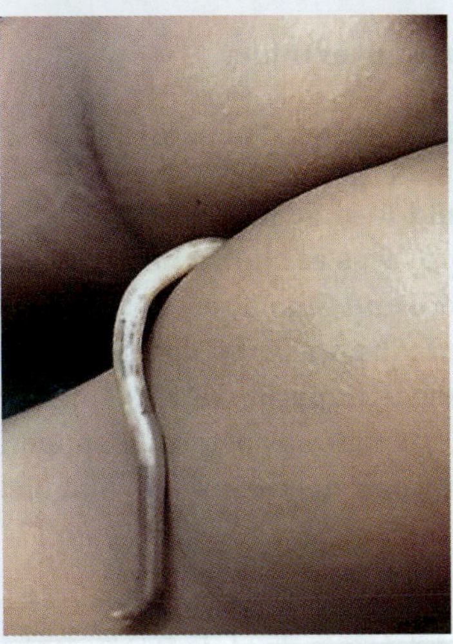

A. What is possible diagnosis?
B. What are common clinical manifestations of the condition?
C. What are the complications of this condition?
D. What is the drug of choice and its dosage?

Q-10. A 8-year-old girl from Bihar presented with complaints of fever (102– 103°F) for 3 months. She had weight loss of 3 kg in last 2 months. She had Liver 3 cm below right costal margin and spleen 12 cm, no lymphadenopathy. Investigations for malaria, tuberculosis, enteric fever, brucellosis and malignancy negative. She had pancytopenia. USG abdomen showed huge splenomegaly and mild-to-moderate hepatomegaly, no ascites. The clinical photographs are as below. Bone marrow aspiration confirmed the diagnosis.

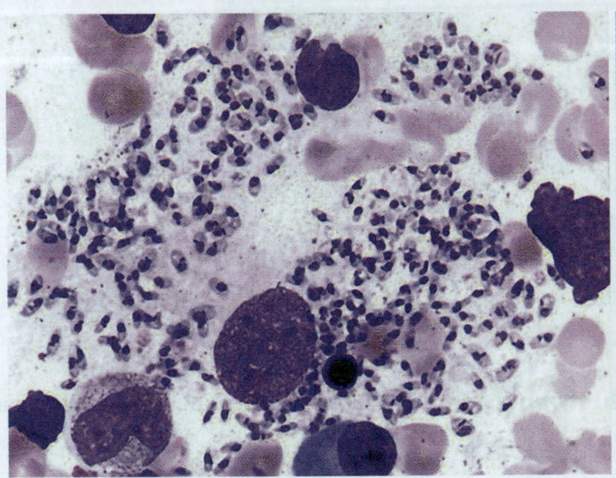
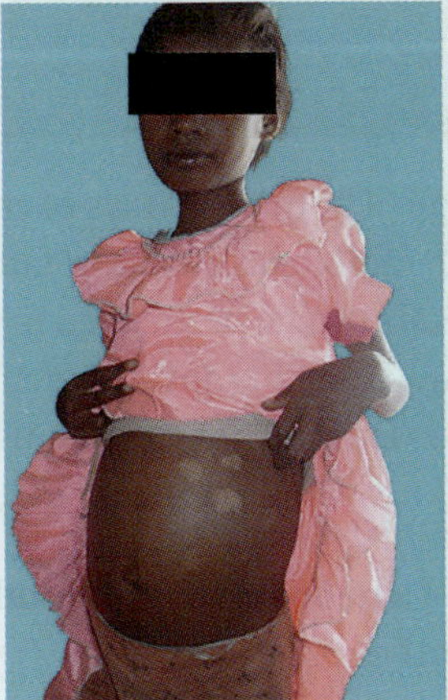
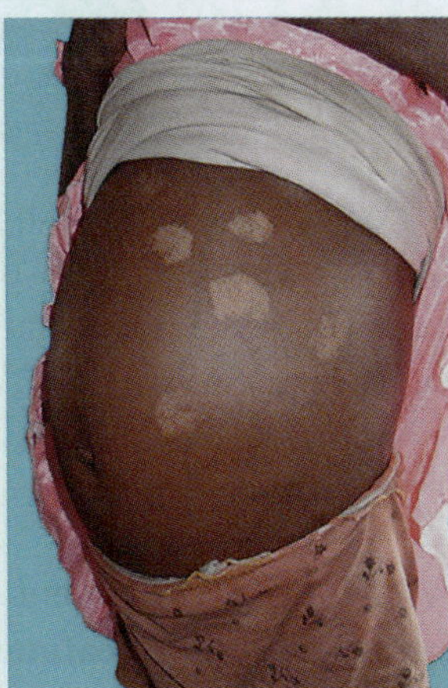

A. What is probable diagnosis?
B. What are differential diagnosis?
C. What are laboratory investigations for confirmation of diagnosis?
D. What is the line of treatment?

Q-11. **A 2-year-old girl presented with fever and cough of 3 weeks duration. She also had significant weight loss. Her chest X-ray showed right side paratracheal enlarged lymph nodes. GeneXpert of her gastric aspirate was positive for *Mycobacterium tuberculosis* complex, rifampicin resistance not detected. Anti-tuberculous drugs started. What is schedule for follow-up? What should be checked on each follow-up? How will you monitor the patient?**

Q-12. **Define anti-tuberculous drug-induced liver injury.**

Q-13. **Management of anti-tuberculous drug-induced hepatitis.**

Q-14. **A 7-year-old girl presented with mild-to-moderate fever, cough and weight loss of 2 months duration. She was almost cachexic. Her chest X-ray was as shown in below picture. Mantoux Test was positive. Sputum examination showed presence of AFB and GeneXpert was reported as positive for *Mycobacterium* complex, rifampicin resistance not detected. She was HIV negative. She was treated with isoniazid, rifampicin, pyrazinamide and ethambutol along with pyridoxine in appropriate dosage with good compliance. After 8 weeks of therapy, she was afebrile, cough was persistent, appetite improving and gaining the weight. The repeat chest X-ray was performed by parents themselves and picture was as follow. The patient responded to same anti-tuberculous drugs on follow-up.**

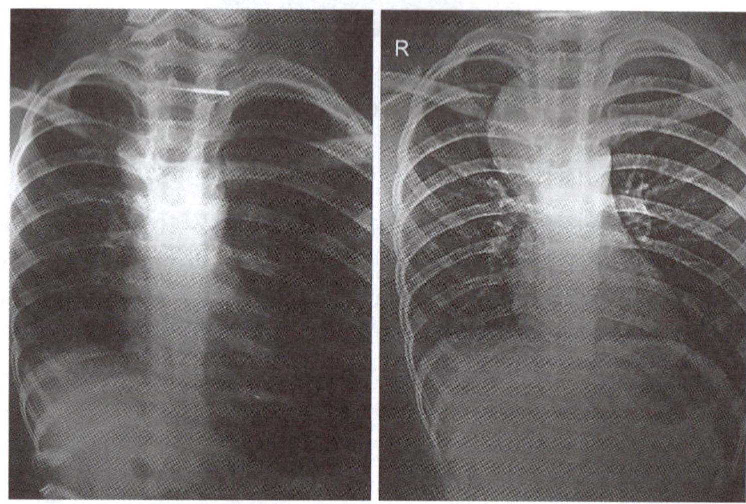

A. What is the interpretation of both the X-rays of chest?
B. What are possibilities on radiological interpretation of these X-rays of chest?
C. What further investigations can be performed in this type of situation?
D. The patient responded well on same anti-tuberculous drugs. What is likely possibility? What is the explanation of increasing tuberculous lesions in spite of anti-tuberculous drugs and ultimately responding to same anti-tuberculous drugs?

Q-15. **What is the management of a neonate born to mother who is suffering from pulmonary tuberculosis and on anti-tuberculous treatment?**

Q-16. **A 14-month-old girl had fever, 102–103°F, difficulty in breathing, stridor and drooling copious. She was toxic and keeping the neck flexed. Edema neck and lymphadenopathy were noted on right side of neck. Total WBC count was 18,400/cumm with polymorphs 90%.**

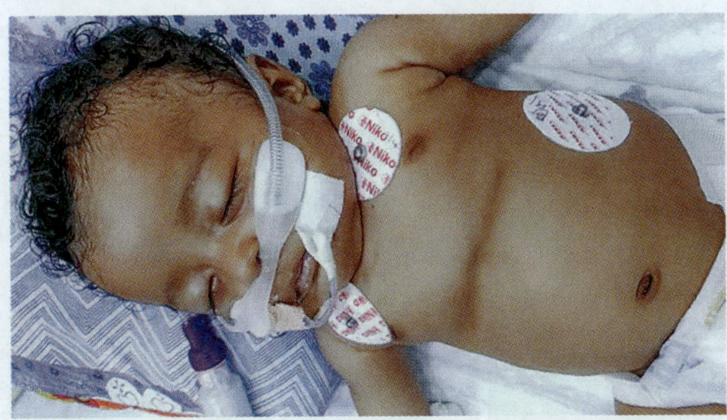

A. What is the probable diagnosis?
B. What is most common age for this disease?
C. What are common organisms responsible for this disease?
D. What are principles of treatment?
E. What should be choice of empirical antibiotics?

Q-17. The 7-year-old boy brought with complaints of fever of 3 weeks duration. He had pharyngotonsillitis and puffy eyes, treated with amoxicillin. Next day, he developed macular rashes. On physical examination, he had generalized lymphadenopathy and hepatosplenomegaly. CBC showed some characteristic findings favoring the diagnosis?

A. What is probable diagnosis?
B. What group of lymph nodes involvement is characteristic of this disorder?
C. What are the characteristics on CBC in this disorder?
D. What serological test is confirmatory for this disease?
E. Which organ rupture may be a fatal complication of this disease?

Q-18. This boy had fever, coryza, headache and diarrhea. He developed these skin rashes over face and circumoral pallor on 4th day of fever. Parents noted reappearing these rashes on exposure to sunlight and on exercise.

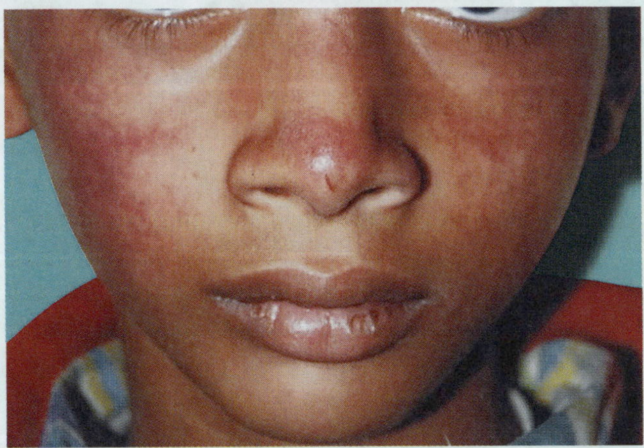

A. What is the probable diagnosis?
B. What are other manifestations of this disease?
C. What is another name of this disorder?
D. What is the line of treatment recommended?

Q-19. A child presented with low-grade fever, inflamed oropharynx and these type of skin lesions over different parts of body.

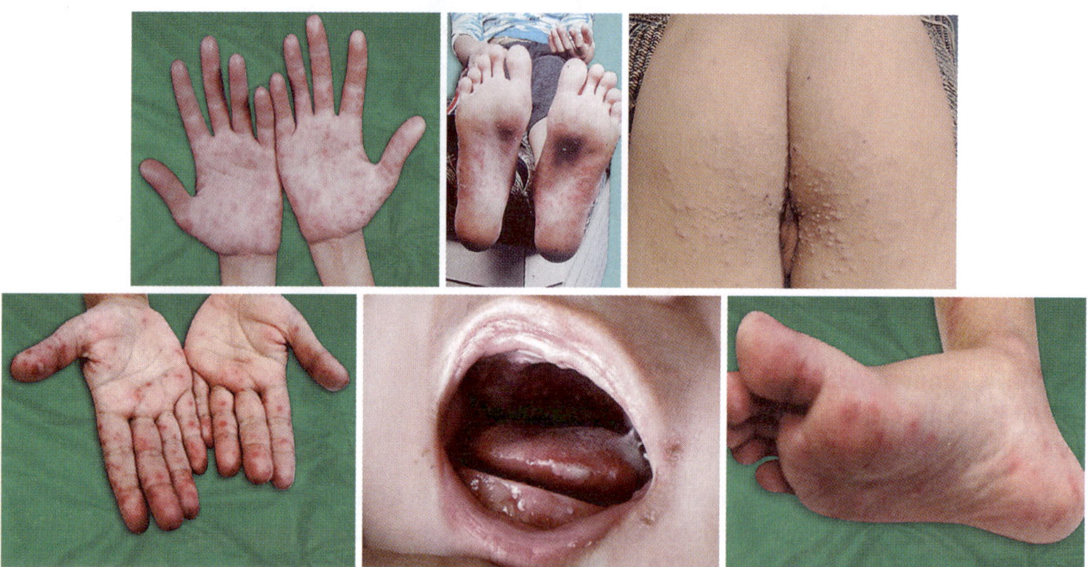

A. What is probable diagnosis?
B. Which organisms are known to cause it?
C. What are known complications of this disease?
D. Which specific serotype is responsible for these complications?

Q-20. This disease is known to present with high-grade fever, blanchable, erythematous rash measly look. Catarrh and typical characteristics of respiratory virus is missing. Retro-orbital pain, headache, backache and arthralgia are common symptoms of this disease. Shock and bleeding tendency are life-threatening complications of this disease.

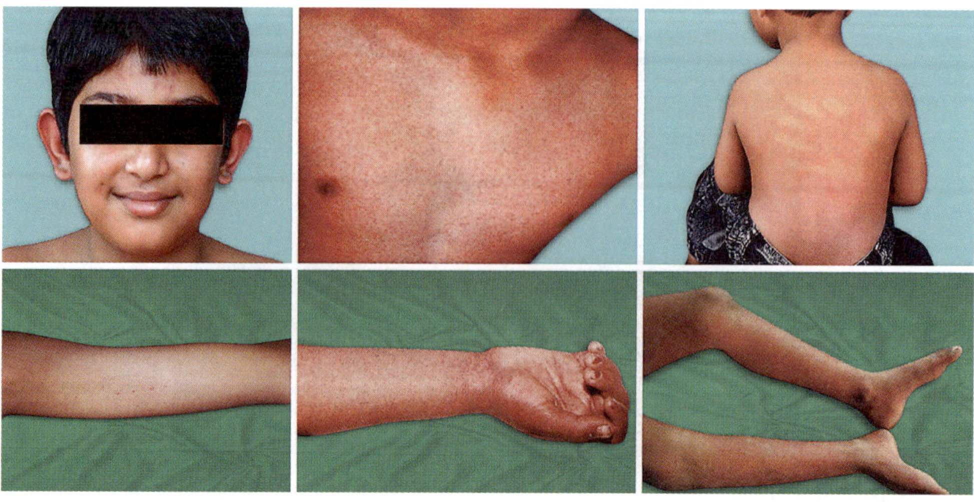

A. What is probable diagnosis?
B. What mechanism is responsible for shock in this disease?
C. Which vector is known to transmit the disease?
D. Which antigen test is useful in diagnosis at its early phase?
E. What are clinical parameters for its monitoring?

Q-21. A 3-month-old infant was brought with complaints of fever high-grade, cough-cold and irritability. It was diagnosed as bronchiolitis by a treating pediatrician and treated with amoxicillin and bronchodilators by nebulizer. Child developed the skin rashes all over body with hyperpigmentation of skin. Mother had illness 10 days back due to same disease

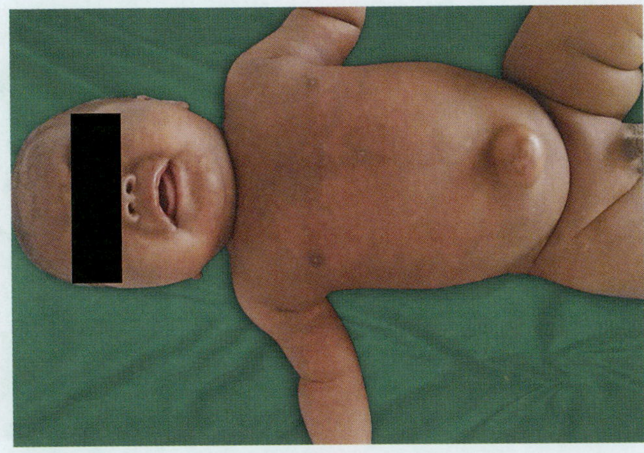

A. What is probable diagnosis?
B. Why is there hyperpigmentation of skin in this condition?
C. What investigations can confirm the diagnosis?
D. What vectors transmit the disease?

Q-22. A 6-year-old boy had fever and cough of 10 days duration. He also had chest pain and chest X-ray was reported pneumonia. Multiple CBC were showing WBC count within normal limits. The pneumonia was not responding to routine antibiotics. He developed skin rashes as shown in the picture.

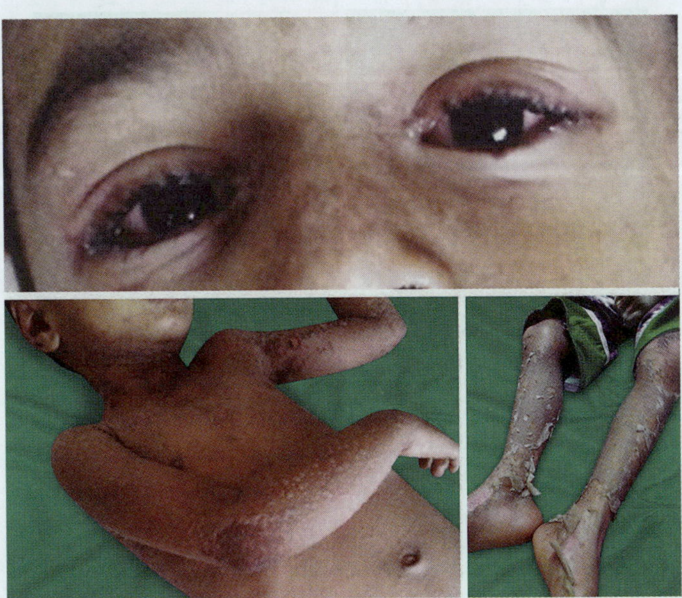

A. What is probable diagnosis?
B. What investigations should be performed to confirm the diagnosis?
C. What is antibiotics of choice for this disease?
D. What are extrapulmonary manifestation in this disease?

Q-23. A 11-year-old girl had high-grade fever and throat pain. She developed erythematous rashes on next day of fever, first around the neck and spread over trunk and extremities. The rashes were rough on touch. The tongue was red and throat examination revealed exudative pharyngitis. After 4 days, rashes started to fade and desquamation was seen.

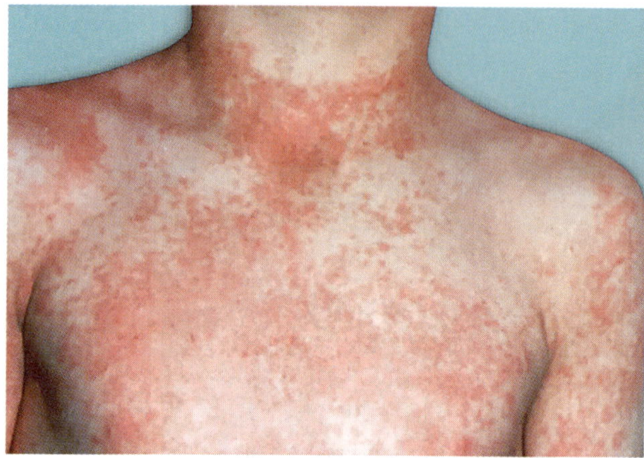
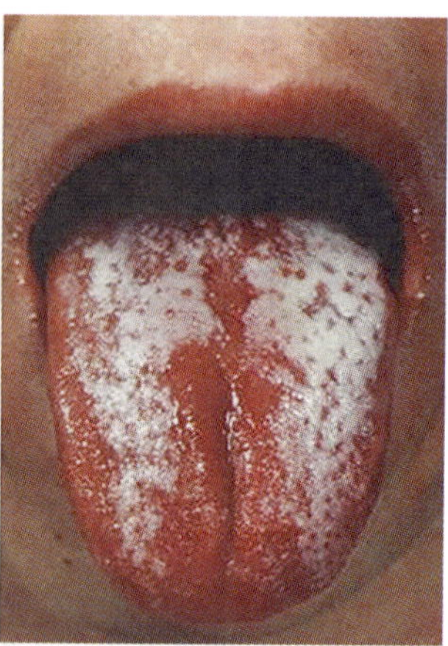

A. What is the probable diagnosis?
B. What is causative agent?
C. Which toxin is considered as responsible for skin rashes?
D. What are common differential diagnosis?

Q-24. A boy had fever, headache, myalgia and anorexia. He also had pain in abdomen, vomiting and diarrhea. He developed maculopapular rash over legs and arms, rapidly spreading all over body including palms and soles. His general condition deteriorated and developed gangrenous patches over buttocks and fingers.

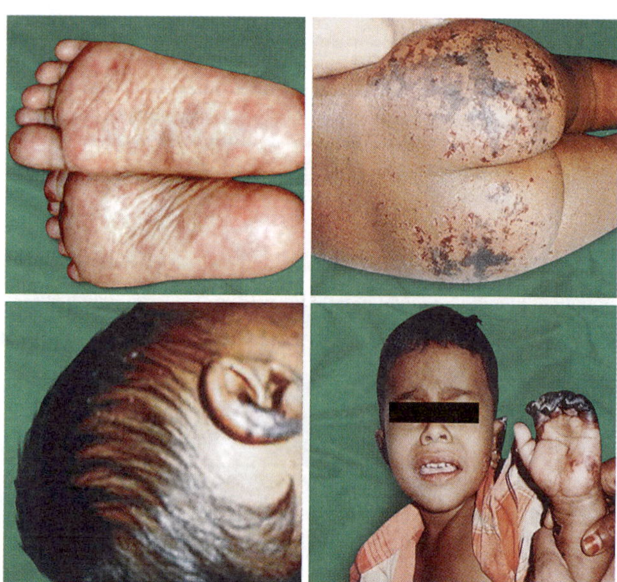

A. What is the probable diagnosis?
B. What history may favor your diagnosis?
C. What is pathognomonic sign which one should search for?
D. What is the Gold Standard test for the condition?
E. What is the drug of choice in this disease? What are alternative antibiotics?

Q-25. A child developed fever following varicella. He developed acutely pain and swelling over thigh and trunk. The swelling was tender, tight, shining and warm. It was very painful. The child was toxic and deteriorated very fast leading to shock.

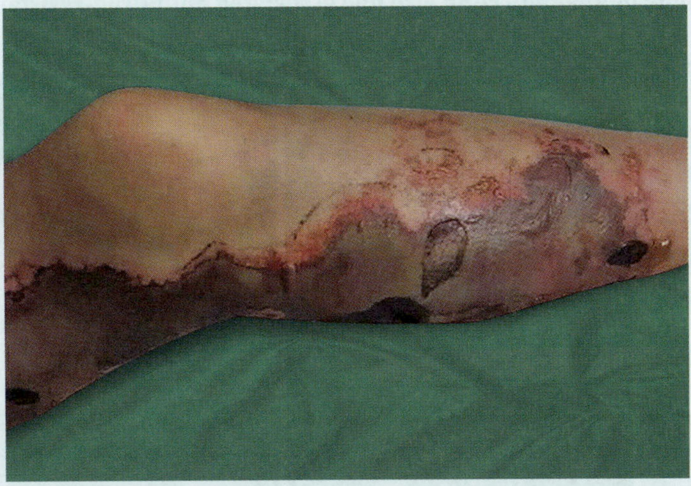

A. What is the probable diagnosis?
B. What is the most common organism causing this condition following varicella?
C. What other organisms are known to cause this disease?
D. What is line of treatment?
E. What antibiotics should be of choice in this condition?

Q-26. This child had high-grade fever, irritability, vomiting and diarrhea. He developed these type of skins lesions rapidly over few hours and started to deteriorate leading to poor perfusion, oliguria and sensorial changes. It is vaccine preventable disease.

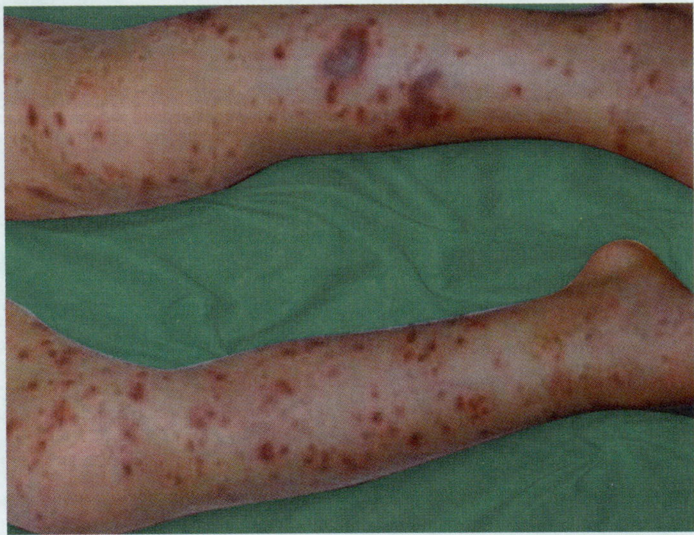

A. What is probable diagnosis?
B. What investigations should be performed for confirmation of diagnosis?
C. What are complications of this disease?
D. What should be antibiotic of choice for meningitis due to this organism? Duration of antibiotics?

Q-27. A 10-month-old boy presented with fever, cough, breathlessness and failure to thrive. He had multiple swellings over neck, axillae and inguinal region. He was consulted by a dermatologist for skin lesions and itching, was diagnosed as scabies. Further investigations for child and mother confirmed some congenital infection. Both of them, mother and child also had associated multidrug-resistant infection.

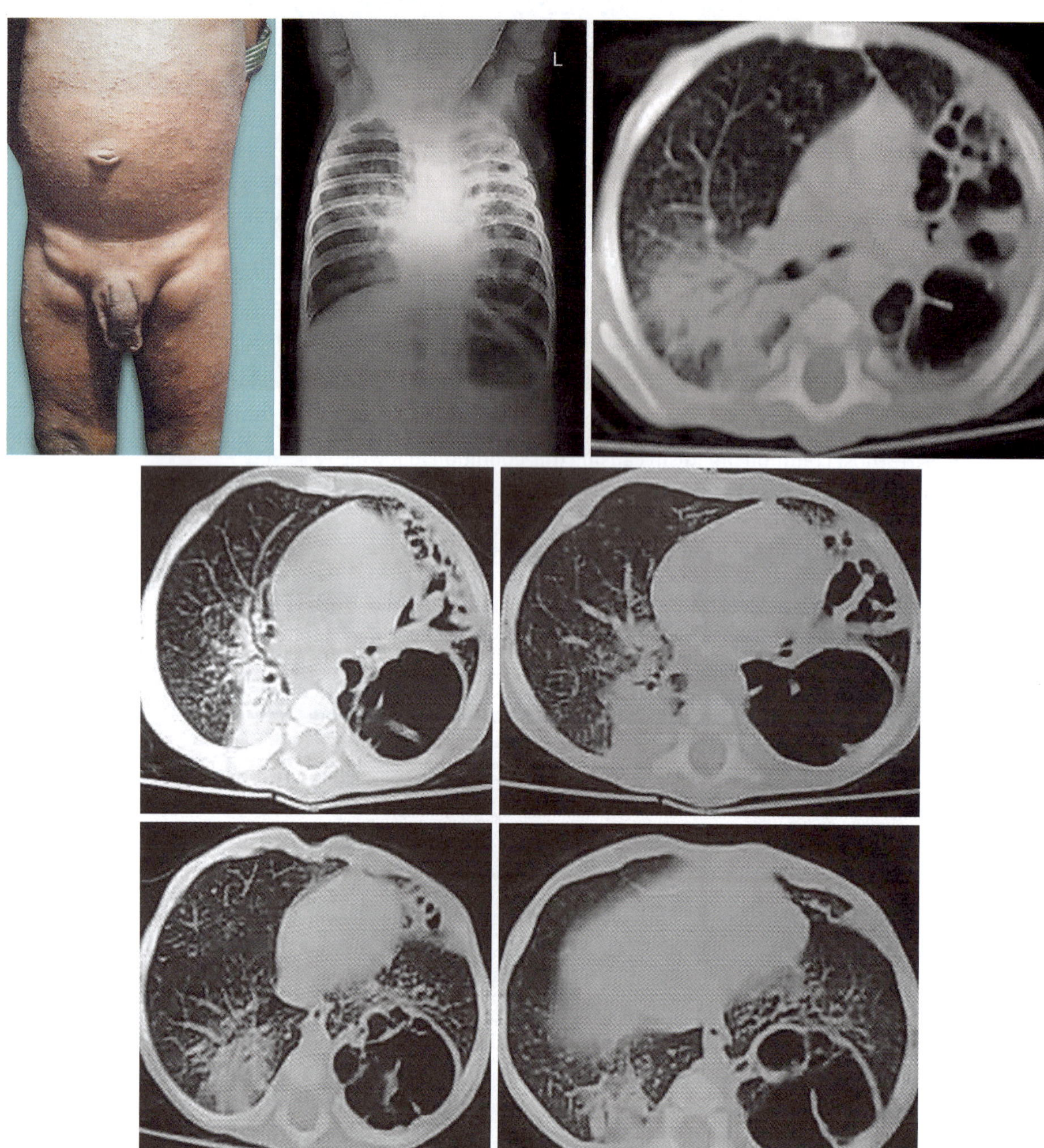

A. What is probable diagnosis?
B. What type of scabies is known to occur with this disease?
C. What investigations should be performed for the child and mother?
D. What type of skin diseases are associated with this disease?

Q-28. Define following therapeutic uses of antibiotics with illustrations.

A. Pre-emptive
B. Empirical
C. Definitive

Q-29. How will you clinically differentiate viral and bacterial infections?

Q-30. Classify the following organisms as per their growth on culture, fastidious, cannot be grown and slow grower.

A. *Brucella, Mycobacterium tuberculosis*
B. *H. Influenza B, Streptococcus pneumoniae*
C. Rickettsia, *Mycobacterium leprae, Mycoplasma*

Q-31. Answer the following questions pertaining to blood culture.

A. How the volume of blood for culture is calculated?
B. What should be ratio of blood to media for blood culture?
C. What is the importance of maintaining ratio of blood to media for blood culture?
D. If it is not possible to send blood sample for culture immediately, how should it be stored in refrigerator?
E. Which specimen of culture should be stored in refrigerator and others to be kept at room temperature?

Q-32

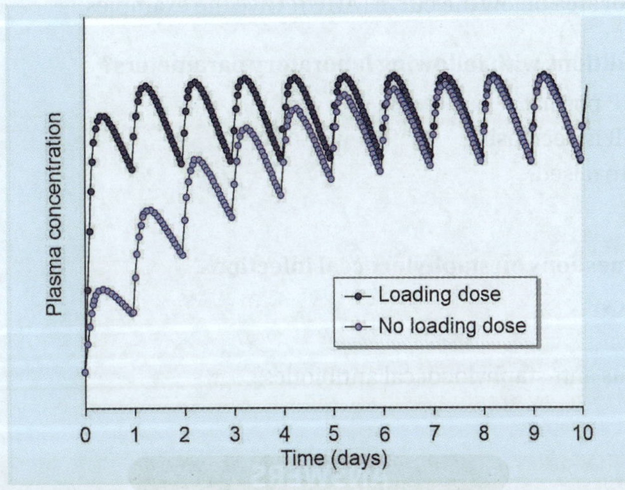

A. What does this graph show regarding pharmacokinetics of antibiotics?
B. What are the benefits of this principle in antibiotic practice?
C. Which property of antibiotics warrants to follow this principle in practice?
D. Examples of antibiotics to be given by this principle.

Q-33. Answer the following questions pertaining to MERINO (2018) trial, a study on antibiotics.

A. What was studied in this trial?
B. What was the conclusion of this study?
C. What should be antibiotic of choice in a case of neonatal meningitis due to extended-spectrum beta-lactamase (ESBL) *E. coli*?

Q-34. Answer the following questions on antimicrobial stewardship (AMS).

A. Define antimicrobial stewardship.
B. When antimicrobial stewardship week is celebrated every year?
C. What are the goals of AMS?

Q-35.

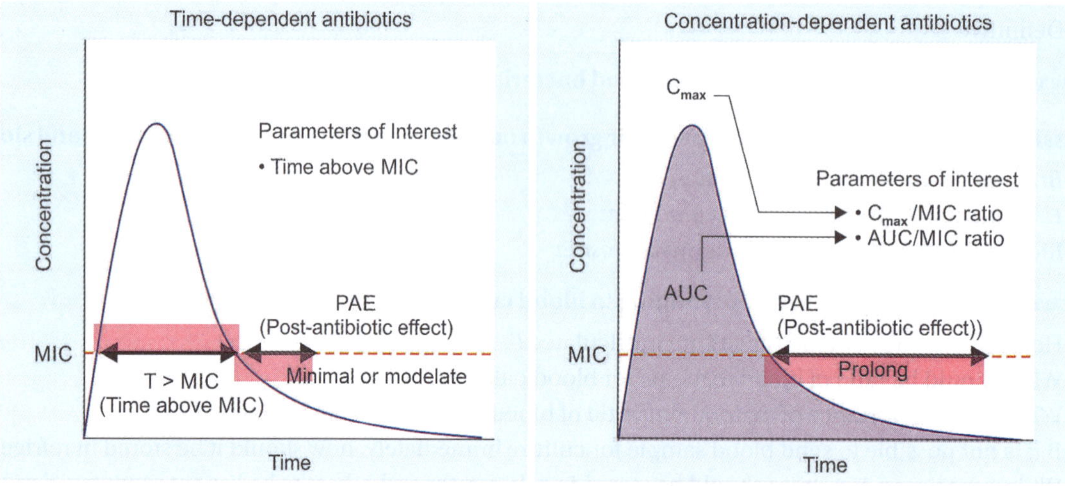

A. What are the characteristics of time-dependent antibiotics? Give examples.
B. What are the characteristics of concentration dependent antibiotics? Give the examples.
C. What is the concept of area below the curve (AUC)? Give the examples.

Q-36. What are probable conditions with following laboratory parameters?

A. ESR is raised and CRP normal.
B. CRP is raised and ESR is decreasing.
C. ESR and CRP both are raised.
D. INR is more than 1.5.

Q-37. Answer the following questions on staphylococcal infections.

A. Anti-MRSA antibiotics
B. Anti-MSSA antibiotics
C. Role of clindamycin as anti-staphylococcal antibiotics

ANSWERS

A-1. A Blood culture

B.

- Operator must clean and dry the hands.
- Use of sterile gloves
- 70% isopropyl alcohol or iodine tincture as antiseptic solutions
- About 3 cm^2 of skin should be disinfected.
- Disinfectant requires 1–2 minutes of contact time for complete action. Allow it to dry.
- Avoid touching and recontamination

A. Volume of blood for culture

- *Neonates:* 1–2 mL
- *Infants:* 1–3 mL
- *Children:* 3–5 mL
- *Adolescents:* 10–20 mL

B. Keep it at room temperature, not in refrigerator.

A-2. A. *Chlamydia trachomatis* Pneumonia
B. Chest X-ray findings in *Chlamydia* infections are hyperinflation with minimal interstitial or alveolar infiltrates.
C. Azithromycin

A-3. A. Staphylococcal-scalded skin syndrome
B. Nikolsky sign
C. Epidermolytic toxins (exotoxin–exfoliation)
D. Cloxacillin + clindamycin or
Vancomycin + clindamycin

A-4 A. HIV/AIDS
B. Norwegian scabies
C. Ivermectin 0.2 mg/kg as single dose
D. *Sarcoptes scabiei* var. hominis

A-5. A. Generalized tetanus
B. *Risus sardonicus*
C. Intractable spasms of buccal and facial muscles
D. Laryngeal muscle spasm causing asphyxia
E. Penicillin

A-6. A. Hand–Foot–Mouth disease (HFMD)
B. Coxsackie virus A16
C. Coxsackie A, Coxsackie B, Enteroviruses, ECHO viruses
D. Myocarditis, pericarditis, shock, encephalomyelitis, pulmonary hemorrhage. More common with Enterovirus 71

A-7. A. Peri osteitis and osteitis
B. Congenital syphilis
C.
- *Treponema pallidum* Hemagglutination Test (TPHA)
- Fluorescent Treponemal Antibody Absorption (FTA–ABS) Test

D. Penicillin

A-8. A. Tuberculous pleural effusion
B.
- Type III (Hypersensitivity reaction)
- Tuberculin protein

C. Positive
D.
- Erythema nodosum
- Phlyctenular conjunctivitis
- Tuberculous lymphadenitis

E. 25%

A-9. A. Ascariasis
B.
- *Pulmonary manifestations:*
  - Fever, cough, dyspnea, wheezing
  - Urticaria
  - Eosinophilia

- *Intestinal manifestations:*
  - Abdominal pain and distention
  - Vomiting
  - Diarrhea
  - Protein energy malnutrition
  - Vitamin A deficiency

C.
- Poor growth and deficiency of protein, vitamin A and others
- Intestinal obstruction
- Obstructive jaundice following obstruction to sphincter of oddi
- Cholecystitis
- Peritonitis
- Pancreatitis
- Passing through various orifices like nose, mouth, rectum, vagina, etc.

D. Albendazole 400 mg orally as single dose

A-10. A. Leishmaniasis (Kala-azar)

B.
- Malaria
- Enteric fever
- Tuberculosis
- Schistosomiasis
- Brucellosis
- Lymphoma
- Leukemia

C. *Investigations for leishmaniasis:*
- Serological tests
- Demonstration of LD bodies in tissue specimens like lymph node, splenic pulp, bone marrow aspiration, etc.
- Culture of tissue biopsy or aspirates

D. *Treatment:*
- Pentavalent antimony compounds
- Amphotericin B deoxycholate or liposomal amphotericin B
- Paromomycin

A-11. A.
- An initial visit after 2 weeks.
- Every month till completion of treatment.
- Every 6 months till 2 years after completion of the course.

B.
- After 2 weeks on follow-up, to check that the patient is on correct dosage and combination and is tolerating drug as desirable.
- *Appropriate therapy:*
  - Has received correct combination in correct dose.
  - Is accepting and tolerating all drugs.
  - Counsel about need to complete therapy and not missing doses, to inform in case the doses are missed for any reason.

- *Response to therapy:*
  - Symptomatic response
  - Assessment of adherence
  - Adverse effects of drugs
  - Weight measurement (may need dose revision)
- Microbiological
  At end of intensive phase and end of treatment
- *Follow-up radiographs:*
  - If slow resolution of symptoms (>4 weeks) or persistent symptoms at end of intensive phase.
  - Any deterioration at any time
  - Not required in children who are improving except at the end of continuous phase.
- *Treatment of comorbid conditions:*
  - HIV
  - Severe acute malnutrition
  - Anticonvulsant and other drugs in neurotuberculosis
- *Adherence to therapy:*
  - Pill count
  - Social support, family support.
  - Supervision of therapy.

A-12. *Presence of at least one of the following criteria:*

- Rise of >5 times the upper limit of normal levels of SGPT even when has not symptoms.
- Rise of SGPT >3 times when has nausea, vomiting, diarrhea
- Rise of level of serum total bilirubin >1.5 mg/dL

A-13. Stop hepatotoxic anti-tuberculous drugs and start ethambutol, streptomycin and levofloxacin

↓

Repeat SGPT after 7 days

↓

SGPT <2 times of upper normal limits

↓

Start Rifampicin in full dose

↓

Repeat SGPT after 3 days

↓

SGPT <2 times of upper normal limits

↓

Add INH full dose

↓

Repeat LFT after 3–7 days

↓

SGPT <2 times of upper normal limits

↓

Add pyrazinamide in full dose

A-14. A. First chest X-ray shows right side paratracheal glandular opacity which is considered as highly suggesting tuberculous etiology in a given case scenario. Positive Mantoux test is supporting it. Therefore, it is a case of presumptive tuberculosis. It was confirmed with presence of AFB and positive GeneXpert report.

Second chest X-ray was taken after 8 weeks of ATT with appropriate dosage and good compliance. Still, it shows increased in size of right paratracheal gland.

B.
- Immune reconstitution inflammatory syndrome (IRIS) or paradoxical reaction
- Multidrug resistant tuberculosis
- Other possibilities like lymphoma

C. Lymph node biopsy and histopathological examination

D.
- Immune reconstitution inflammatory response (IRIS) or paradoxical upgrading reactions in tuberculosis
- What is IRIS?
  - Enlargement of old lesions or unexpected appearance of new lesions during apparently adequate ATT.
  - Usually occurs 3–12 weeks after beginning of treatment, most frequently after 6–7 weeks of treatment.
  - Lasts for approximately 2 months.
  - Generally, self-limiting, resolves without sequelae, regresses by same ATT
  - May occur post-treatment as late as 2 years
- Mechanism of IRIS

  Active TB can result in depression of immunity

  After successful ATT, focal immune response improves

  Accumulation of inflammatory exudates at previously invisible microscopic tuberculous foci elsewhere appearing as new lesions.
- Types of paradoxical reactions
  - Increases in size of mediastinal or lymphnode or areas of infiltration with primary tuberculosis
  - Appearance of new lung infiltrates in patients with extrapulmonary tuberculosis
  - Development of tuberculous pleural effusion
  - Increase in size of effusion or appearance of effusion on contralateral side
  - Appearance of new lymphnodes or enlargement of original lymphnodes
  - Increase in size and number of tuberculomas, infarcts or hydrocephalus

A-15.
- *Evaluation of the neonate for presence of tuberculous disease:*
  - *Clinical examination:* Examination of vitals, signs of respiratory distress, hepatosplenomegaly, lymphadenopathy, CNS meningitis
  - Chest X-ray
  - Other investigations like gastric aspirate for Ziehl-Neelsen stain, GeneXpert and MGIT culture. Liver biopsy
- *Prevention of disease, if has no evidence of disease:*
  - INH, 10 mg/kg for 6 months, pyridoxine supplementation 10 mg/day
  - Close observation for development of disease
  - Close observation and no prophylaxis in case of MDR-TB to mother.
- Separation is not required.
- Mother's cough hygiene and etiquette are important.
- Isolation may be required when mother is not adhering to treatment, infectious XDR or MDRTB.
- Breastfeeding is safe and should be continued. In a case of isolation, expressed breast milk can be used.

A-16. A. Retropharyngeal abscess

B. Less than 5 years, as the retropharyngeal lymph nodes involute after 5 years of age

C. *Polymicrobial:* Group A Streptococcal, Staphylococcal, anaerobic

D.
- Incision and drainage of abscess
- IV antibiotics

E.
- Amoxicillin–Clavulanic acid
- Cloxacillin
- Clindamycin

A-17. A. Infectious mononucleosis (Epstein–Barr viral infection)

B. Posterior cervical and epitrochlear group of lymph nodes

C.
- Leukocytosis
- Lymphocytosis
- Atypical lymphocytes on peripheral smear examination
- Thrombocytopenia

D.
- Viral capsid antigen for EBV (VCA-IgM for EBV)
- PCR

E. Spleen rupture

A-18. A. Parvo virus Infection (Erythema infectiosum)

B.
- Arthropathy
- Nonimmune hydrops fetalis
- Transient aplastic crisis in those with chronic hemolytic disorders
- Chronic pure red cell aplasia in immunocompromised individuals
- Myocarditis
- Renal disorders

C.
- Fifth disease
- Slapped cheek syndrome

D. Intravenous Immunoglobulin

A-19. A. Hand foot and mouth disease (HFMD)

B. Coxsackie virus A16, A5, 7, 9 and 10

C. Neurological disease—encephalitis, pulmonary hemorrhage and shock

D. Enterovirus 71

A-20. A. Dengue fever

B. Increased capillary permeability and leaking of fluid

C.
- *Aedes aegypti*
- *Aedes albopictus*

D. NS1 antigen for dengue virus

E. Pulse, respiratory rate, blood pressure, weight and urine output

Clinical Monitoring in a case of dengue fever:

- *Pulse:*
  - *Tachycardia:* Leaking of fluid resulting in hypovolemia or development of myocarditis as complication
  - *Bradycardia:* Common in recovery phase when fluid is returning to vascular compartment
- *Respiratory rate:* Tachypnea may be due to pleural effusion or development of acidosis

- *Blood pressure:* Narrow pulse pressure in leaking phase and decreased intravascular fluid volume
- Weight gain due to edema
- *Urine output:*
  - Scanty and dark-colored urine due to decreased intravascular fluid in leaking phase
  - Increased urine output and light color urine indicates return of fluid in recovery phase

A-21. A. Chikungunya in an infant
B. Petechial hemorrhages in the skin causes hyperpigmentation
C. IgM antibodies and PCR for chikungunya virus
D. *Aedes aegypti* and *Aedes albopictus* mosquitoes

A-22. A. *Mycoplasma* infection
B.
- Cold agglutination test
- IgM antibodies against mycoplasma by ELISA
- PCR from respiratory secretions

C.
- Azithromycin, 10 mg/kg in one dose on first day and then 5 mg/kg in one dose for 4 days
- Clarithromycin, erythromycin and doxycycline are other alternatives.
- Increasing resistant to azithromycin has been reported recently.

D.
- Skin manifestations
- Erythematous macular rashes, morbilliform rash, papulovesicular exanthem, erythema nodosum
- Erythema multiforme
- Stevens–Johnson syndrome
- Neurological manifestations like encephalitis, aseptic meningitis, transverse myelitis, peripheral neuropathy
- Involvement of heart, kidney and joints

A-23. A. Scarlet fever
B. Group A streptococci
C. Exotin (Erythrognenic toxin)
D.
- Kawasaki disease
- Viral exanthema
- Drug reactions
- Staphylococcal associated scarlatiniform rash

A-24. A. Rickettsial disease
B. History of travel to endemic area or visit to forest
C. Eschar–Painless at initial sites of tick attachment
D. Indirect immunofluorescent assay
E.
- Doxycycline is drug of choice 4.5 mg/kg/day in 2 divided doses for 3–5 days
- Azithromycin and chloramphenicol are other alternative antibiotics.

A-25. A. Necrotizing fasciitis
B. Group A streptococci—*S. pyogenes*
C. *Polymicrobial infection is more common Gram-positive organisms:* Group A streptococci, staphylococci *Gram-negative organisms: Klebsiella, E. coli* anaerobic organisms
- Supportive

- Surgical debridement
- Appropriate antibiotics

D. *Gram-positive organisms:* Ceftriaxone, vancomycin, linezolid, daptomycin, clindamycin
Gram-negative organisms: Piperacillin, tazobactam

A-26. A. Meningococcemia

B.

- Blood culture
- CSF culture
- Antigen test

C.

- Adrenal hemorrhage
- Meningococcal meningitis
- Coagulopathy

D. Ceftriaxone

A-27. A. HIV and MDR Tuberculosis

B. Norwegian scabies

C.

- *Investigations for HIV:*
  - ELISA test for mother
  - PCR test for the child
- *Investigations for tuberculosis:*
  - Chest X-ray of baby and mother
  - Sputum for Ziehl-Neelsen stain and GeneXpert for mother
  - Gastric aspirate for Ziehl-Neelsen stain and GeneXpert for baby
  - Culture of sputum and gastric aspirate
  - Lymph node biopsy

A-28. A. *Preemptive:* Antibiotics are started on basis of probable infection on clinical grounds, but not proven, e.g., amoxicillin with diagnosis of bacterial tonsillitis

B. *Empirical:* Infection most likely exact organism and sensitivity not known, e.g., urinary tract infection diagnosed on basis of positive dipstick test like leukocyte esterase and nitrites. Urine culture report is pending.

C. *Definitive:* Proven pathogen with or without antibiotic susceptibility available, e.g., Blood culture—*Salmonella* positive enteric fever and starting cefixime 20 mg/kg/day.

A-29.

Viral infection	*Bacterial infection*
High at onset fever, gets better by day 3 or 4	Moderate at onset and peak on day 3 or 4
Nontoxic	Toxic
Child is normal during interfebrile period, playful, taking feeds	Child is sick—not well during interfebrile period, nonactive, does not like to take food
Dissemination of infection (URTI + LRTI) is common, Fever, cough–cold, diarrhea and vomiting	Localization of infection is common
Multiple members in family or community involved	No sick contact

A-30. A. Slow grower

B. Fastidious

C. Can not be grown

A-31. A. 1% circulating blood volume. The blood volume in 10 kg weighing child would be (80 mL × 10) 800 mL. 1% of 800 ml would be 8 mL. Therefore, 8 mL of blood should be collected for culture in 10 kg weighing child.

B. Ratio of blood to media is 1:5.

C. By dilution the effect of defense components of blood (WBC, immunoglobulins, complements) preventing growth of organisms can be minimized.

D. Blood culture specimen should be kept at room temperature, not in refrigerator.

E.

- Samples from contaminated sites like urine and stool should be kept in refrigerator.
- Samples from sterile sites like blood, CSF, ascites fluid, etc. should be kept at room temperature.

A-32. A. loading dose of antibiotics

B.

- Loading dose (LD) helps in achieving the desired therapeutic level quickly.
- It is important for drugs with long half-life.
- Important for critically ill patients to achieve desired level of drugs from beginning.
- It also prevents development of resistance.

C. Drugs with longer half-life should be used with loading dose.

D. Vancomycin, aminoglycosides like gentamicin, etc.

A-33. A. Piperacillin–tazobactum versus meropenem for the treatment of ceftriaxone resistant *E. coli* or *Klebsiella pneumoniae* bloodstream infections

B. Piperacillin–tazobactum is not a suitable definitive treatment for bloodstream infections caused by ceftriaxone resistant *E. coli* or *Klebsiella* species. Meropenem should be used instead.

C. Meropenem

A-34. A. Antimicrobial stewardship is a systematic approach to improve how healthcare professionals prescribe and use antimicrobial medicines like antibiotics to achieve the best patient outcomes while minimizing harms such as adverse effects, development of antimicrobial resistance and harm to the society. It involves coordinated interventions like education, guidelines and monitoring to ensure the appropriate selection, dose, duration and route of administration for antibiotics

B. November 18 to 24

C. Goals of AMS

To maximize treatment benefit and to minimize harm to patients and community. It can be achieved by:

- Antibiotics prescription only when needed
- Ensuring that antibiotics are prescribed in right diagnosis, right dose, right duration and right route

A-35. A.

- Time-dependent killing means concentration of antibiotics remains above MIC (T >MIC)
- It should be at least 50% of the dosing interval.
- It has minimal post-antibiotic effect.
- For example, beta-lactam antibiotics

B. Concentration dependent antibiotic killing where the peak level concentration (Cmax) is important and capitalizes on the postantibiotic effect of the drug. Aminoglycoside and fluroquinolones are examples of this principle.

C. In AUC, these drugs have both time-dependent killing and concentration-dependent killing. For these drugs, it is shaded area below the curve (AUC) over the MIC which is important. Vancomycin, linezolid, clindamycin and azithromycin are examples of this group.

A-36. A. Systemic lupus erythematous (SLE)

B. Hemophagocytic lymphohistiocytosis (HLH)

C. Inflammatory conditions may be infections or noninfective conditions like JIA.

D. Acute liver failure

A-37. A. Anti-MRSA antibiotics
- Vancomycin
- Telcoplanin
- Linezolid
- Clindamycin
- Daptomycin
- Tigecycline

B. *Anti-MSSA antibiotics:*
- Cloxacillin
- Cefazolin
- Cephalexin
- Clindamycin
- Co-trimoxazole

C. Clindamycin is useful for following reasons as anti-Staph. agent:
- PVL-like toxins are suppressed.
- Biofilm inhibitions
- Effective tissue penetration

CHAPTER 13

Gastroenterology

QUESTIONS

Q-1. An 11-year-old male child was admitted for jaundice and high-colored urine of 3 months duration. Clinically, vitals were stable, afebrile, icterus noted, no pallor, no lymphadenopathy, Liver 4 cm, firm, spleen 2 cm firm. Eye examination was contributory. S. bilirubin 4.5 mg%, direct type, SGPT 670 U/L. CBC, coagulation profile normal. Seromarkers for viral hepatitis negative. The child was born of a consanguineous parents. His elder sister died at the age of 7 years due to similar illness.

A. What is your most probable diagnosis?
B. What would be finding on eye examination?
C. Name three confirmatory laboratory investigations for this disease.
D. Specific treatment of the condition
E. Dietary advice

Q-2. A 3-month-old male child was referred with frequency of stool 15- 20/day, watery since birth. He was full-term baby with birth weight 2.9 kg. He was found with severe dehydration, hypokalemia, hypochloremia and metabolic alkalosis.

A. What is your diagnosis?
B. What is the basic defect in this condition?
C. What finding is common in antenatal USG study in this disorder?

Q-3. This investigation was performed in an infant who presented with vomiting, irritability and FTT. The investigation was favoring the condition.

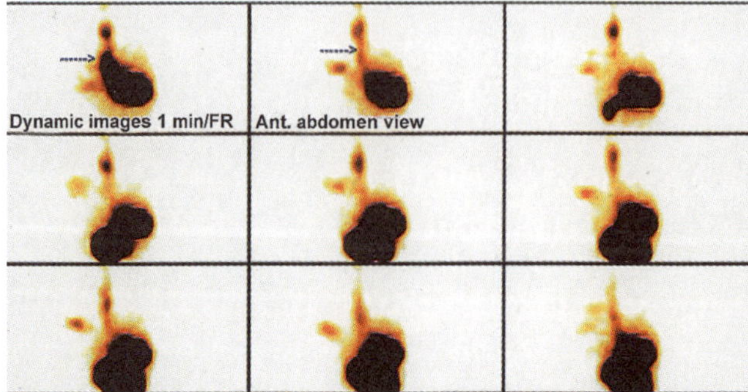

A. Name the investigation and condition.
B. Due to what the child is irritable and having arching in this condition?
C. What are other investigations for diagnosis of this condition?
D. What pharmacotherapy is considered as most potent at present?

Q-4. A 2-month-old male infant presented with complaints of non-bilious, projectile vomiting for one month. He required hospitalization for neonatal hyperbilirubinemia. The baby was not gaining the weight. On physical examination, moderate dehydration was noted. Arterial blood gas analysis showed pH 7.55, HCO_3 44 and SPO_2 98%. Below is the picture of upper GI contrast study.

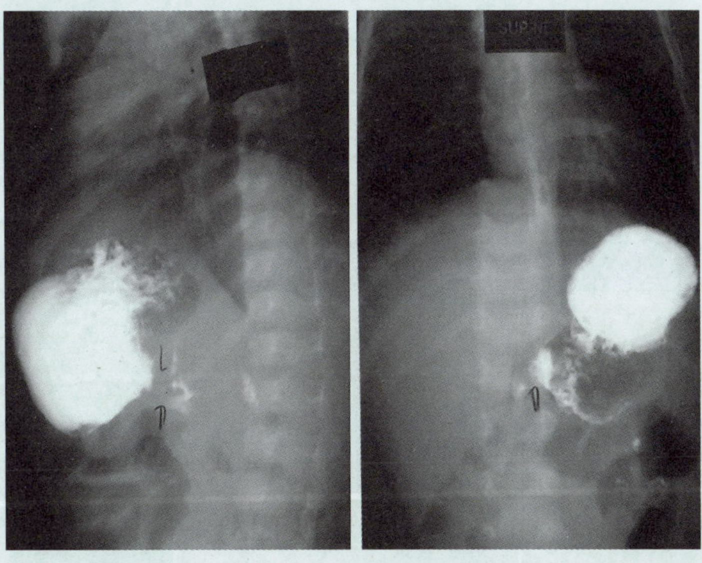

A. What is the interpretation of ABG?
B. What are radiological findings?
C. What is probable diagnosis?
D. What other diagnostic modality is sensitive for diagnosis?
E. What is the surgical treatment?

Q-5.

Type 1	Separate hard lumps, like nuts (hard to pass)
Type 2	Sausage-shaped but lumpy
Type 3	Like a sausage but with cracks on the surface
Type 4	Like a sausage or snake, smooth and soft
Type 5	Soft blobs with clear-cut edges
Type 6	Fluffy pieces with ragged edges, a mushy stool
Type 7	Watery, no solid pieces, entirely liquid

A. What is the name of this chart?
B. What is its clinical application?
C. How it helps in diagnosis of various conditions?

Q-6.

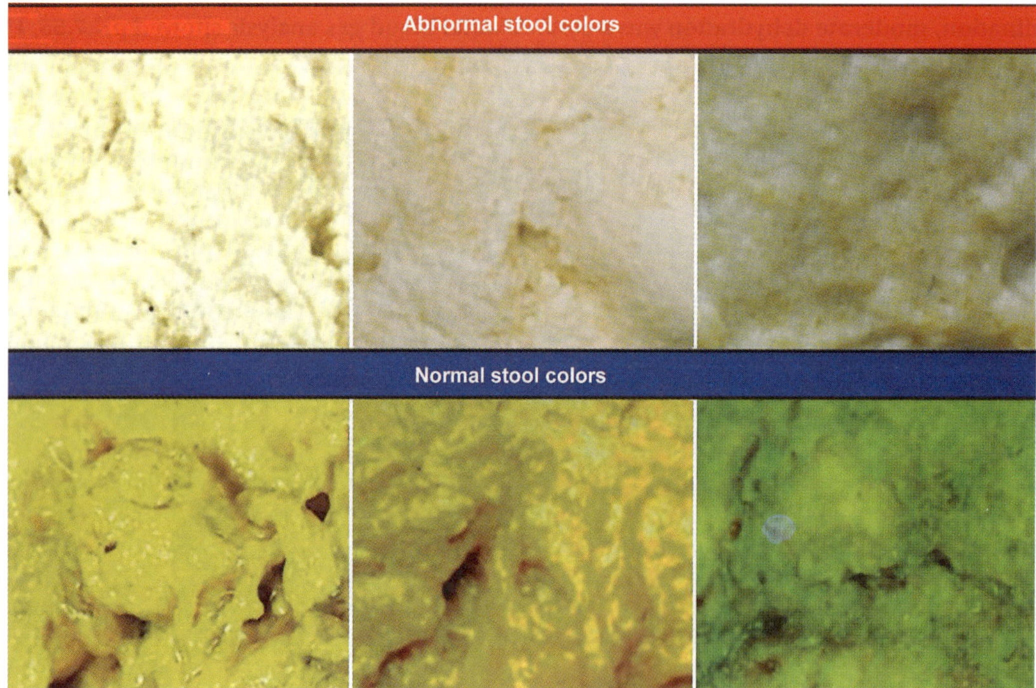

A. This card is prepared for identification of change in color of stool of infants. What is the name of this card?
B. What is the interpretation of this card? Why is there abnormal color of stool in this condition?
C. Which condition can be suspected from abnormal color of stool?
D. What is the reliability of this test?

Q-7. A newborn was born with following abdominal wall defect:

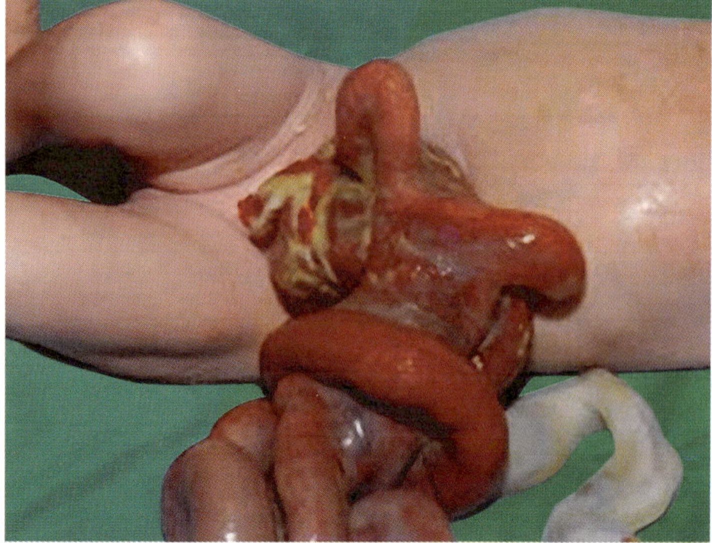

A. What is probable diagnosis?
B. What are the clues for the condition?
C. What are the contents of this swelling?

Q-8. A newborn was delivered with the below given congenital defect in the abdomen.

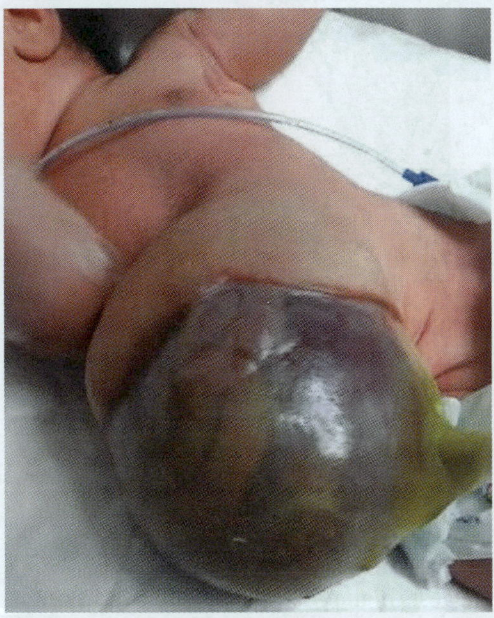

A. What is the probable diagnosis?
B. What are the differential diagnosis?
C. How will you differentiate it from other conditions?
D. What tests should be performed for antenatal diagnosis?
E. What is the immediate management?
F. What is the final management of the lesion?
G. What are the associated anomalies/syndrome known with this condition?

Q-9.

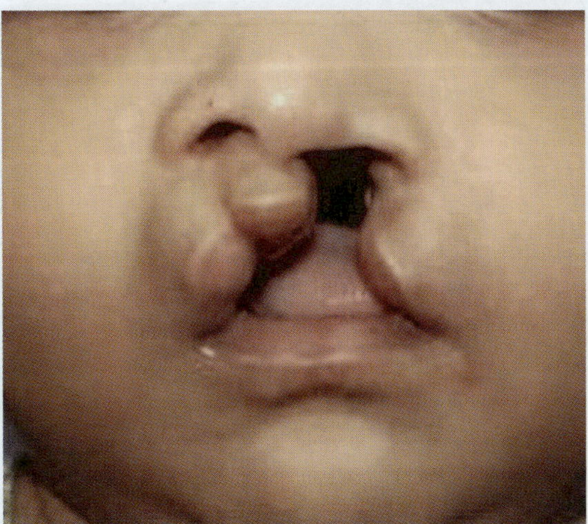

A. Name the condition.
B. What is its classification?
C. What are the clinical problems with this disorder?
D. What is the currently recommended treatment schedule of this condition?

Q-10. A 2-year-old child presented with constipation since almost birth. There was history of delayed passage of meconium, more than 72 hours. The radio-imaging study was performed as shown below in the picture.

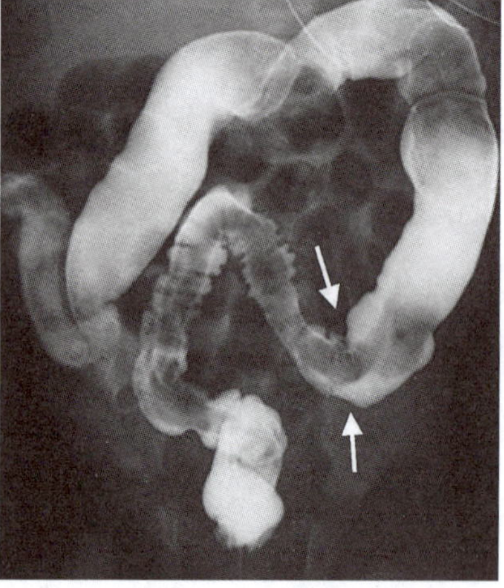

A. What radio-imaging study is it?
B. What is the diagnosis?
C. What clinical examination suggests high probability of the condition?
D. What investigations can be performed in this disease? What is the final confirmatory investigation?
E. What is the line of treatment?

Q-11. A 3-year-old boy from Rajasthan was referred for chronic diarrhea, failure to thrive and bilateral pedal edema. The diarrhea started at the age of 1 year. On clinical examination, he had severe anemia, bilateral pedal edema and multiple vitamin deficiency, despite of good appetite and dietary intake.

A. What is probable diagnosis?
B. What are differential diagnosis?
C. What tests should be performed for confirmation of diagnosis?
D. What treatment should be advised?

Q-12.

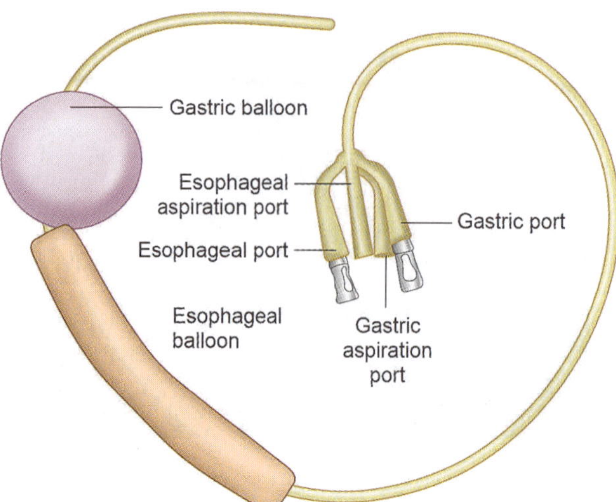

A. Identify the instrument.
B. What are the indications for its use?
C. What is the mechanism of its actions?
D. What complications are known to occur on its use?

Q-13.

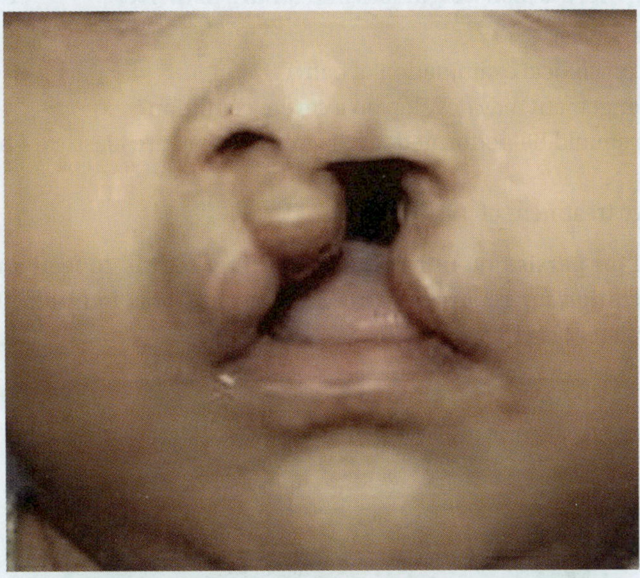

A. What is the diagnosis?
B. What is the embryologic basis of this defect?
C. If the baby has not any other anomaly and healthy, at what age, are these defect repaired?

Q-14. An infant had viral acute diarrheal disease, mild fever and vomiting. He was treated with various drugs including antibiotics by a family physician. He was referred for persistent, large quantity, watery diarrhea, distention of abdomen and perianal redness as shown in following picture.

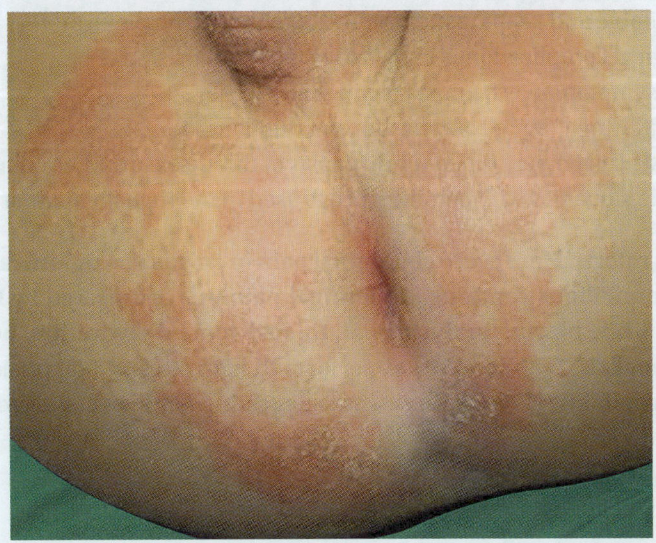

A. What is the diagnosis?
B. What is the pathophysiology of diarrhea in this condition?
C. What are the types of this disease? Which one is common?
D. What findings on stool examination favor the diagnosis?
E. Which test is used in older children for this disease?
F. What is the management in breastfed infants with this disease?

Q-15. A first born male child presents at 5 weeks of age with projectile, nonbilious vomiting. The baby is very hungry after vomiting. There is also weight loss and failure to thrive.

A. What is probable diagnosis?
B. What do you expect on clinical examination of baby?
C. What metabolic derangement may develop on a severe condition?
D. What radio-imaging should be performed for diagnosis? What are classical findings in the radio-imaging in this condition?
E. What is the corrective treatment of this condition?

Q-16. An infant was referred for persistent, non-bilious vomiting, refusal to feed and irritability. The child also needs frequent nebulization for recurrent wheeze. The child was found in the position as shown in the picture below with persistent crying.

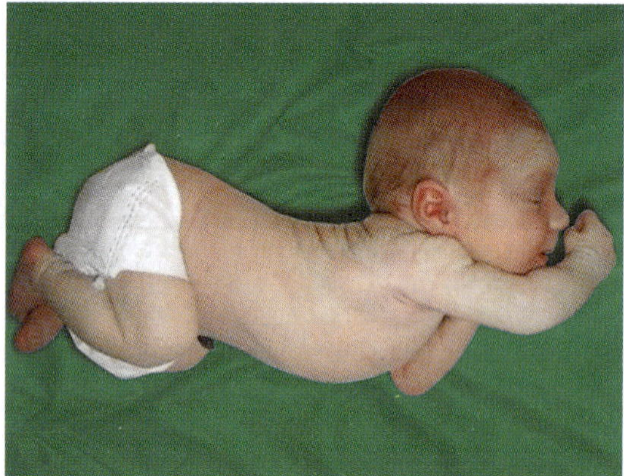

A. What is the probable diagnosis?
B. Why is the child irritable and keeping the posture as shown in the picture?
C. What rare neurological complication is known to occur in this disorder?
D. What neurological symptom may be mistaken in this disease?
E. What are possible life-threatening complications of this condition?
F. What diagnostic tests can be performed for diagnosis of this disease and its complication?
G. Mention therapeutic strategies with common drugs used in the management of this condition.

Q-17. An 8-year-old boy was referred for severe abdominal pain in epigastric region, radiating to back. He also had multiple episodes of nonbilious vomiting. Abdominal pain was aggravated by food intake. He had history of abdominal trauma while playing in the school. He had some dehydration, but hemodynamically stable without any sign of shock. USG abdomen was performed with clinical diagnosis of appendicitis. Appendix and kidneys were normal, but USG findings were suggesting some other condition, known to present as acute abdomen.

A. What is the probable diagnosis?
B. What clinical signs are supporting the diagnosis?
C. What investigations should be performed to confirm the diagnosis?
D. What is the most specific test for this disease?
E. What are the complications of this disease?
F. What is the management?

Q-18. A 7-year-old boy presented in emergency room with complaints of blood containing vomiting and black-colored stool. There was no history of fever or ingestion of any drug. He had similar episode 6 months back

which was treated in hospital with one PCV, IV fluid and supportive therapy. He had no any complaint between the two episodes. On examination, he had severe pallor and 1 cm palpable spleen. He had no jaundice, no hepatomegaly or ascites.

A. What is probable diagnosis?
B. What points should be derived in the history in this disease?
C. What are common presentations of this disease?
D. What does black-colored stool indicate? How will you confirm it? What is the interval between upper GI bleeding and black-colored stool? What is the interval between control of upper GI bleeding and normal stool from black-colored stool?
E. What investigations should be performed to confirm the disease?
F. How will you manage the upper GI bleeding in this disease?

Q-19. A 3-month-old breastfed infant was brought with complaints of frequent passage of stool with fresh blood and mucus. Antenatal, natal and postnatal periods were uneventful. Birth weight was 2.7 kg. Weight gain of baby was not adequate. The baby also had infantile eczema over cheeks. CBC, PT, APTT and stool examination reports were normal.

A. What is the probable diagnosis?
B. What are the differential diagnosis?
C. How to confirm the diagnosis of this disorder?
D. What is the treatment?

Q-20. A 2-year-old girl was referred for chronic diarrhea, repeated lower respiratory infections and failure to thrive. There was history of meconium ileus in neonatal period. Her elder sibling died due to same illness.

A. What is the probable diagnosis?
B. What are the confirmatory tests?
C. What replacement therapy is recommended for chronic diarrhea in this disease?
D. What is the dose and how to titrate the dose of replacement drug?

Q-21. A 10-month-old healthy boy presented with acute onset, intermittent, screaming with colicky pain and vomiting. The mother noticed red-colored stool without fecal matter. He had history of viral upper respiratory infection few days back. On abdominal palpation, a mass was noted.

A. What is probable diagnosis?
B. What is the most common triad of symptoms with this condition?
C. What clinical examination is important in a suspected case of this disease?
D. What investigations should be performed to confirm the diagnosis?
E. What are the treatment modalities in this condition?

Q-22. These are specimens of ascitic fluid collected from different patients with various clinical conditions. They are from left to right, straw, hemorrhagic, watery, xanthochromic and milky.

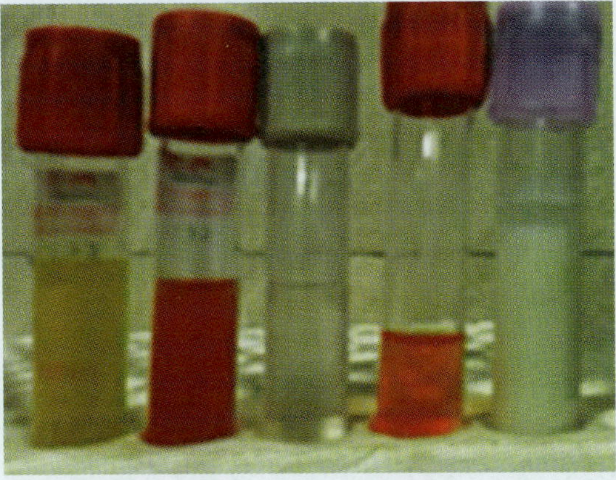

A. Identify probable conditions with each ascitic fluid specimen and its color.
B. What is serum ascites albumin gradient (SAAG)?
C. How is SAAG classified? Give classical examples with each type.

Q-23. A 3-year-old boy presented with sudden onset of pain and redness of right scrotum as shown in following picture

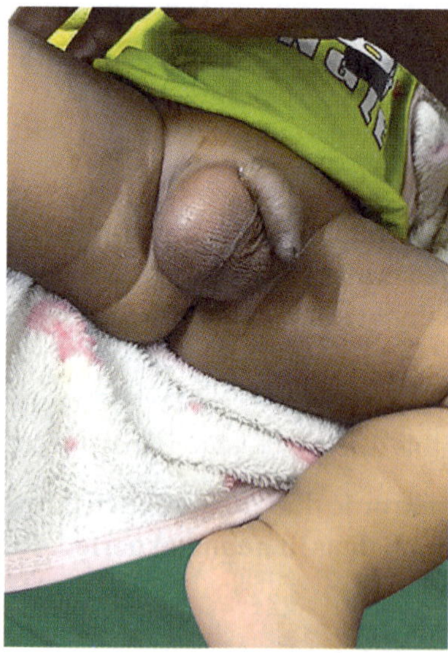

A. What is the probable diagnosis?
B. Name the important clinical sign to look for.
C. What are the differential diagnosis?
D. What investigations should be performed in this patient?
E. What are systemic diseases known to present with this condition as the complication?
F. What is the treatment of this condition?

Q-24. A 40-day-old male infant is referred for persistent jaundice. He had uneventful antenatal, natal and postnatal periods. Birth weight was 2.8 kg. His urine is high colored, staining the diaper and stool is clay colored. On examination, the baby is alert, active and taking breastfeeding. His liver is 5 cm, firm in consistency, no ascites, no splenomegaly or features of coagulopathy.

A. What is the most probable diagnosis?
B. What is the definition of conjugated hyperbilirubinemia in neonatal period?
C. What are differential diagnosis of this disorder?
D. What is the Gold Standard test for this disorder?
E. What is the management of this condition?

Q-25. Answer the following questions on ascites in children.

A. What is the serum ascites albumin gradient (SAAG) in portal hypertension?
B. What are the causes of high gradient and low gradient ascites?
C. What is the neutrophil cut-off in spontaneous bacterial peritonitis (SBP)?
D. What is the most common organism responsible for SBP in nephrotic syndrome?
E. What is the characteristic of secondary bacterial peritonitis?
F. What type of cardiac procedures may result in refractory ascites?

ANSWERS

A-1. A. Wilson's disease

B. Kayser-Fleischer ring

C. Serum ceruloplasmin (<20 mg/dL)

Urinary copper excretion (>100 µg/day, often >1000 µg/day)

Hepatic copper content (>250 µg/g dry weight)

D.

- D-penicillamine 20 mg/kg/day
- Zinc 25 mg three times a day
- Restriction of copper (<1 mg/day)

E. Avoid copper containing foods like liver, shellfish, nuts and chocolates. Avoid storing or cooking in copper or brass vessels

A-2. A. Chloride losing diarrhea

B. Defective transport mechanism of chloride/bicarbonate at distal ileum and colon

C. Maternal polyhydramnios

A-3. A. Milk scan for GERD

B. Esophagitis

C. Contrast radiographic (barium) study, esophageal pH monitoring, endoscopy

D. Proton pump inhibitors.

A-4. A. Metabolic alkalosis

B. *Radiological findings (upper GI barium study):*

- Elongated pyloric channel (string sign)
- A bulge of pyloric muscle into the antrum (shoulder sign)
- Parallel streak of barium seen in the narrowed channel (Double track sign)

C. Congenital hypertrophic pyloric stenosis

D. Ultrasonography (95% sensitivity)

E. *Surgical procedure*: Pyloromyotomy, called Ramstedt operation

A-5. A. Bristol stool chart

B. The patient with constipation can identify his stool pattern from this chart. This information helps the clinician to suspect the condition.

C. Can help to differentiate whether it is normal consistency of stool or constipation. Pasty stool is seen in Hirschsprung disease and large or hard stool in functional constipation.

A-6. A. Infant stool color card

B. On this card, first 3 colors (1 to 3) are abnormal, clay color, paly yellowish and light yellowish, whereas the other 3 (4 to 6) are labelled as normal, yellowish, brown and greenish. This abnormal color helps parents to suspect biliary atresia at the earliest, 4 weeks.

C. Biliary atresia

Normal stool has a brownish color due to the presence of stercobilin. In biliary atresia, stercobilin synthesis is markedly decreased as bilirubin cannot reach the intestine.

D. The sensitivity of this test is almost 90% and specificity 99%.

A-7. A. Gastroschisis

B. *Clues for diagnosis:*

- Abdominal wall defect arising outside the umbilical ring
- Herniated bowel not covered by peritoneum
- Defect lies right to umbilicus

C. *Contents of gastroschisis:*
- Intestines
- Stomach
- Urinary bladder
- Uterus

A-8. A. Omphalocele (Exomphalos)

B. *Differential diagnosis:*
- Exomphalos
- Hernia of umbilical cord
- Gastroschisis

C. Omphalocele is the herniation of intestine from the base of umbilicus covered by intact skin differentiates from gastroschisis. If the width of umbilical ring is less than 4 cm, it is called umbilical hernia

D. *Tests for antenatal diagnosis:*
- Ultrasound study
- Karyotyping by amniocentesis or chorionic villus sampling for chromosomal study. Chromosomal abnormalities is found in 40% of cases.

E. *Immediate management:*
- The baby should be nursed in supine position with the sac supported on both sides.
- Diluted povidone iodine or mercurochrome may be applied to surface to facilitate epithelization.

F. Surgical repair

G. *Associated anomalies:*
- Congenital heart disease
- Genitourinary defects
- Craniofacial, musculoskeletal, vertebral or limb anomalies
- Beckwith-Wiedemann syndrome
- Trisomy 13
- Trisomy 18

A-9. A. Cleft lip and cleft palate

B. *Classification:*
- Isolated cleft lip or isolated cleft palate, unilateral or bilateral, complete or incomplete
- Combined cleft lip or combined cleft palate, unilateral or bilateral, complete or incomplete syndrome

C. *Clinical problems:*
- Feeding problems
- Nasal regurgitation and aspiration
- Middle ear infection
- Speech problems
- Psychosocial problems
- Dental problems

D. *Treatment schedule:*
- *Birth:* Initial assessment, presurgical evaluation and orthodontics
- *3–6 months:* Primary lip repair
- *9–12 months:* Palate repair (before speech develops)
- *2 years:* Speech assessment
- *3–5 years:* Lip revisions
- *8–9 years:* Initial intervention orthodontics
- *10 years:* Alveolar bone grafting
- *16 years:* Nasal revision
- *12–20 years:* Orthodontics surgery

A-10. A. Barium enema study

B. Hirschsprung disease

C. Per rectal examination is important for suspected Hirschsprung disease. On rectal examination, the rectum is felt to be empty, and on withdrawal of the examining finger, there is an explosive passage of flatus and feces.

D. *Investigations for Hirschsprung disease:*

- Barium enema reveals a narrow aganglionic segment and a cone-shaped colon at the junction of the ganglionic and aganglionic segments
- Anorectal manometry
- Full thickness rectal biopsy is the final confirmatory test. It will show absence of ganglionic cells.

E. Removal of the aganglionic segment of colon by surgery is the line of treatment.

A-11. A. Celiac disease

B. *Differential diagnosis:*

- Giardiasis
- Cystic fibrosis
- Lymphangiectasis
- HIV
- Tuberculosis

C. *Investigations for celiac disease:*

- CBC and peripheral smear examination to confirm refractory iron deficiency anemia
- *Serological tests:*
  - Tissue transglutaminase– IgA (TTG–IgA)
  - Anti-endomysial antibodies
  - Upper GI endoscopy and biopsy

D. Gluten-free diet for life time and supportive therapy

A-12. A. Sengstaken-Blakemore tube

B. It is used to control variceal bleed which is refractory to both pharmacological and endoscopic interventions.

C. It has two inflatable balloons, which can mechanically compress both gastric and esophageal varices.

D. *Complications on use of Sengstaken-Blakemore tube:*

- Aspiration
- Esophageal rupture
- Esophageal ulcers
- Airway obstruction

A-13. A. Left side cleft lip and palate (unilateral)

B.

- Hypoplasia of mesenchymal layer resulting in failure of medial nasal and maxillary process to join result in cleft lip.
- Cleft palate is due to failure of palate halves to fuse.

C. Cleft lip is repaired at 3 months and cleft palate by 9–12 months, before development of speech.

A-14. A. Lactose intolerance

B. Any condition (commonly viral infections) which causes intestinal mucosal damage can cause lactose intolerance. This is because the lactase enzyme is present at the tips of intestinal villi and is often among intestinal disaccharidases to be lost in the event of mucosal injury. It causes impaired digestion of disaccharide lactose. Undigested lactose draws more fluid in the intestine, resulting in watery diarrhea. It also causes acidic pH of stool and gas due to fermentation of lactose by bacteria. Gas causes gaseous distention of abdomen and acidic pH of stool causes perianal excoriation.

C. *Two types of lactose intolerance:*
- *Primary lactose intolerance:* Congenital deficiency of lactase enzyme, extremely rare. It presents with diarrhea since birth. It remains permanent and does not improve with time.
- *Secondary lactose intolerance:* It is more common and transient following intestinal mucosal injury.

D. Stool examination in lactose intolerance
- Stool pH less than 5.5.
- Stool reducing substance more than ++. Liquid component of stool should be examined.

E. A lactose hydrogen breath test is used in older children.

F. *Management of secondary lactose intolerance:*
- Reducing or completely avoiding lactose containing food for 48–72 hours.
- Non-lactose milk formula like soya-milk may be used. Do not stop breastfeeding in infants.

A-15. A. Infantile hypertrophic pyloric stenosis

B. *Common findings on clinical examination:*
- Looking alert and hungry
- Dehydration may be present due to persistent vomiting.
- May have slow and shallow breathing due to metabolic alkalosis.
- Left-to-right pulsations may be seen, especially after feeding the baby.
- In 70% of cases, palpable tumor or mass on upper abdomen is found.

C. Hypokalemic, hypochloremic metabolic alkalosis may develop due to persistent vomiting in a severe case.

D. *Radio-imaging studies:*
- USG abdomen shows thickened pylorus and also shows reverse peristalsis on the stomach.
- Contrast study with barium shows a large stomach, delayed emptying, string sign and gastritis.

E. Ramstedt pyloromyotomy is the desired procedure, may be done by open or laparoscopic approach.

A-16. A. Gastroesophageal reflux disease (GERD)

B. Due to reflux esophagitis, the child is irritable with arching of back and extension of neck.

C. Sandifer's syndrome is rare neurological complication known to occur in GERD. It is an unusual movement disorder characterized by spasmodic torsional dystonia with arching of back and opisthotonus posture.

D. Sandifer's syndrome may be mistaken as seizures disorder

E. Life-threatening complications known to occur in GERD:
- Apnea due to laryngospasm caused by nasopharyngeal micro-aspiration.
- Sudden infant death syndrome (SIDS)

F. Following diagnostic tests are performed:
- *Upper gastrointestinal study:*
  - To assess anatomical abnormalities
  - To rule out hiatal hernia, stricture and malrotation
- *24-hours esophageal pH study:*
  - To detect acid reflux in esophagus
  - To correlate acid reflux and extraesophageal manifestations
- *Endoscopy and biopsy:*
  - To diagnose esophagitis and Barrett's esophagus
  - To rule out gastritis, peptic ulcer and eosinophilic gastritis
  - To dilate esophageal stricture
- *Impedance study:*
  - To detect acid and nonacid reflux in the esophagus
  - To correlate acid and nonacid reflux and extra esophageal manifestations

G. *Therapeutic strategies and medicines for GERD:*
- *Changes in lifestyle:*

- Positioning
- Avoidance of smoking exposure
- Weight reduction in children with obesity
- Dietary changes
- *Antacids:*
  - Aluminum hydroxide/Magnesium carbonate 10–20 mL as needed.
  - Aluminum hydroxide/Magnesium hydroxide 10–20 mL as needed.
- *H_2 receptor antagonists:*
  - *Ranitidine*: 6–8 mg/kg/day, divided two doses. Maximum 300 mg/day
  - *Famotidine:* 1 mg/kg/day divided in two doses. Maximum 40 mg/day
- *Protein pump inhibitors (PPI):*
  - Omeprazole 1–3 mg/kg/day. Maximum 40 mg/day
  - Lansoprazole 1–3 mg/kg/day. Maximum 60 mg/day
  - Pantoprazole 20–40 mg/day
  - Esomeprazole 10 40 mg/day
  - Rabeprazole 10–40 mg/day
- *Surgery:* Fundoplication

A-17. A. Acute pancreatitis

B. *Clinical signs of acute pancreatitis:*
- *Cullen's sign:* Bluish discoloration in periumbilical area due to intraperitoneal hemorrhage is highly suggesting acute pancreatitis. It is called as Cullen's sign.
- *Grey Turner's sign:* Bluish discoloration in the loin due to intraperitoneal hemorrhage in a case with such clinical presentation is highly suggesting acute pancreatitis.

C. *Investigations for acute pancreatitis:*
- Serum amylase and serum lipase. Serum lipase is more useful in children for diagnosis of acute pancreatitis.
- Serum trypsin is most accurate investigation for diagnosis of acute pancreatitis, but routinely not available.
- USG abdomen
- CT scan of abdomen with contract

D. Serum lipase is considered as specific test compared to serum amylase for diagnosis of acute pancreatitis. Serum amylase is sensitive, but non-specific test.

E. *Complications of acute pancreatitis:*
- Necrosis
- Pancreatic pseudocyst

F. *Management of acute pancreatitis:*
- Nil orally
- IV fluid
- Analgesics
- No role of prophylactic antibiotics

A-18. A. Extrahepatic portal hypertension

B. *Important points in history in a suspected case of extrahepatic portal hypertension:*
- History of intra-abdominal infection, umbilical sepsis or umbilical catheterization. It can cause portal phlebitis and portal venous obstruction.
- History of hematemesis and melena in the past. Recurrent such episodes are known to occur due to esophageal variceal bleeding

C. In extrahepatic portal hypertension, almost 85% of children present with upper GI bleeding due to variceal hemorrhage and 15% may present with only splenomegaly.

D.

- Black-colored stool in such a case, indicates melena. Passage of black, tarry, sticky and offensive stool is termed melena. Melena suggests upper GI bleeding.
- It can be confirmed by testing stool for occult blood for three consecutive days.
- It takes about 14 hours for blood to be broken down within the intestinal lumen. Therefore, if transit time is more than 14 hours, the patient will have melena.
- Melena can persist for 4–7 days after control of bleeding.

E. *Investigations:*

- Doppler USG—portal cavernoma on USG confirms EHPVO (94– 100% sensitivity and 96% specificity)
- CT angiography or MR portovenogram, if Doppler USG is not useful.
- Liver function tests

F. *Management of upper GI bleeding:*

- *Supportive:* PCV and IV octreotide
- Upper GI endoscopy
- If patient continues to bleed in spite of PCV and octreotide, Sengstaken-Blakemore tube
- Pharmacotherapy
- Emergency surgery

A-19. A. Cow milk protein Allergy (CMPA)

B. *Differential diagnosis:*

- Late hemorrhagic disease
- Dysentery
- Ulcerative colitis

C. The Gold standard for diagnosis of CMPA is elimination and challenge test. The symptoms stop after withdrawal of milk and recur within 48 hours of milk intake. Goldman suggested three such positive challenges for making the definite diagnosis.

D. Elimination of animal milk and milk products in baby's and mother's diet is the management of CMPA.

A-20. A. Cystic fibrosis

B. *Tests for cystic fibrosis*

- *Sweat chloride test:* > 60 mEq/L is diagnostic.
- *Molecular test:* Identification of 2 CFTR (Cystic Fibrosis Transmembrane Conductance Regulatory) mutation. More than 2000 different mutations exist.

C. Pancreatic enzyme replacement therapy

D.

- Infants generally require 450–900 lipase units/g of fat or 2000 to 4000 lipase units/120 mL of formula or when breastfeeding.
- Older children and adults generally require 500–4000 lipase units/g of fat or 500–2500 lipase units/kg/meal and 250–1250 lipase units/kg for snack.
- Doses of enzyme exceeding 2500 lipase units/kg/meal or 400 lipase units/g of fat warrant further investigation. Decreased the frequency of stool and its fat contents, gaining the weight, less episodes of infections indicate sufficient doses.

A-21. A. Intussusception

B. Incessant cry due to intermittent colicky pain, vomiting and bleeding per rectum are classical features of intussusception

C. *Important clinical signs of intussusception:*

- On abdominal palpation, a banana-shaped mass with concavity towards umbilicus
- The mass may be felt on per rectal examination.
- Red currant jelly stool without fecal matter

D. *Investigations for intussusception:*
- *USG abdomen:* Pseudo-kidney sign/Doughnut sign or bowel in bowel sign
- Doppler study
- *Barium enema:* Coiled spring or claw sign

E. Pneumatic reduction, hydrostatic reduction and surgical reduction are modalities for treatment of intussusception.

A-22. A.
- *Straw:* Tuberculosis and cirrhosis of liver
- *Hemorrhagic:* Pancreatitis, malignancy
- *Deep yellow or dark brown:* Biliary ascites
- *Milky or chylous:* Intestinal lymphangiectasia, tuberculosis

B. SAAG is calculated by subtracting the value of ascitic fluid albumin from the serum albumin estimated concurrently

C.
- SAAG is classified as high gradient ascites (>1.1) and low gradient ascites (<1.1).
- High gradient ascites (>1.1) is seen in portal hypertension with a diagnostic accuracy of 97%. Other conditions with high SAAG are Budd–Chiari Syndrome, portal vein thrombosis, acute liver failure and hypothyroidism.
- Low gradient ascites is seen in tuberculous peritonitis, pancreatitis ascites, biliary ascites, nephrotic syndrome and serositis.
- SAAG may be falsely high in chylous ascites since lipid interferes with albumin estimation.

A-23. A. Right side testicular torsion

B. Absence of cremasteric reflex is the sign suggestive of torsion of testis

C. *Differential diagnosis of acute scrotum:*
- Torsion of testis
- Epididymo-orchitis
- Traumatic hematocele

D. *Investigations:*
- Doppler ultrasound to see the blood flow
- Radioisotope scan
- Exploration is recommended in doubtful cases

E. Mumps orchitis and Henoch-Schönlein purpura are known to present with this complication.

F.
- Exploration and orchiopexy, if testis is viable. It may require orchidectomy if blood flow is not reversible.
- Opposite testis should also be orchiopexy done.

A-24. A. Neonatal cholestasis syndrome, most probable biliary atresia

B. Conjugated hyperbilirubinemia is defined as direct bilirubin level more than 1 mg/dL when total serum bilirubin is less than 5 mg/dL or more than 20% of bilirubin, if total bilirubin is more than 5 mg/dL

C. *Differential diagnosis of neonatal cholestasis:*

Hepatocellular causes:
- Neonatal hepatitis: TORCH infection, sepsis, UTI, malaria
- *Metabolic causes:*
  - Galactosemia
  - Tyrosinemia
  - Storage disorders
  - Hemochromatosis

- *Others:*
  - Inspissated bile syndrome
  - Progressive familial intrahepatic cholestasis
  - Hypothyroidism
  - Down syndrome

Obstructive causes:
- Biliary atresia
- Choledochal cyst

Syndromic conditions:
- Alagille syndrome
- Down Syndrome

D. Perioperative cholangiogram with liver biopsy are Gold Standard for biliary atresia

E. *Management of biliary atresia:*
- Supportive therapy with injection vitamin K, oral vitamins A, D, E supplementation
- Nutrition
- Kasai portoenterostomy
- Liver transplantation

A-25. A. In portal hypertension, SAAG is high gradient, ≥1%. Its accuracy is 97%.

B.
- *High gradient ascites (SAAG ≥1.1):*
  - Portal hypertension
  - Budd-Chiari syndrome
  - Portal vein thrombosis
  - Acute liver failure
  - Hypothyroidism
- *Low gradient ascites (SAAG <1.1)*
  - Tuberculous peritonitis
  - Pancreatic ascites
  - Nephrotic syndrome
  - Serositis
  - Biliary ascites

C. Neutrophils ≥250 in SBP

D. *Streptococcus pneumoniae*

E. *Multiple organisms are implicated in SBP:* Fontan and bidirectional Glenn shunt and procedures which involve right ventricular ventriculostomy like tetralogy of Fallot intracardiac repair.

CHAPTER 14

Pulmonology

QUESTIONS

Q-1. A 2-year-old boy presented with persistent high-grade fever, cough and breathlessness following measles, not responding to oral amoxi-clavulanic acid. His Hb was 9.6, TLC 31,300 with polymorphs 81%, platelets 10,48,000. His chest X-ray showed right lower zone pneumonia as shown below. Injection ceftriaxone was started. Patient was deteriorating very fast. His repeat CBC showed Hb 9.4, TLC 3600, Polymorphs 40%, lymphocytes 56%. Repeat chest X-ray showed some complication. CT thorax was as below:

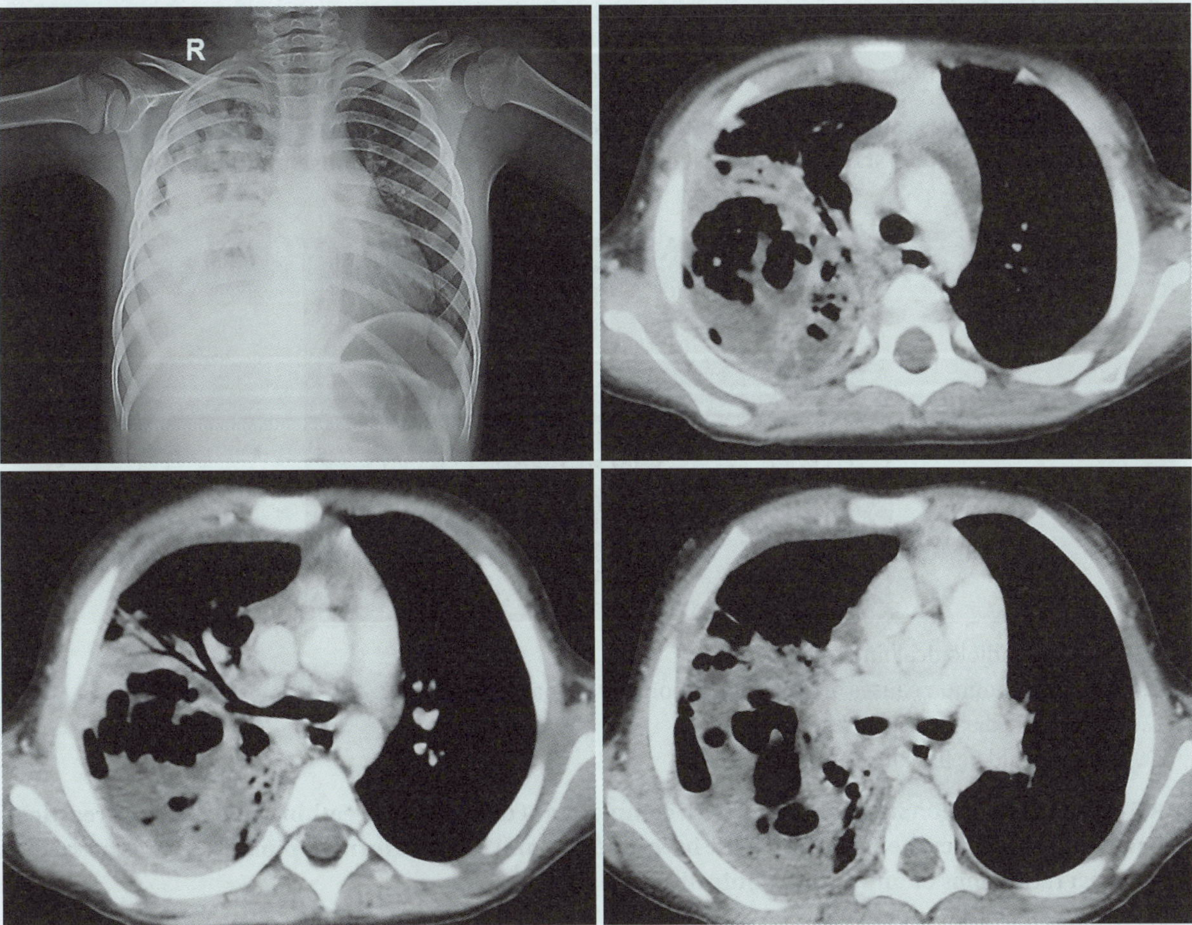

A. What are X-ray chest findings?
B. What are findings of CT thorax?
C. What is probable diagnosis?
D. What is most common organism in such cases?
E. What should be line of treatment?
F. What are antibiotics of choice? Why?

Q-2. A 2-day-old female infant was brought with complaints of difficulty in breathing and bluish discoloration of lips and nails while taking breastfeeding. On discontinuation of breastfeeding and crying, baby becomes pink with normal breathing. Her CT scan of upper airway is below:

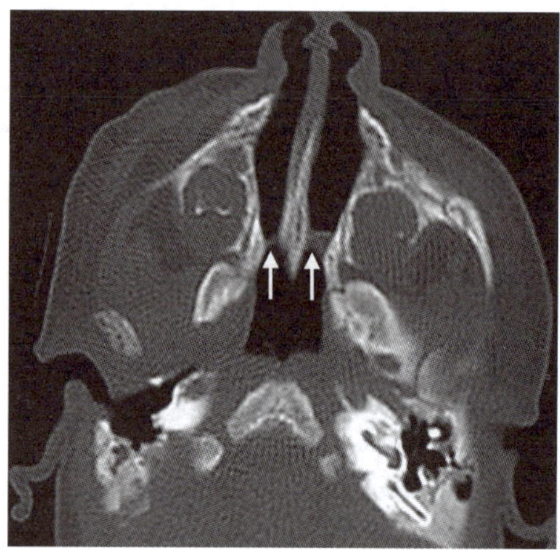

A. What is the diagnosis?
B. What will you do bedside suspicious of the condition? What examination may directly show the pathology?
C. What other conditions are known to be associated with this disorder?

Q-3. A 7-year-old boy presented with complaints of swelling and pain right lower eyelid and mild fever. He also had complaint of blood-stained nasal discharge on right side. X-ray of nose and paranasal sinuses was as below:

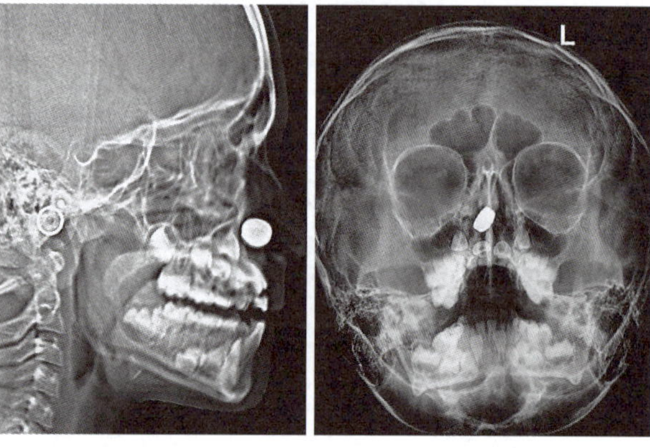

A. What are radiological findings?
B. What are common causes of unilateral bloodstained nasal discharge?
C. What is the diagnosis of present case?
D. What should be line of treatment?

Q-4. A 5-day-old male neonate was brought with complaints of difficulty in breathing while taking breastfeeding, becoming blue. Once, he stops to take the breastfeeding and cries, he turns to pink. There was no tachypnea, no chest retractions or any sound. Clinically normal.

A. What is the diagnosis?
B. What other anomalies are associated with this condition?
C. What are the diagnostic investigations?
D. What is the line of treatment?

Q-5. A 2.5-year-old boy presented with cough for almost 10 days. He also had mild fever off and on. There was no weight loss or history of tuberculous contact. CBC was performed multiple times and found within normal limits. His chest X-rays were as follows:

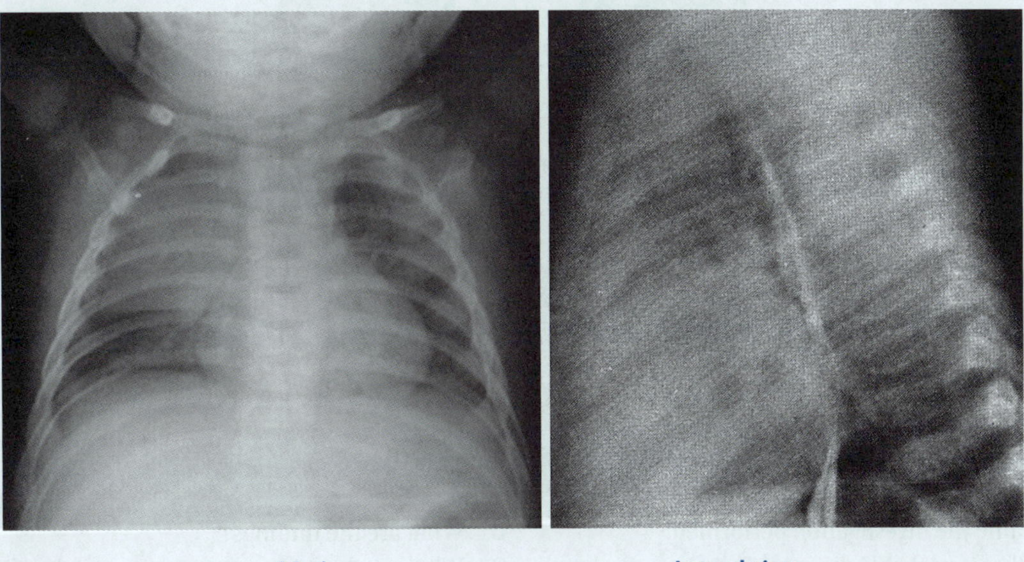

PA view Lateral view

A. What is the interpretation of X-rays of chest?
B. In which mediastinum the shadow is seen in lateral view of chest X-ray?
C. What are the normal anatomical contents in the mediastinum in which opacity is seen in lateral view?
D. What are the possibilities with these shadows in X-rays of chest?

Q-6. What are probable possibilities in different patterns of cough as shown in below picture?

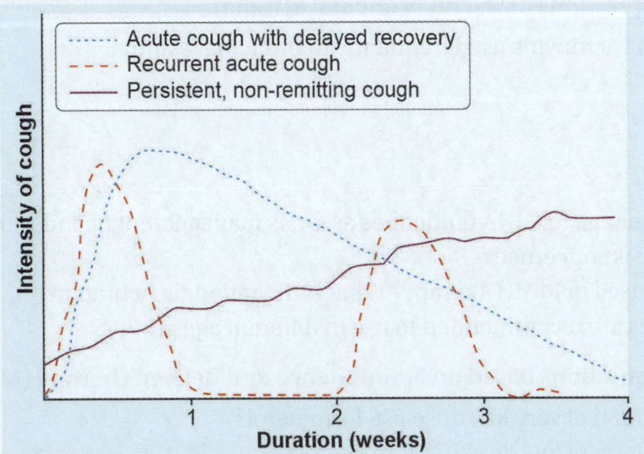

A. Acute cough with delayed recovery
B. Recurrent acute cough
C. Persistent, non-remitting cough

Q-7. A 9-month-old child was referred for recurrent pneumonia which gets resolved with antibiotics. There was also history of recurrent vomiting. Further evaluation was as shown in following picture:

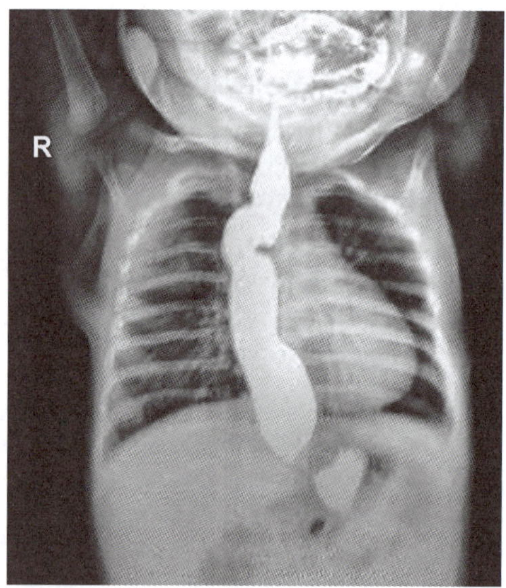

A. Name the investigation performed.
B. What are the findings?
C. What is probable diagnosis?
D. What are the common symptoms of this disease?
E. What is the treatment of this disorder?

Q-8. A 2-year-old girl presents with fever, cough and fast breathing. The respiratory rate is 70/min. The child has subcostal and intercostal indrawing. She is lethargic and not taking feeds.

A. What is probable diagnosis?
B. What are cut-off values of respiratory rate for tachypnea at different age groups?
C. What are the signs of increased work of breathing?
D. What is the classification of severity of this disease as per acute respiratory tract infection (ARTI) control program?

Q-9. Answer the following questions based on bronchial asthma:

A. Expand the following acronyms used frequently in bronchial asthma:
   - GINA
   - ICS
   - MART
   - ART
B. What is the recent change in GINA guidelines as far as management of children between 6 and 11 years with intermittent wheeze is concerned?
C. What are the drugs used in MART therapy? What is the rationale behind it?
D. What inhaler devices are recommended to use in different age groups?

Q-10. Answer the following questions based on Maintenance and Reliver Therapy (MART).

A. What is the composition of very low dose ICS formoterol?
B. What is the composition of low dose ICS formoterol?
C. What is the maximum dose of ICS formoterol in adolescents when used as reliver?
D. What is the maximum dose of ICS-formoterol in children 6–11 years when used as reliver?

Q-11. Name and elaborate the components of scoring system for acute tonsillitis.

Q-12. A 6-year-old girl was brought with complaints of fever and persistent cough of 4 weeks duration. Mother also noted loss of weight. The father is on antituberculous drugs since 4 months for pulmonary tuberculosis.

A. What is your presumptive diagnosis?
B. What are the points for presumptive diagnosis in this child?
C. What is tuberculous contact?
D. What initial specific investigations would you perform in this case?

Q-13. A 12-year-old girl presented with complaints of mouth-breathing, snoring and decreased attention with deteriorating school performance. On clinical examination, she was obese, having short neck and some craniofacial abnormalities.

A. What is probable diagnosis?
B. What are the symptoms and signs of this disorder?
C. What is the scoring system for tonsillar size?
D. What investigation should be performed in this patient for confirmation of diagnosis?
E. What is the management of this disease?
F. What are the criteria for tonsillectomy?

Q-14. Name and elaborate components of scoring system for acute croup.

Q-15. A 6-month-old child presented with recurrent lower respiratory tract infections, chronic diarrhea with sticky, offensive stools, failure to thrive. There was history of one sibling death at the age of 1 year due to similar illness. Clinical examination showed FTT, multiple vitamin deficiencies and dehydration. Investigations showed hyponatremia, hypokalemia, hypochloremia and metabolic alkalosis. It was diagnosed as Bartter syndrome by previous consultant. Urinary electrolytes were within normal limits.

A. What is this syndrome with metabolic alkalosis and electrolytes derangements, but urinary electrolytes normal?
B. What is most probable diagnosis in this patient?
C. What are the diagnostic tests for this disease?
D. Which newborn screening test can make one to suspect this disorder?

Q-16. A 10-year-old child came in OPD with complaints of fever, purulent nasal discharge, more on left side, nasal block and headache. Clinical examination elicited maxillary sinus tenderness. X-ray of paranasal sinuses was as below:

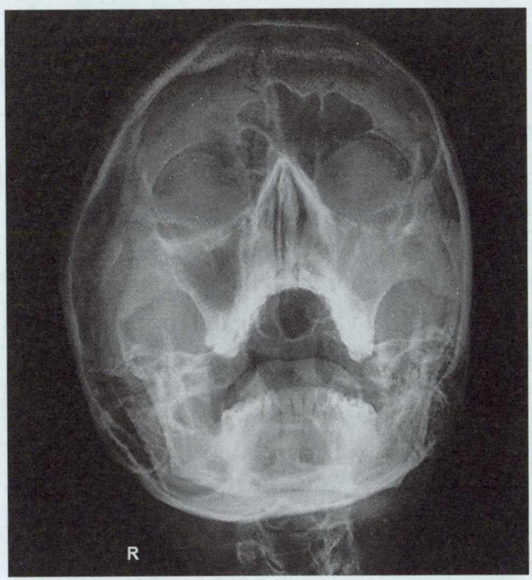

A. What are the findings on this X-ray?
B. What is the diagnosis?
C. What are common bacterial infections causing this disease?
D. What fungal infection in this disease are known to occur with intracranial extension?
E. What are predisposing factors for fungal infection in this disorder?

Q-17. Answer the full forms of acronyms commonly used in the practice.

A. Explain the full form of acronyms commonly used in the practice.
- CT
- HRCT
- CECT
- MDCT

B. What are the indications of various CT thorax modalities in children?
- CT thorax
- HRCT
- CECT
- MDCT

Q-18. A 10-year-old boy came with purulent nasal discharge, nasal block for 10 days and headache 4 days. On examination, there was maxillary sinus tenderness on both sides.

A. What is the diagnosis?
B. What is the classification of sinusitis based on duration?
C. What is the choice of antibiotics in uncomplicated mild-to-moderate acute bacterial sinusitis?
D. What is the age for development of various paranasal sinuses?

Q-19. Answer the following questions on pneumonia:

A. Define persistent pneumonia.
B. Define recurrent pneumonia.
C. Conditions presenting as persistent pneumonia.
D. Conditions presenting as recurrent pneumonia.
E. What is walking pneumonia?

ANSWERS

A-1. A. Right midzone and lower zone opacity suggesting pneumonia
B. CT thorax shows right side opacity with multiple air-filled spaces, suggesting pneumonia with necrosis of lung tissues, replaced by air filled cavities
C. Necrotizing pneumonia
D. *Staphylococcus aureus, Klebsiella pneumoniae, Acinetobacter*, etc.
E. Antibiotics and surgical intervention like video-assisted thoracoscopy (VATS)
F. MRSA is most common organism, leukopenia indicates liberating PVL toxin. Therefore, antibiotics of choice should be vancomycin and clindamycin.

A-2. A. Bilateral choanal atresia
B.
- Passing a firm catheter through each nostril may not be possible beyond 3–4 cm in the nasopharynx.
- Fiberoptic rhinoscopy may show atretic plate.

C. *Associated conditions:*
- CHARGE (Coloboma, Heart defects, Atresia choanae—Choanal atresia, Growth retardation, Genital abnormalities and Ear anomalies) syndrome
- Treacher–Collins syndrome
- Kallmann syndrome
- VATER (Vertebral defects, Imperforate anus, Tracheoesophageal fistula, and renal defects) syndrome

A-3. A. A radiopaque foreign body is seen in the right nostril. It is rounded in shape, may be a coin or a button cell.

B. Unilateral blood-stained nasal discharge may be due to:
- Foreign body
- Nasal diphtheria
- Congenital syphilis
- Epistaxis from Little's area

C. Right nasal radiopaque foreign body

D. To remove with forceps and nasal specula by an ENT surgeon

A-4. A. Bilateral choanal atresia

B. CHARGE

Coloboma, Heart disease, Atresia choanae, Retarded growth and development, or CNS anomalies or both, Genital anomalies or hypogonadism or both and ear anomalies or deafness or both

C.
- Fiberoptic rhinoscopy
- CT scan

D. Transnasal repair

A-5. A.
- X-ray chest PA view shows a homogeneous opacity in right upper zone, air bronchogram is not seen.
- Lateral view of chest X-ray shows, opacity in posterior mediastinum

B. Posterior mediastinum

C. Normal anatomical structures in posterior mediastinum:
- Thoracic duct
- Descending thoracic aorta
- Veins
- Sympathetic chains
- Spinal column
- Nerve roots

D. Pathological conditions known to occur in posterior mediastinum:
- Neuroblastoma
- Neurofibroma
- Neurilemmoma
- Ganglioneuroma

A-6. A. Viral upper respiratory tract infection like adenovirus, respiratory syncytial virus, etc.

B. Bronchial asthma, hyper-reactive airway disease

C. Tuberculosis

A-7. A. *Barium study:* Esophagogram

B. Gross dilatation of esophagus with narrowing at lower end

C. Achalasia cardia

D. *Common symptoms of achalasia cardia:*
- Non-bilious vomiting

- Recurrent lower respiratory tract infections due to aspiration
- Failure to thrive

E. *Management of achalasia cardia:*
- Medical management with oral medicines like nitrates, calcium-channel blockers and *S. phosphodiesterase* inhibitors for temporary relief of symptoms
- *Surgical management:* Heller's myotomy with anti-reflux procedure.

A-8. A. Severe pneumonia

B. Tachypnea for different age groups
- *0 to 2 months:* >60/min
- 2 months to 1 year: >50/min
- 2 to 5 years: >40/min
- >5 years: >30/min

C. *Signs of increased work of breathing:*
- Tachypnea
- Chest retractions (subcostal/intercostal/suprasternal)
- Use of accessory muscles of respiration (sternocleidomastoid)
- Various sounds (wheezing/stridor/grunting)
- Tracheal tug (inward movement of trachea during inspiration)
- Flaring of alae nasi
- Head bobbing
- Cyanosis

D. *Classification of severity of pneumonia as per ARI program:*
- *No pneumonia:* Cough–cold, no fast breathing
- *Pneumonia:* Fast breathing as per criteria for tachypnea, with or without indrawing
- *Severe pneumonia:*
  - Tachypnea
  - Lower chest indrawing
  - Unable to drink or breastfeed
  - Lethargy
  - Cyanosis
  - Convulsions
  - Unconscious

A-9. A. *Expand acronyms used in bronchial asthma:*
- *GINA:* Global Initiative for Asthma
- *ICS:* Inhaled Corticosteroid
- *MART:* Maintenance and Reliever Therapy
- *ART:* Anti-inflammatory Reliever Therapy

B. Give ICS whenever inhaled short-acting beta agonist is given" is the recent and very important change.

C.
- *MART therapy:* Use of inhaled steroid combination with long- acting beta 2 agonist formoterol in the same pressurized meter dose canister is MART therapy.
- Other long-acting beta 2 agonists do not have shorter time of onset of action like formoterol and hence MART therapy is always only with formoterol with ICS in the same canister.

D. *Inhaler devices and their use in different age groups:*
- *Up to 3 years:* PMDI + Spacer + facemask or nebulizer
- *4 to 6 years:* PMDI + Spacer +/– facemask
- *>6 years:* PMDI +/– Spacer or dry powder inhaler

A-10. A. *Very low dose:* Formoterol 6 μg + 100 μg ICS either budesonide or beclomethasone

B. *Low dose:* Formoterol 6 μg + 200 μg of ICS either budesonide or beclomethasone

C. *MART—reliever in adolescents:* Maximum 12 doses/day

D. *MART—reliever in children 6–11 years:* Maximum 8 doses/day

A-11.

Criteria	*Points*
Age 3–14 years	1
Tonsillar swelling or exudate	1
Tender/Swollen anterior cervical lymph nodes	1
Fever (Temperature/38°C–100.4°F)	1
Absence of cough	1

- The Centor score assesses the likelihood of Group A *Streptococcus* (GAS) bacterial infection in tonsillitis by assigning 1 point for each of the clinical criteria.
- The clinical criteria for centor score are fever, tonsillar, exudate, tender anterior cervical lymphadenopathy and absence of cough.
- Centor score of 3 or 4 suggests a higher probability (40–60%) of bacterial infection and warrants further investigation or treatment.
- Centor scores of 0, 1, 2 indicate a low probability of bacterial infection and should be given symptomatic treatment.

A-12. A. Tuberculosis

B. *Points for presumptive tuberculosis:*

- Persistent, documented fever of more than 2 weeks duration without a known cause
- Unremittent cough for more than 2 weeks
- Significant weight loss. It is defined as more than 5% weight loss compared to highest recorded in last 3 months despite adequate nutrition, or failure to gain weight in last 3 months.

C. Tuberculous contact is defined as contact with a person with any form of active tuberculosis within last 2 years.

D. Chest X-ray

A-13. A. Obstructive sleep apnea (OSA)

B. *Symptoms and signs of OSA:*

- Habitual snoring (≥3 nights/weeks)
- Restless sleep
- Excessive sweating
- Hyperextended neck during sleeping
- Observed episodes of apnea
- Mouth-breathing
- Headache
- Recurrent ear infections
- Learning problems
- Obesity
- Adenoidal faces
- Tonsillar hypertrophy
- Craniofacial anomalies

C. *Mallampati scoring for tonsillar size:*
- *Tonsil 0:* Tonsils fit within tonsillar fossa
- *Tonsil 1+:* Tonsils <25% of space between the pillars of oropharyngeal width
- *Tonsil 2+:* Tonsils <50% of space between the pillars of oropharyngeal width
- *Tonsil 3+:* Tonsils <75% of space between the pillars of oropharyngeal width
- *Tonsil 4+:* Tonsils >75% of space between the pillars of oropharyngeal width

D. Investigation for OSA is polysomnography (PSG). It is noninvasive test involving the measurements of a number of physiologic functions overnight including EEG, pulse oximetry, oronasal airflow, abdominal and chest movements, partial pressure of carbon dioxide and video recording.

PSG will demonstrate not only the presence or absence of OSA, but also its severity.

E. *Management of OSA:*
- Adenotonsillectomy
- Non-invasive positive pressure ventilation CPAP or BAPP
- Supplemental oxygen
- Craniofacial reconstructive procedures
- Weight loss in a case of obesity
- Intranasal corticosteroids or leukotriene modifier therapy

F. *Paradise criteria for tonsillectomy:*
- Minimum frequency of sore throat episodes 7 or more episodes in the preceding year (OR)
- 5 or more episodes in each of the preceding 2 years (OR)
- 3 or more episodes in each of the preceding 3 years

Clinical features (sore throat + presence of one or more qualifies as a counting episode)
- Temperature >38°C (OR)
- Cervical lymphadenopathy (tender lymph node or >2 cm) (OR)
- Tonsillar exudate (OR)
- Positive culture for group A beta-hemolytic streptococci

Treatment: Antibiotics administered in conventional dosage for proved or suspected streptococcal episodes

Documentation:
- Each episode and its qualifying features substantiated by contemporaneous notation in a clinical record (OR)
- If not fully documented, subsequent observance by the clinician of 2 episodes of throat infection with patterns of frequency and clinical features consistent with the initial history
- Sleep apnea due to adeno tonsillar hypertrophy

A-14. Westley Croup scoring system

Symptom	***Score***
Level of consciousness:	
• Normal (including sleep)	0
• Disoriented	5
Cyanosis:	
• None	0
• Cyanosis with agitation	4
• Cyanosis at rest	5
Stridor:	
• None	0
• When agitated	1
• At rest	2

Contd...

Contd...

Symptom	*Score*
Air entry:	
• Normal	0
• Decreased	1
• Markedly decreased	2
Retractions:	
• None	0
• Mild	1
• Moderate	2
• Severe	3

- *Scores ≤2:* Mild croup
- *Scores 3 to 7:* Moderate croup
- *Scores ≥8:* Severe croup

A-15. A. Pseudo-Bartter syndrome
B. Cystic fibrosis
C.
- Sweat chloride test. Sweat chloride more than 60 mEq/L is diagnostic.
- Genetic study for mutation

D. Immunoreactive trypsin is newborn screening test for cystic fibrosis

A-16. A. Opacification is seen on left maxillary sinus
B. Acute left side maxillary sinusitis
C. Common bacterial infections for sinusitis
- *Streptococcus pneumoniae*
- *Hemophilus influenzae*
- *Moraxella catarrhalis*

D. Common fungal sinusitis is due to *Aspergillus* and mucor, it is known to cause intracranial extension.
E. Predisposing conditions for fungal sinusitis are diabetes mellitus, immunosuppressive therapy, malignancy, bone marrow transplantation, etc.

A-17. A. *Acronyms related to CT scan:*
- *CT:* Computed tomography
- *HRCT:* High-resolution computed tomography
- *CECT:* Contrast-enhanced computed tomography
- *MDCT:* Multi-detector computed tomography

B. *Indications of various CT Thorax modalities in pediatrics:*
- *CT thorax:* Interstitial lung disease, cystic fibrosis, lung abscess, bronchiectasis, bronchiolitis obliterans
- *HRCT thorax:* Diffuse interstitial lung disease, bronchiectasis, cystic fibrosis, chronic airway disease
- *CECT thorax:* Necrotizing pneumonia, lung abscess, cystic fibrosis, Interstitial lung disease, tumor or mass
- *MDCT thorax:* Airway abnormalities, pulmonary arterial hypertension, Thoracic aortic abnormalities, foreign body aspiration

A-18. A. Acute bilateral maxillary sinusitis
B. Classification of sinusitis based on duration
- *Acute:* <30 days
- *Subacute:* 1–3 months
- *Chronic:* >3 months

C. Amoxicillin 40–50 mg/kg/day for 2 weeks

D.

- Maxillary and ethmoid sinus are present at birth.
- Sphenoidal sinus develops at 3–5 years of age.
- Frontal sinus develops at 7–8 years of age

A-19. A. Persistent pneumonia is defined as persistent of symptoms and radiographic abnormalities in a child with lower respiratory tract infection for more than a month despite a course of adequate antibiotic therapy.

B. Recurrent pneumonia is defined as at least two distinct episodes of radiologically established pneumonia within the same year or three or more such episodes over any period of time. There must be complete resolution of clinical and radiological findings between episodes.

C. *Persistent pneumonia:*

- Cystic fibrosis
- Tuberculosis
- Bronchiectasis
- Structural lung abnormalities like bronchogenic cyst, pulmonary sequestration, etc.

D. *Recurrent pneumonia:*

- Cystic fibrosis
- Immune deficiency disorders
- Congenital anomaly like agenesis of lung
- Foreign body in airways

E. *Mycoplasma pneumonia* is also called as walking pneumonia.

CHAPTER 15

Cardiology

QUESTIONS

Q-1. Medical treatment of cyanotic spell in a case of Fallot's tetrad.

Q-2. Prophylaxis for prevention of recurrence of rheumatic fever.

Q-3. An 8-year-old boy was brought for upper respiratory symptoms and was diagnosed as adenoiditis. His pulse examination showed some significant problem. His ECG is as follows:

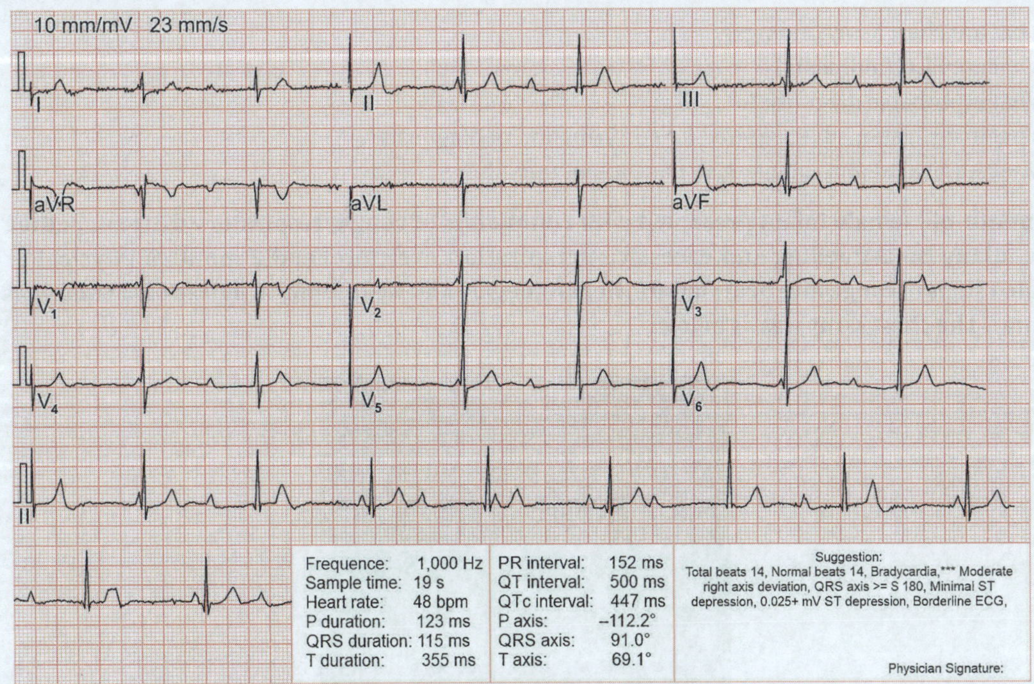

A. What are the ECG findings?
B. What is the diagnosis?
C. What complications can occur in this condition?
D. What treatment should be advised?

Q-4. A 2-month-old male infant was brought with complaints of cough, respiratory distress, restlessness, irritability and perspiration for 1 month. Physical examination revealed signs of heart failure without cardiac murmur and cyanosis. His chest X-ray and ECG were as below:

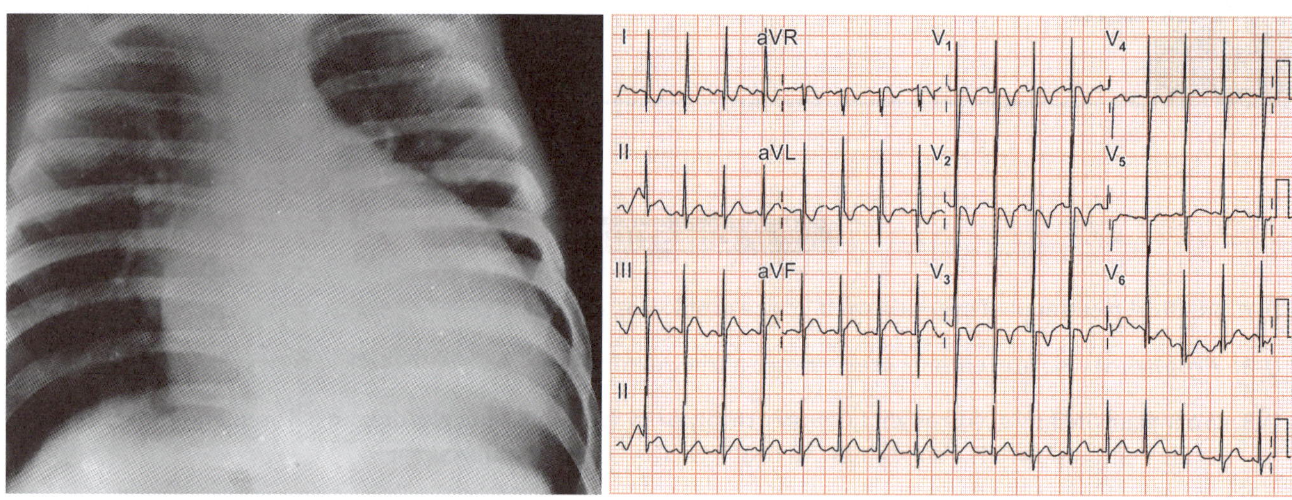

A. What are chest X-ray findings?
B. What are ECG findings?
C. What is probable diagnosis?
D. What investigations are required for confirmation of diagnosis?
E. What surgical treatment may give permanent remedy?

Q-5. A 4-month-old female infant presented with complaints of cough, respiratory distress, getting exhausted while taking breastfeeding and excessive perspiration over forehead 2 months. Physical examination revealed signs of congestive heart failure, hepatomegaly and weak femoral pulsations. There was no cardiac murmur. The chest X-ray was as below:

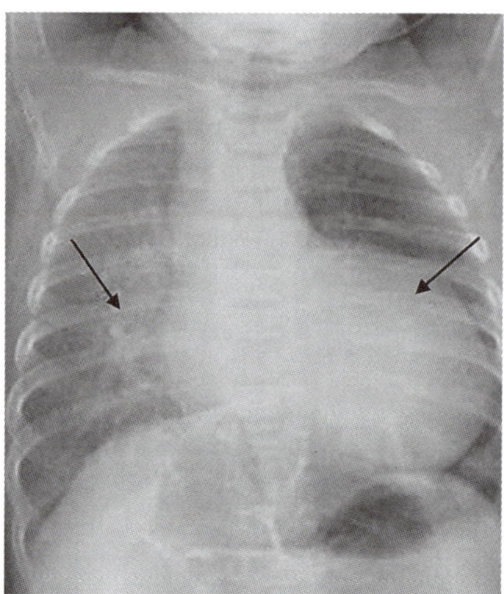

A. What are the chest X-ray findings?
B. What is the probable diagnosis?
C. What investigations can confirm the diagnosis?
D. What treatment can be lifesaving in a neonate with severe condition?
E. What invasive procedure may offer remedial solution?

Q-6. These nodules were found over occiput in a 12-year-old boy suffering from acquired heart disease.

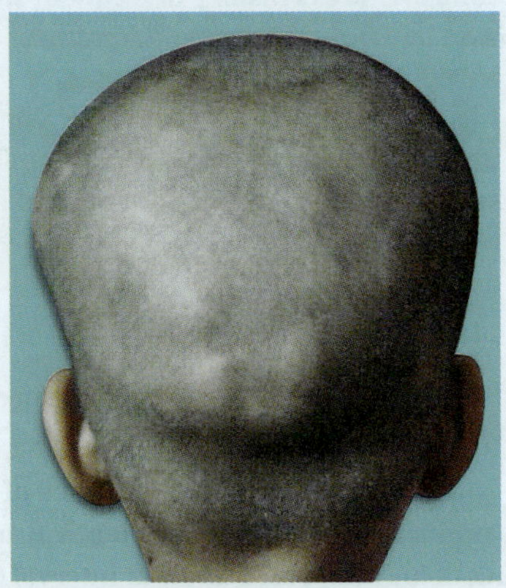

A. What do you call it?
B. In which disease, they are found?
C. What is the clinical description of these lesions?
D. What is the importance of their presence in this condition?

Q-7. A patient of acute renal failure presented with generalized weakness and irregular pulse. An urgent ECG was performed.

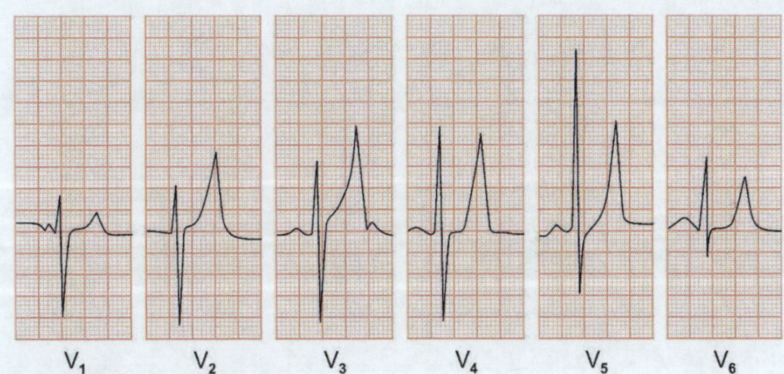

A. Describe ECG abnormality.
B. What does it suggest?
C. What are other ECG changes of the condition?
D. Mention the line of treatment.

Q-8.

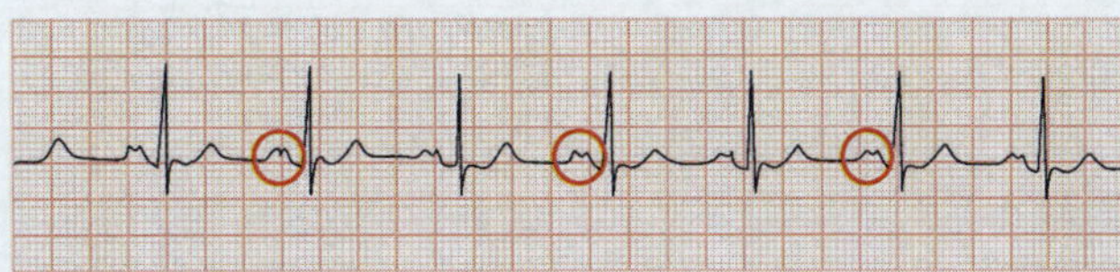

A. Name the ECG abnormality.
B. What does it indicate?
C. What are other ECG criteria for its diagnosis?

Q-9. A 7-year-old boy presented with history of sudden-onset giddiness and fall with transient loss of consciousness and recovers within few seconds. There is history of frequent such episodes. His clinical examination was normal. His ECG was as below:

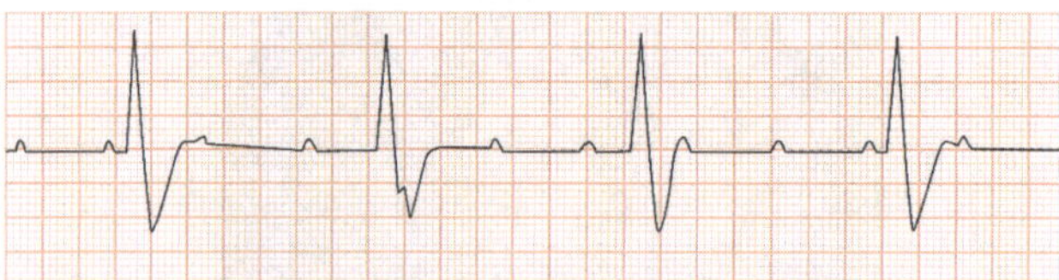

A. What is the diagnosis?
B. What is the drug of choice for this condition?
C. What are two non-pharmacological treatment options?

Q-10. A 10-year-old boy was brought with history of multiple episodes of transient unconsciousness and falls, MRI brain and EEG reported as normal. He was on antiepileptic drugs with diagnosis of clinical epilepsy. There was history of sudden death of his father and uncle at interval of 2 years, presumed to be myocardial infarction. His clinical examination was noncontributory. His ECG recording was as follows:

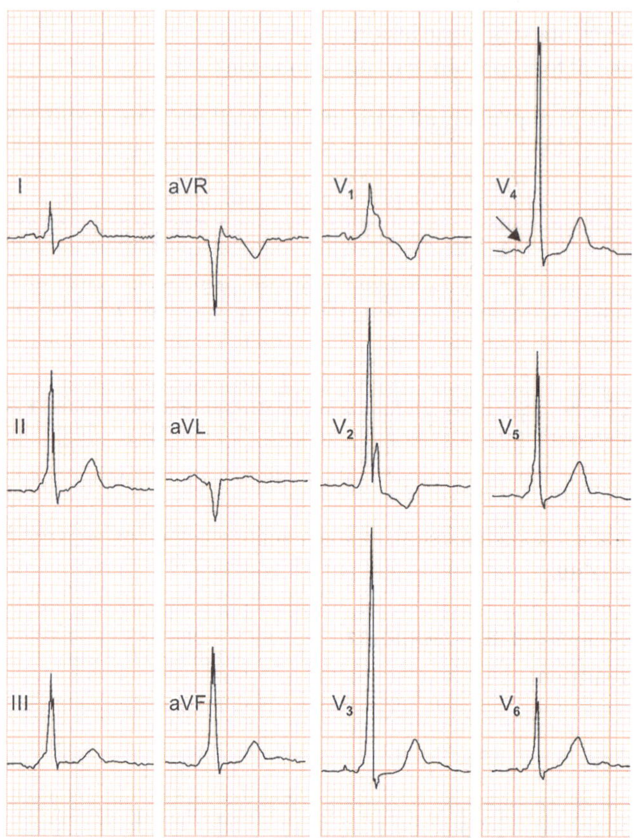

A. What are ECG findings?
B. What is probable diagnosis?
C. What is the basic defect in this condition?
D. Which drugs should be avoided in this disease?
E. What is the long-term treatment of this disorder?

Q-11. A 3-day-old neonate is brought with cyanosis and hyperpnea and acidotic breathing. Clinical examination revealed single second heart sound and no sign of cardiac failure. Chest X-ray showed oligemic lung field and ECG was as follows:

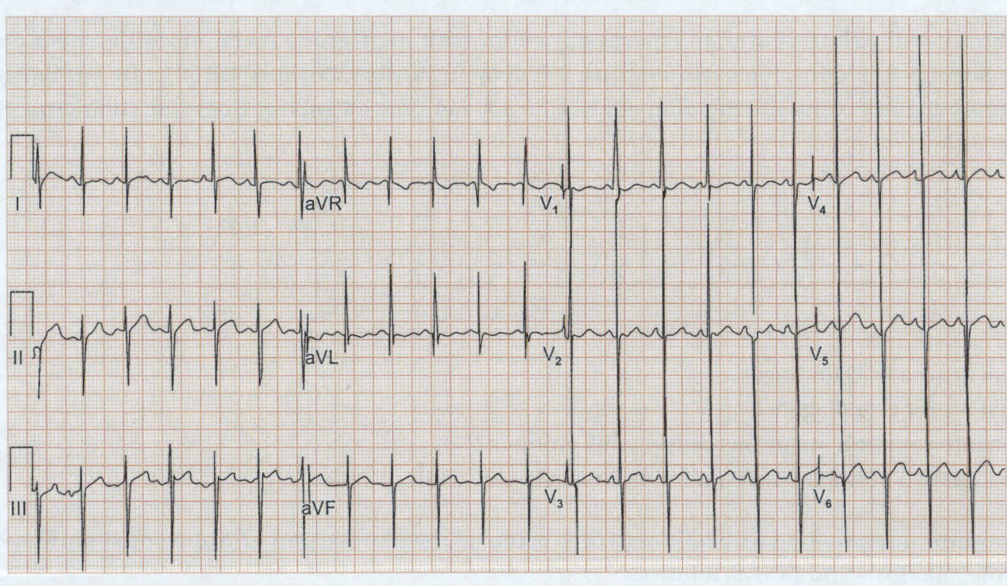

A. What are ECG findings?
B. What is probable diagnosis?
C. What drug may be lifesaving in this disorder in a neonate presenting at birth with severe cyanosis and low arterial oxygen saturation? What is the dose of drug?

Q-12. A resident doctor found significant bradycardia in a neonate on routine examination. The baby was asymptomatic. Echocardiography excluded any structural heart defect. The ECG of baby was as follows. On further work-up, it was confirmed due to some maternal illness.

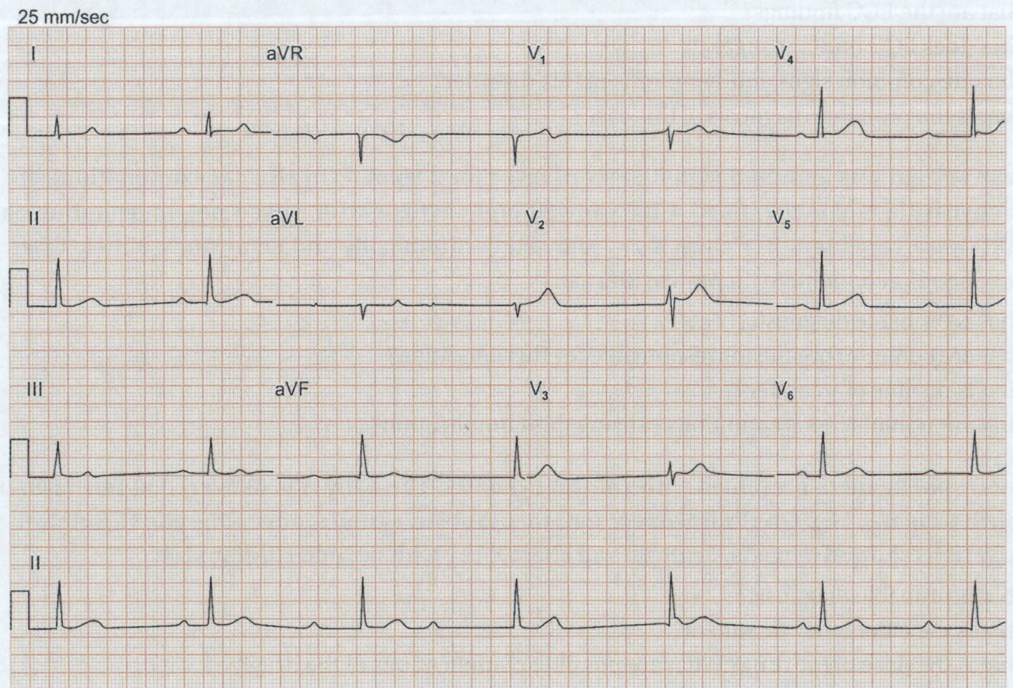

A. What are the ECG findings?
B. What is the probable maternal illness responsible for this cardiac problem in a baby?
C. What cardiac management may be required in such babies in further?

Q-13. A 20-month-old girl presented to emergency room with high-grade fever, breathlessness and excessive crying. She was fully conscious, temperature 103°F, tachycardia (220/min) RR 60/min, muffled heart sounds and engorged neck veins and hepatomegaly. Chest X-ray showed enlarged cardiac silhouette. ECG findings were as follows:

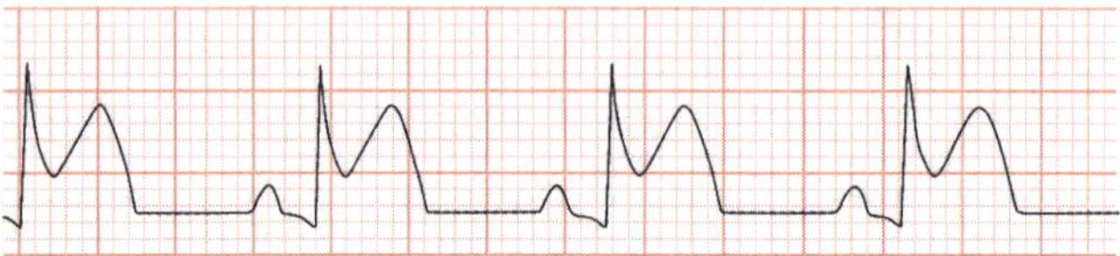

A. What are the ECG findings?
B. What is probable diagnosis?
C. What are common organisms causing this problem?
D. Mention two non-infective conditions known to cause this disorder.

Q-14. A 18-month-boy presented with failure to thrive, muscle weakness, polyuria and constipation. ABG showed metabolic alkalosis and ECG as follows:

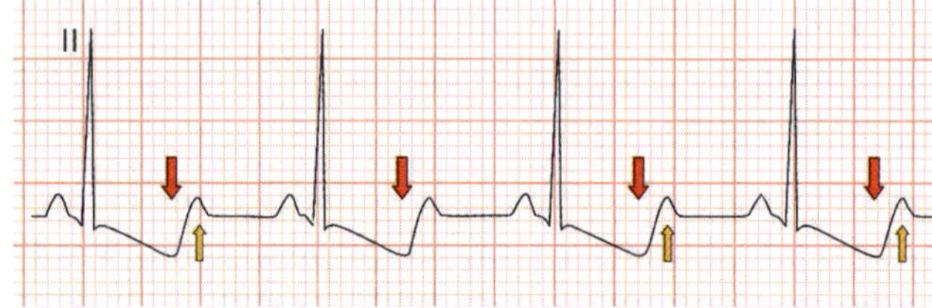

A. What are the ECG findings?
B. What does ECG findings suggest?
C. What are common signs and symptoms of this disorder?
D. What is the probable diagnosis of this case?

Q-15. A 5-year-old girl was admitted with history of fever for 2 weeks. On clinical examination, she was febrile, had tachycardia and tachypnoea. CBC showed leukocytosis with raised polymorphonuclear cells. ESR and CRP were very high. Her chest X-ray showed cardiomegaly and echo study of heart was reported as heterogeneous echogenicity in pericardial sac.

A. What is probable diagnosis?
B. What are common organisms responsible for this condition?
C. What is the line of treatment?
D. What are noninfectious conditions causing this complication?

Q-16. A 70-hour-old neonate presented with central cyanosis. The baby was delivered at full-term uneventfully with birth weight 3.2 kg. On clinical examination, cyanosis, systolic murmur grade II, Single S_2 were noted. Investigations showed hypoxia, acidosis and chest X-ray with normal cardiac size.

A. What is probable diagnosis?
B. What is the emergency treatment?
C. What is the dose of the drug? What are possible complications of the drug?

Q-17. Match the following:

A. Down syndrome	Supravalvular aortic stenosis
B. Turner syndrome	Hypertrophic cardiomyopathy
C. Marfan syndrome	AVSD
D. William syndrome	Coarctation of aorta
E. Tuberous sclerosis	Dissecting aneurysm
F. Pompe disease	Aortic arch anomaly
G. DiGeorge syndrome	Cardiac rhabdomyoma

Q-18. A 12-year-old boy has bicuspid aortic valve, detected in early childhood incidentally. He is referred for persistent fever of 4 weeks duration and fatigue off and on, routine investigations did not reveal any diagnosis, persistent leukocytosis and raised acute phase reactants.

A. What is most probable diagnosis?
B. What are clinical manifestations of this condition?
C. What investigations should be performed to confirm the diagnosis?
D. What are most common organisms responsible for this disease?
E. What treatment regimen is ideal?

Q-19. A 13-year-old boy presented with exertional dyspnea. He was diagnosed to have some congenital heart disease in his infancy, but did not follow advice of a pediatrician for further evaluation and management. Parents ignored the problem. On examination, bluish discoloration was noted at toes, oxygen saturation was 97% in upper limbs and 80% in lower limbs. P_2 was loud and early diastolic murmur was noted in pulmonary area. His chest X-ray was as below:

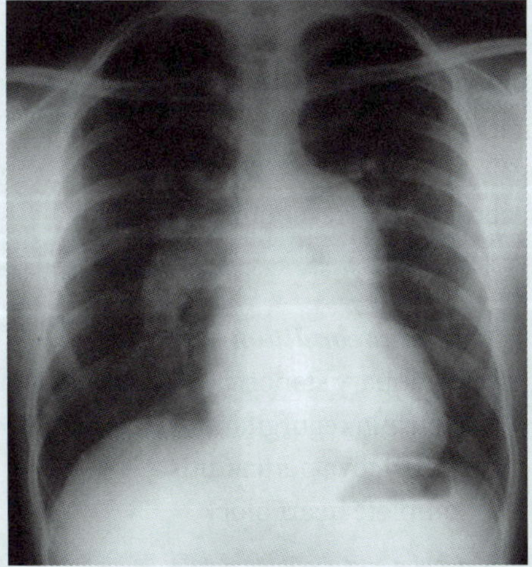

A. What is the explanation for quite significant difference in oxygen saturation in upper limbs and lower limbs? Give another example where upper limbs are cyanosed and lower limbs pink.
B. What does P_2 loud suggest?
C. What are the X-ray findings?
D. What is the probable diagnosis?

Q-20. Match the following:

Heart sounds	***Possible cardiac disease***
A. Loud S_1	Pulmonary valve stenosis
B. Loud P_2	Mitral stenosis

C. Soft P_2	Pulmonary hypertension
D. Reversed splitting of S_2	Aortic regurgitation
E. Soft S_1	Thyrotoxicosis
F. S_3	Aortic stenosis

Q-21. Answer the following questions pertaining to ventricular septal defect (VSD).

A. What are types of VSD?

B. What factors make a child vulnerable to develop recurrent lower respiratory tract infections and pneumonias?

C. What is the classification VSD based on its size?

D. What is the timing of VSD closure as per its size?

Q-22. True or false for physiological (innocent) murmurs:

A. May be associated with thrill.

B. More common in infants who are small for their gestational age.

C. Heard hardly in children.

D. Changes in intensity and quality with position of the child.

Q-23. A 3-week-old baby was brought with complaints of refusal of feeds for 2 days and breathlessness for 1 day. Baby was delivered by LSCS and was given to mother for breastfeeding soon after birth. Baby and mother were discharged after 4 days. Birth weight was 2.4 kg. On clinical examination, general condition of baby was poor with mild subcostal indrawing. Heart rate was 170/min, RR 70/min, capillary refill time was more than 3 seconds. Femoral and dorsalis pedis pulsations were very weak. Soles were dusky in color. Right upper limb NIBP was 84/62 mm of Hg. Capillary blood glucose was 82 mg/dL. It was diagnosed as shock, started IV saline boluses 5 mL/kg. Still, there was no improvement, dorsalis pedis very weak and enlargement of liver.

A. What is probable diagnosis?

B. Why is there sudden deterioration in this baby at 3 weeks of age?

C. Which drug can be lifesaving?

D. Name structural cardiac defects that can present in this way?

Q-24. Match the following:

JVP abnormality	*Cardiac condition*
A. Canon ‘a’ wave	Pulmonary stenosis
B. Giant ‘a’ wave	Tricuspid regurgitation
C. Large ‘v’ wave	Constrictive pericarditis
D. Steep ‘y’ descent	Complete heart block

Q-25. A 7-week-old baby was referred with complaints of breathlessness for 1 week, difficulty in taking breastfeeding for 3 days. The baby was also not gaining the weight. There was no history of fever or cough-cold. Antenatal and natal periods were uneventful, was delivered by LSCS and birth weight was 2.8 kg. On clinical examination, HR 170/min, RR 70/min and SpO_2 98% in room air. BP was normal and perfusion was good. Systolic murmur noted at left lower parasternal area, grade IV/VI. Chest X-ray showed cardiomegaly with plethoric lung fields. Echo cardiography was performed.

A. What is probable diagnosis?

B. What are differential diagnosis with structural cardiac lesions?

C. What is the initial immediate line of treatment of this baby?

D. What cardiac defects having similar clinical presentation, do not manifest at this age?

Q-26. A 5-year-old boy was brought for second booster doses of vaccines. While examining, grade 2 systolic ejection murmur was noted clearly in second intercostal space (ICS) on left side.

A. What are differential diagnosis?
B. What are auscultatory findings in a case of ASD?
C. What are types of ASD?
D. What are characteristic ECG changes in ASD?
E. Which associated conditions should be ruled out in children with ASD and moderate-to-severe pulmonary hypertension?

Q-27. A baby was delivered at hospital by normal vaginal route at 36 weeks following labor pain, cried soon after birth and birth weight was 2.450 kg. Antenatal period was uneventful. Mother noted fast breathing and mild retractions at about 7 hours of life. The treating pediatrician performed chest X-ray with possibility of hyaline membrane disease. Chest X-ray was as below. Baby was treated with surfactant therapy along with supportive therapy. However, baby's condition did not improve and baby was intubated. SpO_2 did not pick up and remained at 82% despite FiO_2 >90%.

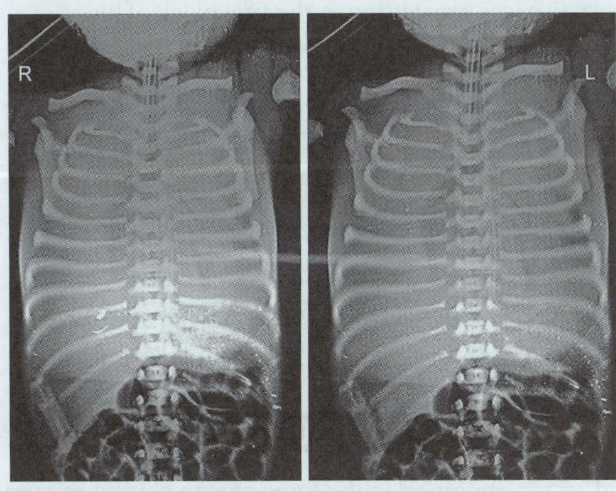

A. What are the chest X-ray findings?
B. What cardiac condition should be suspected in a given scenario, if patient does not improve and X-ray findings remain the same after surfactant therapy?
C. What are respiratory and cardiac differential diagnosis in newborns with this type of X-ray findings?
D. What should be next action of a treating pediatrician?
E. What is the definite management of this patient, if suspected cardiac lesion is confirmed?
F. What drugs are contraindicated in this cardiac anomaly?

Q-28. A term infant was referred for sudden development of cardiac failure on 8th day of life. The baby was pink, pulses were collapsing and noncardiac murmur. Chest X-ray showed cardiomegaly. Echo study of heart was reported as normal heart, normal great vessels and PDA closed.

A. What is most probable diagnosis?
B. What are other manifestations of this condition?
C. What investigations can confirm the diagnosis?
D. What are treatment options available?

Q-29. A 5-day-old boy is on ventilatory support. He was born at 31 weeks gestations uneventfully. His birth weight was 1.8 kg. He has continuous murmur, bounding peripheral pulses and hyperdynamic precordium. Echo study of heart revealed large patent ductus arteriosus (PDA) without any other associated cardiac anomaly.

A. What clinical manifestations would make one to think PDA?
B. What are the complications of PDA?
C. What is pharmacological closure of PDA, medication and dosage?

Q-30. A term infant was delivered uneventfully with birth weight of 3.8 kg. The baby developed cyanosis after 2 hours of birth. The clinical examination showed central cyanosis, heart rate 160/min and respiratory rate 60/min, SpO_2 70% in the right hand and 75% in the foot with 100% FiO_2 via hood oxygen therapy. There was no murmur. Chest X-ray was normal.

A. What is probable diagnosis?
B. What are differential?
C. Describe hyperoxia test.
D. What are the causes of differential cyanosis and reversed differential cyanosis?

Q-31. The resident doctor noticed one-day-old baby dusky during breastfeeding. He started oxygen via nasal canula and after 3 hours, the baby developed tachypnea. On clinical examination, HR 170 beats/min, RR 76/min and BP on right arm 50/30 mm of Hg. Right leg BP 54/32 mm of Hg and SpO_2 90% on oxygen. Echo study of heart confirmed hypoplastic left heart syndrome (HLHS).

A. Describe clinical examination findings of CVS?
B. What was wrong in management of this patient?
C. Mention congenital heart diseases presenting in the first week of life
D. What is the emergency management of this patient?

Q-32. What are the components of following variable of tetralogy of Fallot (TOF)?

A. Tetralogy of Fallot
B. Pentalogy of Fallot
C. Pink TOF
D. Trilogy of Fallot
E. Diology of Fallot
F. Monology of Fallot

Q-33. Explain the following clinical signs in cardiovascular system.

A. Tapping apex beat
B. Heaving apex beat
C. Hyperdynamic apex beat
D. Double impulse

ANSWERS

A-1.
- Patient should be placed on the abdomen in the knee chest position or over the shoulder of mother in the case of an infant.
- Administration of oxygen
- Injection morphine 0.2 mg/kg by subcutaneous route or injection ketamine 3–5 mg/kg/dose by intramuscular route
- Injection sodium bicarbonate 1–2 mL/kg, 1:1 dilution IV
- Injection propranolol 0.2 mg/kg IV
- Correction of hypovolemia (10 mL/kg DNS)
- Keep the child warm
- PCV SOS (If Hb <12 g/dL)
- Monitoring for heart rate and blood pressure
- Vasopressors and mechanical ventilation SOS

A-2. Benzathine penicillin (Penidure-LA) 1.2 million units IM at interval of 3 weeks in children with weight >30 kg and 0.6 million units IM at interval of 3 weeks in children with weight <30 kg.

OR

Penicillin V 250 mg twice orally

OR

Sulfadiazine 500 mg twice orally, if weight is >30 kg or 250 mg twice orally if weight is <30 kg

OR

Erythromycin 250 mg twice daily

Duration

- The risk is greater within the first 5 years after primary acute rheumatic fever (ARF). American Heart Association recommends life-time prophylaxis for patients with residual rheumatic heart disease.
- *Practical recommendations are:*
  - For at least 5 years or until the child reaches 18 years whichever is later.
  - For patients of carditis, for 10 years after the last attack or at least until age of 25 years, whichever is longer.
  - More severe valvular diseases or post-valvular surgery for life time.

A-3. A.
- Heart rate is 50/min.
- Atrial contraction and ventricular contractions are independent, autonomous.
- Indicates A–V node block.

B. Complete heart block (third degree heart block)
C. Syncope, hypotension, hemodynamic instability and death
D. Pacemaker implantation

A-4. A. *Chest X-ray:* Cardiomegaly, left ventricular type
B. *ECG changes:* Deep Q waves, inverted 'T' were elevated ST segment
C. Aberrant left coronary artery originating from pulmonary artery (ALCAPA)
D.
- 2D Echo with color Doppler confirms diagnosis in most cases.
- CT or MRI can confirm the origin of coronary artery.

E. Detaching the anomalous coronary artery from the pulmonary artery and anastomosing it to the aorta establish normal myocardial perfusion.

A-5. A. Cardiomegaly and pulmonary congestion
B. Coarctation of aorta
C. Echocardiography, Doppler study may confirm the diagnosis. CT and MRI may require in other cases.
D. Prostaglandin E_1
E.
- Primary angiography
- Primary stent placement

A-6. A. Subcutaneous nodules
B. Acute rheumatic fever
C.
- Nodules of varying in size from pinhead to almond size.
- Nontender
- Common on bony prominences such as shin of tibia, wrist, elbow, knee, ankle, spine and occiput.

D.
- Rheumatic fever with subcutaneous nodules always have carditis.
- Persistence of nodules is associated with chronic carditis.

A-7. A. Tall, peaked, tented T-waves
B. Hyperkalemia
C. ST segment depression
Prolonged P–R interval
Flattening of P wave
Widening of QRS complex
D. 10% calcium gluconate 0.5 to 1 mL per kg diluted IV slowly under cardiac monitoring.

A-8. A. P Mitrale
B. Left atrial hypertrophy
C. Wide and notched P-wave in second lead, biphasic P-wave in V_1, P-wave duration prolonged (>0.1 sec)

A-9. A. Prolonged QT syndrome
B. Propranolol
C.
- Pacemaker
- Implanted defibrillator

A-10. A.
- Short PR interval
- Prolonged QRS complex
- Slurred delta wave

B. Wolf–Parkinson–White syndrome (WPW syndrome)
C. Congenital accessory pathway, also called pre-excitation syndrome
D. Calcium-channel blockers like adenosine and verapamil and betablockers like propranolol should be avoided.
E. Catheter ablation: Radiofrequency ablation

A-11. A.
- Q wave in leads 1 and aVL
- Left axis deviation
- Left ventricular hypertrophy

B. Tricuspid atresia
C. Prostaglandin E1 (PGEI)
Starting dose 0.05 μg/kg/min and gradually reducing to 0.02 μg/kg/min provided desired oxygen saturation is maintained.

A-12. A. Complete heart block (third degree heart block)
B. Systemic lupus erythematosus (SLE)
C. Pacemaker

A-13. A. Low QRS voltage, ST elevation, depression of P-R segment
B. Acute pericardial effusion
C. *Staphylococcus aureus*
Streptococcus pneumoniae
D. Juvenile idiopathic arthritis, SLE, hypothyroidism, uremia

A-14. A.
- ST segment sagging
- T-wave depression
- U-wave elevation

B. Hypokalemia
C.
- Muscle weakness, cramping, fasciculations
- Paralytic ileus
- Hypoventilation and hypotension with severe hypokalemia
- Bartter syndrome

A-15. A. Pericardial effusion (pyopericardium)
B. Common organisms causing pericardial effusion or pyopericardium
- *Bacteria: Staphylococcus aureus, Klebsiella pneumoniae, Streptococcus pneumoniae, E. coli, Salmonella*
- *Viral:* Common in infants by coxsackie virus
- *Mycobacterium tuberculosis*
- *Fungus: Candida* and *Aspergillus*

C. Line of treatment:

- Ceftriaxone and vancomycin for *Staphylococcus aureus*
- ATT for tuberculosis
- Antifungal for fungal infections
- Pericardiocentesis as therapeutic or diagnostic purpose

D. Noninfectious causes for pericardial effusion are hypothyroidism, rheumatological conditions like SLE, JIA, chronic renal failure, malignancies, etc.

A-16. A. Duct-dependent cyanotic heart disease, most common D-TGA with intact interventricular system or pulmonary atresia with intact interventricular septum.

B. IV Prostaglandin E_1 infusion

C. *Dose:* Starting dose 0.05 µg/kg/min IV infusion, titrated dose between 0.01 and 0.1 µg/kg/min based on response. It should be tapered slowly.
Complications: Hypotension, apnea, flushing, bradycardia

A-17. A. *Down syndrome:* AVSD

B. *Turner syndrome:* Coarctation of aorta

C. *Marfan syndrome:* Dissecting aortic aneurysm

D. *William syndrome:* Supravalvular aortic stenosis

E. *Tuberous sclerosis:* Cardiac rhabdomyoma

F. *Pompe disease:* Hypertrophic cardiomyopathy

G. *DiGeorge syndrome:* Aortic arch anomaly

A-18. A. Infective endocarditis (IE)

B. *Clinical manifestations of IE:*
- Fever with chills or rigors, loss of appetite, weight loss, arthralgia, night sweats, malaise and weakness
- Clinical examination of CVS may be normal. One should look for signs of cardiac failure, presence of murmur or development of new murmur.
- Embolic episodes presenting with stroke, hematuria from renal infarct, splenic infarct, GI bleeding
- Regurgitant murmurs due to damage to aortic or mitral valves
- Features of immunological responses like arthralgia, myalgia, clubbing, splenomegaly, microscopic hematuria, splinter hemorrhages, petechiae over skin, Roth spots on eye examination, Osler nodes—tender nodes on pulp of fingers, Janeway lesions—nontender erythematous patches over palms and soles

C.
- *CBC:* Normocytic, normochromic anemia, leukocytosis, thrombocytopenia
- Raised ESR and CRP
- Microscopic hematuria
- *Echocardiography:* Presence of vegetations
- Blood culture may show growth of organisms.

D. *Most common organisms for IE:*
- *Streptococcus viridans*
- *Staphylococcus aureus*
- Rarely fungal endocarditis
- *E. coli* and *Pseudomonas* are rare.

E. *Treatment options for IE:*
- Penicillin/Ceftriaxone + Aminoglycoside (Gentamicin, Amikacin, Streptomycin)
- Cloxacillin/Vancomycin + Aminoglycoside
- Amphotericin B for fungal infection

A-19. A. Lower limb SpO_2 85% and upper limb SpO_2 97%, suggests differential cyanosis. As congenital heart disease was detected in his infancy and remained untreated, now presenting with differential cyanosis, it is likely PDA with pulmonary hypertension. Due to pulmonary hypertension, now there is reversal of shunt and therefore, unoxygenated blood is mixing with oxygenated blood in descending aorta leading cyanosis in lower limbs, while upper limbs are not affected.

The condition with upper limb cyanosis and lower limb normal is called as reversed differential cyanosis. Reversed differential cyanosis is found in transposition of great vessels (TGV) with pulmonary hypertension.

B. Loud P_2 suggests pulmonary hypertension.

C. Chest X-ray shows dilated main pulmonary and central pulmonary arteries with decreased peripheral vasculature.

D. PDA with Eisenmenger syndrome.

A-20. A. *Loud S_1:* Thyrotoxicosis

B. *Loud P_2:* Pulmonary hypertension

C. *Soft P_2:* Pulmonary valve stenosis

D. *Reversed splitting of S_2:* Aortic stenosis

E. *Soft S_1:* Mitral stenosis

F. *S_3:* Aortic regurgitation

A-21. A. *Types (classification) of VSD as per anatomical location:*

- *Perimembranous (subaortic):* 80%
- *Muscular (Swiss-cheese type):* 5–20%
- *Outlet VSD (subpulmonic):* 5–7%
- *Inlet defects (endocardial cushion type):* 8%

B. *Factors leading to LRTIs or pneumonias in a case of VSD:*

- Pulmonary venous hypertension (PVH) causes exudation of fluid into interstitium and alveoli leading to peribronchial edema
- Pulmonary arterial hypertension (PAH) causes dilatation of pulmonary artery leading to compression of bronchi and bronchioles. It causes air and mucus trapping favoring bacterial growth and ciliary dysfunction.
- Infants cannot bring out sputum and secretions.
- Associated syndromes like Down syndrome aggravates the situation
- Associated problems like malnutrition, GERD and immunodeficiency contribute for further problems

C. *Classification of VSD based on size:*

- *Small VSD:* <1/3 of aortic root, orifice area <0.5 cm^2/m^2
- *Moderate VSD:* 1/3 to 2/3 of aortic root, orifice area 0.5–1 cm^2/m^2
- *Large VSD:* >2/3 of aortic root, ≥1 cm^2/m^2

D. *Timing of VSD closure:*

- Large VSD with severe PAH: 3–6 months
  Uncontrolled congestive heart failure
- Moderate VSD with moderate PAH: 1–2 years of age
  - *With one LRTI/FTT:* Earlier
  - *With no PAH:* 2–4 years of age
- *Small outlet VSD:* Yearly follow-up
  - With aortic valve prolapse: 2–3 years of age
  - With aortic regurgitation: As soon as possible
- *Small VSD with aortic valve prolapse with no/mild AR:* Yearly follow-up
- Small VSD with ≥1 episode of bacterial endocarditis as soon as possible.
- *Certain facts on spontaneous closure of VSD:*
  - 10% of large VSDs die in first years of age mainly due to CHF.
  - Spontaneous closure is rare in large VSD.
  - 30–40% moderate or small VSDs close spontaneously, majority by age of 3–5 years

A-22. A. False

B. False

C. False

D. True

A-23. A. Duct dependent cardiac defect

B. In duct dependent CHD, the newborn has a severe obstruction preventing adequate blood flow to either systemic circulation or pulmonary circulation. Immediately after birth, the conditions are dependent upon PDA for maintenance of circulation. Because the PDA naturally closes after birth, these conditions present as life threatening and require immediate diagnosis and management.

C. Prostaglandin E_1 infusion is life-saving drug because it keeps PDA open.

D. *Duct-dependent cardiac defects:*

- *Obstruction to systemic circulation:*
  - Severe coarctation of aorta
  - Hypoplastic left heart syndrome
  - Interrupted aortic arch
  - Critical aortic stenosis
- *Obstruction to pulmonary circulation:*
  - Pulmonary atresia

A-24. A. *Canon 'a' wave:* Complete heart block

B. *Giant 'a' wave:* Pulmonary stenosis

C. *Large 'v' wave:* Tricuspid regurgitation

D. *Steep 'y' descent:* Constrictive pericarditis

A-25. A. Left to right shunt in form of VSD or PDA. VSD is more likely.

B. Left to right shunts lesions such as VSD, PDA.

C. Anti-congestive therapy is important initial management. Digoxin, enalapril, furosemide and spironolactone with restriction of fluid should be started.

D. Atrial septal defect (ASD) and partial anomalous pulmonary venous drainage do not manifest in neonatal period.

A-26. A. Differential diagnosis in a case with systolic murmur in second left ICS.

- ASD
- Pulmonary stenosis (PS)
- Aortic stenosis (AS)
- Coarctation of aorta
- Increased pulmonary blood flow

B. *Auscultatory findings in ASD:*

- Soft, wide, fixed splitting of second sound
- Ejection systolic murmur at second left ICS
- Diastolic murmur at lower left parasternal border due to increased blood flow at tricuspid valve.

C. *Types of ASD:*

- Ostium primum
- Ostium secundum
- Persistent foramen ovale
- Sinus venosus ASD
- Coronary sinus ASD

D. *ECG changes in ASD:*

- Right bundle branch block (RBBB) (rsR pattern)
- Right axis deviation
- Right atrial and right ventricular enlargement

E. Conditions with ASD and pulmonary hypertension

- Large ASD
- ASD + TAPVC

- ASD + PAPVC
- Cotriatrum

A-27. A. Ground-glass like opacification of both lung fields, also called as white out lungs in newborn.
B. Obstructed total anomalous pulmonary venous connection (TAPVC)
C. Causes of white out lung fields or ground-glass opacification of both lung fields in newborns
- *Respiratory:*
  - Hyaline membrane disease (HMD)
  - Meconium aspiration syndrome (MAS)
  - Pneumonia
  - Pleural effusion
- *Cardiac:*
  - TAPVC
  - Pulmonary edema
  - Cardiomyopathy
  - Congestive heart failure

D. Opinion of cardiologist and urgent echo study of heart
E. Emergency cardiac surgery
F. Oxygen and prostaglandin are contraindicated in TAPVC.

A-28. A. Arteriovenous (AV) fistula
B. *Manifestations of AV fistula:*
- Congestive heart failure
- Hemorrhagic stroke, seizures
- Head swelling
- Prominent veins

C. CT angiography/MR angiography
D. *Treatment options:*
- Interventional radiology: Catheter-guided coils to close it off from inside.
- Surgery: Use clips to close abnormal connections

A-29. A. *Clinical manifestations of PDA:*
- Preterm baby
- Tachycardia, tachypnea, bounding peripheral pulsations
- Respiratory distress
- Hyperdynamic precordium
- Continuous murmur
- Not gaining the weight

B. *Complications of PDA:*
- Necrotizing enterocolitis
- Intracranial hemorrhage
- Ventilatory dependency
- Bronchopulmonary dysplasia

C. *Pharmacological therapy for PDA:*
- *Indomethacin:* 0.2 mg/kg/dose 3 doses 12 hours apart by IV or oral route
- *Ibuprofen:* 10 mg/kg on first day, followed by 5 mg/kg for next 2 days.
- *Paracetamol:* 15 mg/kg 6 hourly for 3 days.

A-30. A. Transposition of great arteries (TGA)
B. *Differentials:*
- TGA

- Persistent pulmonary hypertension (PPHN)
- Fallot's tetralogy
- Pulmonary atresia
- Hypoplastic left heart syndrome

C. *Hyperoxia test in newborn:*
- The hyperoxia test helps to determine the cause of cyanosis, cardiac or pulmonary.
- Partial pressure of oxygen ($PaCO_2$) in an arterial blood gas (ABG) is measured before and after administering 100% oxygen for 10–15 minutes.
- A significant rise in PaO_2 (PaO_2 >150 mg) suggests a pulmonary cause, while marginal increase in PaO_2 indicates cyanotic heart disease.

D.
- *Causes of differential cyanosis (oxygen saturation is higher in upper limbs than lower limbs):*
  - Persistent pulmonary hypertension (PPHN) with PDA
  - Interrupted aortic arch
  - Severe coarctation of aorta with VSD and PDA
- *Causes of reversed differential cyanosis (oxygen saturation is lower in upper limbs than lower limbs):*
  - TGA with PDA with pulmonary hypertension
  - Supracardiac total anomalous pulmonary venous connection (TAPVC) with PFO and PDA
  - TGA with PDA and preductal coarctation of aorta or aortic interruption

A-31. A. HLHS is duct-dependent cardiac defect. The cardiac findings would be poor pulses, signs of shock, hyperdynamic precordium, palpable, loud single P_2 and no murmur. Poor systemic perfusion may cause metabolic acidosis.

B. Oxygen therapy is contraindicated in this condition. Oxygen causes pulmonary vasodilatation, compromising systemic perfusion.

C. *Congenital heart disease presenting in first week of life:*
- Transposition of great arteries (TGA)
- Coarctation of aorta
- Infradiaphragmatic TAPVC
- Hypoplastic left heart syndrome
- Aortic stenosis
- PDA
- Large VSD

D. Prostaglandin E_1 (PGE_1) to keep PDA open

A-32. A. Obstruction to right ventricular outflow tract (RVOT) (pulmonary stenosis/supravalvular obstruction/pulmonary artery stenosis) + overriding of aorta + Subaortic VSD + Right ventricular hypertrophy

B. TOF + Atrial septal defect (ASD)

C. *Pink Fallot:* RVOT obstruction is minimal.

D. Pulmonary stenosis + Right ventricular (RVH) + Atrial septal defect (ASD)

E. Pulmonary stenosis + Over-riding of aorta

F. Under development of pulmonary infundibulum

A-33. A. *Tapping apex beat:* It is forceful, sharp and not sustained. It is found in right ventricular hypertrophy.

B. *Heaving apex beat:* It is forceful, broad, diffuse and well sustained. It is the characteristic of left ventricular hypertrophy.

C. *Hyperdynamic apex beat:* It is forceful, very rapid and normal in duration. It is produced in conditions with volume overload like VSD, PDA, anemia, etc.

D. Double impulse is seen in hypertrophic cardiomyopathy.

CHAPTER

16

Neurology

QUESTIONS

Q-1. A 6-year-old boy is finding difficulty in getting up as shown in picture below:

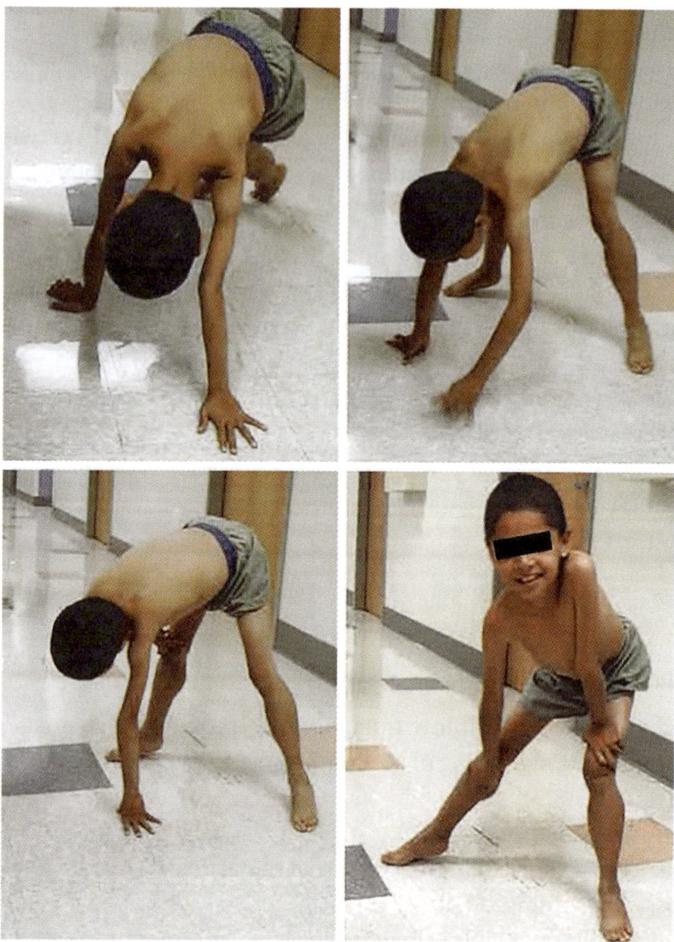

A. Name the sign.

B. At what age, this sign is fully expressed? At what age, it may be evident?

C. What deficiency is responsible for the disease?

D. Which clinical syndrome in girls has been found with full clinical picture of this disease?

E. At what age usually they die? What are the common causes of death in this group?

Q-2. An 8-year-old boy presented with illness of 18 months duration in form of headache and vomiting, gradually increasing, difficulty in vision and no fever. He was proportionate short and fundus examination showed papilledema. His CT brain was as below:

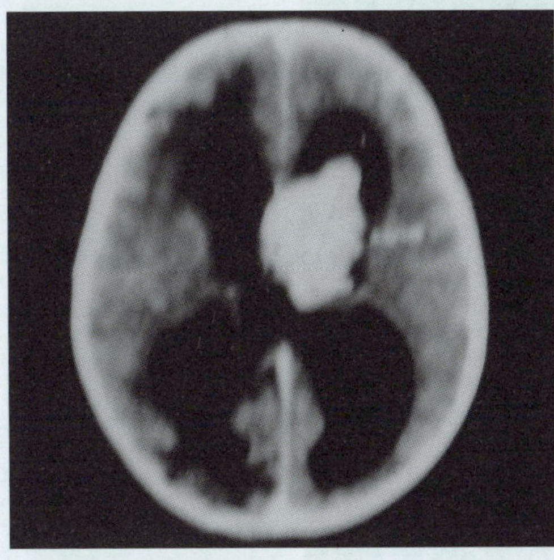
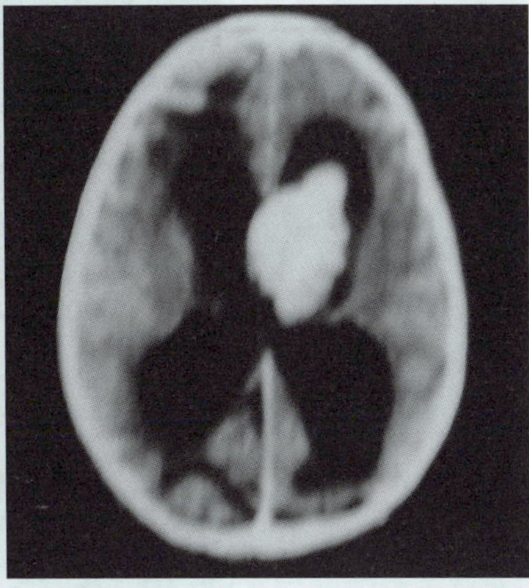

A. What is your diagnosis?
B. What are CT brain findings?
C. What embryonal structure is represented in this disorder?
D. What endocrinal disorders are known to occur in this disease?

Q-3. A 9-year-old boy presented with complaints of easy fatigability and diplopia. The second picture was taken after administration of some drug by IV route.

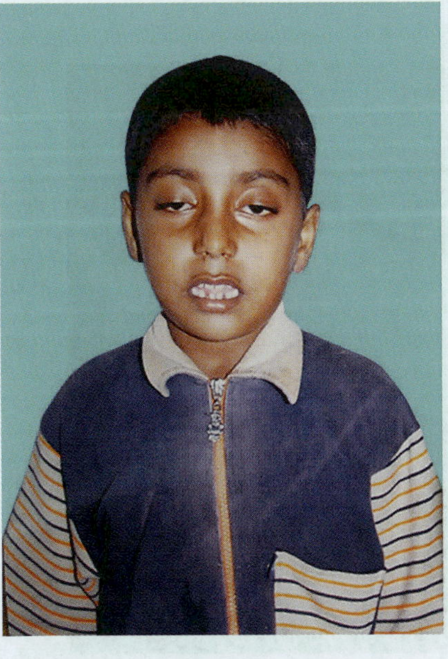
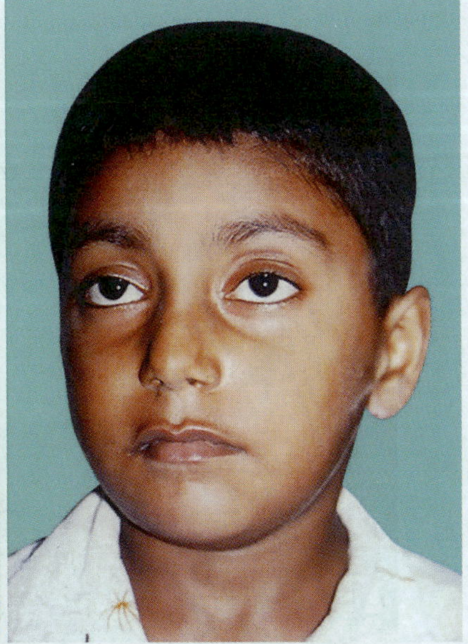

A. Name the condition.
B. What is the site of lesion in nervous system?
C. Which drug is administered for clinical testing? What is diagnostic dose?
D. Which drug should be available in a syringe ready for IV administration at bedside during the clinical test? What is its dose?

Q-4.

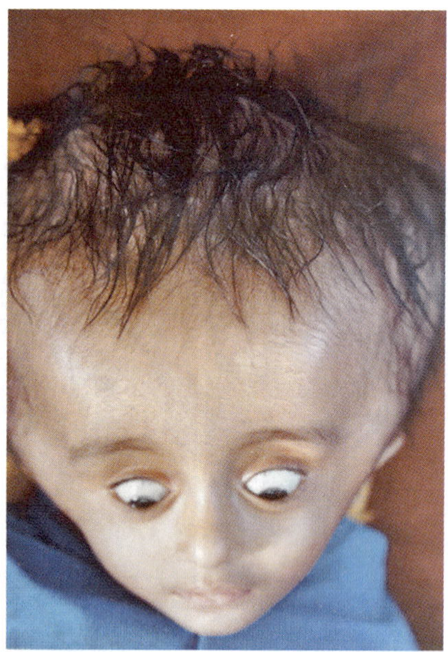

A. Name the clinical eye sign.
B. What is the mechanism of this sign?
C. Name the sign elicitable on percussion of skull in this condition beyond 2 years of age.
D. Which regular follow-up examination often indicates this condition at the earliest?

Q-5. There was history of decreased movements of this baby in utero. This infant also had fasciculation of tongue.

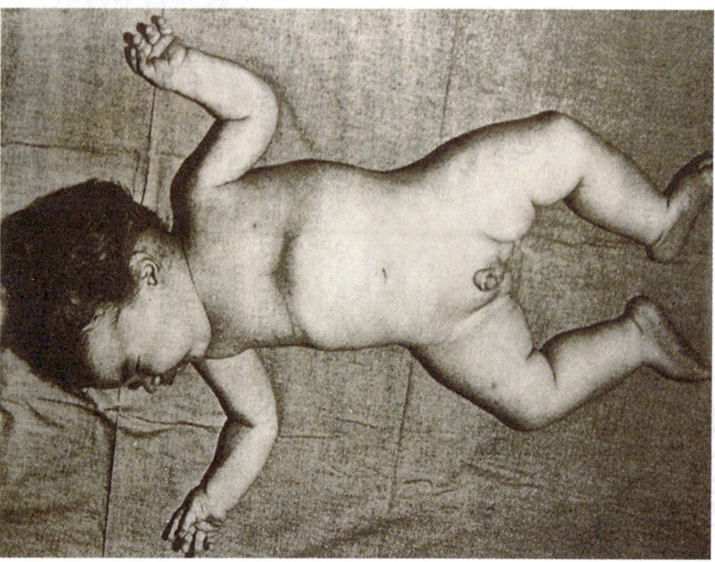

A. What is your diagnosis?
B. Which structure of nervous system is affected in this disorder?
C. What testes can be performed to confirm the diagnosis?
D. How is CPK affected in this disorder?

Q-6. A 10-year-old boy, born of nonconsanguineous parents, with normal birth and developmental history, presented with complaints of painless progressive bilateral vision loss, more on left than on right side for 1 month. He had history of recurrent episodes of transient ischemic attacks and seizures 5 years back. His MRI of brain and MR angiography are as below:

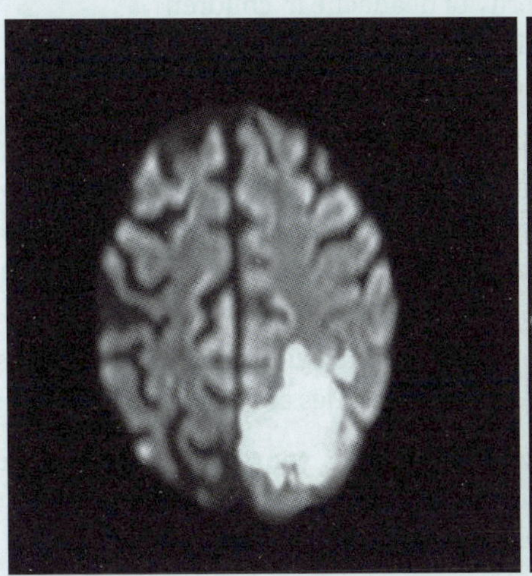

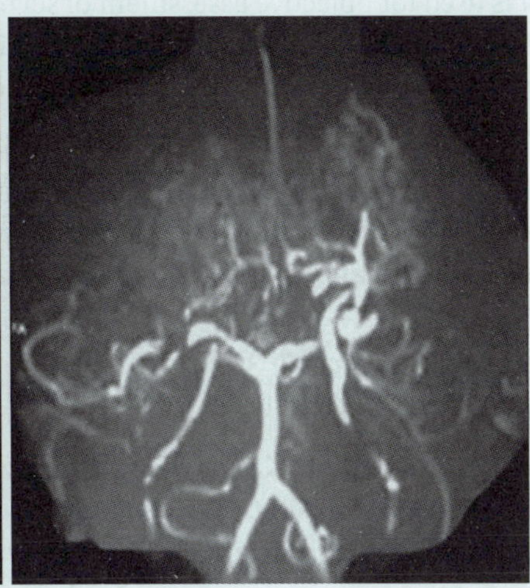

A. What are the findings of MRI brain and MR angiography?
B. What is called the appearance of such MR angiography? How is the name derived?
C. What are common causes of this disorder?

Q-7.

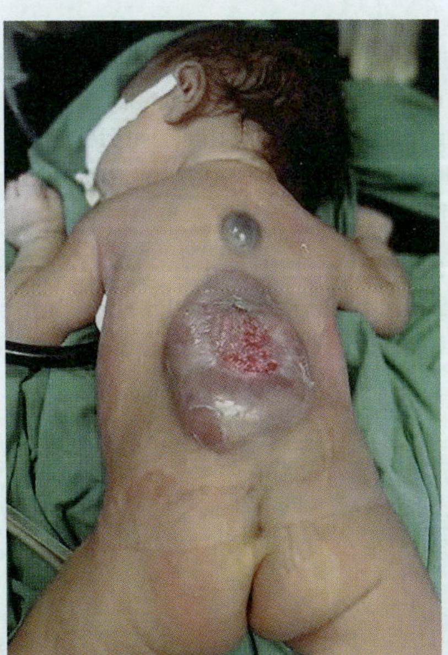

A. Identify the condition.
B. What congenital anomalies of central nervous system are called neural tube defects (NTDs)?
C. What factors are considered responsible for NTDs?
D. What investigations are useful for antenatal diagnosis?
E. What are the indications, dosage and duration of folic acid supplementation for primary and secondary prevention of NTDs?

Q-8. A 10-year-old girl presented with episodic headache for past one year. The frequency of episodes is 3–4 in 9 months, lasting for 20 minutes to an hour. The headache is associated with photophobia, phonophobia, nausea and occasionally vomiting. Each episode is relieved with rest. Her mother also has similar problem.

A. What is the diagnosis?
B. What test is used for objective assessment of severity of headache in children?
C. What is the treatment of an episode of headache in this disorder?
D. What investigation would like to do to confirm the diagnosis?
E. What is long-term management?

Q-9. A 12-year-old obese girl was referred for intermittent headache for 8 months. An episode of hedache was also associated with blurring of vision and vomiting, no photophobia or phonophobia. There was no history of headache in family. Fundus examination showed bilateral papilledema. MRI brain was reported as normal.

A. What is probable diagnosis?
B. How would you confirm the diagnosis?
C. How will you treat this condition?
D. Which drugs are known to cause this order?

Q-10. A 6-year-old girl presented with swaying while walking from 3 years of age. She has unsteady gait and problem is gradually increasing. She also has history of frequent lower respiratory tract infection. Her eye examination revealed an important clinical clue for diagnosis of the condition.

A. What is probable diagnosis?
B. What is likely eye examination finding giving an important clue for the diagnosis?
C. What is the mode of inheritance of this disease?

Q-11. A 5-year-old boy was referred for failure to thrive, anemia, unsteady gait and progressive swaying. The child also had loose stools bulky, sticky and oily.

A. What is probable diagnosis?
B. What is the characteristic finding on blood peripheral smear examination in this disorder?
C. What biochemical test gives an important clue towards the diagnosis of this condition?
D. What ophthalmological finding may be found in this disorder?
E. What anatomical part of CNS involvement is responsible for neurological manifestation?
F. What is the treatment of this disease?

Q-12. An 11-year-old boy presented with frequent falls, unsteady gait and intention tremors gradually progressive over 8 months. On CNS examination, he had pyramidal signs but deep tendon reflexes were sluggish and bilateral planters extensors. Echo study of heart revealed changes of cardiomyopathy. His foot deformity was as shown in the picture.

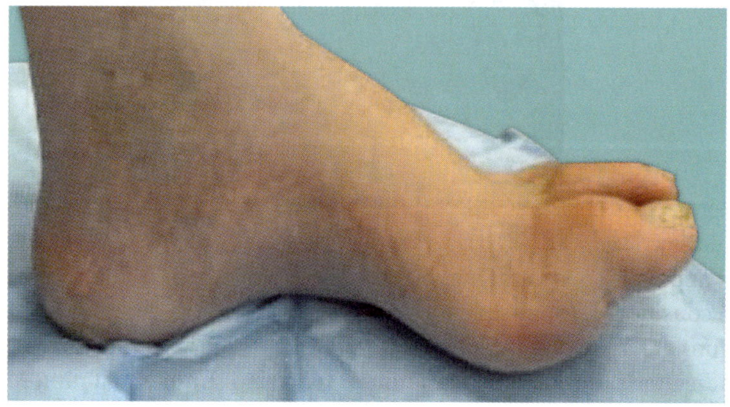

A. Identify the foot deformity.
B. What is the diagnosis?
C. What is the mode of inheritance of this condition?
D. What endocranial disorder should be screened in this disease?
E. What is the most common cause of death in this disorder?

Q-13. A 12-year-old adolescent girl presented with involuntary, jerky dance like movements of limbs and they are absent during sleep. She also had emotional lability.

A. What is probable diagnosis?
B. What is the characteristic triad of this condition?
C. What other signs would you like to elicit to confirm the diagnosis?
D. What investigation should be performed in this patient?
E. What is the treatment?

Q-14. A 10-year-old girl presented with change in hand writing, behavioral changes and intermittent abnormal twisting posture of limbs and rapid involuntary jerky dance like movements of limbs for 8 months. Her young sibling died at the age of 4 years due to jaundice and hepatic encephalopathy without any obvious reason.

A. What is the probable diagnosis?
B. What ophthalmic examination finding would be an important clue to diagnose the condition?
C. What is the mode of inheritance of this disease?
D. What is the gene implicated in this condition?
E. What biochemical test would you like to perform?
F. What are expected findings on MRI brain of this patient?
G. What is the treatment of this disorder?

Q-15. A 10-year-old boy was referred for gradual worsening school performance, behavioral problems and congnitive decline for 6 months. He also has complaints of frequent falls and sudden jerks with injury marks over forehead for last 4 months. The child also had seizures. EEG was performed by a pediatric neurologist and was reported with some specific changes leading to a diagnosis.

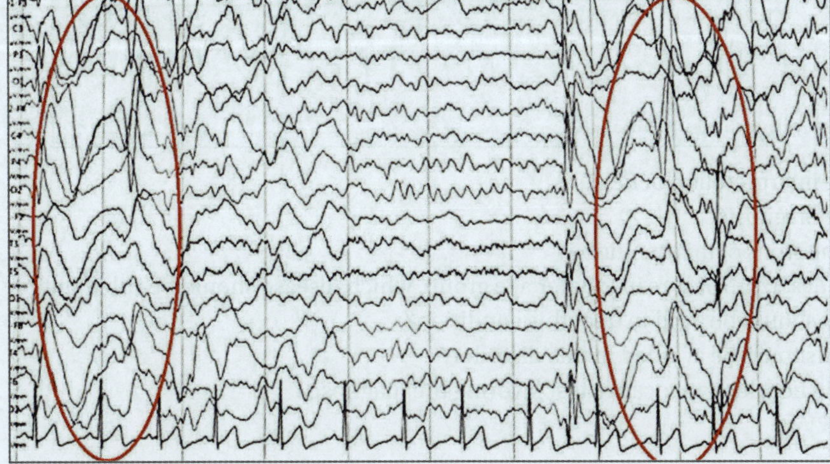

A. What is probable diagnosis?
B. What specific past history may favor the diagnosis?
C. What is the specific EEG finding expected favoring the diagnosis?
D. What is the confirmatory investigation?

Q-16. A 10-month-old child presented with afebrile encephalopathy for 2 days followed by vomiting and running nose for a day only. His development was normal prior to this illness. The child had frequent dystonia which was observed on admission. MRI brain showed symmetrical basal ganglia and brainstem T2 hyperintensities with diffusion restriction. Magnetic resonance spectroscopy (MRS) gave an important etiological clue.

A. What is the probable diagnosis?
B. What is expected MRS finding, an important etiological clue?
C. What is the confirmatory test?
D. What is the treatment?

Q-17. A 2.5-year-old male child born to third degree consanguineous parents presented with encephalopathy and seizurs. His development was delayed. Perinatal period was normal. On clinical examination, alopecia and seborrheic dermatitis were obvious findings. He lost his elder sibling at 7 months of age due to similar illness and refractory seizures. Investigations for HIV were negative.

A. What is the probable diagnosis?
B. What is the mode of inheritance of this condition?
C. What investigations would confirm the diagnosis?
D. What is the treatment of this disease?
E. Is there any risk of recurrence of this disorder in the next pregnancy?

Q-18. A 6-year-old boy was bought in OPD by parents after teacher complained of episodes of starting in the classroom and occasionally drop of pencil. EEG image was as below.

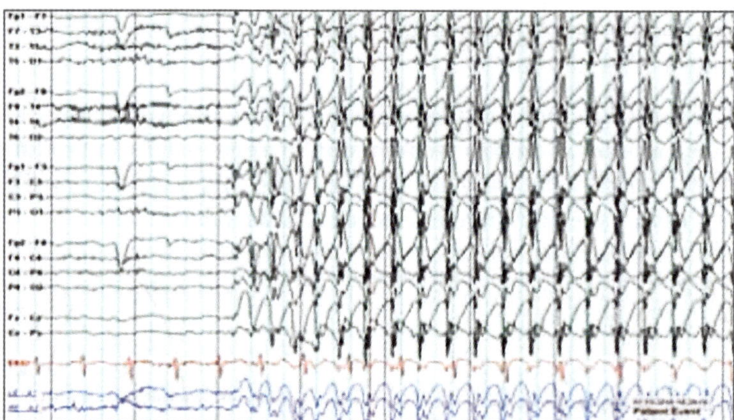

A. What is the interpretation of EEG?
B. What is the diagnosis?
C. What are the types of this condition?
D. If this type of seizure occurs in toddler age group, which disease should be ruled out?
E. What drugs should be used to treat this condition?
F. What drugs should be avoided in this disorder?
G. Which is the bedside provocative test favoring the diagnosis?

Q-19. A 10-month-old infant is brought by parents with complaints of multiple episodes of sudden forward bending of body, arms and legs for few seconds, followed by a pause of 5–10 seconds followed by similar episode of clusters. EEG was as below:

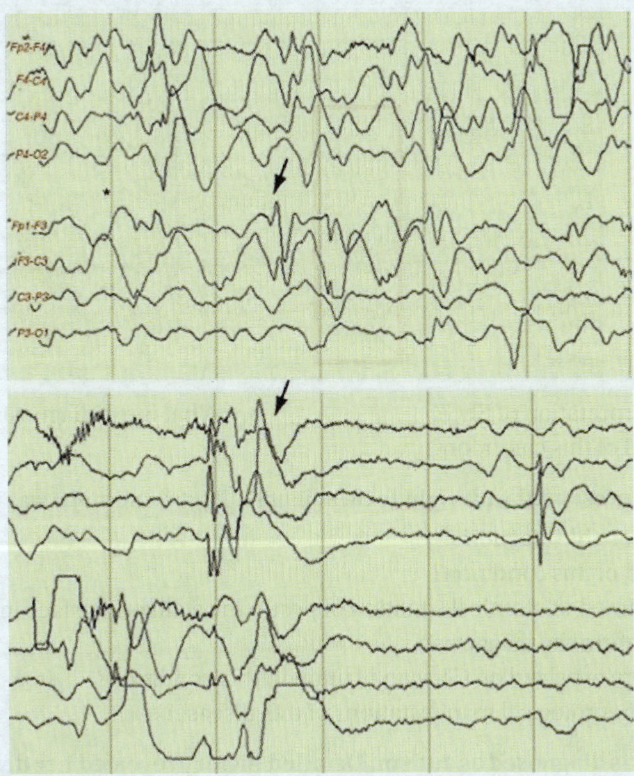

A. Identify EEG abnormality in the image.
B. What is the diagnosis?
C. What are the clinical manifestations?
D. What is the treatment?

Q-20. A 4-year-old boy presented with status epilepticus in emergency. He also has cognitive issues and behavioral problems. The child had first seizures at 4 months of age following vaccination. Later on, he had fever provoked focal seizures frequently and generalized tonic–clonic seizures after 2 years of age. He has seizures once in every 2–3 months and started to share unrpvoked seizures after 2.5 years along with fever provoked seizures intermittently. He also develops intermittent brief blank episodes lasting for few seconds. Perinatal period was normal. MRI brain is reported as normal.

A. What is the probable diagnosis?
B. What is the most common gene implicated in this condition?
C. What is the most common pattern of inheritance?
D. What anticonvulsant drugs are used to control seizures in this condition?
E. Which anticonvulsant drugs to be avoided by this disease?

Q-21. A 4-year-old boy presented with delayed development, multiple seizures in form of vacant stares and sudden jerks, recurrent head drops and falls. EEG was as below:

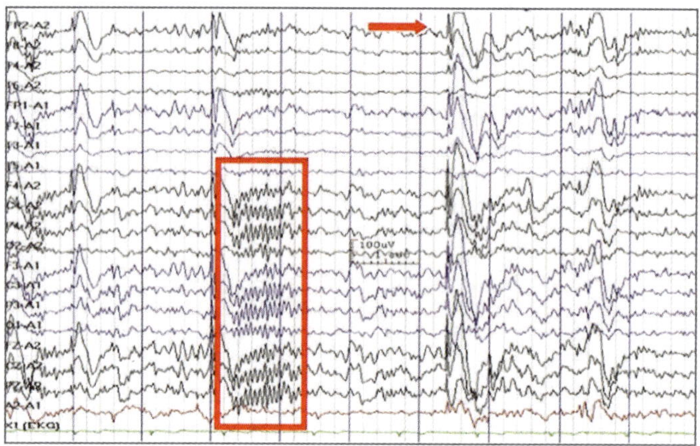

A. What is the interpretation of EEG?
B. What is the diagnosis?
C. What is the triad of this condition?

Q-22. A 4-year-old child presented with right focal seizures. Port-wine stain was noted on left side of face.

A. What is most probable diagnosis?
B. What is the triad of this condition?
C. What is the common anatomical situation of port-wine stain on the face in this disorder?
D. How do you confirm the diagnosis?
E. What findings are expected on CT scan of brain in this condition?
F. What are other neurological manifestations of this disease?

Q-23. A 3-year-old girl was diagnosed as autism. Detailed history revealed her development normal till 10 months of age, then gradually started to develop cognition regression, autistic features and loss of purposeful hand movements and abnormal gait. She also had microcephaly.

A. What is probable diagnosis?
B. What is the most common pattern of inheritance?
C. What is the most common gene implicated in this condition?
D. What is the common cause of death in this disease?

Q-24. A 5-year-old boy presented with neuro-regression, stopped walking, standing and sitting, non-ambulatory by 4 years of age. His development was normal till 2 years of age. On examination, spasticity and pyramidal signs were noted, but ankle jerk was diminished. He had no seizures. MRI brain was done and picture was as shown below.

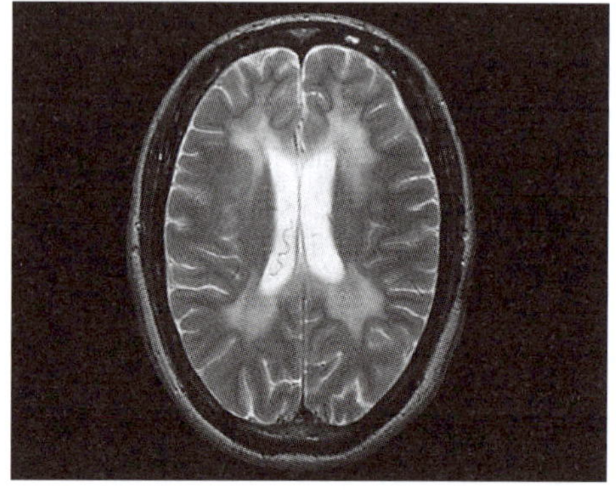

A. What is the interpretation of MRI brain?
B. What is most likely diagnosis?
C. What is the enzyme deficient?
D. What is the mode of inheritance?
E. Why is the ankle jerk diminished in this condition?
F. What is the risk of recurrence in next pregnancy?

Q-25. An 18-month-old male child presented with regression in developmental milestones since 10 months of age and cognition regression since 1 year of age. Child had severe pallor, hypopigmented sparse hairs, and hyperpigmented knuckles. He was predominantly breastfed only.

A. What is probable diagnosis?
B. What are other clinical features of this condition?
C. What hematological abnormalities are commonly detected in this disorder?
D. What is the treatment of this disease?

Q-26. A 10-month-old male child presented with delayed head control, vision impairment and epileptic spasms. The child had macrocephaly and central hypotonia. Fundus examination revealed optic atrophy. MRI brain was as below.

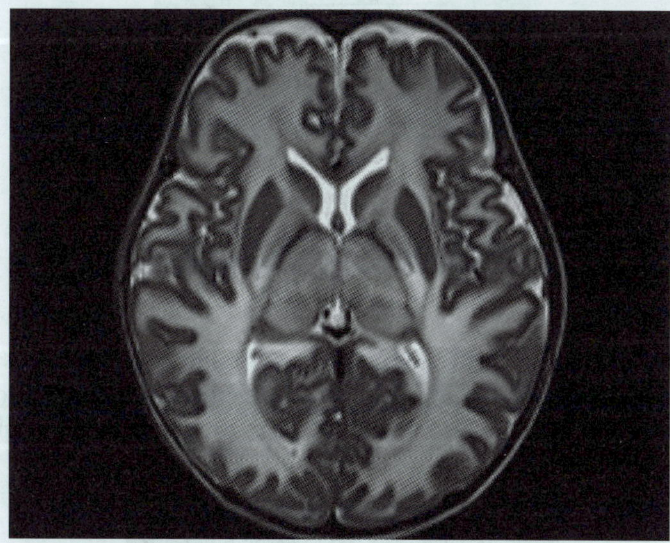

A. What is the interpretation of MRI brain?
B. What is most probable diagnosis?
C. What is the enzyme deficient?
D. What is the mode of inheritance?
E. What classical finding is expected in MRI spectroscopy examination of brain in this condition?

Q-27. A 15-month-old child presented with motor and cognitive neuroregression noted since 8 months of age. He also had seizures and vision regression since 10 months of age along with progressive dystonia. Parents noted exaggerated response to noise. There was no organomegaly.

A. What is probable diagnosis?
B. What fundus examination finding will be an important due to diagnosis?
C. What enzyme deficiency causes this disease?
D. What is the mode of inheritance?

Q-28. A 9-month-old male child presented with delayed head control, neuroregression, opisthotonic posturing and huge splenomegaly.

A. What is probable diagnosis?
B. What enzyme is deficient in this condition?
C. What are the types of this disorder?
D. How will you confirm the diagnosis?
E. What is the mode of inheritance?

Q-29. Below image is the sagittal section of MRI of spine.

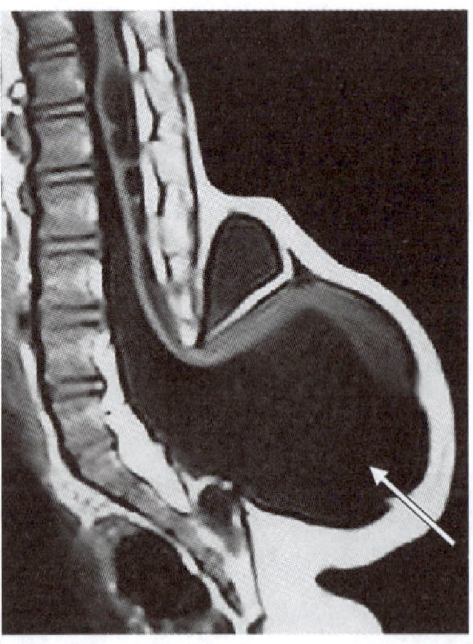

A. Spot the diagnosis.
B. What are the risk factors to develop this condition?
C. What are the indications and timing of surgery?
D. What are the long-term complications?
E. What is Chiari crisis? What are the manifestation of this condition? What is its management?

Q-30. A 12-year-old boy was brought from the school with complaints of weakness on right side of body and aphasia of sudden onset while playing on the ground. He also had similar such episodes 3 times in last 2 months. He recovered within few days by himself every time. MRI angiography was done, the image is shown below.

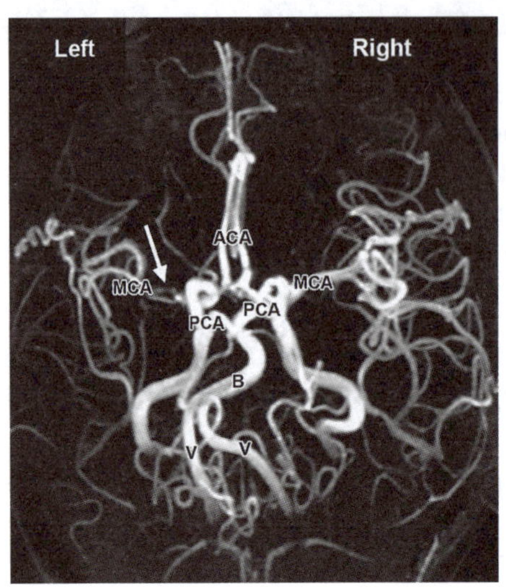

A. Identify the MRI sequences in above image.
B. What is probable diagnosis?
C. What is radiological sign in angiography?
D. What are the conditions associated with this disorder?
E. What are the treatment options?

Q-31. A 10-year-old boy presents with frequency and urgency of micturition and constipation of insidious onset with 18 months duration. He also had urinary tract infection twice in past. He also has low back pain and difficulty in walking. He is found to have asymmetry in feet and arching of feet.

A. What is probable diagnosis?
B. What are cutaneous markers associated with this condition?
C. What congenital spinal anomalies are known to present with this type of disorder?
D. What is the management?

Q-32. A 2-year-old child developed generalized tonic–clonic seizures with fever lasting for 5–7 minutes. Neurological examination was normal.

A. What is probable diagnosis?
B. What are the indications of lumbar puncture in such a presentation?
C. Is radioimaging indicated in this patient?
D. What are the indications for prophylaxis in this disorder?
E. What are the risk factors for recurrence of this condition?
F. What are the risk factors for epilepsy with this condition?

Q-33. A 3-year-old girl presented with high-grade fever for 5 days, irritability and vomiting for 2 days and altered sensorium followed by seizures. Signs of meningeal irritation were present. Child has received vaccines as per national immunization program.

A. What is probable diagnosis?
B. What are most common etiological organisms for acute bacterial meningitis?
C. What should be empirical antibiotics in this patient?
D. What are contraindications of lumbar puncture in this child?
E. What are the indications for neuroimaging in this scenario?
F. What is duration of antibiotics, if the probable diagnosis is confirmed?

Q-34. Spot the MRI findings and diagnosis given in images A to C.

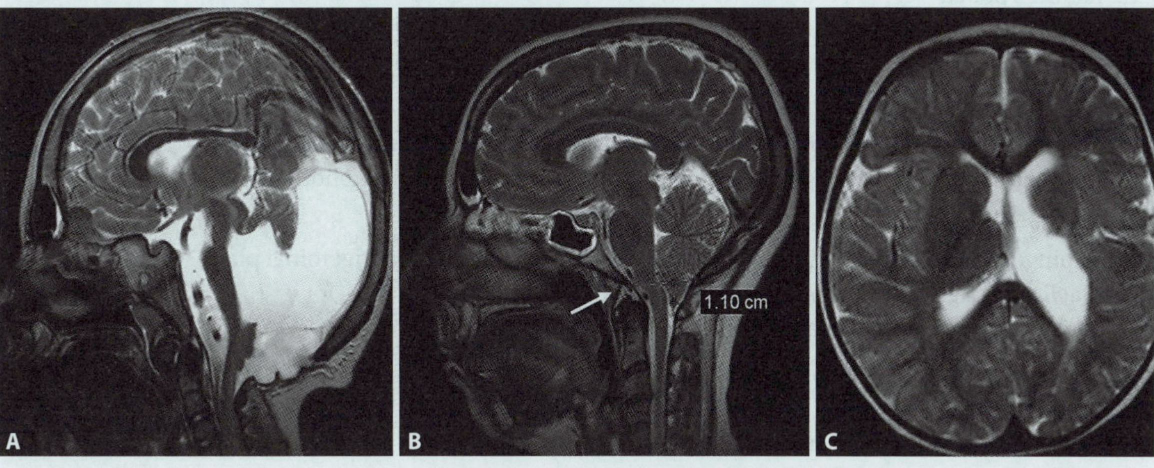

Q-35. Spot neuroimaging and their diagnosis given in images A to C.

A. Basal ganglia calcification
B. Temporal calcifications
C. Periventricular calcification
D. Scattered calcifications

Q-36. What are clinical features suggestive of hypotonia of central origin?

Q-37. In a case of traumatic brain injury, following signs may be present. What does each sign suggest?

A. Battle sign
B. Racoon eyes
C. CSF rhinorrhea
D. Setting sun sign (may be present late)
E. Fundoscopy examination may show________

Q-38. What is the management of raised intracranial pressure?

Q-39. Answer the following questions pertaining to Guillain-Barré syndrome (GBS):

A. What are the features strongly suggesting GBS?
B. Which features that should raise the doubt about diagnosis of GBS?
C. Why is there albumin cytology dissociation?
D. What are the predictors of bad prognosis in GBS?

Q-40. Answer the following questions pertaining to acute flaccid paralysis (AFP).

A. Define AFP.
B. What investigation should be performed? Within what time frame?
C. What is the duration of follow-up of the patient of AFP? what to follow?

ANSWERS

A-1. A. Gowers' sign
B. 5 years
3 years
C. Dystrophin
D. Turner syndrome
E. 18–20 years age.
Respiratory failure, Intractable heart failure, airway obstruction

A-2. A. Craniopharyngioma
B. Cystic swelling with calcification in suprasellar area, with development of hydrocephalus
C. Rathke's pouch
D. Hypopituitarism, precocious puberty, Diabetes insipidus

A-3. A. Myasthenia gravis
B. Neuromuscular junction
C. Edrophonium chloride (Tensilon), 0.1–0.2 mg/kg (maximum 10 mg)
D. Atropine sulfate, 0.01 mg/kg, to block acute muscarinic effects of edrophonium

A-4. A. Setting-Sun eye sign
B. Impingement of the dilated suprapineal recess on the tectum (Quadrigeminal plate)
C. MacEwen's sign (Cracked pot sound), 2–18 years of age
D. Serial measurements of head circumference

A-5. A. Werdnig-Hoffmann disease (Spinal Muscular Atrophies Type 1)
B. Anterior horn cells
C. Electromyography (EMG), muscle biopsy
D. CPK remains normal in this disorder.

A-6. A.

- MRI brain shows subacute infarct in the left occipital region.
- MR angiography shows complete occlusion of right supraclinoid internal carotid artery and severe narrowing of the left supraclinoid internal carotid artery with collateral formation.

B. Moyamoya disease. It is progressive cerebrovascular disease caused by blocked arteries at the base of the brain. Moyamoya means 'puff of smoke' in Japanese language and is used to describe the tangled appearance of tiny vessels compensating for the blockage.

C. *Common causes of Moyamoya:*

- Moyamoya disease (idiopathic or primary)
- *Moyamoya syndrome (secondary):*
  - Sickle cell anemia
  - Neurofibromatosis
  - Trisomy 21
  - William syndrome
  - Alagille syndrome
  - Hyperthyroidism

A-7. A. Meningomyelocele

B. Embryological defects and NTDs

Embryological defects	***NTDs***
Defect of neural folding and formation	Meningomyelocele, anencephaly
Disordered post-neurulation development	Encephalocele
Incomplete dysjunction	Dermal sinus, dermoid and epidermoid tumors
Premature dysjunction	Spinal cord lipomas
Disorders of gastrulation	Split cord malformation, neurenteric cysts
Disordered secondary neurulation	Thickened filum terminale, myelocystocele
Failure of development of caudal neuraxis	Sacral agenesis

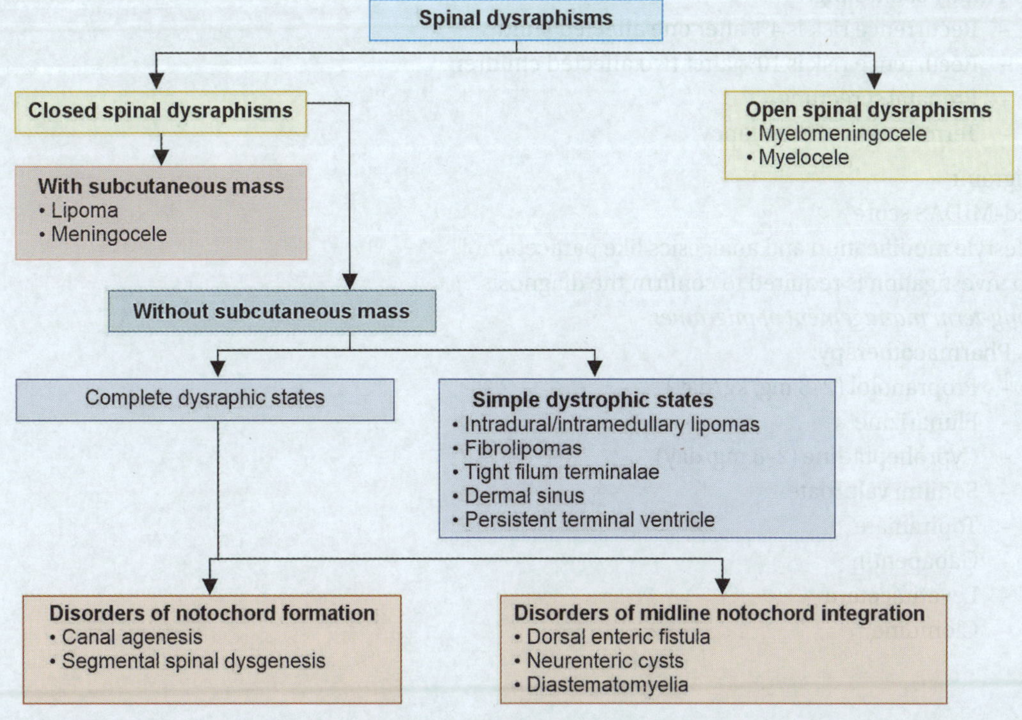

C. *Etiological factors for NTDs:*
- Genetic predisposition (Multifactorial trait)
- *Environmental triggers:*
  - Maternal diabetes mellitus
  - Maternal vitamin B_{12} status
  - Pesticides
- Role of folic acid
- *Teratogens:*
  - Retinoic acid
  - Antiepileptic drugs (Valproic acid, carbamazepine)

D. *Antenatal diagnosis:*
- Maternal serum alpha-fetoprotein
- Ultrasound examination
- Amniotic fluid acetylcholinesterase

Investigations after birth:
- X-ray chest and spine
- Ultrasonogram
- CT scan
- MRI
- Karyotyping
- Renal scan

E. *Prevention of NTDs:* Periconceptional folio acid supplementation
- *All prospective mothers:*
  Dose: 0.4 mg/day
  2 months prior to conception and 3 months after conception
- *Prospective mothers with previous child with NTD:*
  Dose: 4 mg/day
  When: 2 months prior to conception and 3 months after conception
- *Family counseling:*
  - Recurrence risk is 4% after one affected child
  - Recurrence risk is 10% after two affected children
  - Prenatal screening
  - Termination of pregnancy

A-8. A. Migraine
B. Ped-MIDAS score
C. Lifestyle modification and analgesics like paracetamol
D. No investigation is required to confirm the diagnosis.
E. *Long-term management of migraine:*
- Pharmacotherapy:
  - Propranolol (2–3 mg/kg/day)
  - Flunarizine
  - Cyproheptadine (2–8 mg/day)
  - Sodium valproate
  - Topiramate
  - Gabapentin
  - Levetiracetam
  - Clonidine

- To avoid exertion, lack of sleep, hunger
- Bright-light, loud noise should be avoided.
- Nuts, Chinese food or any trigger detected, should be avoided.

A-9. A. Idiopathic intracranial hypertension (Pseudotumor cerebri)
B. CSF manometry to measure CSF opening pressure
C. Therapeutic lumbar puncture to remove CSF and oral acetazolamide
D. Tetracycline, nalidaxic acid,steroids, lithium like drugs are known to cause this disorder.

A-10. A. Ataxia telangiectasia B. Telangiectasia in bulbar conjunctiva
C. Autosomal recessive

A-11. A. Abetalipoproteinemia
B. Acanthocytes—irregular margin of cell wall of RBCs on blood peripheral smear examination is the characteristic of abetolipoproteinemia.
C. Lipid profile—decreased levels of serum cholesterol and triglycerides
D. Retinitis pigmentosa on eye examination
E. Posterior columns of the spinal cord and spinocerebellar tracts
F. Vitamin E

A-12. A. Pes cavus and hammer toes
B. Friedreich's ataxia
C. Autosomal recessive
D. Diabetes mellitus
E. Hypertrophic cardiomyopathy leading to congestive heart failure

A-13. A. Sydenham's chorea
B. Chorea, hypotonia and emotional lability is the triad of Sydenham's chorea.
C. *Other signs of Sydenham's chorea:*
- Hypotonia
- Pronator sign
- Milkmaid grip
- Jack in the box tongue
- Hung-up ankle jerk
- Halted speech
- Changing hand writing

D. ASO titer, ESR, CRP, ECG and Echo study of heart.
E.
- To control chorea drugs like valproate, carbamazepine and dopamine receptor antagonists
- Long-term penicillin prophylaxis

A-14. A. Wilson disease with neurological presentation
B. Kayser–Fleischer (KF) ring
C. Autosomal recessive
D. *ATP7B* gene
E. Serum ceruloplasmin, 24 hours urinary copper and genetic testing
F. Bilateral basal ganglia involvement. There may be presence of "Face of giant panda sign".
G. Chelation therapy with d-penicillamine and copper restricted diet are mainstay of treatment. Oral zinc supplementation is also required.

A-15. A. Subacute sclerosing panencephalitis (SSPE)
B. Past history of measles

C. Periodic complexes
D. CSF antimeasles antibodies and EEG are confirmatory tests for SSPE.

A-16. A. Leigh's disease
B. Double inverted lactate peak
C. Genetic testing is confirmatory.
D.
- *Mitochondrial cocktail drugs:* Carnitine, Thiamine, Riboflavin, Biotin, etc.
- *Treatment for dystonia:* Trihexyphenidyl, physiotherapy and stimulation.

A-17. A. Biotinidase deficiency
B. Autosomal recessive
C. Biotinidase enzyme assay and genetic testing are confirmatory investigations for this disease.
D. Biotin supplementation
E. Yes, 25% in each pregnancy

A-18. A. EEG shows 3 Hz spike-wave discharge suggestive of typical childhood absence epilepsy.
B. Childhood absence epilepsy
C. Typical, atypical and juvenile absence seizures, typical absence occurs in childhood absence epilepsy, atypical absence occurs in Lennox-Gastaut syndrome and juvenile absence occurs in juvenile myoclonic epilepsy.
D. Glucose transporter 1 (GluT1) deficiency
E. Ethosuximide and sodium valproate should be used.
F. Carbamazepine and phenytoin should be avoided.
G. Hyperventilation

A-19. A. EEG shows hypsarrhythmias (chaotic mixture of asynchronous, very high voltage polymorphic delta slowing and multifocal spikes)
B. West syndrome
C. Infantile spasms with developmental delay or regression
D. Injection ACTH or steroids. When it is associated with tuberous sclerosis, vigabatrin is drug of choice.

A-20. A. Dravet syndrome
B. *SCN1A*
C. Autosomal dominant
D. Sodium valproate, clobazam, levetiracetam should be used.
E. Phenytoin, carbamazepine and lamotrigine should be avoided.

A-21. A. EEG shows diffuse slow spike wave discharge <2.5 Hz occurring in repetitive sequences
B. Lennox-Gastaut syndrome
C. Psychomotor delay/regression, refractory multiple seizures types and classical EEG is the triad of Lennox-Gastaut syndrome.

A-22. A. Sturge-Weber syndrome
B. Facial port-wine nevus, leptomeningeal angiomatosis and glaucoma are the triad of Sturge-Weber syndrome
C. Ophthalmic division of trigeminal nerve is the site for port-wine nevus.
D. MRI brain with contrast
E. Tram-track calcification with unihemispheric atrophy
F. Hemiparesis, transient ischemic attacks and headache are other neurological manifestations besides seizures in Sturge-Weber syndrome.

A-23. A. Rett syndrome
B. X-linked dominant
C. *MECP2* gene
D. Cardiac arrhythmia

A-24. A. Symmetrical periventricular white matter T2 hyperintensities sparing the subcortical fibers
B. Metachromatic leukodystrophy (MLD)
C. Arylsulfatase A
D. Autosomal recessive
E. Ankle jerk is diminished due to peripheral neuropathy.
F. 25% recurrence risk is each pregnancy.

A-25. A. Infantile tremor syndrome (ITS) or Anemia tremor syndrome (ATS)
B. Other clinical features are tremors, cry is tremulous (bleating of a goat), skin hyperpigmentation and multiple vitamin deficiencies.
C. Microcytic, macrocytic anemia, hypersegmented neutrophils, macro-ovalocytes in peripheral smear examination.
D. Vitamin B_{12}, iron therapy, folic acid, zinc and magnesium and good complementary feeds

A-26. A. Diffuse symmetrical white matter T2 hyperintensities with prominent subcortical U-fiber involvement
B. Canavan's disease
C. Aspartoacylase
D. Autosomal recessive
E. Giant N-acetylaspartate 9NAA peak

A-27. A. Tay-Sachs disease (GM2 gangliosidosis)
B. Cherry-red spot
C. Hexosaminidase A enzyme
D. Autosomal recessive

A-28. A. Infantile Gaucher's disease
B. Beta-glucocerebrosidase deficiency
C. Types of Gaucher's disease
Type-1: Non-neuropathic form
Type-2: Acute neuropathic form
Type-3: Chronic neuropathic form
D. Enzyme assay and genetic testing
E. Autosomal recessive

A-29. A. Lumbosacral meningomyelocele
B. *Risk factors for meningomyelocele:*
- Folic acid deficiency
- Drugs like trimethoprim, antiepileptics like phenytoin, phenobarbitone and valproate which act as antagonist to folic acid

C.
- Ruptured sac with CSF leak is indication for immediate surgery.
- Other meningomyeloceles should be operated in first few days of life

D. *Long-term complications of meningomyelocele:*
- Neurogenic bladder and bowel
- Hydrocephalus
- Clubfeet
- Contractures of ankles and knees
- Hip subluxation
- Tethered cord

E. *Chiari crisis:* 15% of infants with hydrocephalus and Chiari II malformation develop symptoms of hindbrain (brainstem) dysfunction, including difficulty in feeding, choking, stridor, apnea, vocal cord paralysis, pooling of secretions and spasticity of upper limbs. If it is untreated, can cause death. This crisis is due to downward herniation of the medulla and cerebellar tonsils through the foramen magnum.

A-30. A. Diffusion-weighted imaging (DWI) and MRI angiography

B. *Moyamoya disease:* Chronic, usually bilateral, vasculopathy of undetermined etiology characterized by progressive narrowing of the terminal intracranial portion of the internal carotid artery.
C. Puff of smoke sign (Moyamoya in Japanese)
D. *Conditions associated with Moyamoya disease:*
   - Trisomy 21
   - Tuberculous meningitis
   - Neurofibromatosis Type I
   - Sickle cell disease
   - Noonan syndrome
   - Alagille syndrome
   - Williams syndrome
E. *Treatment options:*
   - *Medical:* Aspirin to prevent recurrent strokes
   - *Surgical:* Definitive treatment
   - Direct vascularization
   - Indirect vascularization

A-31. A. Tethered cord syndrome
B. Dermal sinus, presence of tuft of hair, discoloration of skin, pit, lump or hemangioma at lumbosacral region are markers associated with tethered spinal cord.
C. Congenital spinal malformations associated with tethered spinal cord are:
   - Myelomeningocele
   - Diastematomyelia
   - Syringomyelia
   - Lipoma of the cord
   - Fatty filum terminale
D. Surgery

A-32. A. Typical febrile seizures
B. Indications of lumbar punction in this situation.
   - In infants (<12 months of age) with fever and seizures.
   - Ill-looking babies those who have not received *H. influenza* and pneumococcal vaccines.
C. Not indicated
D. *Risk factors for recurrences:*
   - Complex febrile seizures
   - Associated neurological deficit
   - Family history of epilepsy
   - Febrile status epilepticus
E. Risk factors for recurrence are age less than 1 year, duration of fever <24 hours, low-grade fever.
F. Neurodevelopmental abnormalities, complex febrile seizures, family history of epilepsy are risk factors for epilepsy.

A-33. A. Acute bacterial meningitis
B. *H. Influenza B*, *Strept. pneumoniae* and *Meningococcus* are common organisms for acute bacterial meningitis.
C. Intravenous Injection ceftriaxone 100 mg/kg/day and injection vancomycin 15 mg/kg/dose 6 hourly should be started as empirical antibiotics.
D. *Contraindications of lumbar puncture:*
   - Cardiopulmonary instability
   - Raised intracranial pressure with closed anterior fontanel

- Local skin infection at the site of lumbar puncture
- Thrombocytopenia with platelets count less than 20,000/cumm.

E. *Indications for neuroimaging:*
- If lumbar puncture is contraindicated.
- Suspected complications in a case of acute bacterial meningitis like subdural effusion, hydrocephalus, brain abscess, ventriculitis, etc.
- Focal seizures
- Infarction
- Sinovenous thrombosis
- Raised intracranial pressure

F. Total duration of IV antibiotics is 7–10 days in acute bacterial meningitis.

A-34. A. Dandy-Walker malformation B. Arnold-Chiari malformation C. Periventricular leucomalacia

A-35. A. Japanes Encephalitis B. Herpes Simplex Encephalitis C. Cytomegalo viral infection D. Toxoplasmosis

A-36. *Clinical features suggestive of hypotonia of central origin*
- Dysmorphic facial features
- Global delayed development
- Predominantly axial weakness
- Fisting of hands
- Increased deep tendon reflexes
- Persistent neonatal reflexes
- Pseudobulbar palsy

A-37. A. Fracture of basilar skull bones B. Periorbital ecchymosis is a sign of basal skull bones C. Fracture of cribriform plate D. Raised intracranial pressure E. Retinal hemorrhage

A-38. *Steps for management of raised intracranial pressure*
- Sedation/Analgesia
- Mild hyperventilation
- 30° elevation of head
- Head in neutral position
- Hyperosmolar therapy
- External ventricular drain
- Decompressive craniotomy

A-39. A. *Features strongly favoring GBS:*
- Progression of symptoms over days to 4 weeks
- Symmetry of symptoms
- Areflexia
- Absence of fever at onset of disease
- Bilateral VII nerve palsy
- High concentration of CSF protein with few cells
- Typical electrodiagnostic features

B. *Features that raise the doubt for diagnosis of GBS:*
- Marked persistent asymmetry of weakness
- Bladder or bowel dysfunctions at onset
- Fever at onset

- Raised cells in CSF, polymorphonuclear type
- Sharp sensory level

C. In GBS, the inflammatory response is severe at junction of dorsal and ventral roots at the site of dural attachment. It causes breakdown in the blood brain barrier and transudation of proteins in the spinal CSF resulting in albumin cytology dissociation.

D. *Predictors of bad prognosis in GBS:*
- Obesity
- Malnutrition
- Autonomous nervous system disturbances (tachycardia, hypertension, flushing, sweating)
- Fast progressive disease

A-40. A. AFP is a clinical syndrome characterized by the rapid onset of muscle weakness and loss of muscle tone, progressing to maximum severity within days or weeks. It is not a diagnosis itself but a sign of underlying condition, such as poliomyelitis, GBS, transverse myelitis. Its reporting is mandatory up to age of 15 years and extended to any age when polio is suspected.

B. Two stool samples should be collected at 24–48 hours apart and should be sent to WHO accredited laboratory for polio investigations.
Follow-up for 60 days for any residual paralysis.

CHAPTER 17

Nephrology

QUESTIONS

Q-1. A newborn was delivered with the following lower abdominal defect:

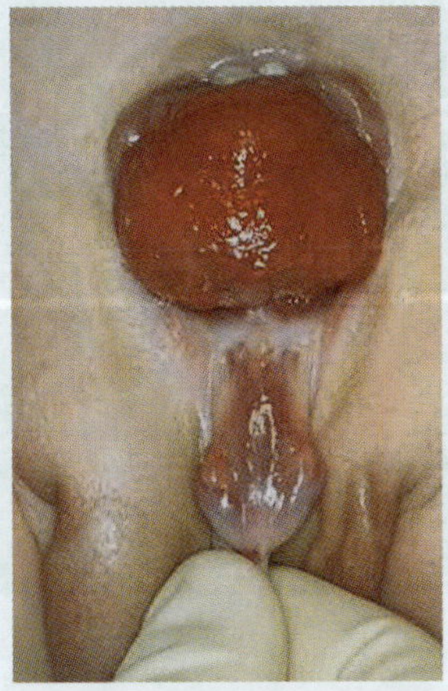

A. What is probable diagnosis?
B. What other anomalies are known to be associated with this?
C. What immediate measures to be taken as a part of management?
D. Which malignancy is common if it is left untreated?

Q-2. A 3-year-old boy presents with sudden severe scrotal pain and swelling on left side. The cremasteric reflex is absent.

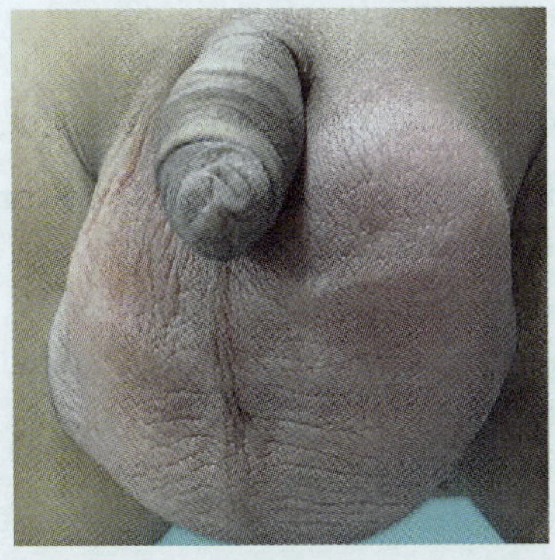

A. What is your diagnosis?
B. What delay in the treatment will decrease the survival of an organ?
C. What contralateral testis need further care?

Q-3. A 6-month-old male child presented with high-grade fever and vomiting. It was diagnosed as urinary tract infection with further work-up as CBC, urine routine and urine culture examinations. After treating urinary tract infection with appropriate antibiotics and sterile urine, the following investigation was performed.

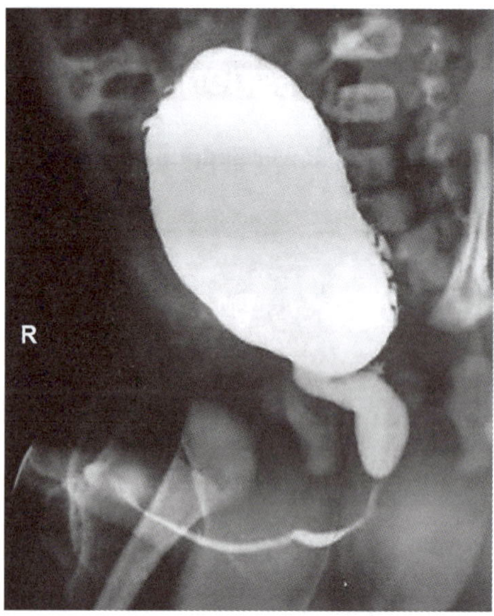

A. Name the investigation.
B. What are the radiological findings?
C. What is the diagnosis?
D. What are the indications of this procedure?
E. What are options for surgical management of this condition?
F. What are complications of this disease, if not treated properly at appropriate time?

Q-4. A 10-month-old girl is diagnosed as tuberculous meningitis. On routine investigations, her serum sodium was 120 and potassium 4.2.

A. What is most likely cause for hyponatremia in this patient?
B. How will your correct hyponatremia?
C. What investigations should be performed to confirm the cause for hyponatremia?

Q-5. A 2-year-old boy was referred for anuria following acute gastroenteritis. His hydration was fair. Investigations showed Hb 7.5, platelets 70,000 and PT 28/20 and APTT 27/30.

A. What is probable diagnosis?
B. What are the characteristic findings on peripheral smear examination of blood film in this condition?
C. What is basic pathology of this disorder?
D. What are the diagnostic criteria for this disease?
E. What is most common etiology for diarrhea associated this disease?

Q-6.

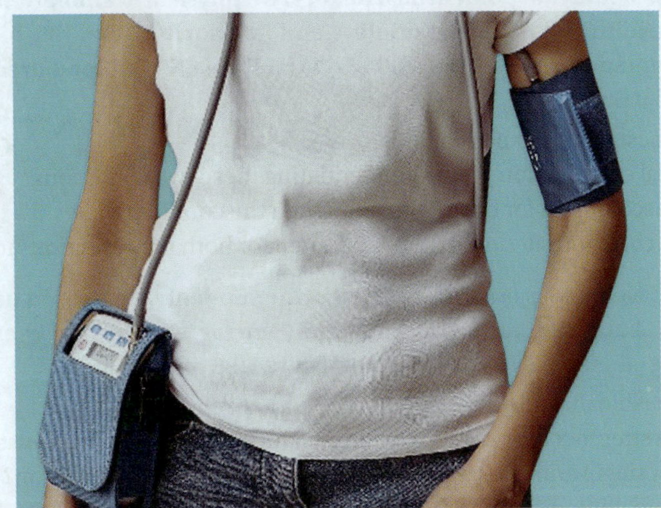

A. What procedure does the picture depict?
B. What are the indications of this procedure?
C. What is white coat hypertension?
D. What percentage of total BP readings measured by this advice above the threshold suggestive of hypertension?

Q-7. A 18-month-old male infant was evaluated for urinary tract infection (UTI) and grade IV vesicoureteral reflux (VUR) was detected on right side. His dimercaptosuccinic acid (DMSA) scan showed 40% function of the right kidney with upper pole scar. Child is on regular follow-up and has no breakthrough UTI.

A. Name the drug of choice for uroprophylaxis with dose in this patient.
B. Mention other drugs for uroprophylaxis with their doses.
C. What are the indications for uroprophylaxis?
D. What is the duration for uroprophylaxis?
E. Is surgery indicated in this patient?
F. Is it indicated repeated micturating cystourethrogram (MCU) in this patient?
G. What other preventive measures for recurrent UTI?

Q-8. A 12-year-old adolescent girl presented with recurrent UTI. She does not urinate in the school and had symptoms of urgency, dysuria and frequency. She also had constipation, passing hard stool at interval of 2–3 days. Her urine examination confirmed UTI and ultrasonography of abdomen was reported with right kidney size 10 cm and left kidney size 10.8 cm, bilateral pelvicalyceal dilatation and post void residual of 50 mL.

A. What is the diagnosis?
B. What radio-imaging investigations are indicated?
C. How should one calculate bladder capacity? What is bladder capacity of this patient?
D. What is the initial management of this patient?

Q-9. An infant born to diabetic mother was referred for hematuria. CBC examination showed Hb 24, HCT 72%, TLC 9100, platelets 65,000. USG abdomen revealed both kidneys enlarged.

A. What is most probable diagnosis?
B. What are differential diagnosis?
C. What investigations will be diagnostic for this condition?
D. What is the treatment of this disorder?
E. What are possible long-term complications of this disease?

Q-10. A 3-year-old girl was brought for abdominal mass detected by mother while bathing her. She has no any other complaint or significant point in past history. On physical examination a mass was noted, arising from right loin and extending up to almost midline and inferiorly 10 cm. Her blood pressure was 140/100 mm of Hg. Urine examination showed 150–200 RBCs/HPF, rest NAD. Blood urea, S. creatinine and electrolytes were within normal limits.

A. What are two most common possibilities?
B. What are clinical examination points differentiating these two conditions?
C. What are the mechanisms for hypertension in both the conditions?
D. What are other common sites other than abdomen for both the conditions to have the lesions?

Q-11. A 8-year-old boy developed gross cola-colored urine suddenly, decreased urine output and edema. He had pyoderma 10 days back and was treated by family doctor. On physical examination, had facial puffiness, mild pedal, pitting edema, old skin lesions and BP 124/96 mm of Hg.

A. What is the probable diagnosis?
B. What serotypes streptococcal infection of throat and skin are known to cause this renal disorder?
C. What is the best single antibody test to confirm streptococcal skin infection?
D. What are life-threatening complications of this disease?
E. What are the indications of renal biopsy in this condition?
F. What is the timeframe to resolve the symptoms in this condition?

Q-12. Answer the following questions:

A. How do you calculate eGFR based on Schwartz formula?
B. What is Stag II chronic kidney disease (CKD) based on eGFR?
C. What is the cause of anemia in CKD?
D. What type of bone problem develops in CKD?
E. What treatment for short stature due to CKD can be given?

Q-13. A 3-year-old boy was brought in OPD with progressive abdominal distention for last few months. Oligohydramnios was reported in antenatal USG study. He was kept in NICU for 7 days for respiratory distress, medical records were not available. Growth chart showed height and weight between 3rd and 10th percentile. His blood pressure was in the 95th percentile. Hepatomegaly and bilateral ballotable kidneys were noted on examination of abdomen. Ultrasonography (USG) of abdomen was reported as echogenic kidney and liver.

A. What is most probable diagnosis?
B. What is Caroli's disease?
C. What hepatic complications are known to occur in this patient?
D. What is the gene involved in this disorder?
E. What are the common causes of abdominal mass or lump in infants?
F. Name associated physical findings to suspect renal disease in children.

Q-14. A 4-year-old male child presented with recurrent episodes of gross hematuria over the last 2 years. He has had three such episodes so far. He had a painless passage of red-colored urine throughout micturition, without any clots, lasting for 3–4 days, subsiding by its own and had a normal growth and activity. Clinical examination was normal, including BP. Urine examination showed 150–200 RBCs/HPF, no pus cells, proteins within normal range. Urine culture did not show growth of any organism. USG abdomen normal.

A. What is most probable diagnosis?
B. What urine test will confirm the diagnosis?
C. What are differential diagnosis?
D. What is the drug of choice for the condition?
E. What is the type of renal tubular acidosis (RTA) associated with nephrocalcinosis?

Q-15. A 14-year-old girl referred for cardiomyopathy, congestive cardiac failure with blood pressure 180/120 mm of Hg in right upper limb. Physical examination revealed weak carotid, brachial and radial pulsations. Bilateral carotid bruits was noted. USG abdomen was reported as bilateral renal artery stenosis. Blood urea and serum creatinine were within normal range. The following investigation confirmed the diagnosis.

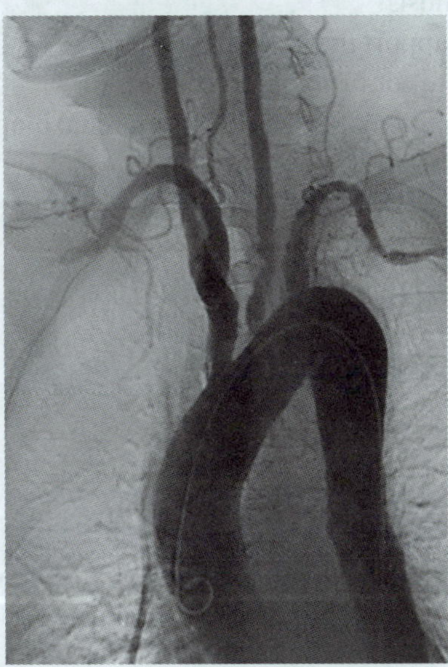

A. What is the investigation performed as shown above? What are your findings?
B. What is the diagnosis?
C. What is the important clinical examination to suspect this disease?
D. What are different clinical presentations of this disease?
E. Which infections are considered possible etiology in this disease?

Q-16. A 2-year-old male child was brought with complaints of failure to thrive, polyuria and polydipsia. He required hospitalization for two times due to acute diarrhea disease and severe dehydration. Laboratory investigations showed CBC within normal limits except moderate anemia. Blood urea and serum creatinine were normal. ABG showed metabolic alkalosis, serum sodium 120 mEq/L, serum potassium 2.5 mEq/L, chloride 94 mEq/L and bicarbonate 36 mEq/L. His blood pressure was normal.

A. What is the probable diagnosis?
B. What other investigations should be performed?
C. What is the management of the disease?
D. What is the long-term renal complication in adulthood?

Q-17. A 3-year-old boy was referred for delayed gross motor milestones, failure to thrive and bony deformities. His weight was 7.5 kg, height 80 cm and had clinical features of rickets, treated with two coursed of oral vitamin D_3 without any response. His investigations showed pH 7.1 on ABG analysis, serum sodium 130 mEq/L, potassium 2.6 mEq/L, Chloride 110 mEq/L and bicarbonate 8 mq/L with anion gap normal, urinary pH 7.5 and urinary anion gap 22. USG abdomen showed nephrocalcinosis.

A. What is most probable diagnosis?
B. What is the interpretation of ABG and electrolytes?
C. How urinary anion gap should be calculated? What is the significance of urinary anion gap?
D. What is the treatment of this disorder?
E. What is Lowe syndrome?
F. What are the causes of nephrocalcinosis?

Q-18. A 9-year-old boy was referred for pain in abdomen and microscopic hematuria. He also required evaluation for hearing problem by an ENT surgeon. His maternal uncle is under care of a nephrologist for chronic kidney disease and he is on dialysis. Physical examination revealed his BP 124/94 mm of Hg. Urine examination showed albumin +2, 30–40 RBCs/HPF and 3–4 WBC/HPF.

A. What is the most probable diagnosis?
B. What other investigations will support the possibility?
C. What test should be performed to confirm the diagnosis?
D. What are characteristic electron microscopic findings on renal biopsy?

ANSWERS

A-1. A. Bladder exstrophy

B.
- Anterior abdominal wall defect
- Exposed urinary bladder
- Epispadias
- Widely separated pubic rami

C.
- Cover the exposed bladder mucosa with plastic wrap to keep it moist
- Do not touch with latex gloves

D. Bladder adenocarcinoma

A-2. A. Torsion of the left testis
B. More than 6 hours
C. Scrotal orchidopexy

A-3. A. Voiding cystourethrography (VCUG) or micturating cystourethrography (MCU)

B.
- Dilatation and elongation of the posterior urethra
- Bladder trabeculations

C. Posterior urethral valve

D. Indications of MCU:
- Evaluation of antenatal hydronephrosis
- Urinary tract infection
- Suspected obstructive anomaly
- Voiding dysfunction
- Neurogenic bladder

E.
- Primary ablation of the valves
- If valve ablation is not possible, vesicostomy

F. *Complications of untreated PUV:*
- Recurrent urinary tract infection
- Secondary vesicoureteral reflux
- Chronic kidney disease (CKD)
- Urinary bladder diverticula

A-4. A. Cerebral salt wasting
B. Serum uric acid and vasopressin acid
C. 3% NaCl

A-5. A. Hemolytic uremic syndrome (HUS)

B. Peripheral smear shows fragmentation of red blood cells as schistocytes, burr cells and helmet cells, characteristic of hemolytic uremic syndrome

C. Basic pathology of HUS is thrombotic microangiopathy in which mixed platelet—fibrin thrombi occur in capillaries, arterioles and sometimes arteries in the absence of vascular inflammation and fibrin deposition. This microvascular injury commonly occurs in kidneys and brain.

D. *Diagnostic criteria for HUS:*
- Microangiopathic hemolytic anemia (Hb <10 g/dL)
- Evidence of hemolysis in peripheral blood smear examination (>2% schistocytes)
- Thrombocytopenia (platelets <1.5 lakhs/cu.mm)
- AKI (>50% rise in serum creatinine)
- Raised LDH

E. 80% cases of diarrhea HUS are caused by Shiga toxin producing *E. coli* (STEC), *Shigella* and *Campylobacter.*

A-6. A. Ambulatory blood pressure monitoring (ABPM). It is a diagnostic test to detect the hypertension by monitoring over 24 hours during normal daily activities.

B. *Indications of ABPM:*
- Stage 1 hypertension over three clinical visits
- High-risk patients with CKD, diabetes mellitus, obesity, obstructive sleep apnea, coarctation of aorta, etc.

C. White coat hypertension is defined as BP >95th percentile on duty or clinical setting, but <95th percentile outside of the working setting

D. 25%

A-7. A. Co-trimoxazole is drug of choice in dose of 2 mg/kg/dose of trimethoprim once daily.

B. *Drugs for uroprophylaxis in children:*

Drug	***Dose (mg/kg/day)***	***Remark***
Cotrimoxazole	2 mg/kg/dose of trimethoprim once daily	Avoid in infants <3 months of age and G-6-P-D deficiency
Nitrofurantoin	1–2	May cause vomiting and nausea. Avoid in infants <3 months of age of G-6-P-D deficiency
Cephalexin	10	Drug of choice for infant 3–6 months of age
Cefadroxil	5	Alternative drug for early infancy

C. *Indications for uroprophylaxis in children:*
- Recurrent febrile UTI
- High-grade VUR
- Infants with low-grade VUR particularly in presence of bowel bladder dysfunction (BBD)

D. *Duration for uroprophylaxis:*
- Until 2 years of age in infancy, at least one year beyond the last UTI
- In older patients, may be continued until resolution of BBD

E. Surgery is not indicated in this patient as there was no breakthrough UTI.

F. Repeat MCU is not indicated in this patient.

G. Other preventive measures for recurrent UTI:
- Circumcision reduces the risk of recurrent UTI in male infants, might be beneficial in patients with high-grade VUR.
- Appropriate management of BBD
- Management of constipation

- Children with neurogenic bladder may require bladder retraining, anticholinergic drugs and/or intermittent clean catheterization

A-8. A. Recurrent UTI with BBD

B. Ultrasonography of abdomen, MCU and DMSA scan should be performed in this patient.

C.

- Calculation of bladder capacity = (Age in years + 1) × 30 mL
- Bladder capacity of this patient = (12 + 1) × 30 = 390 mL

D. *Management of this patient:*

- Uroprophylaxis for recurrent UTI
- *Treatment for BBD:*
  - Fiber-rich diet and water 6–8 glasses/day
  - Polyethylene glycol for constipation
  - Timed and double voiding

A-9. A. Renal vein thrombosis

B. Sepsis, DIC and hemolytic-uremic syndrome are differential diagnosis.

C. USG Doppler study of kidneys is good investigation for renal vein thrombosis.

D. Treatment of predisposing condition like polycythemia, sepsis and heparinization

E. Long-term complications of renal vein thrombosis:

- Systemic hypertension
- Atrophy of the affected kidney

A-10. A. Wilms tumor and neuroblastoma

B. Differentiating points for Wilms tumor and neuroblastoma:

- Wilms tumor arises from kidneys (nephroblastoma), while neuroblastoma originates from neural crest cells, often in adrenal glands.
- Wilms tumor does not cross the midline, neuroblastoma may cross it.
- Wilms tumor commonly presents as abdominal lump, while neuroblastoma as secondary skeletal metastasis.

C. Wilms tumor causes hypertension due to renal ischemia, while neuroblastoma due to increased catecholamine secretion.

D. Wilms tumor causes secondaries in lung and neuroblastoma bones.

A-11. A. Postinfectious (streptococcal) glomerulonephritis (PIGN)

B. Nephritogenic strains of streptococci are type 4 and 12 causing pharyngitis and serotype 49 causing pyoderma

C. Antideoxyribonuclease B level

D. Life-threatening complications of PIGN

- Hypertensive encephalopathy
- Acute left ventricular failure
- Pulmonary edema
- Acute kidney injury (uremia)
- Hyperkalemia
- Metabolic acidosis

E. Indications of renal biopsy in acute glomerulonephritis

- *Systemic features:*
  - Fever, rash, joint pain, pulmonary symptoms, heart disease, history of recurrent disease
  - Absence of serological evidence of streptococcal infection
  - Normal C_3 level
  - Features of both nephritis and nephrotic syndrome
  - High blood urea and serum creatinine, anuria requiring dialysis

- *Delayed resolution:*
  - Oliguria, hypertension and uremia for more than 7–10 days
  - Gross hematuria persistent beyond 3–4 weeks
  - Nephrotic rang of proteinuria beyond 2 weeks
  - Low C_3 level beyond 12 weeks

F.
- PSGN has excellent prognosis in children.
- The symptoms begin to resolve in first weeks of life with loss of edema and fall in BP.
- Gross hematuria and significant proteinuria disappear within 2 weeks.
- Microscopic hematuria and slight proteinuria may persist for several months.
- Hypertension subsides within 2–3 weeks, but rarely may persist for several weeks.
- Renal biopsy is rarely indicated in PIGN.

A-12. A. Schwartz formula for eGFR = $\frac{\text{K} \times \text{Height (cm)}}{\text{Serum creatinine (mg/dL)}}$

Where K is,
- 0.33 for LBW infants <1 year of age
- 0.45 for AGA infant <1 years of age
- 0.55 for children and adolescent females
- 0.70 for adolescent males

B. *Stage II CKD:* eGFR 60–90 mL/kg/1.73 MR

C. *Causes of anemia in CKD:*
- Erythropoietin deficiency
- Iron deficiency
- Blood loss
- Infections
- Hemodialysis
- Nutritional deficits

D. Renal osteodystrophy in CKD due to:
- Phosphorus retention
- Reduced calcitriol
- Decreased calcium
- High levels of parathormone (PTH)

E. Growth hormone is approved treatment for short stature in CKD.

A-13. A. Autosomal recessive polycystic kidney disease (ARPKD)

B. In Caroli's disease, there is cystic dilatation of the intrahepatic bile ducts.

C. Hepatic complications in this disease:
- Poral hypertension
- Ascending cholangitis
- Reversal of portal vein flow
- Thrombocytopenia

D. The polycystic kidney and hepatic disease 1 gene (*PKHDI*)

E. Common causes of abdominal mass or lump in infants:
- Bilateral hydronephrosis
- Multicystic kidney disease
- Polycystic kidney disease
- Horseshoe kidney
- Neuroblastoma
- Wilms tumor

- Hepatoblastoma
- Choledochal cyst
- Teratoma

F. Physical findings to suspect renal disease in children:
- Single umbilical artery
- Hypertension
- External ear anomalies
- Polydactyly and syndactyly
- Imperforate anus
- Other anomalies like CHDs, syndromes and vertebral anomalies

A-14. A. Idiopathic hypercalciuria

B. Urine calcium/creatinine ratio >0.2 is suggesting idiopathic hypercalciuria. It can be confirmed by 24 hours urine calcium, more than 4 mg/kg/day is diagnostic

C. *Differential diagnosis:*
- IgA nephropathy
- Alport's syndrome
- Urolithiasis

D. Hydrochlorothiazide along with alkali therapy. Hydrochlorothiazide increases distal tubular reabsorption of calcium.

E. Distal RTA (dRTA) (RTA Type II)

A-15. A. It is aortic angiography, showing stenosis at both carotids and subclavians.

B. Takayasu disease (Aortoarteritis)

C. Weak or absent peripheral pulsations, right upper limb hypertension, measurement of blood pressure in all the four limbs is an important clinical examination point to suspect Takayasu disease

D. Takayasu may present as:
- Hypertension
- Congestive cardiac failure
- Stroke
- Syncope
- Seizures
- Visual complaints

E. Tuberculosis and syphilis are considered as etiology in some cases.

A-16. A. Bartter syndrome

B. Urinary chloride, urine calcium/creatinine ratio and USG abdomen should be done. Urine chloride is elevated, urine calcium/creatinine ratio is raised indicating calciuria and USG abdomen may show nephrocalcinosis.

C. Potassium supplements as oral potassium chloride and indomethacin 2–4 mg/kg/day.

D. Chronic kidney disease is rare, but known to develop in adulthood.

A-17. A. Distal renal tubular acidosis (dRTA) (RTA Type II)

B. Hyperchloremic, hypokalemic metabolic acidosis with normal anion gap

C.
- Urinary anion gap = (Urinary Na^+ + Urinary K^+) – urinary Cl^-
- Positive urinary gap suggests a deficiency of ammonia genesis and possibility of distal RTA.

D. Alkali therapy. Dose of bicarbonate 2–4 mEq/kg/day

E. *Causes of nephrocalcinosis:*
- Hypercalciuria
- Hypocitraturia
- Vitamin D intoxication
- Furosemide intoxication

F. Lowe syndrome is also called as oculocerebrorenal syndrome characterized by cataracts, Fanconi syndrome and mental retardation

A-18. A. Alport syndrome

B. Hearing assessment to look for high frequency sensorineural hearing loss and ophthalmic examination for anterior lenticonus and macular flecks are almost confirmatory for Alport syndrome.

C. Genetic analysis is the confirmatory test.

D. Electron microscopic examination of renal biopsy.

Thickening and thinning of glomerulus basement membrane (also called as Basket-Weave appearance)

CHAPTER 18

Hematology–Oncology

QUESTIONS

Q-1. An 8-year-old girl presented with fever, pallor and jaundice of acute onset. This was color of her urine. She had fever and cough-cold 2 weeks back.

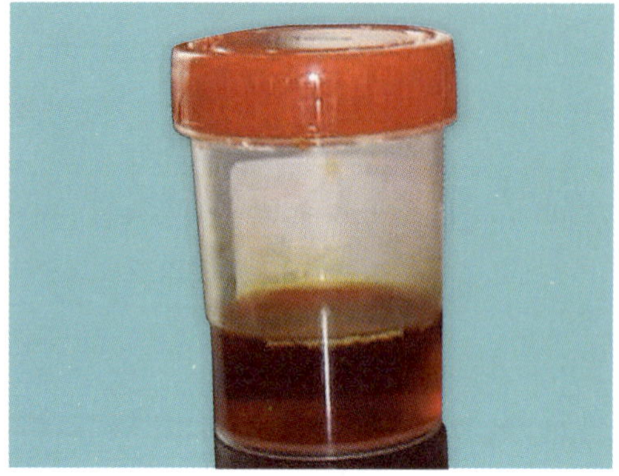

A. What is your diagnosis?
B. What does this color of urine indicate?
C. What investigations should be performed in this case?
D. What are other causes of red-colored urine?

Q-2.

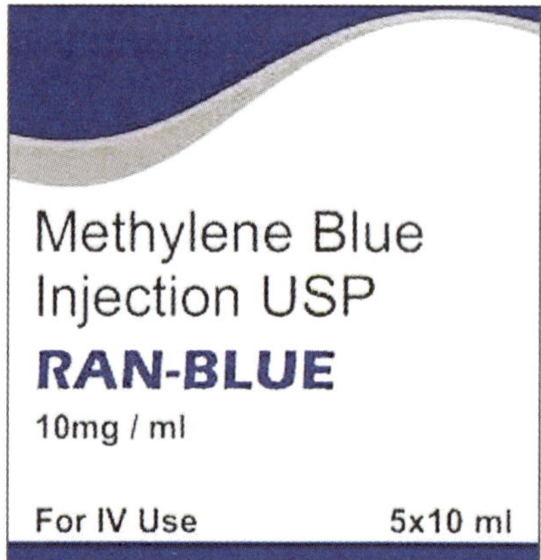

A. Name two indications.
B. Name two contradictions.
C. What is the color of urine when a patient is given methylene blue?

Q-3. Chemoprophylaxis in children with asplenia.

Q-4. A 2-year-old girl presents with ecchymotic patches off and on since birth. There is past history of prolonged umbilical stump bleeding and delayed separation of umbilical cord.

A. What coagulation factor deficiency is likely?
B. What problem is known to occur following surgery in this patient?
C. What observation is the basis for screening tests for deficiency of this factor?
D. What pattern of hemorrhage makes the clinician to suspect the condition?
E. Define delayed separation of the umbilical cord.

Q-5. A known case of Hodgkin's lymphoma presents with sudden onset of cough, dyspnea, hoarseness of voice, stridor, facial edema and drowsiness. All these problems developed within few hours.

A. What complication is likely?
B. What are lifesaving modalities of treatment?

Q-6. A 9-year-old girl presented with high-grade fever of 4 weeks duration. It was diagnosed as brucellosis. She started to deteriorate with high-grade fever and pancytopenia. Bone marrow aspiration confirmed the diagnosis.

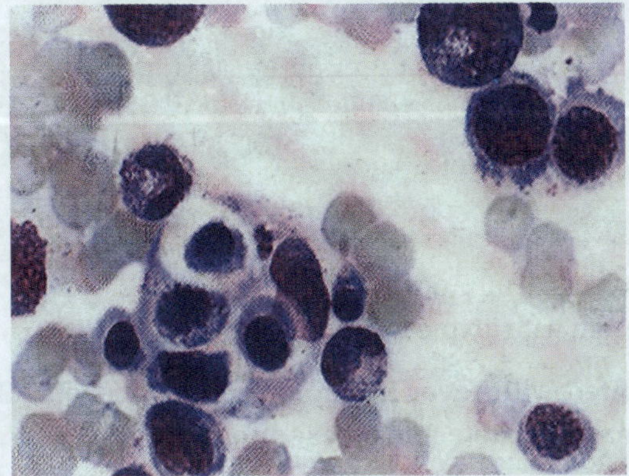

A. Name the condition.
B. Name other two blood investigations included in diagnostic criteria of the condition.
C. Name other similar syndrome associated with autoimmune disease like systemic onset juvenile idiopathic arthritis.

Q-7. A male child was diagnosed as uncomplicated smear positive *P. vivax* malaria and treated with chloroquine. Primaquine was started as radical therapy and returned back with severe anemia and black colored urine as shown in the picture.

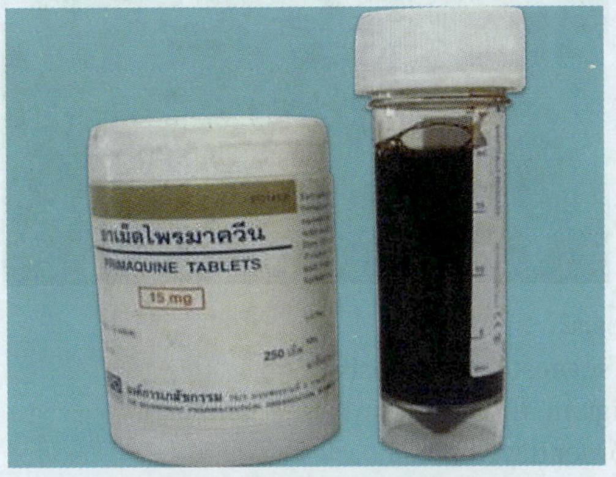

A. What is the possible disorder with the child besides malaria?
B. What is the pattern of inheritance of this disorder?
C. Which antimalarials are known to cause hemolysis in this disorder?
D. What is the cause of black-colored urine in this complication?
E. Why the test does not reveal the diagnosis immediately after an episode of hemolysis?

Q-8. We get the report of peripheral smear examination many a times described as presence of atypical lymphocytes.

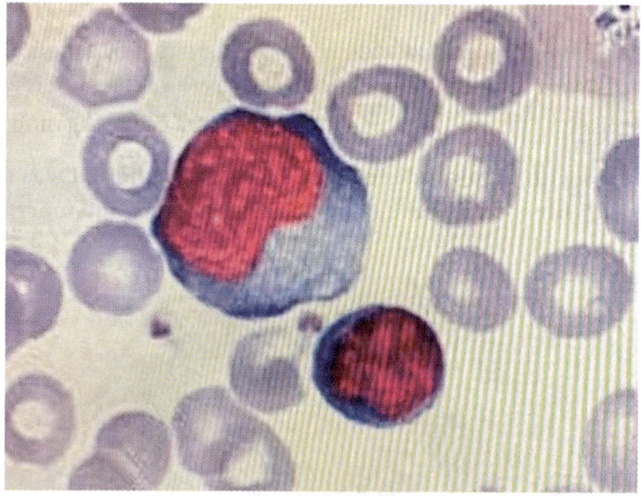

A. What are the features of atypical lymphocytes?
B. Which conditions can present with atypical lymphocytes?

Q-9. A 15-month-old boy presented with fever and marked tachycardia. He also had hypertension. A firm irregular intra-abdominal mass was detected on examination.

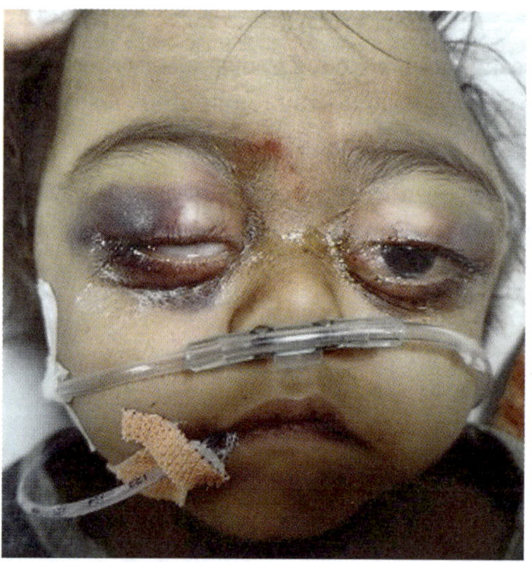

A. What is most likely diagnosis?
B. What are important clues suggesting diagnosis?
C. What is the name of eye sign in this condition?
D. From which cells this disorder develops?

Q-10. A 15-month-old male child was brought for routine vaccination from upper socioeconomical status family. Severe pallor was noted. He was born at full-term uneventfully with birth weight 2.9 kg. Child was consuming 1,600 mL of milk per day by bottle. He was clinically normal except severe pallor. CBC showed Hb 6.5 g/dL, TLC 7,500/cu.mm and platelets 5,80,000/cu.mm S. ferritin was 10 ng/mL. His growth chart was as below:

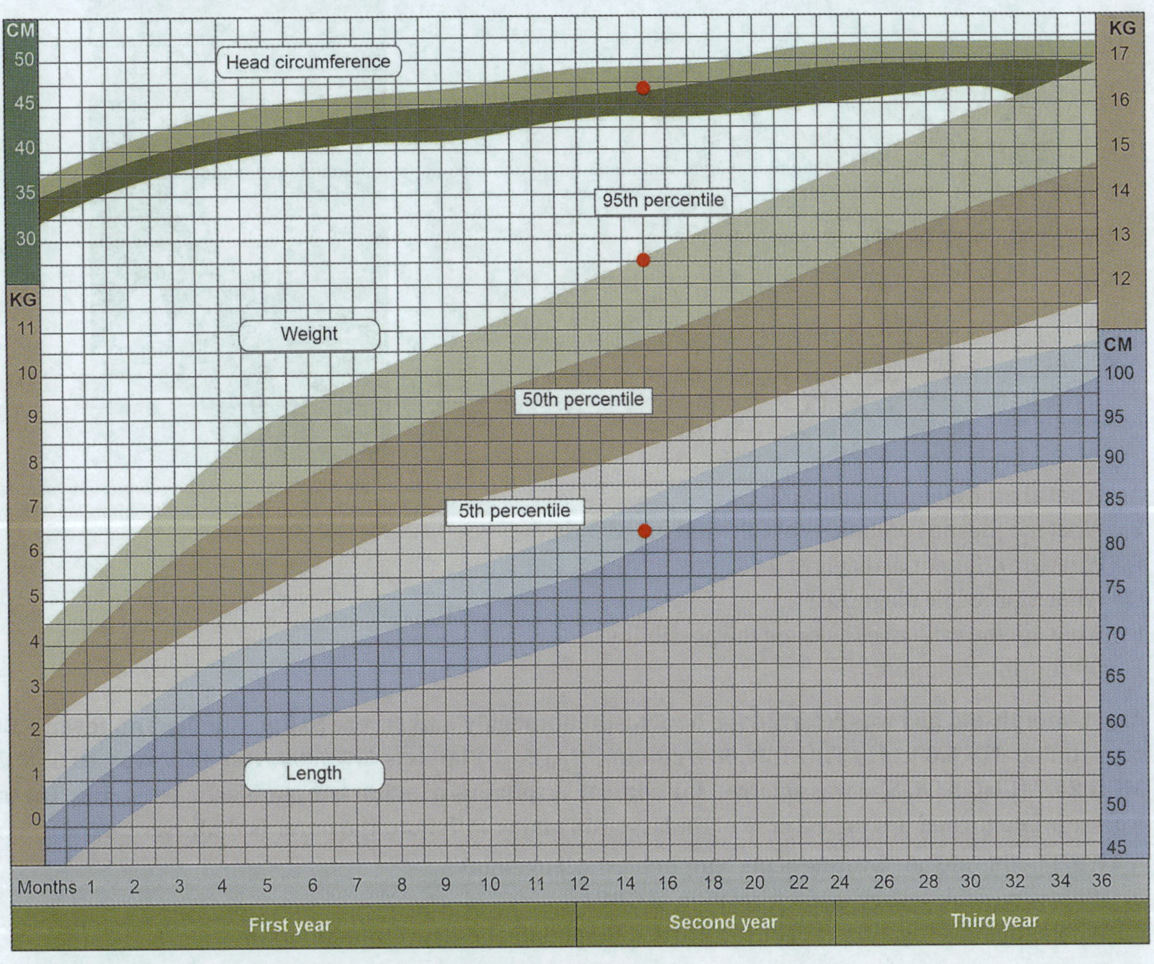

A. What are the interpretations of growth chart and anemia?
B. Which mechanisms are likely responsible for anemia?
C. What should be dietary advice for this child?

Q-11. A 14-year-old girl presented with severe iron deficiency anemia, no response after 8 weeks of oral iron therapy. CBC showed Hb 3.5 g/dl, TLC 4,800, P_{48}, L_{50}, platelets 77,000. HCT 10.9, MCV 112, MCH 33.6, MCHC 32.1, RDW 22.4. Clinical examination was as shown below in pictures:

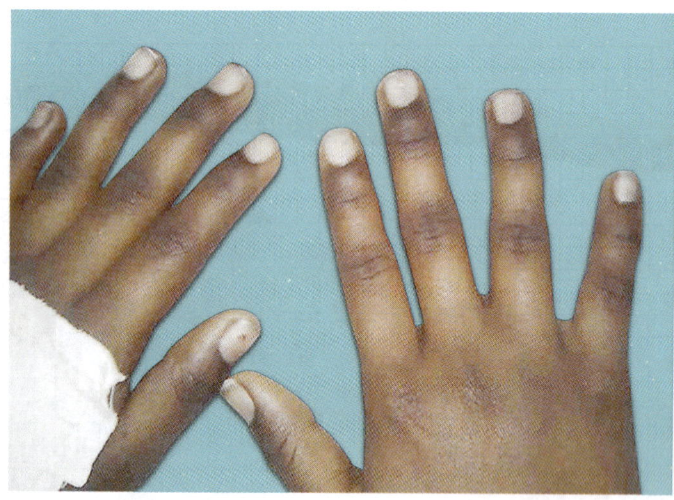
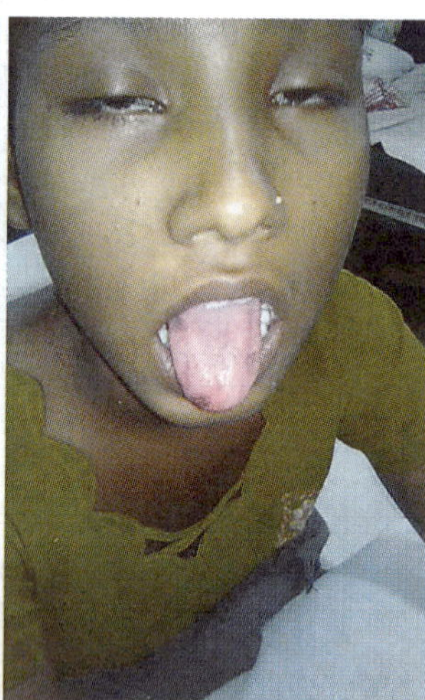

A. What are the clinical findings?
B. What are the interpretations of CBC and blood indices?
C. What are differential diagnosis?
D. What is probable diagnosis?
E. What are the evidences favoring the possibility?
F. Outline the treatment.

Q-12. An 11-month-old girl was referred for hepatosplenomegaly and severe pallor. She had no fever. CBC was reported as Hb 6.6 g/dL, TLC 1,20,000/cu.mm, P_{13}, L_{70}, Platelets 5,73,000. Her PCV was 19.8, MCV 72, MCH 24, MCHC 33.4. She was referred for clinical suspicious of acute lymphoblastic leukemia. On further work-up, she turned out to be a case of thalassemia major with both the parents thalassemia trait.

A. What points are not favoring acute lymphoblastic leukemia?
B. What is possible fallacy in interpretation of CBC?
C. What other investigations will be helpful to differentiate these two conditions?

Q-13. A 5-year-old boy presented with pancytopenia and short stature. He had hyperpigmentation over face and around the neck. A thumb anomaly was noted. On further work-up, renal anomaly was detected.

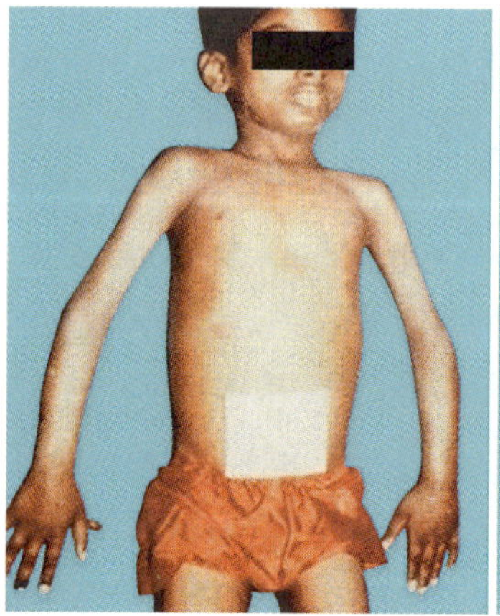
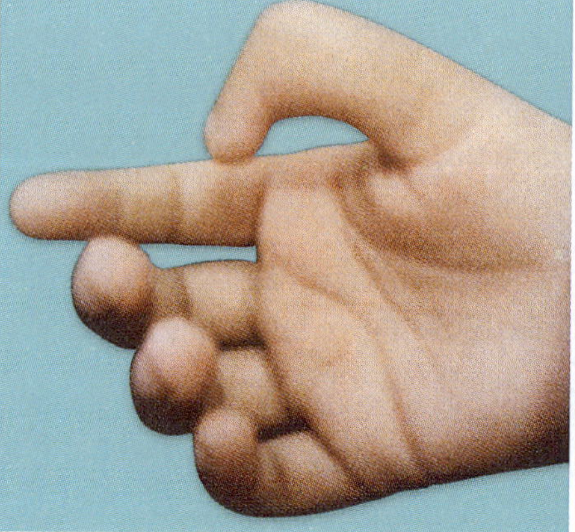
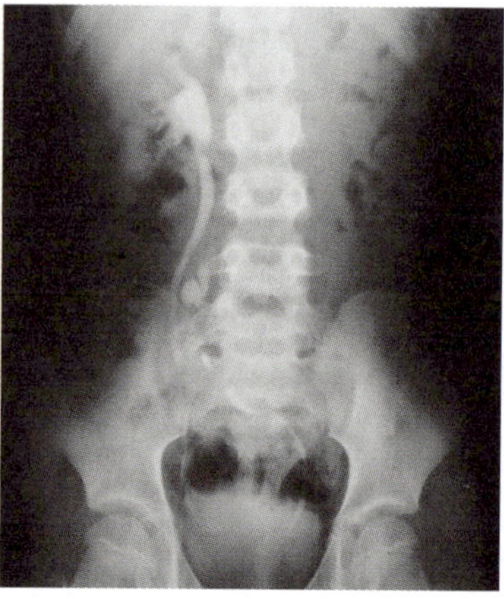

A. What is the probable diagnosis?
B. What type of changes will be seen in peripheral smear examination and bone marrow aspiration and biopsy?
C. What is the confirmatory test for this disease?
D. What are the treatment options?

Q-14. A 2-month-old male presented with severe pallor and hepatosplenomegaly. His Hb was 4.7 g/dL, leukocyte count and platelets were within normal range. Reticulocyte count was low. Both the parents were negative for thalassemia disorder. Bone marrow biopsy confirmed the diagnosis?

A. What is probable diagnosis?
B. What other skeletal manifestations are known to be associated with this disorder?
C. What are points differentiating this condition from thalassemia major?

Q-15. An 8-year-old boy presented with fever, pancytopenia and weight loss. He also had hyperpigmentation around neck, nail and tongue changes with lymphadenopathy. Investigations for HIV and malignancy were negative clinical photographs are as follows:

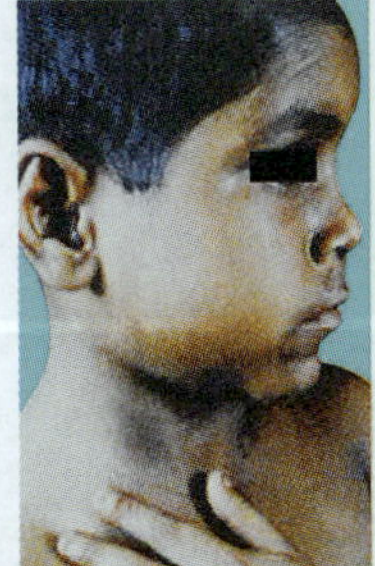
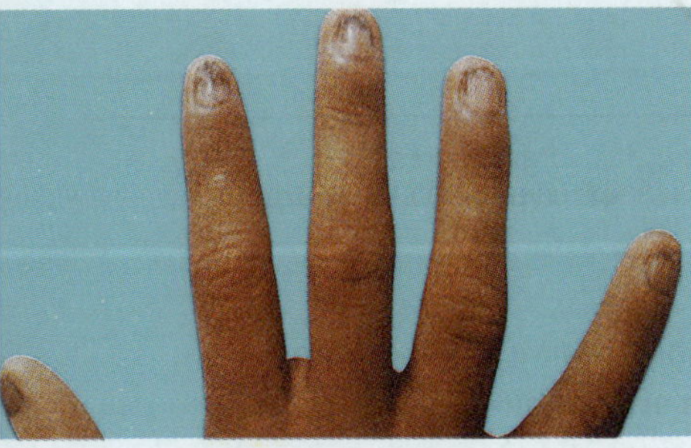
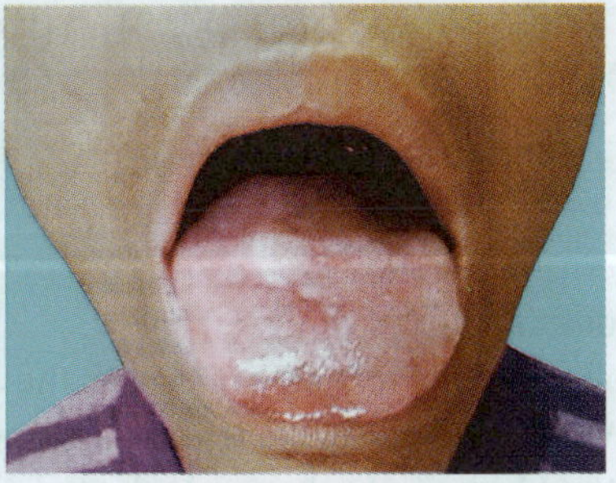

A. What are the clinical findings over nails and tongue?
B. What is probable diagnosis?
C. What are treatment options available?
D. What oncological complications are known to develop in these patients?

Q-16. A 3-year-old child presented with steatorrhea and failure to thrive since infancy. There was history of recurrent bacterial and fungal infections. Anemia, neutropenia and thrombocytopenia were since infancy. HIV, primary immunodeficiency disorders and malignancies were ruled out. Bone marrow failure and pancreatic insufficiency were confirmed.

A. What is probable diagnosis?
B. What endocrinal disorders are known to be associated with this condition?
C. What is pattern of inheritance of this disease?

Q-17.

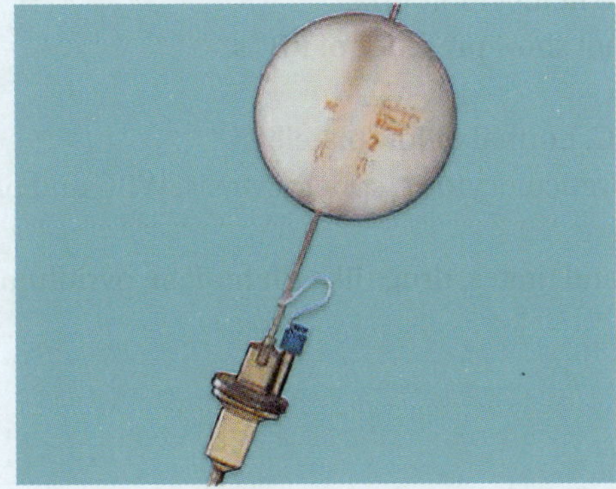

A. Identify the device and its use in the practice.
B. Advantage of using this device.
C. What are other methods to use for the same purpose?

Q-18.

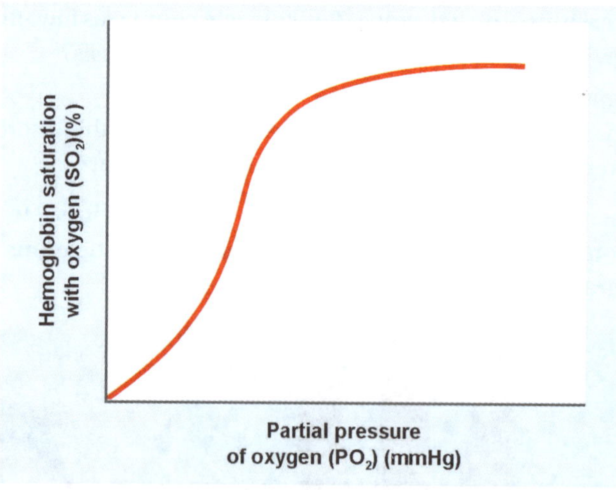

A. Identify the curve.
B. What are the factors which shift the above curve to left or right?
C. What is the normal oxygen content in arterial blood?
D. What is the formula to calculate oxygen content?

Q-19. Answer the questions of febrile neutropenia.

A. What is definition of neutropenia?
B. Classification of neutropenia.
C. What is febrile neutropenia?
D. Which neutropenia granulocyte colony stimulating factor (G-CSF) is used? What is the dose?
E. What antibiotics are recommended in febrile neutropenia?
F. Name congenital neutropenia syndromes.

ANSWERS

A-1. A. Autoimmune hemolytic anemia

B.

- Color of the urine is due to hemoglobinuria.
- Urine examination does not show presence of RBCs.

C.

- *CBC:* Low HB, normal TLC, normal or low platelets
- *PS exam:* Polychromasia, reticulocytosis, spherocytosis, WBC and platelets normal
- Direct Coomb's test positive

D. Pigments in food, beetroots and urates, drugs like rifampicin, pyridium can cause red color of the urine.

A-2. A.

- Antidote for cyanide poisoning
- Drug-induced meth-hemoglobinemia

B.

- G-6-P-D deficiency
- Renal insufficiency

C. Urine and stool turns blue green.

A-3. Asplenia increases risk of fulminant septicemia. Mortality from septicemia is increased 50 fold following splenectomy for trauma and 350 fold due to sickle disease.

Indications:

- Sickle cell disease
- Splenectomy following trauma
- Asplenia with thalassemia, spherocytosis, etc.
- Congenital asplenia

Drugs and dosage:

- In addition to pneumococcal and meningococcal vaccines, influenza vaccine
- Penicillin V 125 mg BD <5 years
- 250 mg BD >5 years,
- At least until 5 years of age or 5 years after surgical removal whichever is longer. Ideally, it should be continued for lifetime.

A-4. A. Factor XIII deficiency (Fibrin stabilizing factor deficiency)
B. Poor wound healing
C. Instability of the clot
D. Delayed hemorrhage (Bruise or hematoma on the next day of trauma)
E. Beyond 4 weeks of age

A-5. A. Superior vena cava syndrome
B. Chemotherapy, radiotherapy

A-6. A. *Infection:* Associated hemophagocytic syndrome (IAHS)
B. S. Triglyceride ↑ (>265 mg/dL)
S. Fibrinogen ↓ (<150 mg/dL)
S. Ferritin ↑ (>500 ng/mL)
C. Macrophage activation syndrome

A-7. A. Glucose-6-phosphate dehydrogenase (G-6-P-D) deficiency
B. X-linked disorder
C.

- Primaquine
- Pamaquine
- Chloroquine
- Quinine

D. Hemoglobinuria
E. Immediately after a hemolytic episode, reticulocytes and young RBCs predominate and they have higher enzyme activity than do older cells and therefore test may fail to diagnose the condition. It should be repeated after few weeks for confirmation.

A-8. A.

- Large in size compared to normal lymphocytes
- More cytoplasm
- Presence of nucleoli and nuclei
- Cytoplasm tends to be indented by RBCs.

B.

- Infection Mononucleosis (EBV)
- Cytomegalovirus
- Toxoplasmosis
- Viral
- Hepatitis B Infection

A-9. A. Neuroblastoma

B.

- Fever
- Irritability
- Bone pain
- Orbital proptosis
- Periorbital ecchymosis

C. Racoon eyes

D. Neural crest cells

A-10. A.

- The weight, length and head circumference are above the 97th percentile, indicating higher than normal growth
- Hemoglobin level indicates severe anemia. S. Ferritin level is also low. Therefore, it is iron deficiency anemia. Total WBC count is normal and higher level of platelets count indicates good bone marrow response. Therefore, it is a case of severe iron deficiency anemia.

B. The discrepancy between growth and iron deficiency anemia indicates selectively iron deficiency. It is possible due to lack of iron from other sources of diet as child consumes mainly milk-based diet.

C. Mechanisms for iron deficiency anemia in children with mainly milk-based diet

- Milk is the poor source of iron.
- Higher content of calcium in animal milk compared to human milk retards absorption of iron.
- Bovine milk protein allergy may cause blood loss from GI tract.
- Due to excessive consumption of milk, iron-containing diet is lacking.

D. Dietary advice

- No milk or milk substitutes initially and then maximum milk 200–300 mL/day
- Encourage for iron-rich food like dates, jaggery, millet, green leafy vegetables, etc.
- Iron supplementation 3 mg/kg/day as elemental iron on empty stomach for 3–4 months for correction of anemia.
- Encourage for cereals and green leafy vegetables and citrus fruits.

A-11. A.

- Severe pallor (Tongue and Nails)
- Hyperpigmented knuckles

B.

- Very severe anemia (Hb 3.5 g/dL)
- Thrombocytopenia
- Low hematocrit

- Raised MCV (macrocytosis)
- Raised RDW

Very severe anemia with raised MCV, RDW, low hematocrit and thrombocytopenia, bicytopenia.

C.

- *Nutritional anemia*: Iron deficiency anemia with vitamin B_{12} and folic acid deficiency
- Bone marrow failure conditions like Fanconi's syndrome
- Acute lymphoblastic leukemia

D. *Nutritional anemia*: Iron deficiency anemia with Vitamin B_{12} and folic acid

E. *Clinically:* Severe anemia
Hypopigmented knuckles

Laboratory evidence:

- Severe anemia
- Thrombocytopenia
- Raised MCV (macrocytosis)
- Raised RDW

F.

- PCV transfusion can be avoided because patient is not in cardiac failure.
- Oral iron 3 mg/kg/day for 2–3 months after hemoglobin normalizes.
- Vitamin B_{12} 500 μg in infants and 100 μg in older children orally for 3 months
- Folic acid 5 mg/day for 3–4 months. Folic acid should be started after 2 weeks of vitamin B_{12} therapy to avoid worsening of clinical manifestation of vitamin B_{12} deficiency.

A-12. A. *Clinically:* No fever, no skin bleeding manifestations and no lymphadenopathy
Investigations: Thrombocytopenia is common in acute lymphoblastic leukemia (ALL), thrombocytosis in the patient, indicates good bone marrow response.

B. In hemolytic anemia, there will be plenty of normoblasts and late normoblasts in circulation. These cells of RBC series are nucleated and larger in size, which will be counted by automatic cell counter as lymphocytes. As a result, it will be reported as leukocytosis and interpreted as ALL.

C.

- Peripheral smear examination for picture of hemolysis and absence of blast cells.
- Reticulocytosis will favor hemolysis
- Bone marrow examination will confirm the condition.

A-13. A. Fanconi anemia

B. Peripheral smear examination shows anemia, macrocytes and reticulocytopenia. Bone marrow is hypoplastic.

C. Next generation sequencing (NGS) is confirmatory test.

D.

- Hematopoietic stem cell transplantation (HSCT) is the only curative therapy.
- Androgens (Danazol and oxymetholone)
- May require transfusion with severe anemia.

A-14.

- Diamond–Blackfan syndrome
- Box-like skull, tripharyngeal thumb or other anomalies of thumb
- *Age:* Diamond–Blackfan syndrome presents in early infancy (2–3 months), while thalassemia major after age of 6 months:
- Reticulocytopenia in Diamond–Blackfan syndrome and reticulocytosis in thalassemia major
- Hypoplastic bone marrow in Diamond–Blackfan syndrome and hyperplasia of bone marrow in thalassemia major

A-15. A.
- Dystrophic nails
- Leukoplakia

B. Dyskeratosis congenita

C.
- Androgens
- Hematopoietic stem cell transplantation (HSCT)

D.
- Myeloid dysplasia syndrome
- Acute myeloid leukemia
- Solid tumors

A-16. A. Shwachman-Diamond syndrome

B.
- Insulin-dependent diabetes mellitus
- Growth hormone deficiency
- Hypogonadism
- Hypothyroidism

C. Autosomal recessive

A-17. A. Bedside leukodepletion filter. It is used to prevent non-hemolytic febrile blood transfusion reactions and transmission of some infections.

B. Advantages of using bedside leukodepletion filter:
- Prevention of non-hemolytic febrile transfusion reactions
- Avoids HLA alloimmunization to some extent
- Prevents CMV infection
- Improved storage of erythrocytes by prior leukodepletion

C. Other methods for leukodepletion:
- Centrifugation can remove 70% of leukocytes in one unit of blood.
- Cell washing or use if deglycerolized red cells can remove more than 95% of contaminated white cells.
- The older microaggregate filters can remove leukocyte contents by 90–93%.
- The third generation leukocyte depletion filters can remove almost 99% of white cells.

A-18. A. Oxygen–Hemoglobin dissociation curve

B. Factors which shift the curve to left:
- High fetal hemoglobin
- Alkaline pH
- Reduction in CO_2
- Hypothermia

Factors which shift the curve to right:
- Low fetal hemoglobin
- Acidic pH
- CO_2 retention
- Febrile illness

C. Normal oxygen content of arterial blood is 20.

D. Formula to calculate oxygen content

$CaO_2 = (1.34 \times Hb \times SaO_2) + (0.003 \times PaO_2)$

A-19. A. Neutropenia is defined as absolute neutrophil count <1500/cu.mm.

B.
- *Mild neutropenia:* Absolute neutrophil count 1000–1500/cu.mm
- *Moderate neutropenia:* Absolute neutrophil count 500–1000/cu.mm
- *Severe neutropenia:* Absolute neutrophil count <500/cu.mm

C. Febrile neutropenia is defined as fever >100.4°F for more than an hour with absolute neutrophil count <500/cu.mm with immunosuppression.

D. Recombinant human granulocyte colony stimulating factor (rhG–CSF) is used in chemotherapy-related neutropenia. Dose is 5–10 μg/kg by subcutaneous route.

E. *Antibiotics in Febrile neutropenia:*
- Ceftazidime or piperacillin-tazobactam and vancomycin as basic combination
- Meropenem in severe infections

F. Congenital syndrome
- Kostmann agranulocytosis
- Cyclic neutropenia
- Shwachman syndrome

CHAPTER 19

Endocrinology

QUESTIONS

Q-1. A 3-year-old girl was referred for precocious puberty and obesity. She also had gelastic seizures.

A. What is the most possible cause of precocious puberty?
B. What is the clinical characteristic of gelastic seizures?
C. What are other clinical manifestations of this disorder?
D. What type of sexual precocity is known to occur in this disorder?

Q-2. A 12-year-old girl presented with obesity (BMI >95th percentile), acne and loss of scalp hairs. Her nape of neck was as shown in figure below.

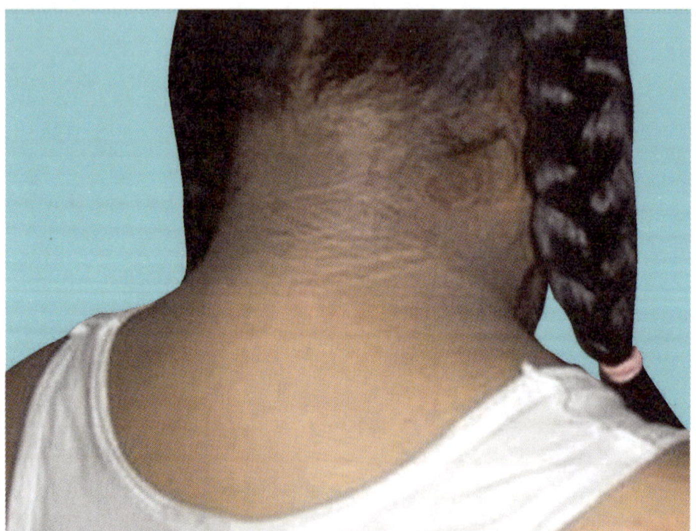

A. What is this clinical sign called?
B. What is the probable diagnosis?
C. What investigations do you suggest?
D. What are increased risks in this condition?

Q-3. A 4.5-year-old boy presented with weight 10.2 kg, height 82 cm. His serum calcium was 5.8 mg/dL, S. phosphorus 7.1 mg/dL, serum alkaline phosphatase 4760 IU/L and serum parathormone raised.

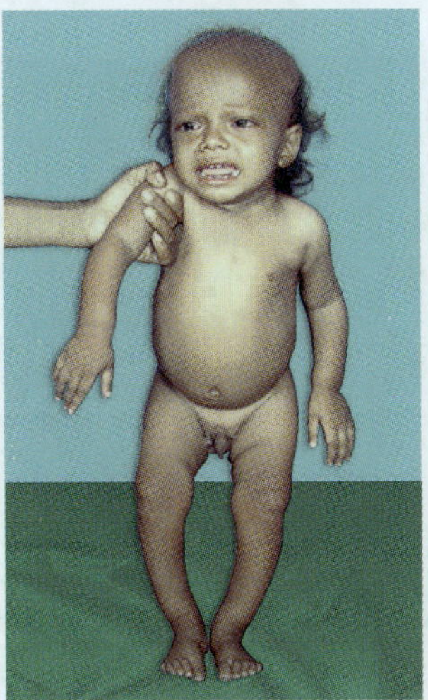

A. What is your clinical diagnosis?

B. What is expected level of 1, $25(OH)_2 D_3$?

C. What is the basic defect in this disorder?

D. What is the pattern of inheritance of this disorder?

Q-4. A neonate was born with these external genitalia. The infant developed vomiting after one month of life and presented with severe dehydration, hyponatremia, hyperkalemia and metabolic acidosis.

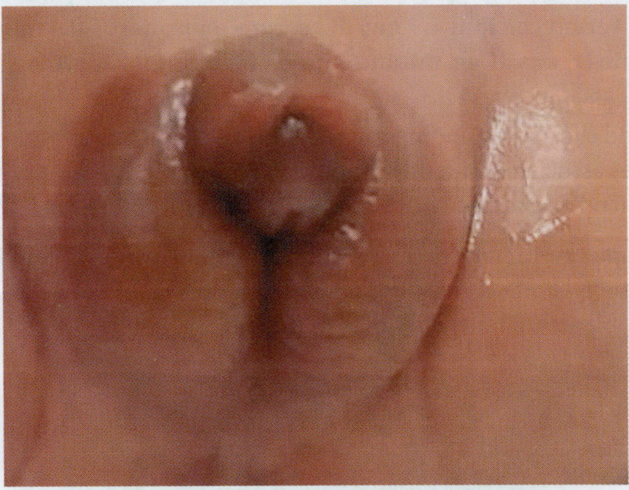

A. What is the probable diagnosis?

B. What is the most common cause for this disorder?

C. Name the definitive biochemical test for confirmation of this condition.

D. Name the drugs used for treatment of this disease.

Q-5. A 3-year-old female had illness of 2 months duration in form of persistent, nonbilious vomiting and pain in abdomen. She also developed constipation. She lost 6 kg weight in 3 months, in spite of excessive eating. She also was drinking water in excess with increased frequency of micturition.

A. What is the probable diagnosis?

B. What investigations would you suggest?

C. What is another presentation of this disease as life-threatening emergency?

Q-6. A 8-year-old boy presented with puffy face, edema feet, weight gain and constipation for 6 months. She had pallor, yellowish skin, but white sclera. CBC and indices showed anemia, high MCV. Serum cholesterol was raised with normal serum albumin and no albuminuria.

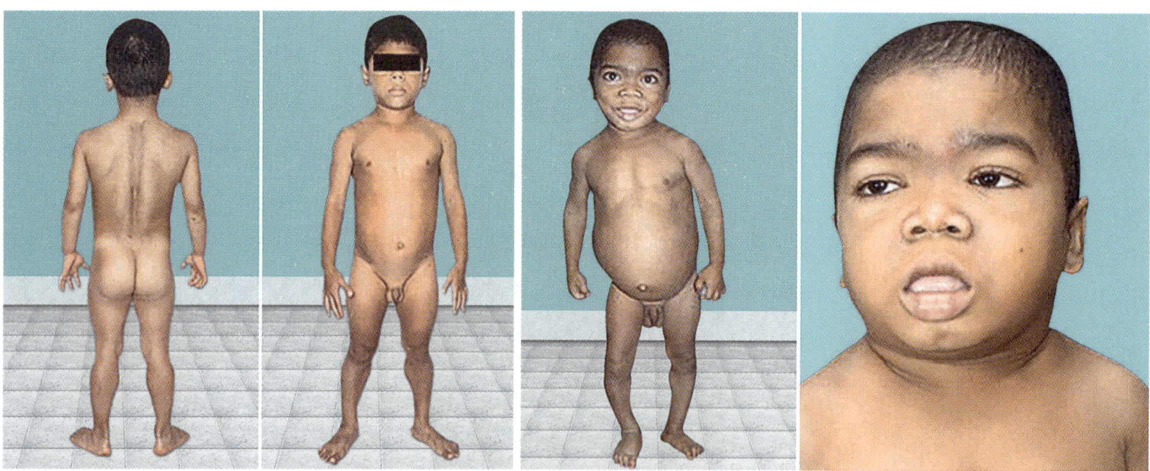

A. What is the probable diagnosis?
B. What investigations should be performed?
C. What is the cause of bradycardia in this disease?
D. What is the name of variant of this disease presenting with prominent calf muscles?

Q-7. A 7-day-old neonate with 3 kg weight presented with seizures. The baby was stabilized and evaluated. The investigations showed serum calcium 4.5 mg/dL, serum phosphorus 8.4 mg/dL, parathormone less than 5 pg/mL 25 (OH) vitamin D_3 was 31 ng/mL and serum creatinine 0.2 mg/dL.

A. What is the probable diagnosis?
B. Mention one ECG and chest X-ray findings one should look for in this infant.
C. Name two syndromes associated with this condition.
D. What is the treatment on discharge?

Q-8. A term neonate developed refractory hypoglycemia. The baby was evaluated and started long-term drug therapy to control hypoglycemia. On follow-up, mother complained of development of some abnormal growth on face and other parts of body as shown in the picture.

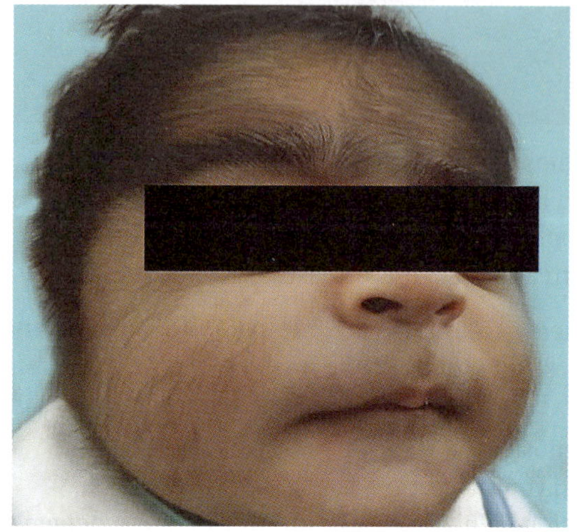

A. What abnormal growth is seen on face of the baby?
B. Name the drug responsible for it.
C. What is the dose of this drug?
D. What are other side effects of this dug?
E. What is the diagnostic investigation for this disorder?

Q-9. A 4-year-old child with type 1 diabetes mellitus is on insulin therapy. He developed a blunt abdominal trauma following a road-traffic accident. His weight is 10 kg. he needs to be taken up for emergency laparotomy. The capillary blood glucose was 320 mg/dL and blood ketone 4 mmol/L.

A. Can this child be taken for surgery?
B. Which fluid should be started in this patient?
C. What is the fluid rate of administration for this child?
D. How frequently blood glucose level should be monitored?
E. What is dose of insulin and route of its administration?
F. What metabolic complications are likely to develop in this patient?

Q-10. A 8-year-old child with type 1 diabetes mellitus (DM) for the past 2 years is brought to you. It is time for him for insulin before breakfast. Please, administer 8 units regular and 14 units isophane (NPH) insulin to this patient. The insulin injections and syringe are presented to you as shown below in the picture. Mention the steps to follow.

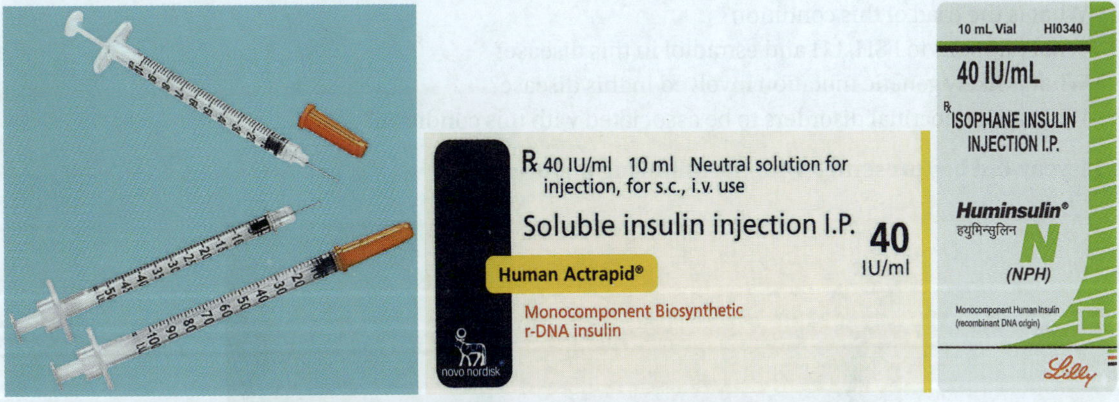

Q-11. Write appropriate interpretations of the followings:

A. HbA_1C 7%
B. Fasting blood sugar 116 mg/dL
C. 2 hour plasma glucose after oral glucose tolerance test of 170 mg/dL
D. Fasting plasma glucose 12 mmol/L
E. HbA_1C 6%

Q-12. A healthy term neonate is screened for congenital adrenal hyperplasia (CAH) by heel prick method. The screening report is 110 nmol/L of 17-hydroxyprogesterone.

A. What is the interpretation of this screening report?
B. What are the next steps to be planned?
C. What disease is identified based on this screening test?
D. What are causes for false-positive this screening test?
E. What are the causes for false-negative this screening test?
F. What problems can be avoided by this screening test?

Q-13. A 4-year-old girl presented with breast stage 3, pubic hair stage 1 and menarche. She had skin lesion as shown below.

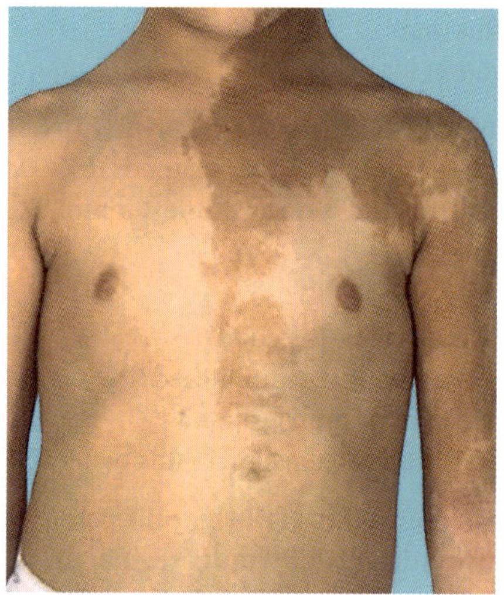

A. Identity the skin lesion.
B. What is most probable diagnosis?
C. What is the triad of this condition?
D. What happens to FSH, LH and estradiol in this disease?
E. What is likely genetic mutation involved in this disease?
F. What are endocrinal disorders to be associated with this condition?

Q-14. A 14-year-old boy presented with the following picture:

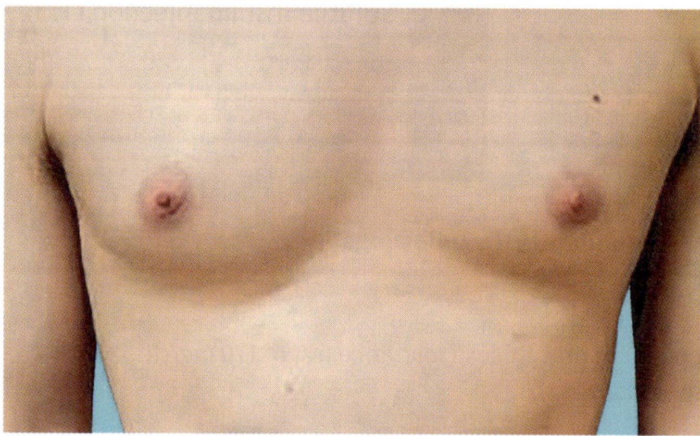

A. What is probable diagnosis?
B. What is the peak age of this phenomenon?
C. What is the Tanner stage when this occurs?
D. What is the testicular volume with this stage?
E. What is the likely course of this condition?
F. What is the cause of this problem?
G. What is the treatment of this disorder?

Q-15. A 9-year-old boy presented as an emergency case with history of polydipsia, polyuria and weight loss. He was in compensated shock. His weight was 30 kg. capillary blood glucose was >500 mg/dL, serum ketone 6 mmol/L and urine ketones high. ABG showed pH 6.9, bicarbonate 6 mEq/L. A diagnosis of diabetes ketoacidosis was obvious. How will you manage the patient immediately?

Q-16. A healthy term neonate is screened for congenital hypothyroidism by heel prick method. The screening report shows thyroid-stimulating hormone (TSH) of 76 mIU/mL. A venous blood sample was tested. It shows Total T_4 4 µg/dL, Free T_4 0.5 ng/dL and TSH 74 mIU/mL.

A. What is the interpretation of screening test?
B. What is the interpretation of venous TSH?
C. What is the interpretation of T_4?
D. What is the interpretation of free T_4?
E. What is the diagnosis?
F. Mention the drug and dose for this baby.
G. Which factors may give rise to false negative screening test?
H. Which cause for this thyroid disorder cannot be identified by screening test?

Q-17. This patient presented in the OPD with neck swelling, tremor, weight loss, irritability and palpation.

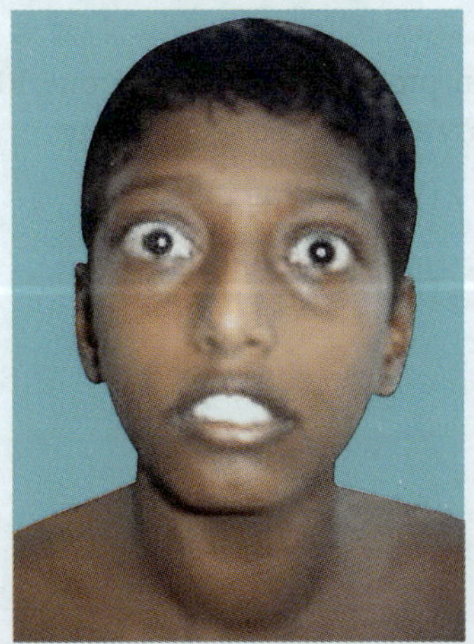

A. Identify the clinical findings in above image.
B. What is the probable diagnosis?
C. What is likely etiology?
D. What biochemical investigation should be carried out to confirm the etiology?
E. What is the first line of treatment?
F. What definitive therapy can be offered in case of large goiter?
G. What pubertal problem is possible in girls with this disease?

Q-18. Complete the following statements with normal, high or low as applicable:

A. Urine sodium in primary polydipsia is __________.
B. Urine sodium in pseudohyponatremia due to hypertriglyceridemia is __________.
C. Serum sodium in cerebral salt wasting is __________.
D. Urine sodium in hypoaldosteronism is __________.
E. The intravascular volume status in cerebral salt wasting is __________.
F. Serum vasopressin level in cerebral diabetes insipidus is __________.
G. The syndrome of inappropriate antidiuretic hormone (SIADH) secretion, the urine sodium is __________.
H. Serum sodium in SIADH is __________.

Q-19. Fill in the blanks:

A. Anti-Mullerian hormone (AMH), inhibin and activin belong to ______ family of growth factors.
B. AMH is secreted by ______ cells of testes.

C. AMH causes regression of _______ ducts.
D. Inhibin is secreted by _______ cells of the ovary.
E. In males, hypogonadism in delayed puberty is identified by measuring _______.
F. _______ stimulates FSH secretion by the pituitary gland.
G. _______ bins activins and inhibits FSH secretion.

ANSWERS

A-1. A. Hypothalamic hamartoma
B. Unnatural crying or laughing
C. Diabetes insipidus, hyperthermia, cachexia
D. Isosexual

A-2. A. Acanthosis nigricans
B. Polycystic ovary disease (PCOD)
C. FSH, LH, prolactin, DHEA, estrogen, progesterone, testosterone, RBS, insulin, lipid profile, thyroid function tests
D. Type II DM, hypertension, coronary artery disease, infertility

A-3. A. Vitamin D dependent rickets type 2 (VDDR Type 2)
B. Elevated
C. End-organ resistance to 1, 25 $(OH)_2 D_3$
D. Autosomal recessive

A-4. A. Congenital adrenal hyperplasia
B. 21 beta-Hydroxylase deficiency
C. Serum 17-hydroxy progesterone
D. Hydrocortisone and fludrocortisone

A-5. A. Diabetes mellitus
B. Blood sugar, serum acetone, arterial blood gas analysis, serum electrolyte, urine examination for sugar
C. Diabetes ketoacidosis

A-6. A. Hypothyroidism
B. Serum T_3, T_4, TSH
C. Decreased basal metabolic rate
D. Kocher-Debre-Semelaigne syndrome

A-7. A. Congenital hypoparathyroidism
B. Prolonged QTC interval in ECG and look for thymus in chest X-ray
C. Syndromes associated with hypocalcemia:
- DiGeorge syndrome
- Kenny Caffey syndrome
- Isolated hypoparathyroidism

D.
- Oral calcium 100 mg/kg/day
- Oral vitamin D_3

A-8. A. Hypertrichosis—excessive growth of hairs
B. Diazoxide
C. 5–15 mg/kg/day
D. *Side effects of diazoxide:*
- Hypertrichosis

- Water retention and edema
- Electrolyte imbalance

E. Serum insulin level >2 μ IU/mL at time of hypoglycemia

A-9. E. As ketones are not significantly elevated, can be taken for surgery
F. 0.45% NS with 5% dextrose and 40 mEq/L potassium chloride is added.
G. 60 mL/hour (1.5 times maintenance fluid rate)
H. 1 hourly glucose monitoring
I. Intravenous insulin in dose of 0.03 units/kg/hour.
J. Hypoglycemia and diabetes ketoacidosis can develop.

A-10.
- Introduction and rapport
- Aseptic and antiseptic precautions, especially hand hygiene
- Make sure that syringe and vials are of same strength. U-40 syringe with U-40 insulin.
- Ensure cold chain.
- Ensure that regular insulin is clear.
- Check the expiry dates.
- Clean the top of the vial with spirit.
- Gently roll the insulin suspension NPH 10–20 times to mix. Do not shake.
- Draw air equivalent to 14 U of NPH required into the syringe, and inject into the vial containing NPH and remove the syringe without taking insulin or air.
- Then draw air equivalent to the 8 U of human insulin R (HIR) insulin required into the syringe and insert in the HIR vial.
- Draw HIR insulin, draw into the syringe.
- Now draw INH into the syringe.
- Remember the sites to choose in the Mock doll (abdomen, thigh, arms)
- Inject by subcutaneous route
- Count for 6–10 after injection. Do not rub.
- Ask the patient to take the breakfast as advised.
- Dispose the sharps in appropriate bin.
- Place insulin back in refrigerator.

A-11. A. Diabetes mellitus
B. Impaired fasting glucose
C. Impaired glucose tolerance
D. Diabetes mellitus
E. Prediabetes

A-12. A. This screening test is positive as 17-hydroxyprogesterone is high (> 37.5 nmol/L).
B. Venous measurement of 17-hydroxyprogesterone and serum electrolytes levels should be performed.
C. Salt wasting type of CAH due to 21-β-hydroxylase deficiency.
D. *False positive screening test:* Sick baby, Preterm and low birth weight baby
E. *False negative screening test:* Maternal corticosteroid therapy
F.
- Salt wasting crisis can be prevented with early identification of disease
- Incorrect sex assignment of the child can be avoided.

A-13. A. Café-au-lait spots
B. McCune-Albright syndrome
C. Café-au-lait spots, precocious puberty and polyostotic fibrous dysplasia
D. FSH and LH are suppressed. Estradiol level is high
E. Activating missense mutation in GNAS-1

F. Cushing syndrome, hyperthyroidism and acromegaly are known endocrinal disorders to be associated with McCune-Albright syndrome

A-14. A. Puberty gynecomastia
B. 13–14 years
C. Tanner stage 3 to 4
D. Testicular volume 5–10 mL
E. Spontaneous resolution with pubertal progress
F. Imbalance between testosterone and estradiol levels
G. No treatment is required.

A-15.
- 300 mL 0.9% NS (10 mL/kg) over a period of one hour in first hour.
- *Second and subsequent hours:*
  - Fluid calculation = Deficit + Maintenance - Bolus
  - Deficit is 8.5%–85 mL/kg → (85 × 30) - 300 = 2,250 mL
  - Maintenance by Holliday–Segar formula, fluid calculation for 48 hours = 1,700 mL × 2 = 3,400 mL
  - Total fluid = 2,250 mL + 3,400 mL = 5,650/47 = 120 mL/hour
- This is administered in beginning as 0.9% NS with 40 mEq/L of potassium chloride. Addition of glucose and adjustment of potassium concentration is titrated as per findings during monitoring for next 48 hours.
- Insulin (50 units regular insulin with 50 mL NS), 25 mL should be flushed out. Start insulin administration at 3 mL per hour to give 3 units/hour at 0.1 unit/kg/hour as an IV infusion.
- Monitor heart rate, respiratory rate, BP, signs of dehydration and sensorium to monitor for development of cerebral edema.

A-16. A. Screening test for congenital hypothyroidism is positive (TSH ≥20 mIU/mL)
B. TSH is elevated. (Venous TSH ≥20 mIU/mL in first 2 weeks and ≥10 mIU/mL beyond 2 weeks is elevated)
C. Low T_4 (Total T_4 <10 μg/dL)
D. Low free T_4 (Free T_4 <1.17 ng/mL)
E. Congenital hypothyroidism
F. Oral levothyroxine 15 μg/kg once a day in the morning
G. Preterm, twins, Sick baby and Trisomy 21 may give rise false negative screening test
H. Central hypothyroidism cannot be diagnosed by screening test.

A-17. A. Signs and symptoms of hyperthyroidism with exophthalmos with goiter
B. Hyperthyroidism
C. Grave's disease
D. Anti-TSH receptor antibody
E. Antithyroid drugs like methimazole or carbimazole
F. Total thyroidectomy
G. Secondary amenorrhea

A-18. A. Normal
B. Normal
C. Low
D. High
E. Low
F. Low
G. High
H. Low

A-19. A. Transforming growth factor-beta (TGF-β)
B. Sertoli cells
C. Paramesonephric duct
D. Theca cells
E. Inhibin B
F. Activin
G. Follistatin

CHAPTER 20

Ophthalmology

QUESTIONS

Q-1. A 9-month-old male infant apparently healthy till the evening of the day of admission was brought with complaints of irritability, vomiting and seizures. There was no history of fever, otorrhea, rash or bleeding from any other site. However, on questioning later, the father admitted to on and off throwing the baby up in the air and catching him as the child enjoyed this form of play. The following is the picture of fundus examination of eye of the patient.

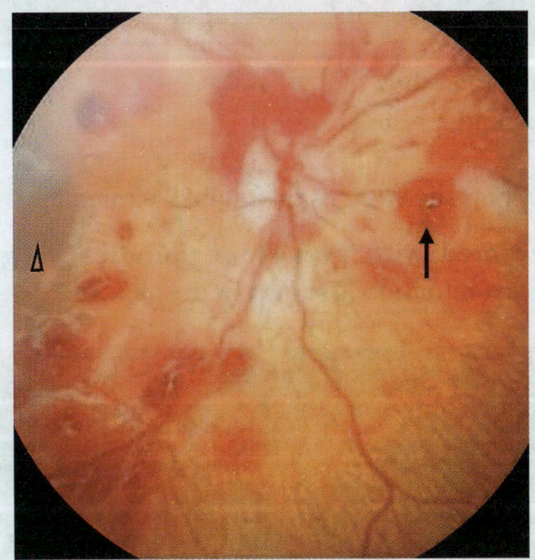

A. What are the findings on fundus examination?
B. What is probable diagnosis?
C. What other investigations of eye may reveal more details of this findings?
D. What other complications are known to occur in this condition?

Q-2. A 7-year-old boy presented as a case of pyrexia of unknown origin of 6 weeks duration with leukocytosis, thrombocytosis, raised ESR and CRP. He also had early clubbing and hepatosplenomegaly. USG abdomen revealed multiple splenic abscesses. His fundus examination is shown in the picture. Echo study of heart confirmed the diagnosis.

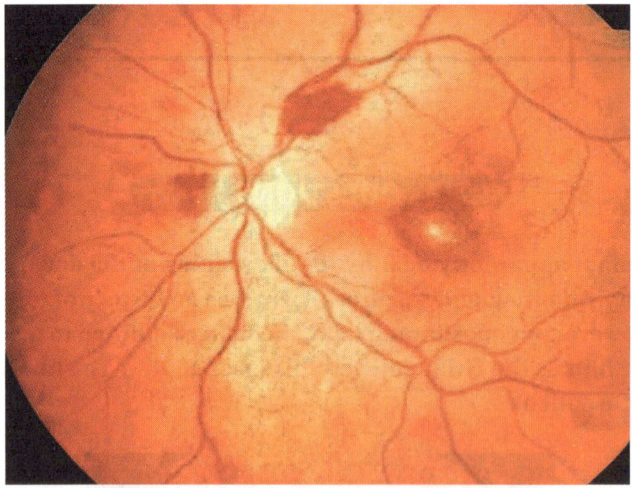

A. What does the fundus examination show?
B. Describe the morphology of fundus lesion.
C. What is the diagnosis?
D. What other conditions may show such lesions on fundus examination?

Q-3. A 3-month-old infant presented with persistent jaundice, large head lymphadenopathy, and hepatosplenomegaly. Fundus examination is shown in the picture.

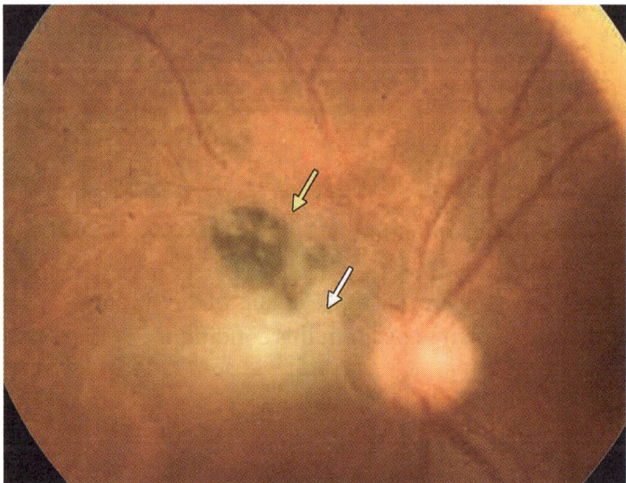

A. What does fundus examination show?
B. What is probable diagnosis?
C. What CT scan of brain findings are common in this condition?
D. What is the triad of this condition?
E. What is the treatment of this disease?

Q-4. A boy presented with skin lesions as shown in Figure 1. His fundus examination revealed lesions as shown in Figure 2. His sister is also diagnosed same condition.

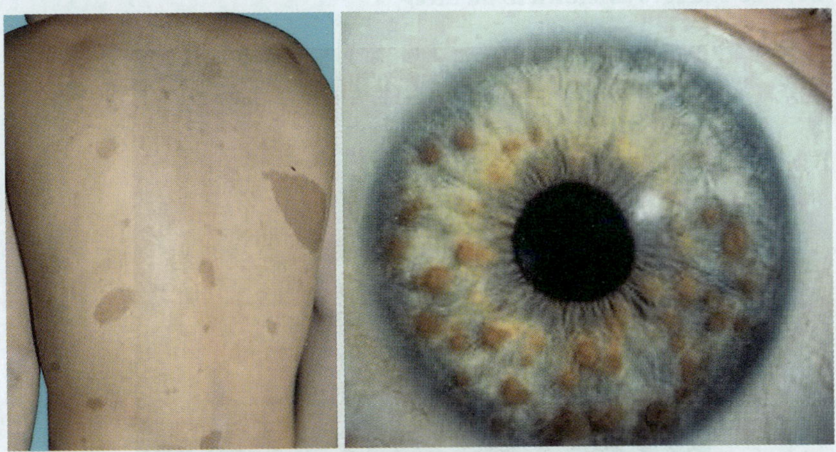

Fig. 1 Fig. 2

A. What is the diagnosis?
B. Name the skin lesions.
C. Describe and name the lesions seen on fundus examination.
D. What tumors are known to occur as the complications in this disorder?

Q-5. A boy was brought with complaints of problems with night vision and tunnel vision (only central vision). He also had obesity, polydactyly and hypogonadism. His fundus examination revealed lesions as shown in the picture.

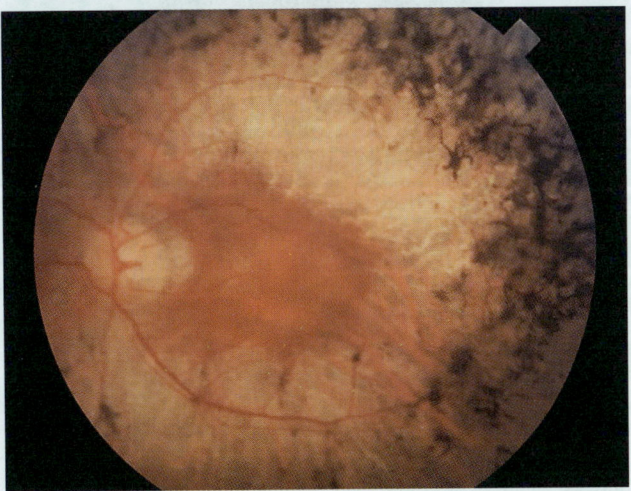

A. What is called as eye lesions as seen on fundus examination?
B. What is the type of inheritance of this eye disorder?
C. Name two conditions associated with these eye lesions.

Q-6. A child was brought with gradual loss of vision. He was already diagnosed as a case of congenital bone marrow failure. He also had hepatosplenomegaly, hearing impairment and facial asymmetry. His fundus examination revealed changes as shown in picture.

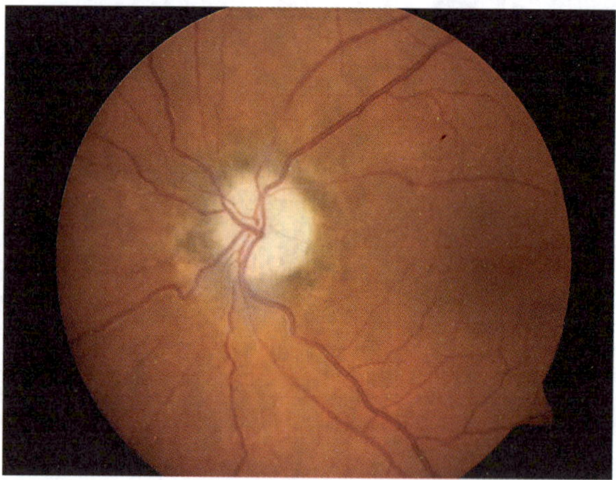

A. What does fundus examination show?
B. What are the common mechanism leading to this eye disorder in children?
C. What is the diagnosis in this patient?
D. Name neurodegenerative disorders causing this eye lesion.

Q-7.

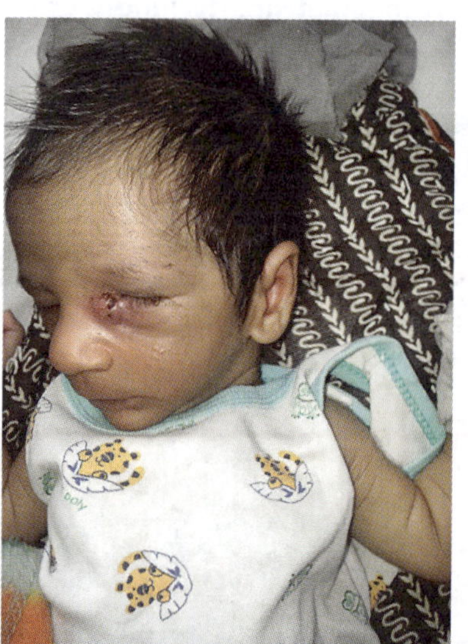

A. What is your diagnosis?
B. What is the primary etiology?
C. How will you manage?

Q-8. Match the following: Systemic conditions and eye disorders

A. Galactosemia	1. Lisch nodules
B. Marfan syndrome	2. Cataract
C. Wilms tumor	3. Aniridia
D. Neurofibromatosis	4. Ectopia lentis

Q-9. A child presents with fever, cough, eye redness, tearing and discharge.

A. What is probable diagnosis?
B. What are the preventive measures to avoid transmission of disease?
C. What are other systemic complications of this disease?

Q-10. Nontender swelling

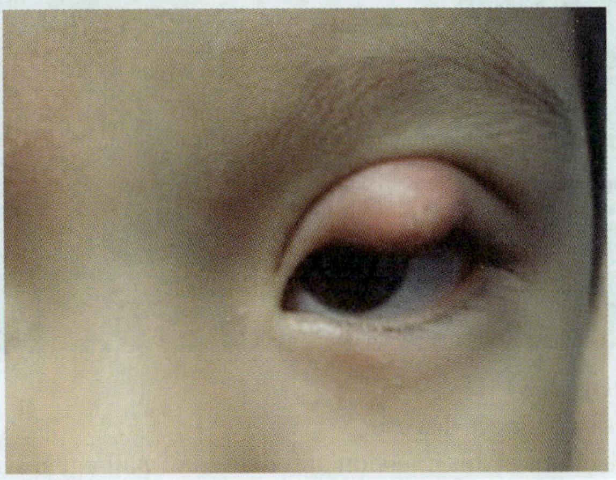

A. What is probable diagnosis?
B. What is the pathogenesis of this condition?
C. What is the outcome?
D. What is the indication of surgery?
E. What is the indication of oral macrolide?

Q-11. Answer the following questions.

A. What is visual acuity of newborn?
B. At what age a child can fixate nearby objects?
C. Up to what age tears are not present while crying?
D. At what age visual acuity reaches 6/6?
E. At what age, eye coordinated is usually achieved?

Q-12.

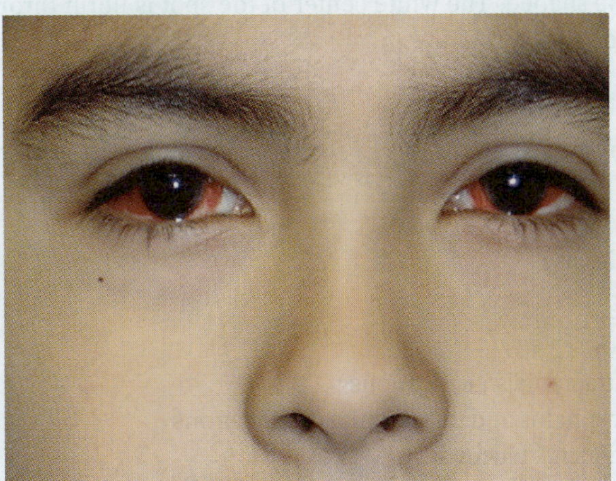

A. What is the diagnosis?
B. What are the causes of this conditions in children?
C. What is treatment?

Q-13. This eye problem is the presentation of hypersensitivity of systemic infection.

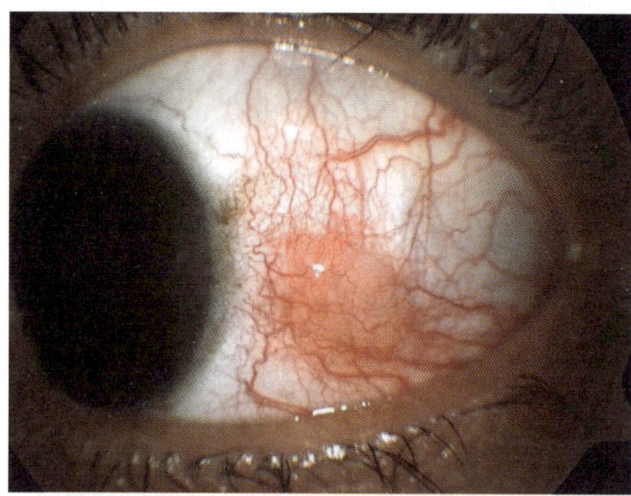

A. What is the probable diagnosis?
B. What is the pathogenesis of this eye disease?
C. What are other manifestations of this infection based on same pathogenesis?
D. What is the treatment?

ANSWERS

A-1. A. Retinal hemorrhage
B. Shaken baby syndrome
C. Slit-lamp examination and fluorescein angiography may reveal preretinal, intraretinal and sub-hyaloid hemorrhage
D. Subdural hematoma and death

A-2. A. Roth spot
B. Roth spots are white-centered retinal hemorrhage. They are caused by a rupture of retinal capillaries and can be round, oval or flame shaped. The white center of the spot is fibrin thrombus at the site of rupture. Roth spots are immunologic.
C. Bacterial endocarditis
D.
- Diabetic retinopathy
- Acute leukemia
- Anemia
- Collagen vascular disease

A-3. A. Chorioretinitis
B. Congenital toxoplasmosis
C. Hydrocephalus and intracranial calcifications
D. Chorioretinitis, hydrocephalus and intracranial calcifications
E. Pyrimethamine, sulfadiazine, leucovorin

A-4. A. Neurofibromatosis type 1

B. Café-au-lait spots, one of the diagnostic criteria, six or more Café-au-lait spots measuring at least 5 mm before puberty or 15 mm after puberty.

C. Iris Lisch nodules. They are melanocytic hamartomas which are highly specific of neurofibromatosis type 1. They appear as dome-shaped pigmented hamartomas on the iris in late childhood, remain asymptomatic and require a slit-lamp examination to be visualized.

D.

- Pheochromocytoma
- Rhabdomyosarcoma
- Breast carcinoma

A-5. A. Retinitis pigmentosa

B. Autosomal recessive

C.

- Usher syndrome
- Laurence–Moon–Biedl syndrome
- Refsum syndrome
- Abetalipoproteinemia
- Cockayne syndrome

A-6. A. Optic atrophy

B. Inflammation of optic nerve, trauma, impaired blood flow, toxins, vitamin deficiencies and tumors

C. Osteopetrosis

D.

- Gangliosidosis
- Metachromatic leukodystrophy
- Krabe's disease
- Canavan disease

A-7. A. Dacryocystitis

B. Congenital nasolacrimal duct obstruction

C. Local antibiotic drops and nasolacrimal duct massage. If abscess formation, drainage of abscess and systemic antibiotics.

A-8. A. 2 B. 4

C. 3 D. 1

A-9. A. Adenoviral infection

B. *Preventive measures to avoid transmission:*

- Frequent washing the hands
- Do not share napkins, towels
- Do not attend school and work place for a week

C. Adenoviral infection can cause pneumonia, hepatitis, encephalitis, nephritis, etc.

A-10. A. Chalazion

B. Due to granulomatous inflammation of meibomian gland

C. Spontaneous resolution in most cases

D. Cosmetic purpose and large enough to distort vision are the indications for surgery.

E. Secondary blepharitis and frequent chalazion should be treated with oral azithromycin.

A-11. A. 6/120
B. 3 months of age
C. 1–3 months of age
D. 2–3 years
E. 3–6 months of age

A-12. A. Bilateral subconjunctival hemorrhage
B. Causes of subconjunctival hemorrhage in children
- Pertussis
- Leukemia
- Scurvy
- Unilateral due to trauma
- Hypertension
- Child abuse

C. Self-limiting, no active treatment is required.

A-13. A. Phlyctenular conjunctivitis
B. Delayed hypersensitivity to tuberculin protein of *Mycobacterium tuberculosis*
C. Other manifestations of delayed hypersensitivity to tuberculin protein:
- Erythema nodosum
- Tuberculous pleural effusion
- Tuberculous lymphadenopathy

D. Anti-tuberculous therapy

CHAPTER 21

Dermatology

QUESTIONS

Q-1. These skin lesions were found due to different reasons as follows. Identify them.

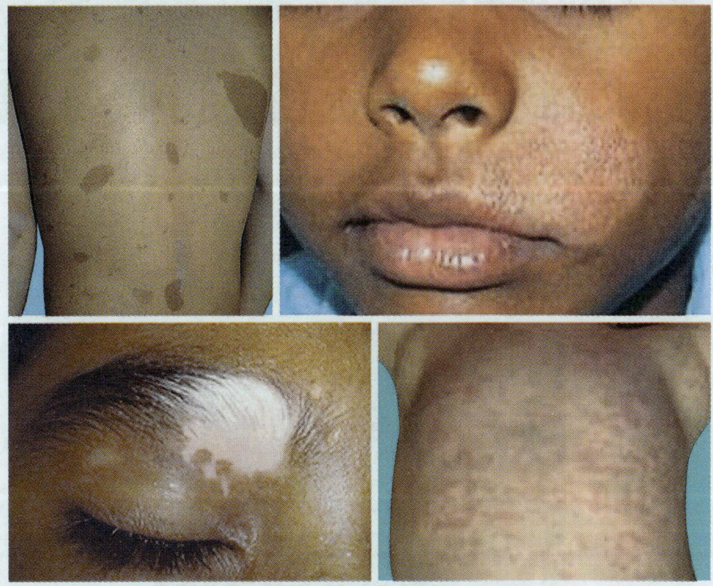

A. It is since birth and associated with neurological disorder.
B. It developed due to some infectious disease and was confirmed by skin biopsy.
C. This skin lesion developed recently. It is considered as autoimmune disorder and having genetic susceptibility.
D. These skin lesions developed following ingestion of amoxicillin.

Q-2. Define following skin lesions.

A. Macules
B. Papules
C. Nodules
D. Vesicles
E. Bullous
F. Pustules
G. Petechiae
H. Purpura
I. Ecchymosis

Q-3. These skin lesions are present since birth, especially with dryness of skin.

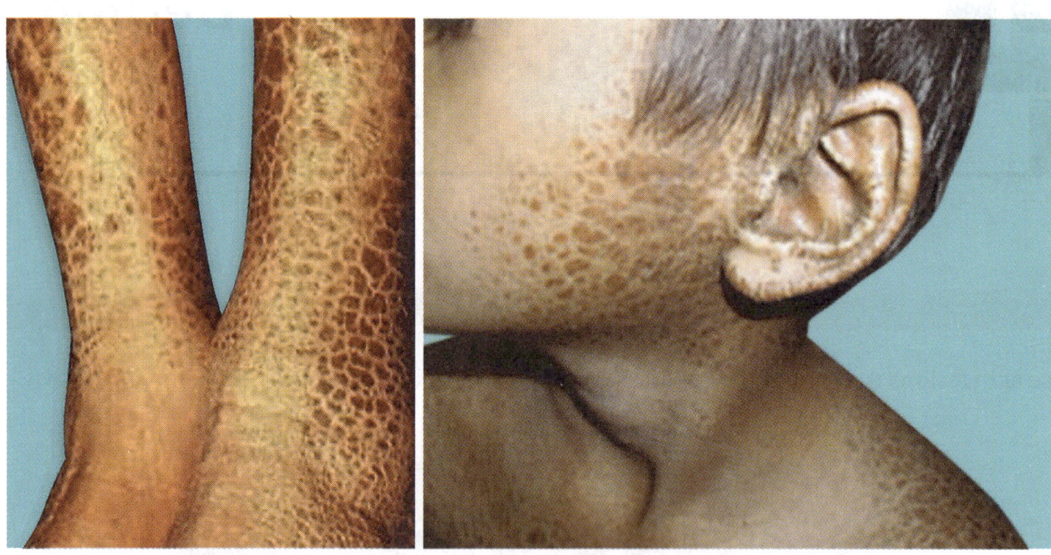

A. What is probable diagnosis?
B. What is the hallmark of the disease?
C. What is the treatment of this disorder?

Q-4.

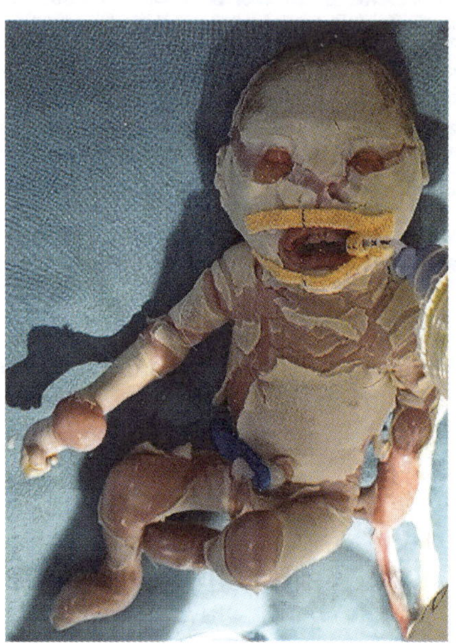

A. What is your diagnosis?
B. How its name is derived?
C. What are common complications of this disease?

Q-5. This baby has tendency to develop blisters even on trivial injury, predominantly at the site of trauma.

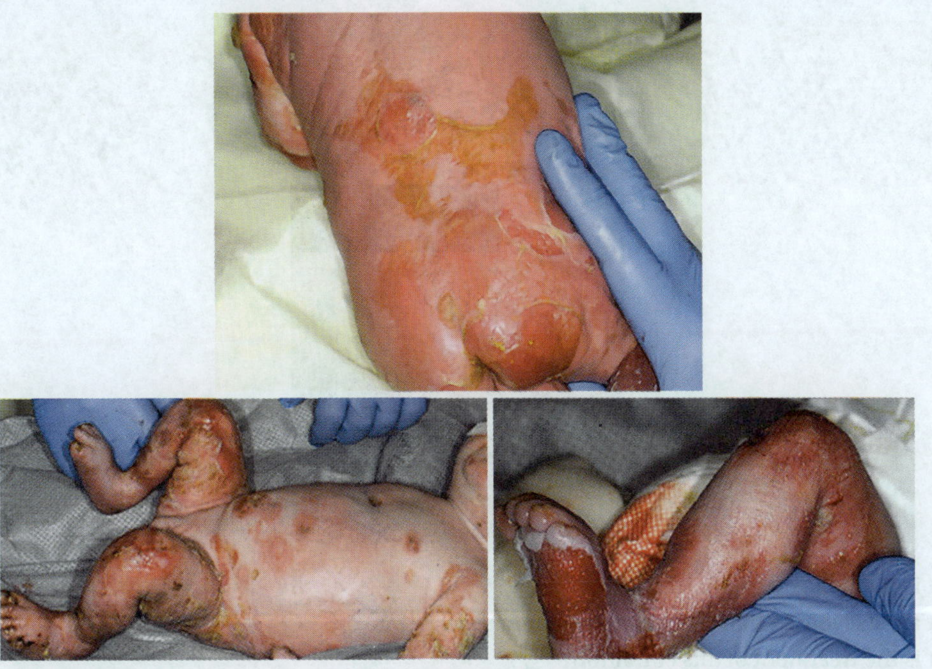

A. What is probable diagnosis?
B. What is the characteristic of skin lesions?
C. What is the basic defect of this disorder?
D. What is the treatment of this disease?

Q-6. A 10-month-old infant had small red-colored skin lesion over left side of forehead, gradually increasing in size and presented with this.

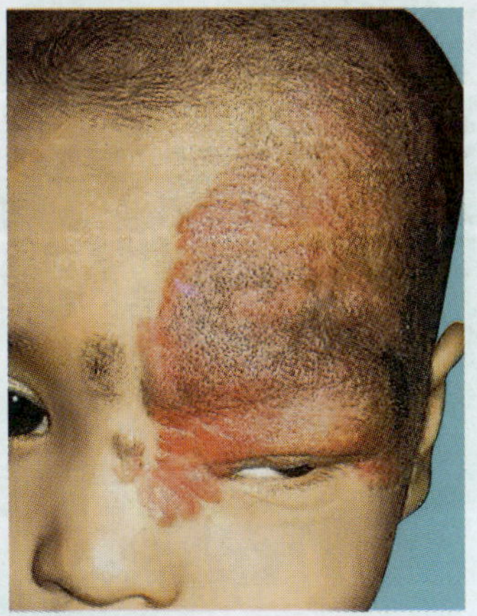

A. What is probable diagnosis?
B. What is the course of this disorder?
C. What are the complications of this disease?
D. What treatment options are available for this condition?

Q-7. This infant presented with itchy, erythematous skin lesions over cheeks since age of 4 months.

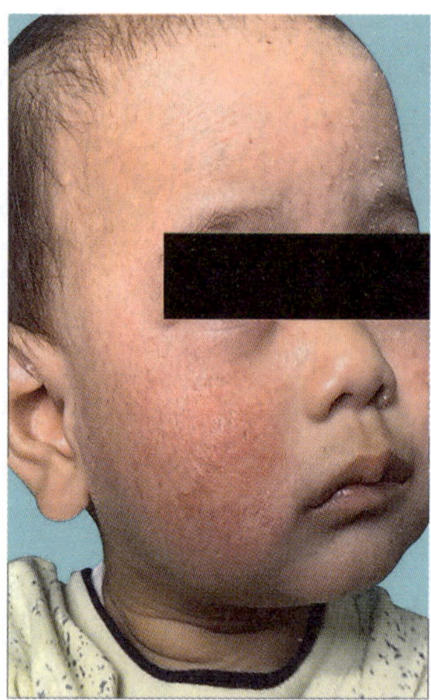

A. What is probable diagnosis?
B. What are its types? What are their different manifestations?
C. What is the treatment of this condition?

Q-8. An infants presented with these skin lesions over buttocks following diarrhea.

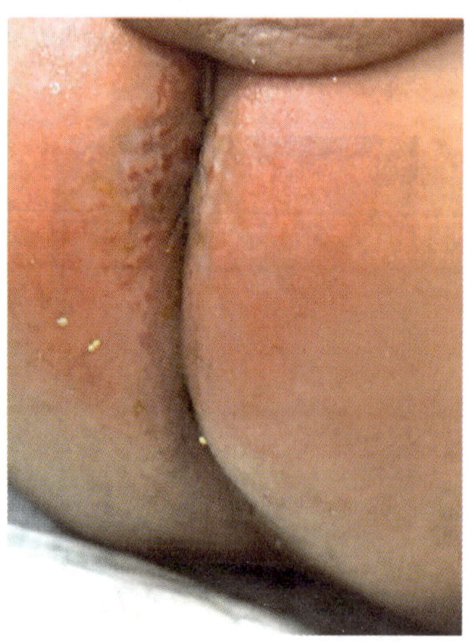

A. What is the diagnosis?
B. What is the mechanism of development of these skin lesions?
C. What is the description of the skin lesions?
D. What is the treatment?

Q-9. A 4-year-old presented with this type of patches over face.

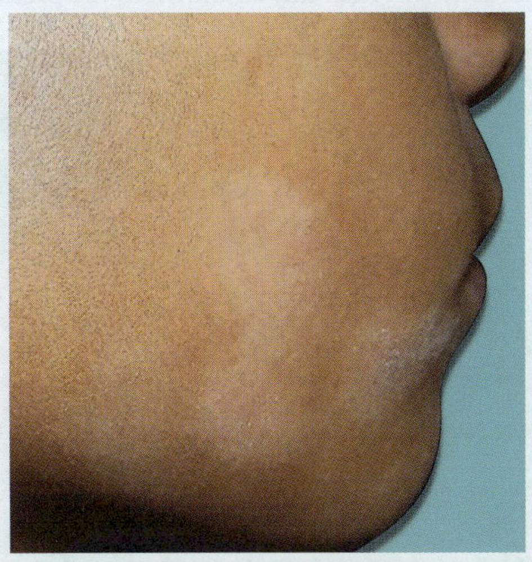

A. What is the probable diagnosis?
B. What are classical features of the condition?
C. What are differential diagnosis?
D. What is the treatment of this disorder?

Q-10. A 13-year-old girl presented with skin lesions on a background of oil skin over face as shown in the following picture.

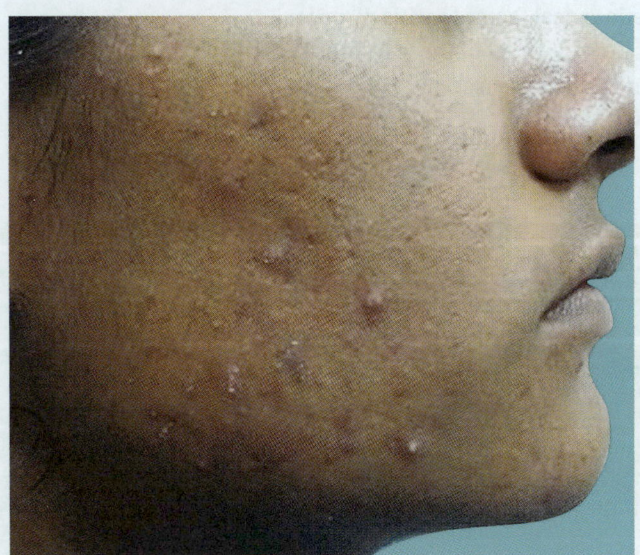

A. What is the probable diagnosis?
B. What is the basic cause of this condition?
C. What is most common age for this disorder?
D. What are the characteristics of skins lesions in this disease?
E. What etiological factors are considered responsible for this disease?
F. What is the management of this disease at different stage of severity?

Q-11. A family doctor prescribed combination of Ibuprofen and paracetamol for fever along with oral amoxicillin, to the child. He developed skin rashes on next day as shown in the picture. He also complained of itching.

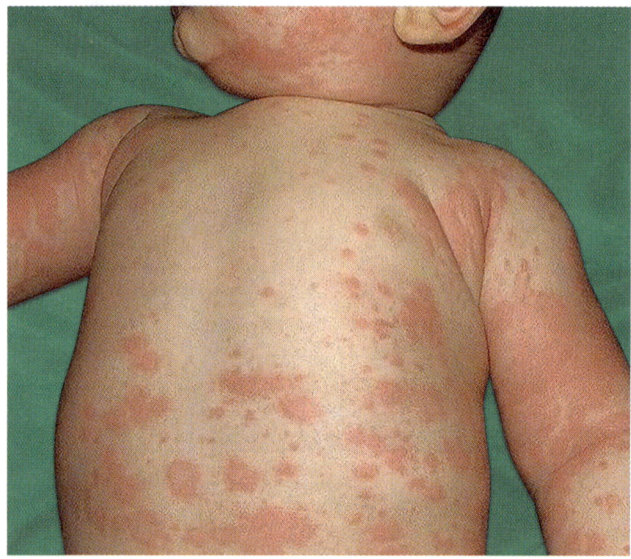

A. What is probable diagnosis?
B. What are the characteristics of this condition?
C. What are common etiological factor for this disorder?
D. What is the basis for development of these lesions?
E. What is the treatment of this disease?

Q-12. Both the children had common condition. First child has skin lesions over face and second on over trunk as shown in pictures.

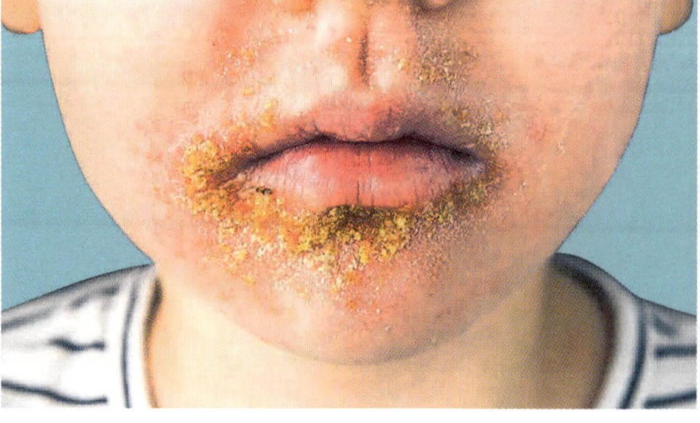

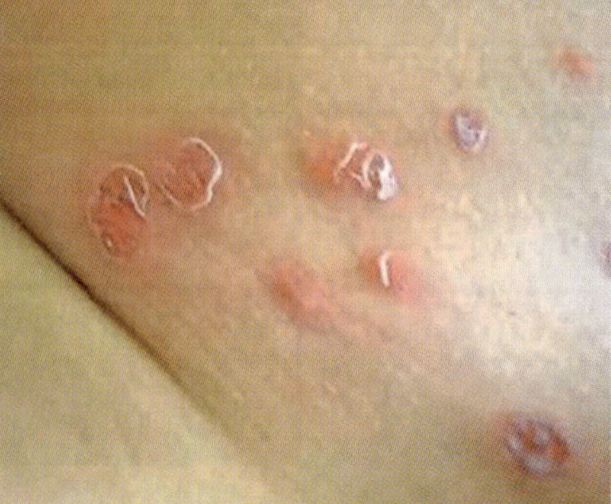

A. What is the probable diagnosis?
B. Name the type of condition in first and second child.
C. Differences between both the types.
D. Treatment of both the types.

Q-13. A girl presented with complaints of hypopigmented lesion over the face for 5 months. She also noticed impaired sensations over the lesion. The skin biopsy confirmed the diagnosis.

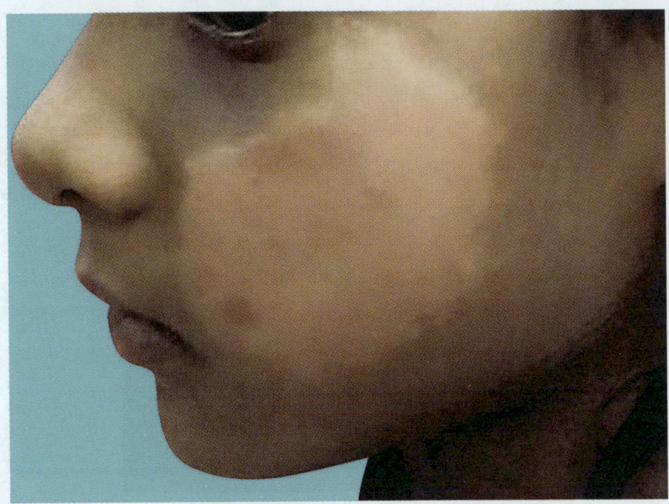

A. What is the probable diagnosis?
B. What investigations can confirm the diagnosis?
C. WHO recommendations for treatment of this disease in children
D. What complications are known to occur in this disorder?

Q-14. A boy presented with this type of skin lesions over face off and on for 2 years. The skin lesions disappear by their own after few months and again new lesions reappear.

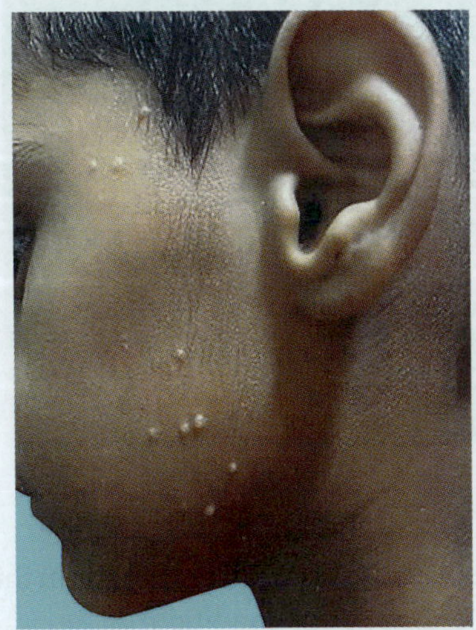

A. What is probable diagnosis?
B. Describe the morphological characteristics of the lesions in this disorder.
C. What treatment options are available?

Q-15. An infant presented with extensive orolabial painful lesions with high-grade fever, irritability, drooling of saliva and refusal to feed. On clinical examination, submandibular lymph adenopathy was detected.

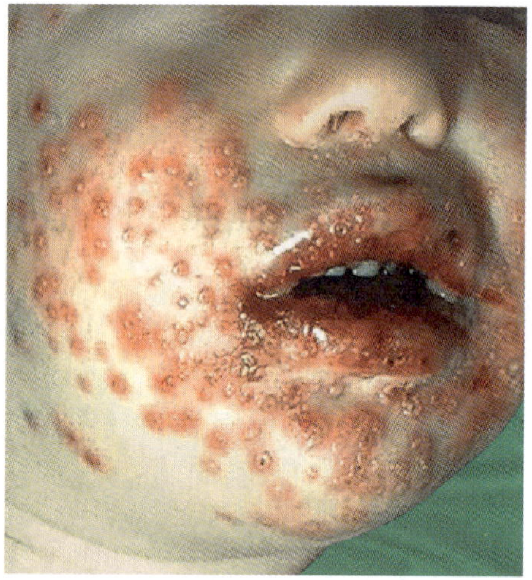

A. What is probable diagnosis?
B. What are different types of this infection with reference to involvement of specific organ?
C. What are different diagnosis?
D. What is the treatment of this disease?

Q-16. These three children presented with skin lesions over face, hands and feet. All of them had itching, worse at night.

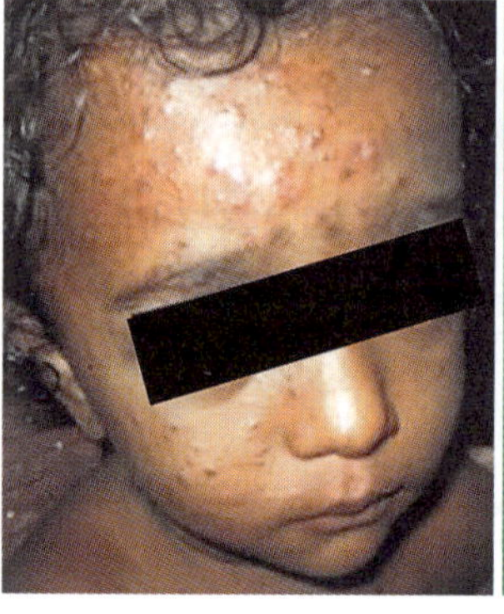

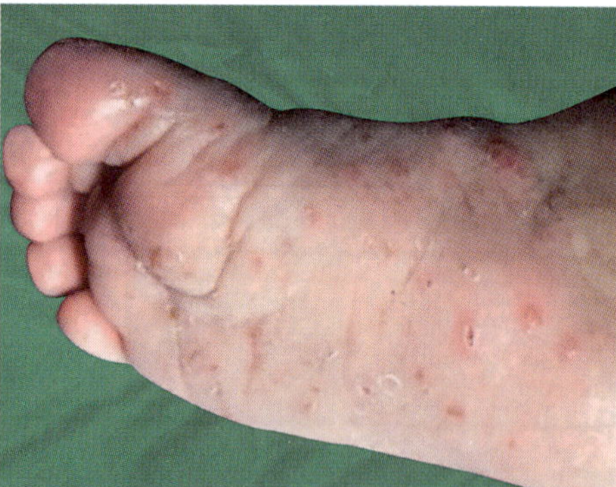

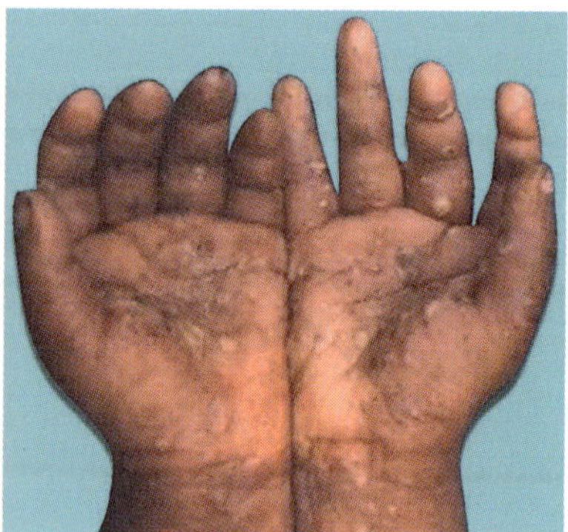

A. What is the diagnosis?
B. Name the organism responsible for this disease.
C. What different morphological skin lesions are known to occur in this disorder?
D. What are common sites for skin lesions in this condition?
E. What are treatment options available for this disease?
F. How will you educate the family for prevention of this disease?

Q-17.

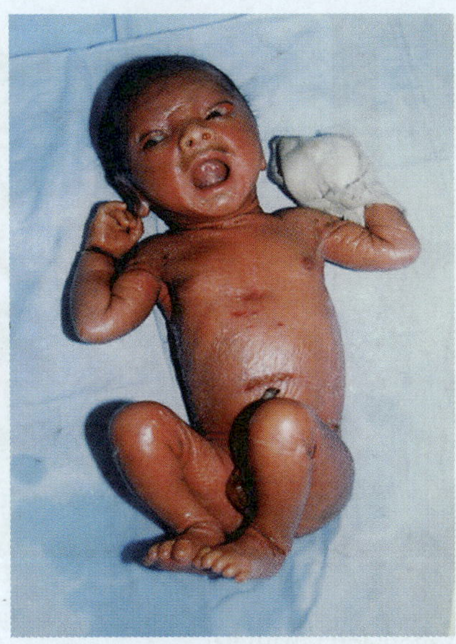

A. What is your diagnosis?
B. Describe the characteristics of the disorder seen in this patient.
C. What morbidities are common in this disorder?

Q-18. The child develops these types of skin lesions on minor trauma or friction since birth. The diagnosis was confirmed by skin biopsy and genetic study.

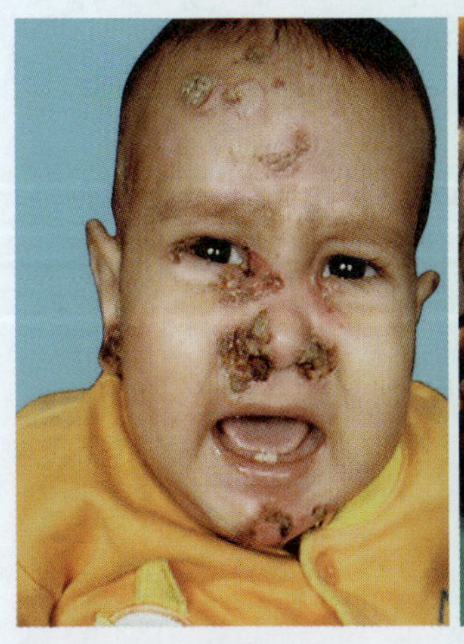

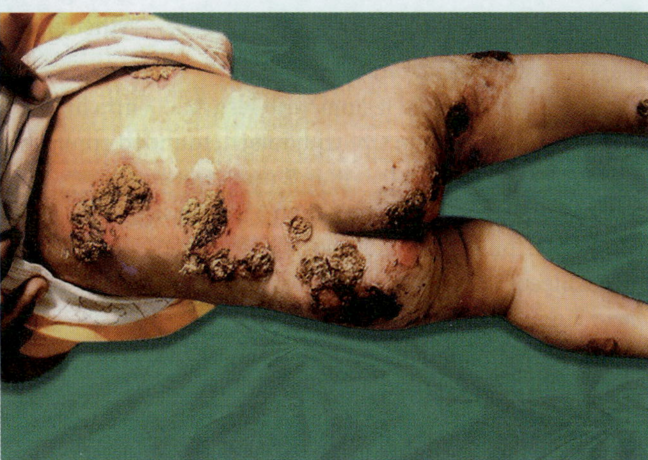

A. Name the condition.
B. What is its pattern of inheritance?
C. What happens to nails and dentition?

Q-19. A 5-year-old boy presented with fever of unknown origin since early infancy.

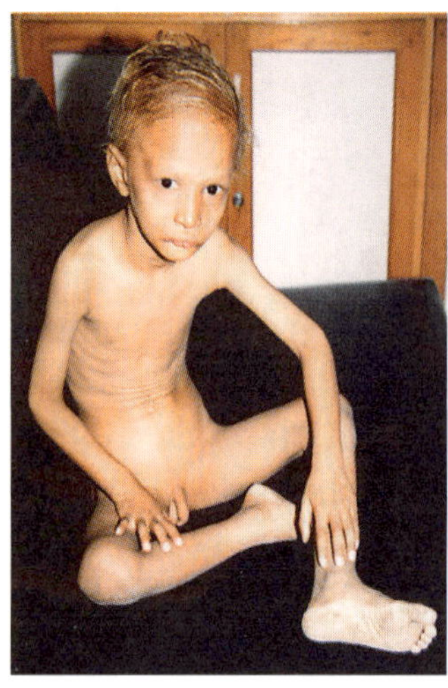

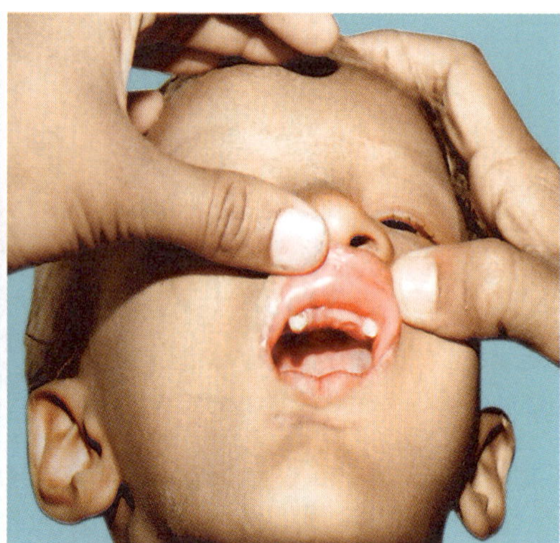

A. Name the condition.
B. Name two disorders commonly associated with it.
C. Name the immunodeficiency disorder associated with it.

ANSWERS

A-1. *Identification of skin lesions:*
A. Café-au-lait spots
B. Hypopigmented patch in leprosy
C. Vitiligo
D. Erythematous rash (Drug rash)

A-2. A. *Macule:* Flat lesions of altered color of skin
B. *Papule:* Raised, flat, topped lesions with less than 5 mm in size
C. *Nodule:* More than 5 mm in size with raised, rounded configuration
D. *Vesicle:* Fluid-filled lesions, less than 5 mm in size
E. *Bullous:* Fluid-filled lesions, more than 5 mm in size
F. *Pustule:* Raised, pus filled skin lesions
G. *Petechiae:* Bleeding into skin lesions, pinhead size, 2 mm. They are not blanchable.
H. *Purpura:* Superficial bleeding skin lesions, 2–5 mm in size
I. *Ecchymosis:* Deep-bleeding skin lesions, more than 5 mm in size

A-3. A. Ichthyosis
B. Hallmark of the disease is fish-like scales
C.
1. Maintenance of hydration
2. Lubrication with petroleum jelly or urea containing creams
3. Keratolytic agents like salicylic acids and propylene glycol
4. Retinoid
5. Topical steroids and antibiotics

A-4. A. Harlequin ichthyosis
B. Its appearance is 'Clown-like' comedy character in Italian street theater. Facial appearance of infants born with this anomaly resembles this character; this is why the disease is called as harlequin ichthyosis.
C. Dehydration, fluid loss, impaired heat balance and sepsis are common complications.

A-5. A. Epidermolysis bullosa

B. The skin lesions are non-hemorrhagic bullae which heal without scarring

C. *Protein defect:* Keratin 5 and 14

D. *Treatment:*

- To avoid friction and trauma
- Wearing soft, well-ventilated shoes
- Gentle handling
- Antibiotics for infected lesions

A-6. A. Infantile hemangioma

B. They usually present as telangiectasia at the times of birth. Over the first few weeks, they become prominent followed by a phase of exponential growth until 9–12 months of age. This culminates into a phase of involution that may last 6–10 years. Some infantile hemangioma resolves completely whereas others leave behind residual changes like telangiectasia, scarring or fibrofatty tissues.

C. *Complications:*

- Ulceration
- Visual compromise
- Auditory canal obstruction
- Cardiac compromise

D. *Treatment:*

- Oral beta-blockers

  Propranolol 2 mg/kg/day in divided doses, duration ranges from 6 to 12 months. Propranolol ideally should be given till the child reaches 1 year of age. The color of the lesion becomes lighter and it becomes softer within 24–48 hours of therapy.

  Common adverse effects of propranolol are bradycardia, hypotension, sleep disruption, acrocyanosis and diarrhea. Most importantly, a watch needs to be kept for hypoglycemia that can be fatal.
- *Oral corticosteroids:*

  Prednisolone 2–3 mg/kg/day (higher dose)
- Lasers
- Treatment of ulcerated infantile hemangioma includes local wound care, saline compresses, antibiotics and analgesics.

A-7. A. Infantile atopic dermatitis

B.

- *Infantile pattern:* Manifests as itchy, erythematous papulovesicular on the face, any time after the age of 3 months. The lesions clear by 18 months of age in 40% and evolve into childhood pattern in the rest.
- *Childhood pattern:* It is characterized by dry, lichenified and crusted plaques seen mainly on antecubital and popliteal fossa, the neck and face. Almost 70% clear by 10 months of age.

C. *Treatment:*

- *General measures:* Avoid contact with irritants like woolens, metals and chemicals. Reduce exposure to house dust mite using barriers on pillows and mattresses, regular vacuuming of rooms, etc. Continue breastfeeding. Dietary restrictions usually, not required.
- *Skin care:* Use of mild soaps and cleaning lotions are used for bathing followed by immediate application of moisturizers.
- Acute lesions can be treated with wet dressing, topical corticosteroids. Antibiotics and antihistamines may be prescribed.

A-8. A. Diaper dermatitis

B. It develops due to prolonged contact with feces and ammonia (produced by the action of urea-splitting organisms in urine), often complicated by superadded *Candida* infection.

C. Diaper dermatitis is characterized by moist, glazed, erythematous lesions on convexity of buttocks, area in contact with diapers. Depth of folds typically spared.

D. *Treatment:*
- Emollient and mild topical corticosteroids with antifungal agents are useful in acute phase.
- Diaper dermatitis can be prevented by keeping area clean and dry and avoiding the use of disposable semiabsorbent occlusive diapers.

A-9. A. Pityriasis alba

B. It typically presents as ill-defined hypopigmented patches with minimal fine scale on the face or trunk. It is benign condition. It is associated with atopic dermatitis.

C. *Differential diagnosis:*
- Hansen disease
- Pityriasis versicolor
- Hypopigmented mycosis fungoides

D. *Treatment:*
- Emollients
- Low-to-moderate patency corticosteroids creams
- Photoprotection

A-10. A. Acne vulgaris

B. The lesions of acne vulgaris develop due to inflammation of the pilosebaceous units (the hair follicles and sebaceous glands)

C. Acne vulgaris occurs in almost all peripubertal children. The most common age is 12–14 years, earlier in females and in about 70% of subjects the lesions subside by the second decade.

D. The skin lesions in acne vulgaris are polymorphic eruptions of open and closed comedones, papules, pustules and nodules on a background oily skin. The lesions usually heal with pitted scars. The lesions typically occur on face and upper trunk.

E. *Etiological factors:*
- Increased sebum secretion due to enhanced sensitivity to circulating androgens
- Microbial colonization
- Occlusion of pilosebaceous orifice by keratin plugs leading to retention of sebum and consequent growth of microbes, setting up a vicious cycle.
- Release of inflammatory mediators
- *Drug-induced acne:* Corticosteroids, androgens, antituberculous and anticonvulsant drugs.

F. *Management of acne vulgaris:*

Severity	*Subtype*	*Drug of choice*
Mild	Comedonal	Topical retinoids like retinoic acid and adapalene
	Papulopustular	Topical retinoids/benzoyl peroxide oral antibiotics, if necessary
Moderate	Papulopustular	Oral antibiotics + Topical retinoids and/or benzoyl peroxide
	Nodular	Oral antibiotics + Topical retinoids and/or benzoyl peroxide *In girls:* Oral anti-androgens + topical retinoids
Severe	Nodular/acne conglobate	Oral retinoids *In girls:* Oral antiandrogens + topical retinoids

Oral medications:
- *Antibiotics:* Tetracycline, doxycycline, minocycline
- *Hormonal therapy:* Anti-androgen medicines

- *Procedures:*
  - Chemical peels
  - Microdermabrasion
  - Laser
  - Corticosteroid injections

Skin care: Gentle cleansing of skin, avoiding harsh scrubbing, keeping skin hydrated
Lifestyle modifications: Diet and exercise

A-11. A. Urticaria

B. It is characterized by development of itchy, evanescent wheals which last for 24–72 hours.

C. Common etiological factors are infections (viral, bacterial, parasitic), cold, heat, foods and food additives, drugs, environmental allergens, insect bites, autoimmune and systemic diseases. Very often, urticaria is idiopathic.

D. It is mediated by histamine like chemicals which are released from mast cells or triggered either immunologically (via IgE, autoimmune) or non-immunologically (by drugs, chemicals, insect bites).

E. *Treatment:*
- Removal of trigger
- Antihistamines
- Oral corticosteroids
- Immunosuppressive drugs like methotrexate, azathioprine and cyclosporine in resistant urticaria
- Montelukast (leukotriene receptor antagonist) and Omalizumab (anti-IgE monoclonal antibody) are used in recalcitrant patients.

A-12. A. Impetigo (Pyoderma)

B. *First child:* Impetigo contagiosa (nonbullous type)
Second child: Bullous impetigo

C.

	Impetigo contagiosa (Nonbullous)	***Bullous impetigo***
Age	Children	Infants
Organisms	*Streptococcus pyogenes*	*Staphylococcus*, MSSA, MRSA
Clinical features	Thin-walled blisters with erythematous halo, ruptures to form honey-colored, yellowish crusts	Thick-walled, blisters on bland skin, rupture only after few days, to leave thin varnish like crusts
Sites of predilection	Face, especially mouth and nose	Face, trunk and other parts of body
Complications	• Post-streptococcal glomerulonephritis • Eczematization	Staphylococcal-scalded skin syndrome

D. *Treatment:*
- *General measures:* Local hygiene, removal of crusts
- Topical antibiotics like mupirocin, fusidic acid
- *Oral antibiotics:*
  - Amoxicillin–clavulanate
  - Clindamycin (for MRSA)
  - Cloxacillin

A-13. A. Leprosy

B. Investigations
- Slit skin smears from the lesions, stained with modified Ziehl–Neelsen method for acid-fast bacilli (AFB)
- *Skin biopsy:* Presence of granuloma and nerve involvement

C.

	Paucibacillary	*Multibacillary*
Definition	5 or less lesions	>5 lesions
Duration of therapy	6 months, to be completed in 9 months	12 months, to be completed in 18 months
Supervised (monthly)	Rifampicin 450 mg	Rifampicin 450 mg + Clofazimine 150 mg
Unsupervised (daily)	Dapsone 50 mg + Clofazimine 25 mg	Dapsone 50 mg + Clofazimine 25 mg

D. *Complications:*
- Trophic ulcers
- Deformities such as claw hand, clawing of toes, footdrop, saddle nose deformity, etc.
- Ophthalmic complications
- Kidney involvement

A-14.

A. Molluscum contagiosum

B. The lesions are multiple, pearly white, dome-shaped papules with central umbilication.
The lesions are seen on any part of body. Axillae, face, neck, lower abdomen and thigh are common sites. The lesions are limited, but may be innumerable in immunocompromised individuals. Large number of lesions are also seen in children with atopic dermatitis.

C. *Treatment options:*
- Topical application of phenol, salicylic acid, lactic acid, etc.
- Electrocautery
- Cryocautery
- Laser treatment

A-15. A. Orolabial herpes simplex viral (HSV) infection

B. *Different types of HSV:*
- Orolabial
- Cutaneous herpes
- Genital herpes
- Ocular herpes
- CNS herpes
- Neonatal herpes

C. *Differential diagnosis:*
- *Orolabial herpes:* Viral or bacterial pharyngitis, herpangina
- *Cutaneous herpes:* Eczema, cellulitis, varicella
- *Genital herpes:* Gonorrhea, impetigo
- *Ocular herpes:* Conjunctivitis
- *CNS herpes:* Viral meningoencephalitis, meningitis
- *Neonatal herpes:* Neonatal sepsis

D. Acyclovir, foscarnet, valacyclovir

A-16. A. Scabies

B. Sarcoptes scabies var hominis

C. *Different morphological skin lesions in scabies:*
- Primary lesion is a burrow, a grey thread like serpentine line with a minute papule at the end
- Papules and papulovesicular
- Pustules

- Nodules
- Urticaria
- Eczematized lesions

D. Common sites for skin lesions in scabies are webs of hands, on wrists, ulnar aspects of forearms, elbows, axillae, umbilical area, genitals, feet and buttocks. Face is usually spared, except in infants in whom face, scalp, palms and soles are also involved. Nodular lesions are common on genitals. Secondary infections are common, especially streptococcal infection which may result in post streptococcal glomerulonephritis.

E. *Treatment of scabies:*

- *General measures:* All close contacts of the patient, even if asymptomatic, should be treated.
- *Specific measures:*
  - Antibiotics for secondary infections
  - Antihistamines for 1–2 weeks to reduce itching
  - The topical scabicide should be applied all over body below the neck with a bath.
- *Scabicides:*
  - *Permethrin 5%:* Overnight single application is treatment of choice in children older than 2 months of age.
- *Crotamiton 10%:* Two applications daily for 14 days for infants less than 2 months of age.
- *Benzyl benzoate 25%:* Three applications 12 hourly intervals.
- *Ivermectin:* Single oral dose of 200 microgram/kg body weight, in children older than 5 years of age is the treatment of choice for epidemics as in orphanages.

F.

- Education of family and treatment of all close contacts is very essential
- All close contacts, even if asymptomatic should be treated.
- Nails should be trimmed.
- Good hygiene should be maintained.
- Individual towel and other clothes should be used.
- All family members and close contacts should be treated simultaneously.

A-17. A. Collodion baby

B. Oiled parchment skin, ectropion, fixation of the lips in an O-shaped configuration

C. Cutaneous infections, aspiration pneumonia, hypothermia, hypernatremic dehydration

A-18. A. Epidermolysis bullosa simplex—generalized

B. Autosomal dominant

C. Nails become dystrophic and dentition is normal.

A-19. A. Anhidrotic (Hypohidrotic) ectodermal dysplasia

B. Atopic disorders and GERD

C. Dysgammaglobulinemia

CHAPTER 22

Radiology

QUESTIONS

Q-1. A 2-year-old child presented with high-grade fever, toxic look and right mid zone pneumonia following measles. Child deteriorated after 5 days of hospitalization. Chest X-ray was taken.

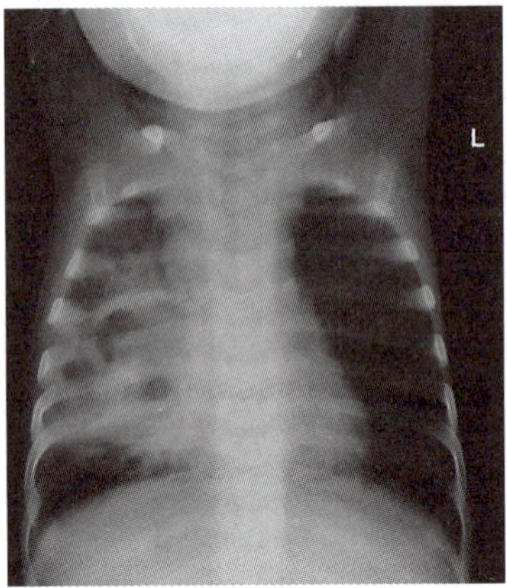

A. What does it show?
B. What is the most common organism responsible for this complication?
C. What will be your choice of antibiotics?

Q-2. Incidentally, chest X-ray showed this picture in a 2-year-old child who was asymptomatic.

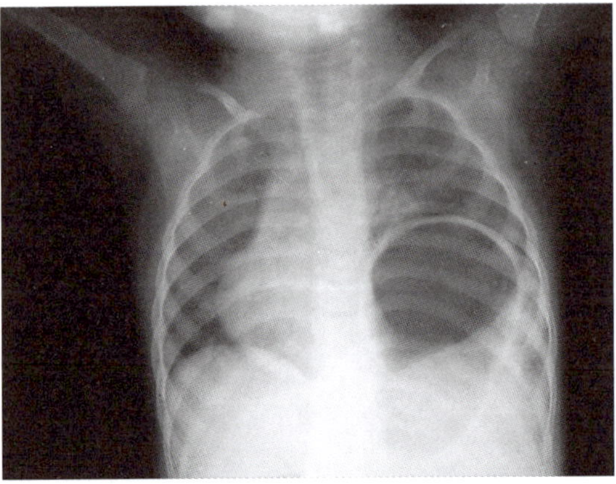

A. Name the condition.
B. What are other differential diagnosis?
C. What other conditions may be associated with its congenital type?

Q-3. X-ray chest of a newborn was taken for respiratory distress.

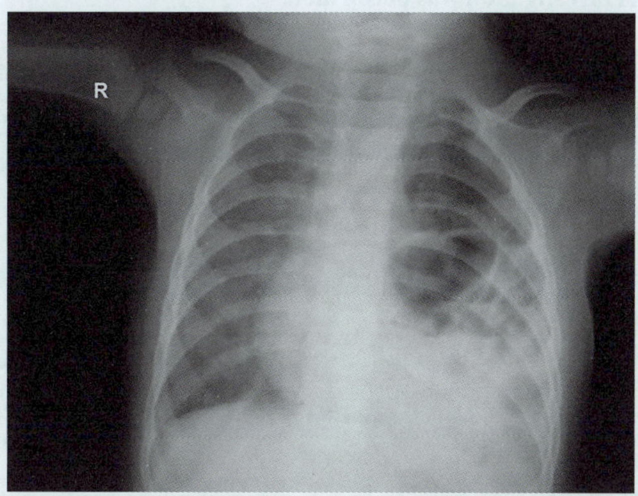

A. Name the condition.
B. What problem is faced by the clinician while resuscitating such a baby for birth asphyxia by bag and mask?
C. What is the line of treatment?
D. What associated condition is a limiting factor for survival of the baby?

Q-4. The child was brought with complaints of cough, chest pain and dyspnea. X-ray chest was taken in erect posture.

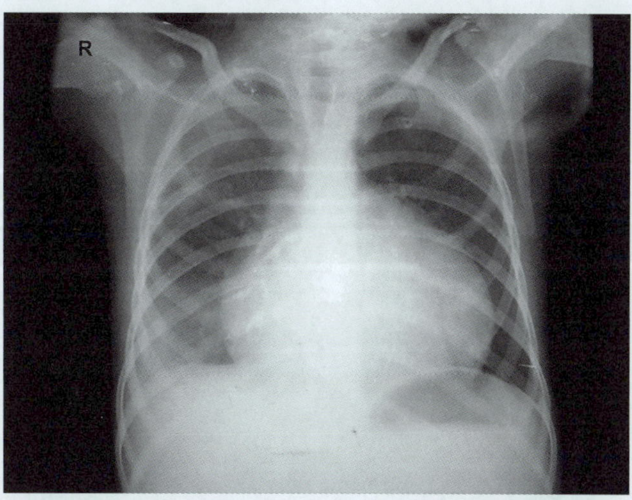

A. What is the cardiac contour?
B. What is your diagnosis?
C. What is the most sensitive diagnostic modality?

Q-5. A 10-month-old child developed severe intermittent pain in abdomen with a mass in right side of abdomen following diarrhea. This investigation was performed.

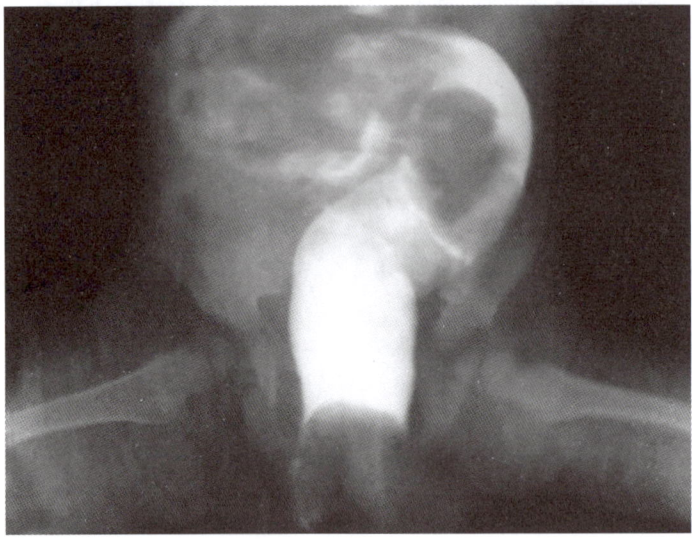

A. Name the investigation.
B. What is your diagnosis?
C. Which clinical examination may be informative on suspicious of this condition?

Q-6. A 2-month-old child presented with marked respiratory distress since birth. X-ray chest was performed.

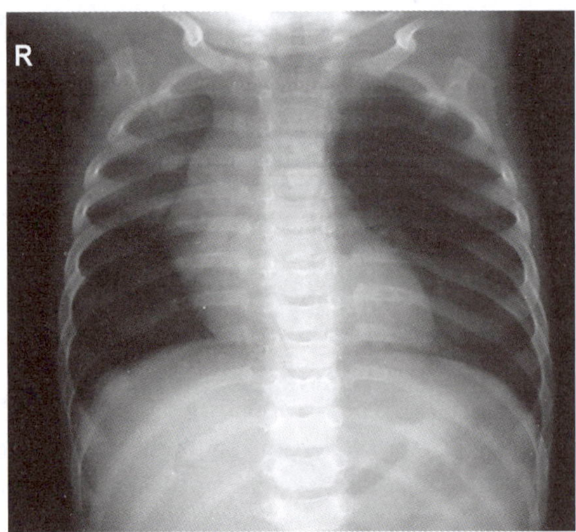

A. What is your diagnosis?
B. What is the most common site of this condition?
C. What is the line of treatment for this disease?

Q-7. A 5-year-old child brought with complaints of cough, chest pain, hemoptysis and no fever. Chest X-ray was taken. USG thorax confirmed the diagnosis.

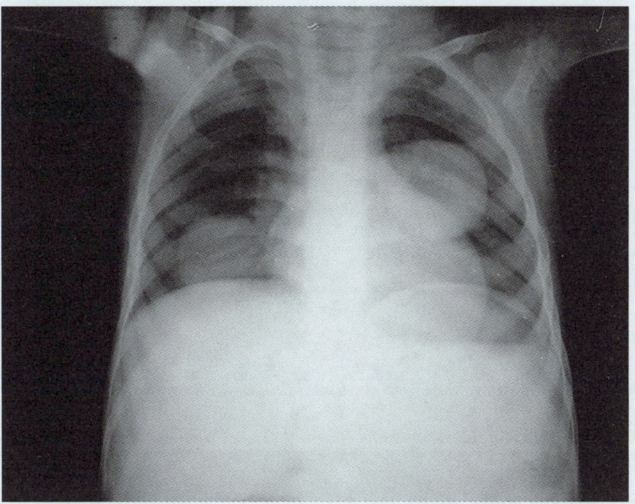

A. Name the condition.
B. What medicine can be given in this disease? What is the dose the drug? What is the duration of therapy?
C. Name the pathogen for this condition.

Q-8. X-ray of a term male infant who presented with bilious vomiting and scaphoid abdomen.

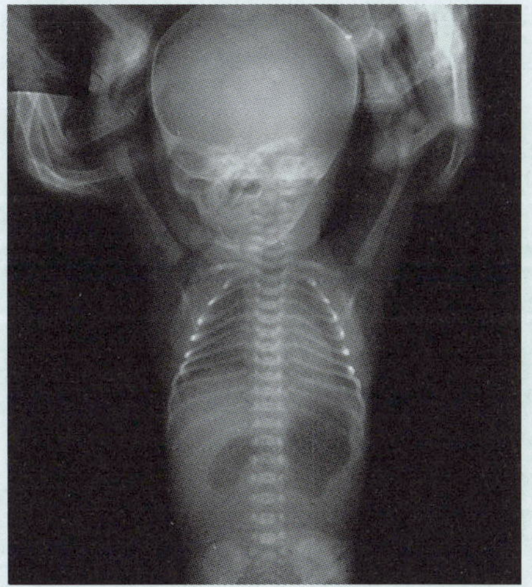

A. Name the abnormality seen.
B. What is the diagnosis?
C. What is the most common chromosomal abnormality associated with this anomaly?
D. What is the most common upper GI tract abnormality associated with this?

Q-9. On routine auscultation of posterior chest of a 5-year-old child, air-entry was found diminished on right side. Barium study was performed.

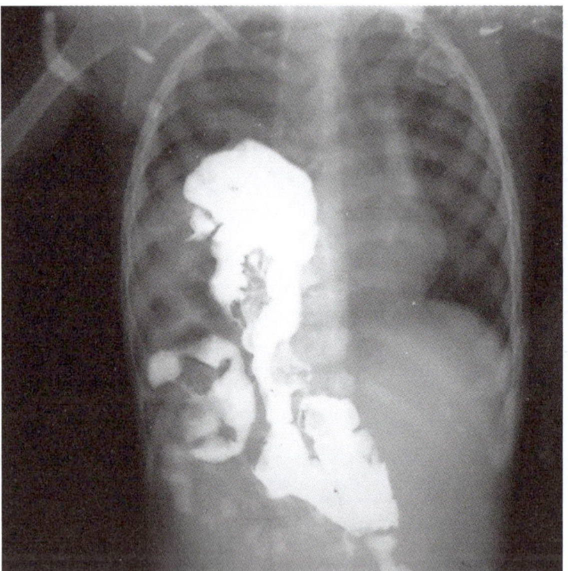

A. Name the condition.
B. What is the name of this type of condition?
C. What is another type of this disorder?

Q-10. A 5-year-old child presented with high-grade fever, cough, mild breathlessness and pain at left shoulder. A left lateral decubitus X-ray chest was taken besides this one and it was diagnostic.

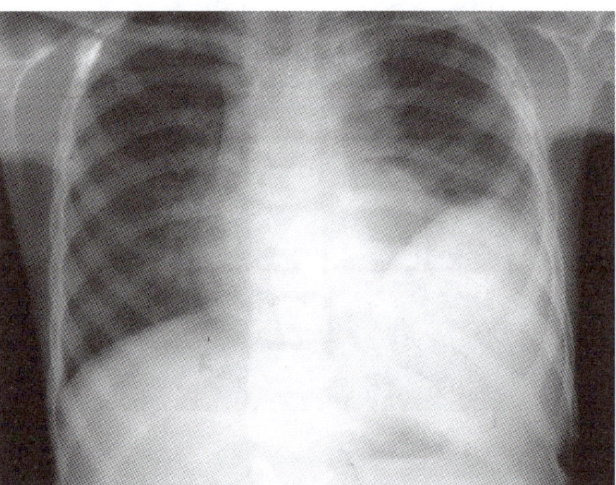

A. What does this X-ray chest show?
B. Which diagnostic test is expected to be positive in this child?
C. What diagnostic procedure should be performed?

Q-11. An infant presented with mild fever, cough and breathlessness since 15 days. On clinical examination, chest signs were minimal and hepatosplenomegaly. Chest X-ray was taken.

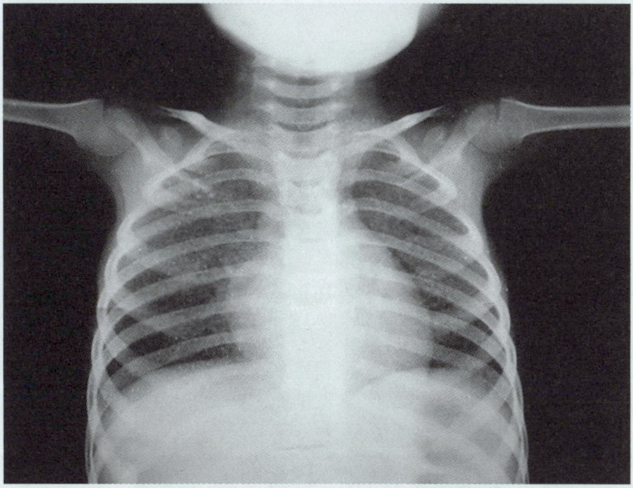

A. What is your diagnosis?
B. Which specific investigations for CNS involvement should be performed in such patients?
C. Which component of lungs is specifically involved in this disease?

Q-12. A 5-month-old infant presented with mild fever, running nose, rattly chest. CBC was normal. Chest X-ray was reported as right upper zone pneumonia, treated with antibiotics for 7 days. Child was asymptomatic and playful. Repeat chest X-ray was reported as persistent right upper zone pneumonia. Lateral chest X-ray was performed.

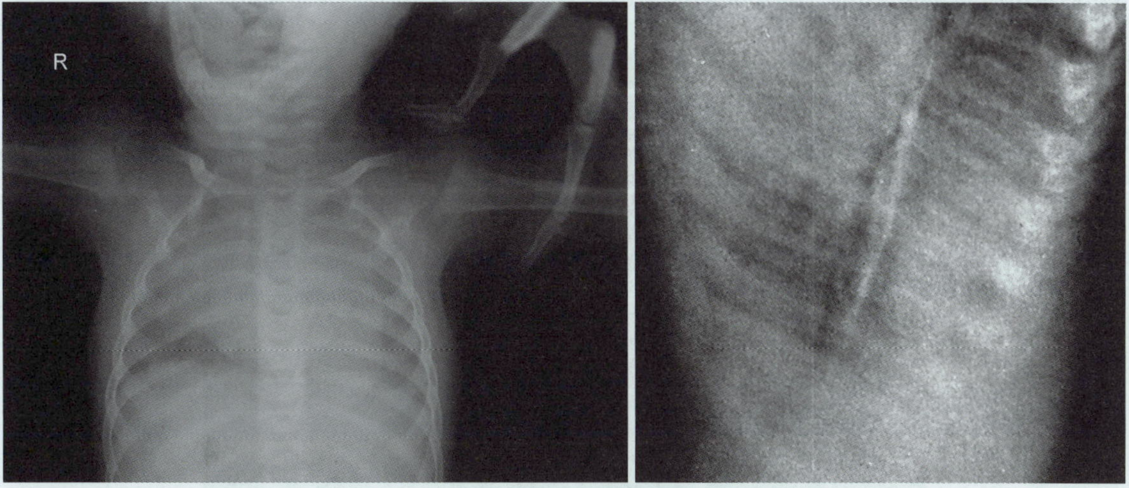

A. What is the anatomical location of an opacity in lateral chest X-ray?
B. What is your diagnosis?
C. In which conditions, this shadow may decrease in size or may be absent?

Q-13. A 10-hour-old girl presented with tachypnea, subcostal and intercostal indrawing and grunting after 4 hours of birth. She was preterm (32 weeks), emergency LSCS born to a diabetic mother. Birth weight was 2.2 kg. There was not history of birth asphyxia. Marked cyanosis was noted. This was chest X-ray.

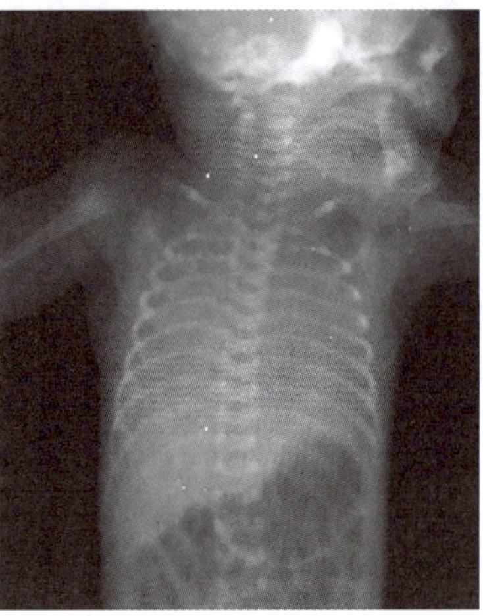

A. What are the radiological findings?
B. What is the diagnosis?
C. What types of different radiological features are known in this condition?
D. What is grunting?

Q-14. A 2-hour-old female infant was brought with fast breathing, noted by the mother. She was delivery by LSCS for pregnancy induced hypertension. Birth weight was 2.6 kg. The baby was alert, respiratory rate 80/min with mild intercostal indrawing. There was no grunting, no cyanosis. SpO_2 was 94% with oxygen support. Baby recovered after a day. The following are chest X-rays of baby taken 36 hours apart.

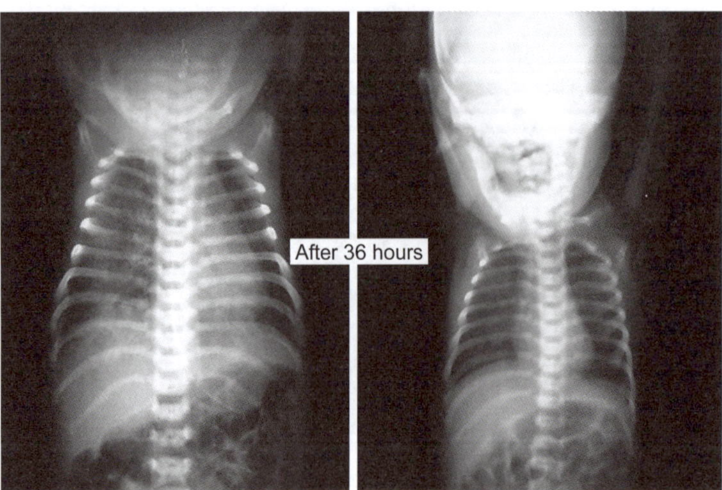

A. What are the radiological findings?
B. What is your diagnosis?
C. Why is it more common in babies delivered by LSCS?
D. Whether surfactant is indicated in this condition?

Q-15. A 10-month-old child had pneumonia. It was managed successfully with antibiotics. Repeat chest X-ray after 2 weeks of antibiotics was as below.

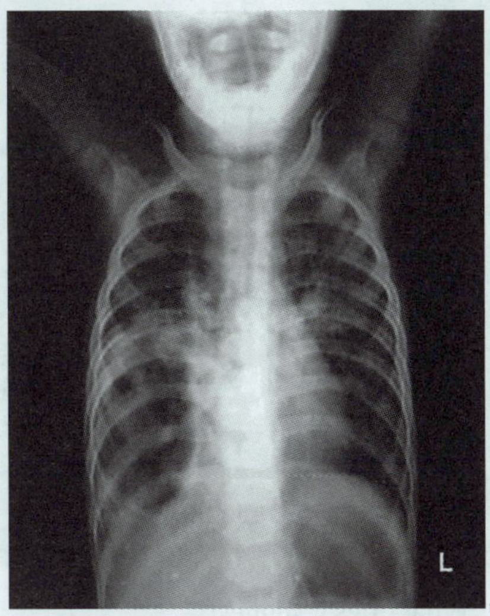

A. Describe the radiological finding. What is called it?
B. What is most common organism causing this lesion?
C. What are possible complications following this lung lesion?

Q-16. An infant had left lower zone post-measles pneumonia, treated by a family physician with oral cefixime. The child was brought with high-grade fever, toxic look and respiratory distress.

This was the chest X-ray.

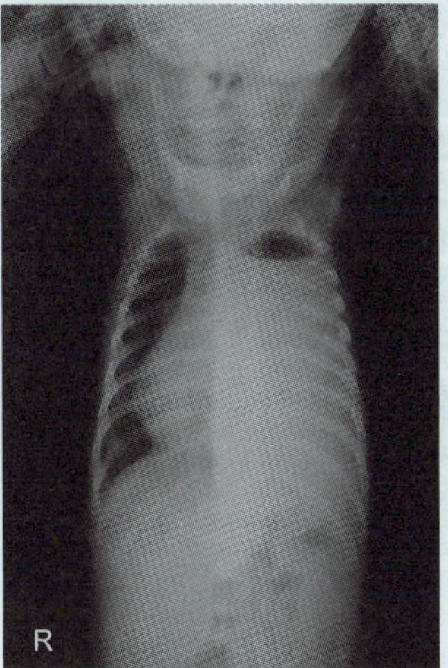

A. Describe the radiological findings.
B. What is probable diagnosis?
C. What is choice of radiological investigation to confirm the diagnosis?
D. What are most common organisms causing this complication?
E. What should be choice of antibiotics?

Q-17.

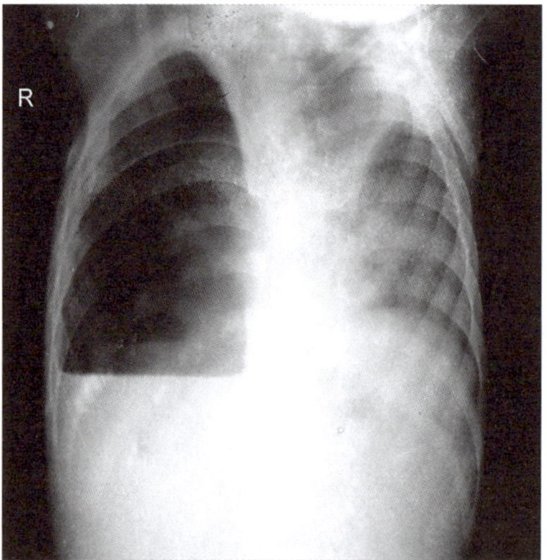

A. What are radiological findings? What does it suggest?
B. What are common organisms responsible for this disorder?
C. What line of treatment is suggested?

Q-18.

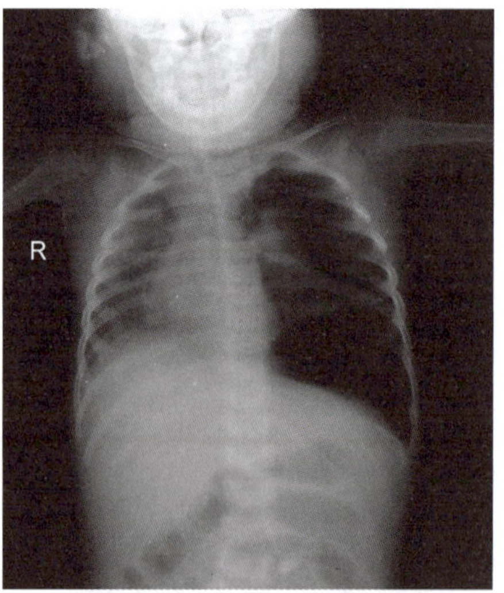

A. What are the radiological findings? What does it suggest?
B. What are common causes for this disorder of lung in children?
C. What is the first line of treatment of this complication?

Q-19. A preterm baby was admitted in NICU for sepsis. In due course of illness, baby developed distention of abdomen, periumbilical redness and suddenly deteriorated. The X-ray abdomen was taken in erect posture. The picture is shown below.

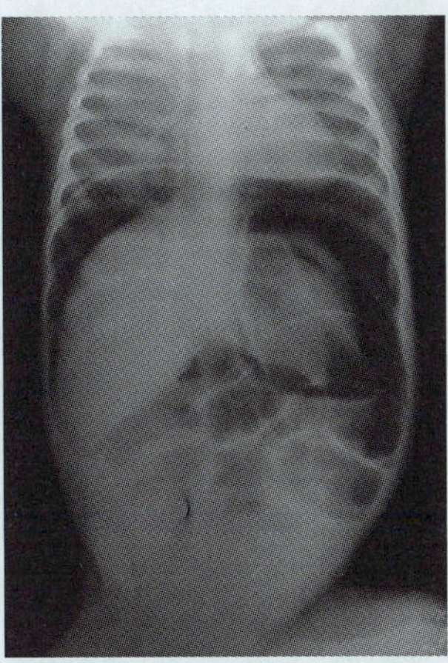

A. What are the X-ray findings? What does it indicate?
B. What is the diagnosis in this baby?
C. What are the common causes for this type of X-ray findings in pediatric practice?
D. What are the complications in this condition?

Q-20. A 2-year-old boy was brought with complaint of persistent cough and breathlessness 5 days. He had no fever. Onset of cough was sudden with choking. The followings were chest X-rays.

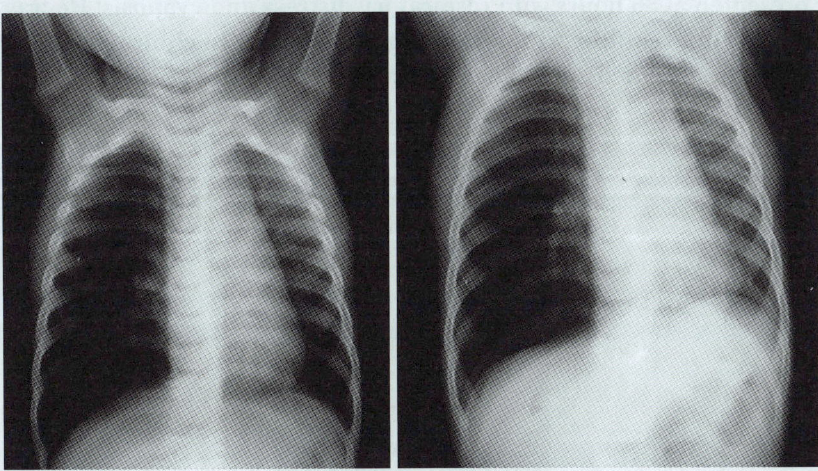

A. What are X-ray findings?
B. What is the probable diagnosis in this case?
C. What are the other causes for such X-ray findings in children?

Q-21. A 3-year-old boy presented with recurrent (3 times) right basal pneumonia in last 1 year. He was treated with multiple antibiotics and anti-tuberculous drugs without any response. He had no history of wight loss. Investigations for tuberculosis were negative. His chest X-ray was as below:

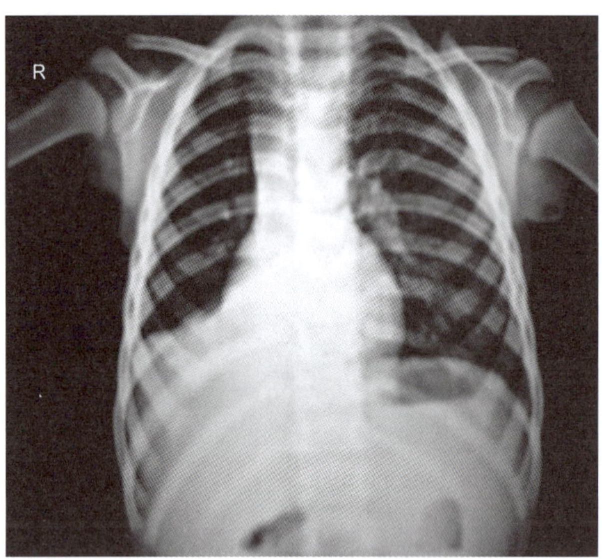

A. What are X-ray findings?
B. What are the possibilities?
C. What investigations are suggested?

Q-22. A male infant presented at 36 hours with respiratory distress and cyanosis. He was born at full-term by normal vaginal route uneventfully with birth weight of 2.7 kg. On clinical examination, tachypnea and absent air entry on left side noted. Abdomen was scaphoid. Chest X-ray was as below:

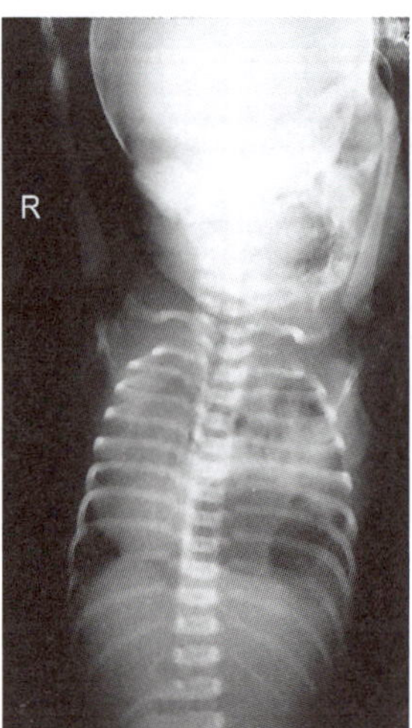

A. What are X-ray findings?
B. What is your diagnosis?
C. What problems are expected in resuscitation of such baby on birth?
D. What is the type of this disorder?
E. Which factor determines outcome after surgery?

Q-23. A neonate was brought with complaints of excessive salivation and drooling. Mother noticed development of cough, choking and bluish discoloration during feeding. Some radiological investigation was performed as below.

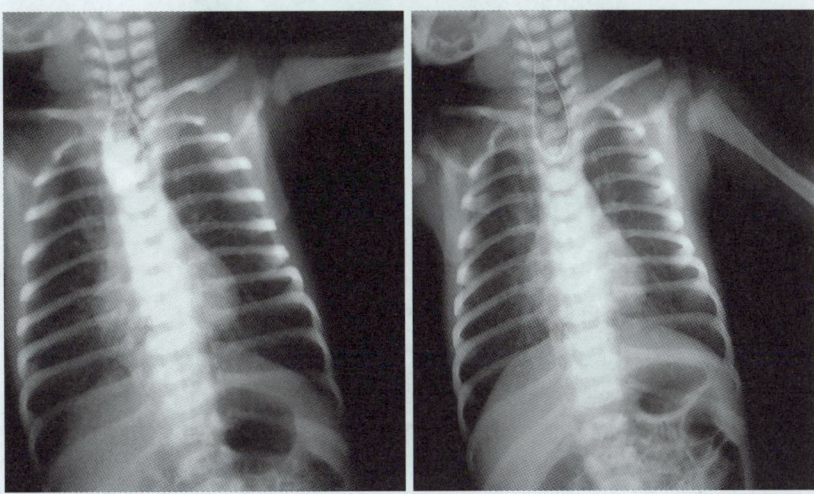

A. What are radiological findings?
B. What is the diagnosis?
C. What antenatal ultrasonographic findings may diagnose this condition?
D. Which type of this disorder may present as recurrent pneumonia and bronchospasms? What investigations will confirm the diagnosis?

Q-24. A 5-week-old male infant presented with nonbilious, projectile, forcible vomiting. There was history of prolonged neonatal jaundice. The infant had severe dehydration and ABG showed metabolic alkalosis. Some radiological investigation was performed as below:

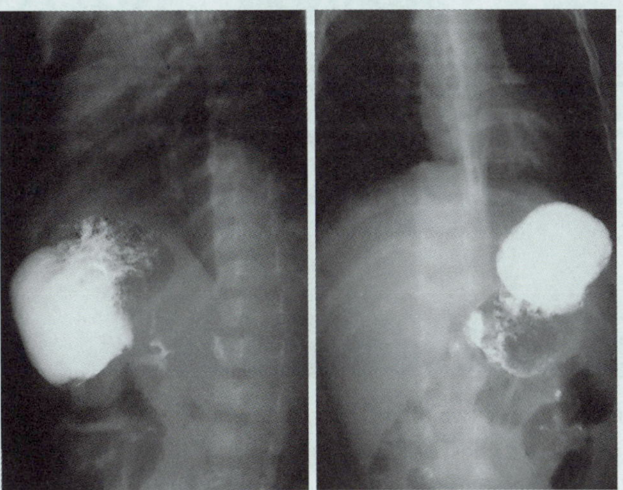

A. What are radiological findings?
B. What is probable diagnosis?
C. What clinical findings are characteristics of the condition?
D. Which diagnostic modality has more sensitivity?
E. What is line of treatment?

Q-25. A diagnosed case of Down syndrome presented with bilious vomiting. The plain X-ray abdomen was as below:

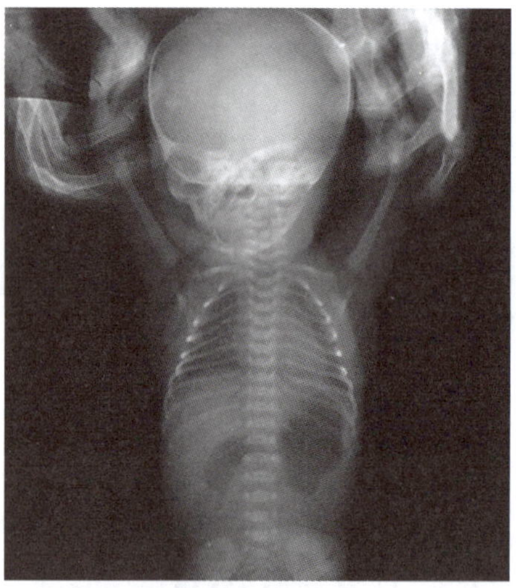

A. What are the radiological findings?
B. What is the diagnosis?
C. What are antenatal ultrasonographic findings suggesting the condition?
D. What anomalies can cause this disorder?

Q-26.

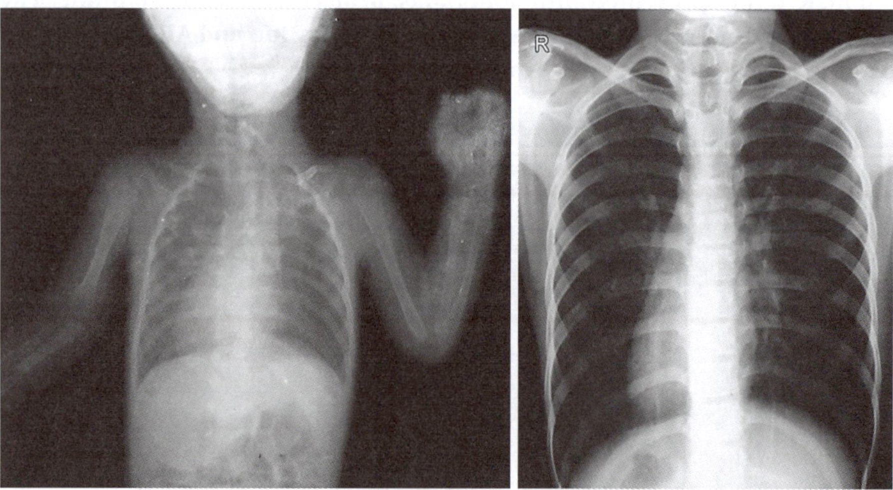

A. What is common finding is these two chest X-rays?
B. What is difference in these two chest X-rays?
C. What other anomalies are known to be associated with this condition?

Q-27. A 20-day-old neonate born as full-term was brought for persistent jaundice. His anterior fontanelle was wide open and posterior fontanelle was also found open. His X-ray knee was as below:

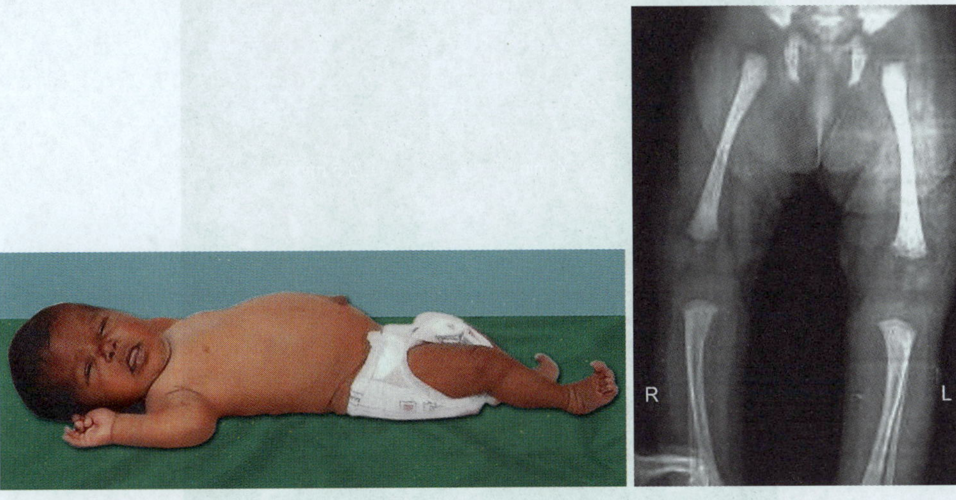

A. What are the X-ray finding?
B. What biochemical tests would you suggest for confirmation of the condition?
C. What are other clinical features of this disorder?
D. What preventive measure is recommended for this disease?

Q-28.

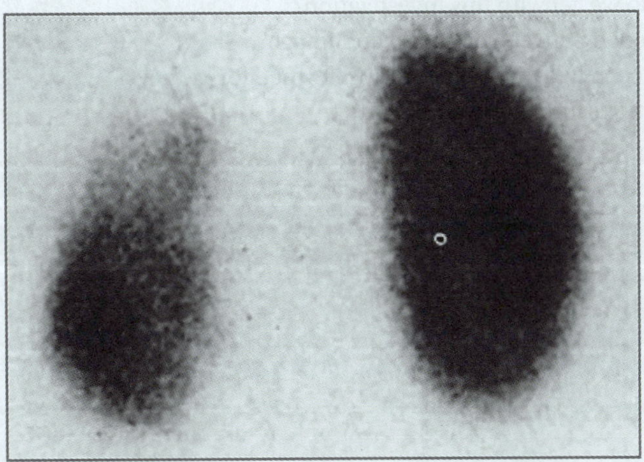

A. Identify the investigation performed for renal system.
B. What is possible diagnosis in this case?
C. Write four indications for this investigation.
D. Is it indicated in a case of urinary tract infection (UTI)? At what time should it be performed following UTI? What do you expect to see?

Q-29.

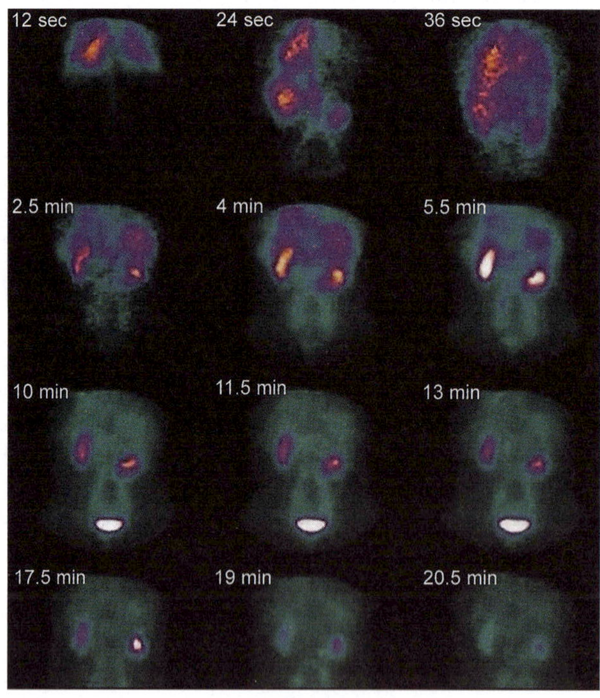

A. Identify the investigation performed for renal disorder.
B. What information do we get with this investigation?
C. How much time needed between injection and image?
D. What is the difference in two different scans performed for kidneys?
E. What are the indications for this investigation?

Q-30. The following investigation was performed in a 6-week-old infant for persistent direct hyperbilirubinemia.

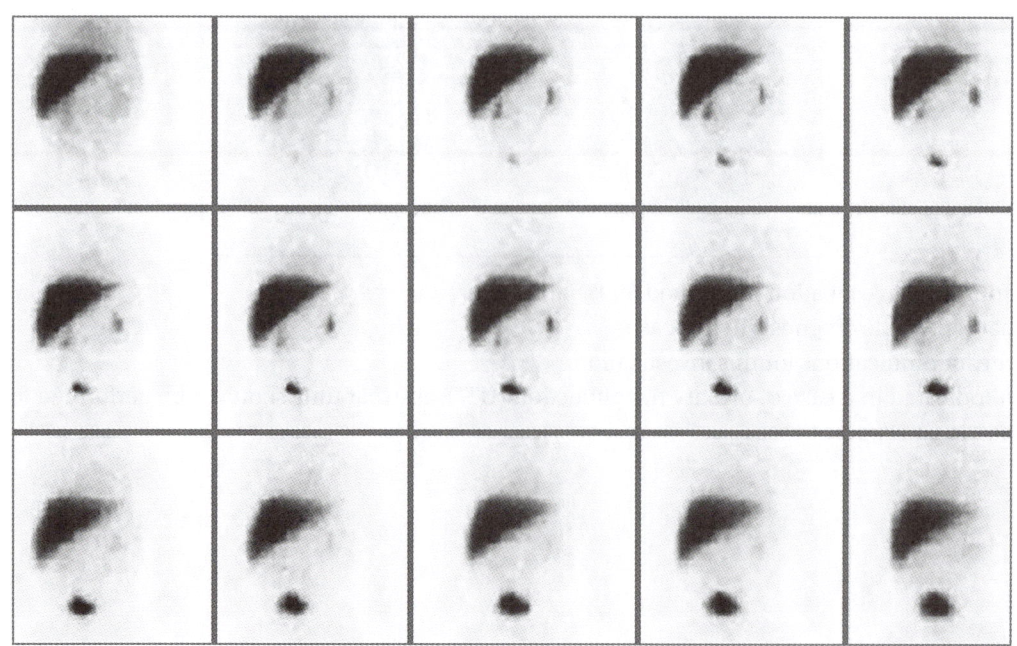

A. Name the investigation.
B. What does it show?
C. What is most likely diagnosis?
D. What dye is used for this investigation?
E. What are prerequisitions before performing this test?
F. What is the golden time for this investigation?
G. List any 5 supplementary medicines indicated for this infant.
H. What is gold standard for diagnosis for this condition?

Q-31. A female with short stature presented with features of Turner syndrome. Her DMSA renal scan pictures are as below:

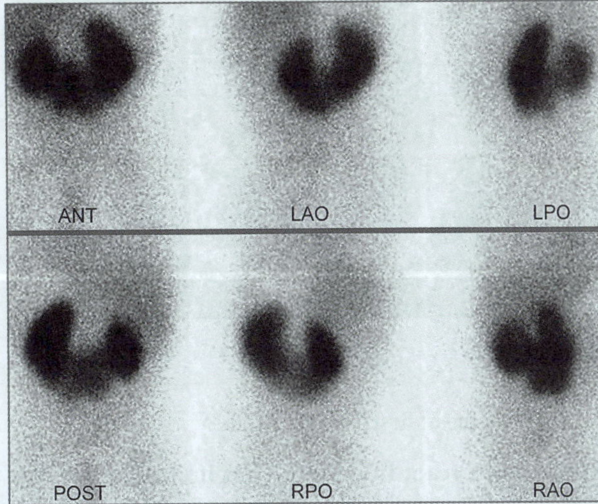

A. What are interpretations of the scan?
B. What is probable diagnosis?
C. What are known complications of this disorder?
D. Mention four conditions associated with this anomaly.

Q-32. An infant was brought with fever, large head, hepatosplenomegaly, jaundice and convulsions. Eye examination revealed bilateral chorioretinitis. CT scan of brain picture is as below:

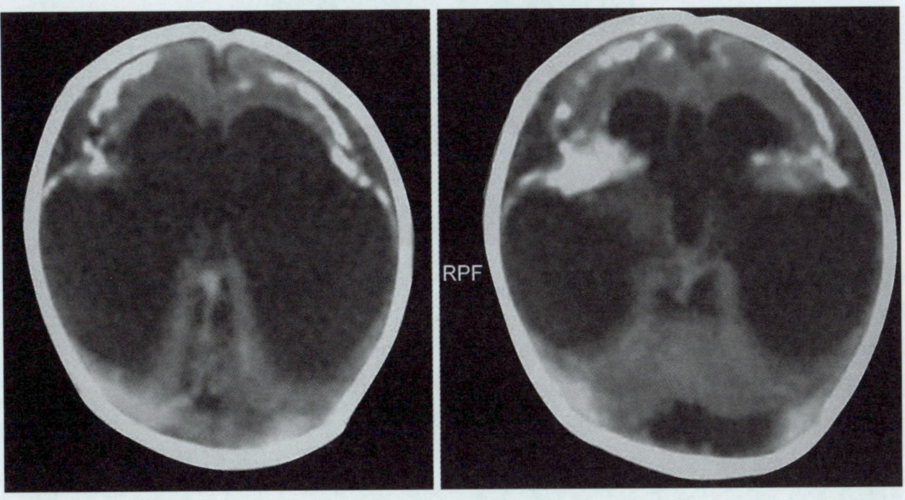

A. What are the CT scan brain findings?
B. What is the probable diagnosis?
C. What is the gold standard for diagnosis of the condition?
D. What is the drug of choice for this congenital disease?

Q-33. An infant presented with IUGR, not gaining weight, persistent jaundice, hepatosplenomegaly and thrombocytopenia. CT scan of brain picture is as below:

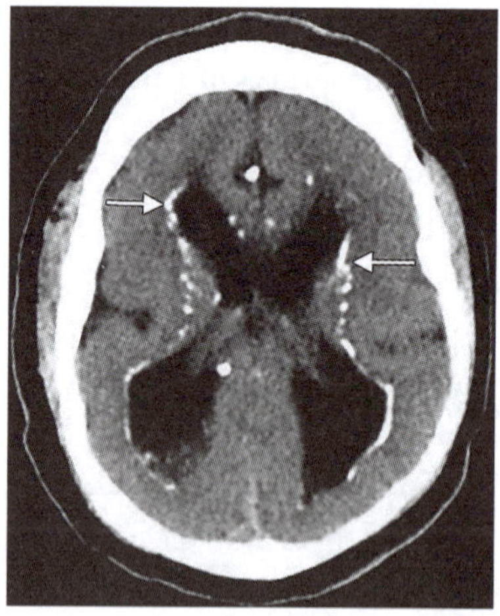

A. What are findings of CT scan brain?
B. What is probable diagnosis?
C. What test can confirm the diagnosis in first 2 weeks of life?

Q-34. A neonate presented with urinary tract infection. This investigation was performed after treating the infection.

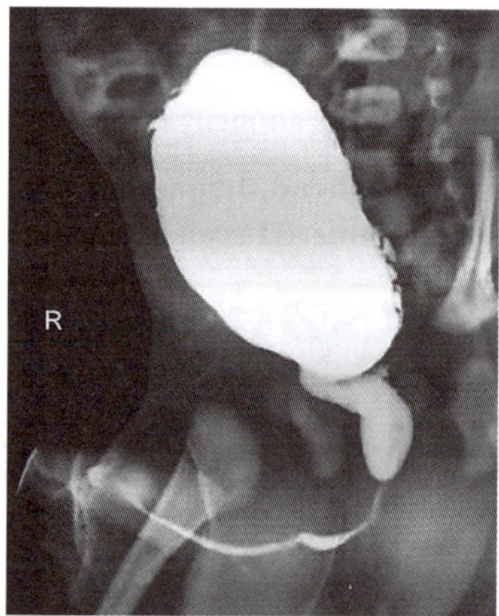

A. Name the investigation.
B. Describe the radio-imaging findings.
C. What antenatal intervention may be indicated in this condition?
D. What surgical procedures can be performed in this disorder?

Q-35. A child presented with recurrent urinary tract infection. Following are the pictures of the investigation which was performed after treating the infection.

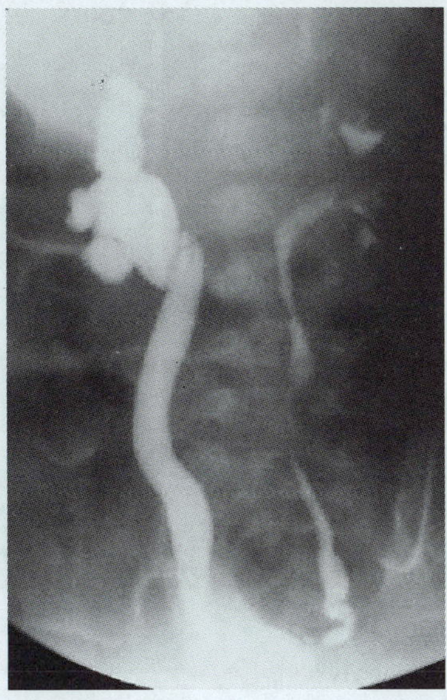

A. Name the investigations.
B. What are the interpretations of this investigation?
C. What are the gradings of this condition on MCU study?
D. What antibiotic is preferred as prophylaxis for prevention of UTI in 4 months of old infant? What is the dose?

Q-36. This infant had deformities of the limbs since birth. X-ray revealed the diagnosis.

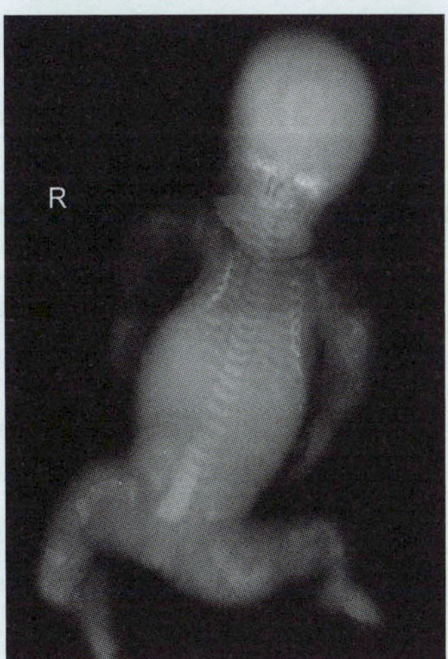

A. Name the condition.
B. What is its inheritance pattern?
C. What is the clinical triad of this disease?
D. What is the biochemical defect?
E. What are the medical treatment options available for this condition?

Q-37. A 45-day-old male child presented with severe anemia, thrombocytopenia, hypocalcemia, hepatosplenomegaly and severe sepsis.

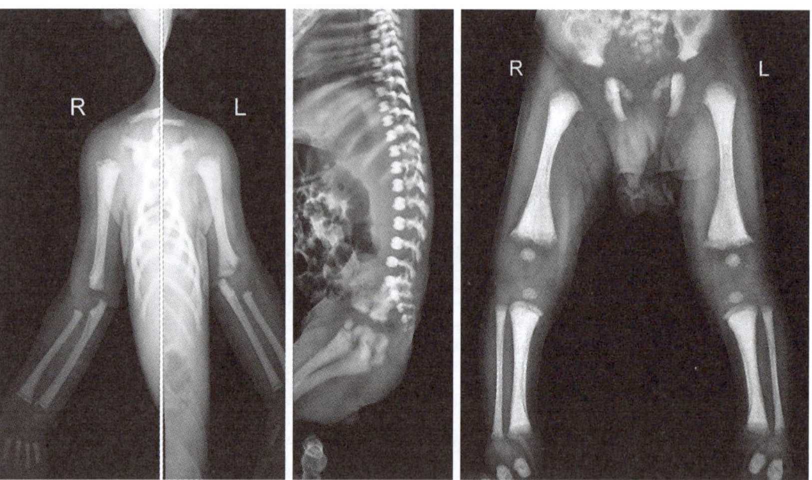

A. What is your diagnosis?
B. What is the cause of hepatosplenomegaly?
C. Why is there dysfunctions of optic nerve and facial nerve?
D. What can be offered as treatment?

ANSWERS

A-1. A. Right midzone lung abscess B. *Staphylococcus aureus*
C. Ceftriaxone and vancomycin

A-2. A. Congenital eventration of left dome of diaphragm
B.
- Diaphragmatic paralysis
- Iatrogenic injury to phrenic nerve after surgery
- Diaphragmatic hernia

C. Pulmonary sequestration, congenital heart disease, chromosomal trisomy

A-3. A. Congenital diaphragmatic hernia (Bochdalek type)
B. Baby becomes more hypoxic with use of bag and mask resuscitation
C. Surgery
D. Pulmonary hypoplasia

A-4. A. Bottle-neck appearance (Erlenmeyer flask) B. Pericardial effusion
C. Echocardiography

A-5. A. Barium enema B. Intussusception
C. Per rectal examination

A-6. A. Congenital lobar emphysema left upper lobe
B. Left upper lobe
C. Excision of the affected lobe

A-7. A. Hydatid cyst
B. Albendazole 15 mg/kg/day in two divided doses (max. 800 mg/day) for 3–6 months
C. *Echinococcus granulosus*

A-8. A. Double-bubble appearance B. Duodenal atresia
C. Down syndrome D. Annular pancreas

A-9. A. Anterior congenital diaphragmatic hernia B. Foramen of Morgagni
C. Bochdalek hernia

A-10. A. Left side subpulmonic pleural effusion B. Mantoux test
C. USG-guided pleural fluid tapping

A-11. A. Miliary tuberculosis B. Lumbar puncture for tuberculous meningitis
C. Interstitial tissues of lung

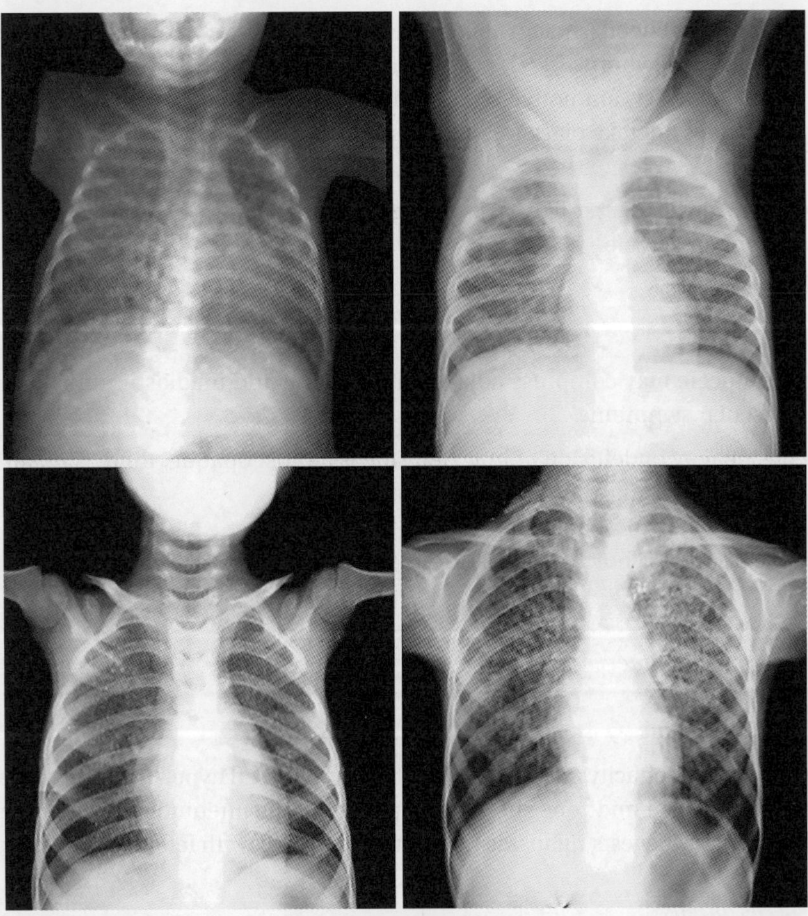

Miliary tuberculosis

- Millet size (2–3 mm) scattered opacities in both the lung fields.
- The spread is by hematogenous route.
- It is more common in immunocompromised children like following measles, severe degree of malnutrition, suffering from HIV, etc.
- It is interstitial lung disease. Child has marked tachypnea, cyanosis but minimal chest signs on auscultation. Hepatosplenomegaly is common. There may be CNS involvement in form of TBM. Therefore, CSF examination should be routinely performed in a case of miliary TB even in absence of signs of meningitis.
- MT may be negative.

With strong clinical diagnosis and absence of miliary shadows on chest X-ray. CT thorax may be diagnostic.

A-12. A. Anterior superior mediastinal compartment
B. Normal thymus gland
C. May decrease in size in response to stress, steroids and cyanotic congenital heart disease, absent in DiGeorge's syndrome.

A-13. A. Ground-glass appearance with air bronchogram in both lung fields
B. Hyaline membrane disease
C.
- White lung
- Granular opacities with air bronchogram
- Heart border cannot be delineated.

A-14. A. First X-ray shows homogeneous opacity in lung fields. Second X-ray chest, taken after 36 hours is normal.
B. Transient tachypnea of newborn (TTN)
C. In a case of normal delivery, amniotic fluid present in alveoli is squeezed out while baby is passing through birth canal, which does not take place in LSCS delivered babies.

A-15. A.
- It is thin-walled, air-filled, cyst-like cavity on right lower zone.
- It is called as pneumatocele.

B. *Staphylococcus aureus*
C.
- Pneumothorax
- Large pneumatocele may compress adjacent lung tissue and mediastinum enough to cause respiratory and cardiovascular symptoms.

A-16. A. A homogeneous opacity on left side of lung, left side is almost opaque, there is no air bronchogram, left CP angle is obliterated and mediastinum is shifted on right side.
B. Left-sided pleural effusion, probably empyema
C. Ultrasonogram of thorax is choice of investigations for fluid in pleural cavity.
D.
- *Staphylococcus aureus*
- *Streptococcus pneumoniae*
- *Klebsiella pneumoniae*

E. Ceftriaxone and Cloxacillin

A-17. A. Right side homogeneous opacity on lower side with sharp line and hyper-translucency above it. Right dome of diaphragm is not seen. Left mid zone shows opacity, suggesting pneumonia. Left dome of diaphragm is seen. Left CP angle is clear. It suggests right side hydropneumothorax with left mid zone pneumonia.
B.
- *Staphylococcus aureus*
- *Klebsiella pneumoniae*
- *Pseudomonas aeruginosa*
- *Acinetobacter*

C.
- Insertion of intercostal drainage tube on right side, at posterior axillary line on lower chest
- Empirical antibiotics—ceftriaxone and vancomycin

A-18. A. Left side is hyper-translucent, collapse lung is seen at hilar region, left dome of diaphragm is flattened and left side of chest is expanded. The mediastinum is shifted on right side. It suggests pneumothorax.
B.
- Penetrating chest injury
- Spontaneous pneumothorax in newborns

- Following vigorous cough in a case of bronchial asthma
- Occasionally in a child with pertussis (whooping cough)
- Staphylococcal-like organisms.

C. Insertion of a needle or chest tube is life-saving treatment.

A-19. A. There is gas under right dome of diaphragm. Right side lung opacity is also noted, suggesting pneumonia. The gas under diaphragm indicates perforation of intestine, likely complication of necrotizing enterocolitis in preterm baby.

B. Perforation of intestine following necrotizing enterocolitis (NEC).

C.

- Hollow viscous perforation is most common cause.
- Endoscopic gastrointestinal procedures and perforation as a complication.
- Peritoneal dialysis
- Mechanical ventilation

D. It can cause peritonitis, shock and death.

Congenital Diaphragmatic Hernias

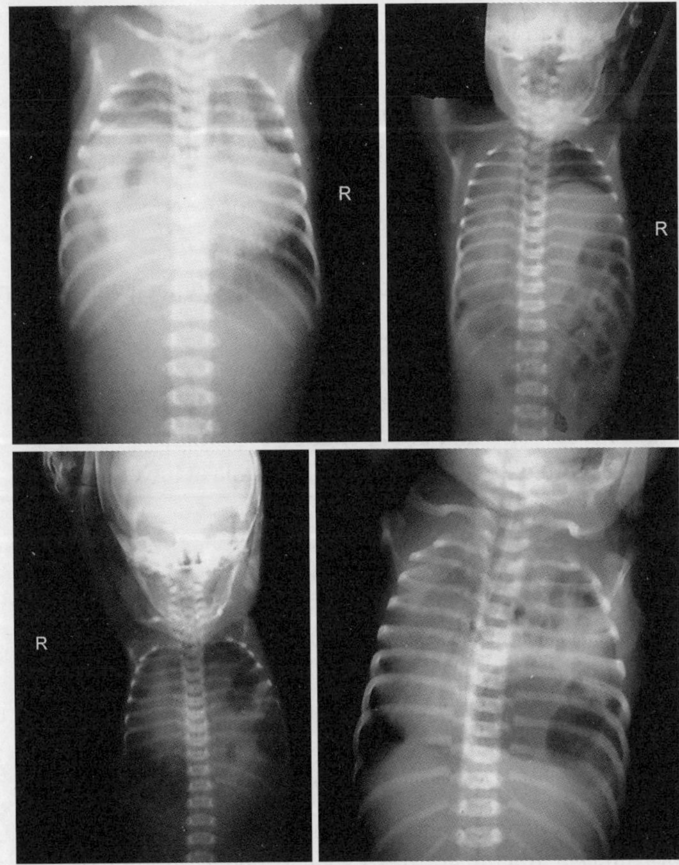

- Most common through posterolateral foramen of Bochdaleck (85–90%) (80% on left side) (bilateral in 5%)
- Anterior or medial foramen of Morgagni
- Central defect is rare.
- Large CDH present with acute, severe respiratory distress at the time of birth, bag and mask resuscitation is contraindicated.
- Antenatal USG study may diagnose.
- Hypoplastic lung is important factor for postoperative outcome.

A-20. A. There is translucency on right side, right dome of diaphragm is flattened, shifting of mediastinum on left side. Splaying of ribs and separation of vascular markings are also other features.

B. Foreign body in right airway with partial obstruction.

C. Any enlarged lymph node due to tuberculosis, sarcoidosis, lymphoma can also cause partial obstruction of the airway from external side and can result in such radiological picture. Any mass pressing over airway can also cause such X-ray findings.

A-21. A.

- Right lower zone collapse of lung.
- Lower mediastinum is pulled on right side suggesting right lower zone collapsed lung.

B.

- Foreign body in right bronchus
- Some lymph node (tuberculosis or lymphoma) or a mass compressing lower bronchus.
- Congenital malformation

C.

- Flexible bronchoscopy to remove a foreign body, if it is there.
- CT scan of thorax for congenital malformation.
- CT angiogram for malformation-like pulmonary sequestration.

A-22. A.

- Left hemithorax is enlarged, filled with multiple cystic lucencies in continuity with those of abdomen, left dome of diaphragm is not delineated. The mediastinum is shifted on right side.
- Left lung hypoplastic.
- Right lung is compressed.

B. Congenital left side diaphragmatic hernia

C. Baby will deteriorate on bag and mask resuscitation as air in stomach will cause more compression of lung.

D. Bochdalek type of hernia

E. Hypoplasia of left lung

A-23. A. An orogastric tube is seen coiled in the upper blind pouch. The presence of gas in stomach and intestine is also noted. Both lung fields are normal. Cardiac shadow is normal.

B. Tracheoesophageal fistula with blind upper pouch and fistula at lower end.

C.

- Polyhydramnios
- Absence of stomach bubble
- Pouch sign

D.

- 'H' type tracheoesophageal fistula
- Bronchoscopy or methylene blue dye study.

A-24. A.

- Upper GI barium study is performed.
- It shows elongated pyloric channel, called as string sign
- Bulge of the pyloric muscle into the antrum is seen, called as shoulder sign.
- Parallel streaks of barium seen in narrowed channel, called as double tract sign.

B. Congenital hypertrophic pyloric stenosis

C. 'Olive' shaped, hard mass on left side of abdomen on palpation, present in 80% cases. This mass develops especially on feeding. The mass is seen moving in form of visible peristalsis from left to right. It disappears after vomiting. Baby is alert, bright looking and hungry.

D. Ultrasonographic study of abdomen

E. Ramstedt's pyloromyotomy, surgery is treatment of choice.

A-25. A. Double-bubble shadow in abdomen, one air bubble is stomach and another in first part of duodenum

B. Duodenal obstruction

C.

- Polyhydramnios
- Dilated stomach and duodenum

D.

- Duodenal atresia
- Duodenal stenosis
- Duodenal web
- Annular pancreas (common in Down syndrome)
- Extrinsic compression by bands and duplication cyst

A-26. A. Both X-rays show dextrocardia.

B.

- Left X-ray shows dextrocardia with situs solitus (liver on right side and stomach on left side as normal)
- Right X-ray shows dextrocardia with situs inversus (liver on left side and stomach on right side, abnormal location)

C.

- Kartagener syndrome
- Asplenia
- Malrotation of intestine

A-27. A. Absence of centers of epiphysis of femur and tibia on both knees. It is expected to be present in full-term baby. It indicates retardation of skeletal age.

B. T_3, T_4, TSH for hypothyroidism.

C. Delayed passage of meconium, constipation, lethargic baby, prolonged neonatal jaundice, excessive weight gain, protrusion of tongue, etc., are other clinical features.

D. Every newborn should be screened for congenital hypothyroidism by performing TSH level by collection blood from heel prick after 72 hours of birth.

Radiological changes in hypothyroidism

- The distal femoral epiphysis, normally present at birth, is often absent
- Retardation of skeletal age
- Epiphyseal dysgenesis (multiple foci of ossification)
- Beaking of verebrae (12th Thoracic and 1st and 2nd lumbar)
- *Skull:*
- Large fontanels
- Wide sutures
- Wormian (intersutural) bones
- Enlarged sella turcica, rarely erosion and thinning
- Delayed eruption of teeth
- Cardiac enlargement and pericardial effusion

A-28. A. DMSA renal scan (demercapto succinic acid scan)

B. Multiple focal cortical defects in the upper and lower poles of the left kidney suggesting diffuse parenchymal abnormality.

C.

- Urinary tract infection
- Renal infarct
- Horseshoe kidney
- Ectopic kidney
- Multicystic dysplastic kidney

D.

- Yes
- After 4–6 months of acute infection
- To detect renal scarring or renal injury

A-29. A. A DTPA (Diethylene triamine penta acetic acid) scan

B.

- Renal blood flow
- Glomerular filtration rate
- Tubular function
- Urinary excretion

C. The scan is started immediately and images are taken for 30 minutes

D. DMSA scan is usually static imaging, while DTPA is usually used by dynamic imaging to assess renal excretion.

E.

- Assessment of GFR
- Acute renal failure
- Obstructive hydronephrosis

A-30. A. Hepatobiliary iminodiacetic acid (HIDA) scan also called as cholescintigraphy.

B. Dye has been taken up by liver, but dye is not reaching the intestine.

C. Biliary atresia

D. Iminodiacetic acid

E.

- Fasting for 2–4 hours before the scan
- Phenobarbitone should be given for 5 days before the investigation

F. Less than 10 weeks

G.

- Vitamin A
- Vitamin D
- Vitamin K
- Calcium, phosphorus and zinc

H. Liver biopsy

A-31. A. All the views show fusion of lower poles of both kidneys, suggesting horse-shoe kidney

B. Turner syndrome (Turner syndrome has associated Horseshoe kidney)

C.

- Pelvic ureteric junction obstruction (most common)
- Vesicoureteral reflux
- Urinary tract infection
- Malignancy

D.

- Turner syndrome
- Edward syndrome
- Down syndrome
- Patau syndrome

A-32. A. Hydrocephalus with multiple, irregular, scattered calcifications.

B. Congenital toxoplasmosis

C. Detection of persisting specific IgG antibodies at the age of 1 year

D. Pyrimethamine

A-33. A. Hydrocephalus and periventricular calcification
B. Congenital cytomegalovirus infection
C. Urinary PCR test

A-34. A. Micturating cystourethrogram (MCU)
B. Dilatation of posterior urethra, suggestive posterior urethral valve
C. In severe PUV obstruction, vesicoamniotic shunting can be done.
D.
- Primary valve fulguration
- Vesicostomy and high ureterostomy

A-35. A. Micturating cystourethrogram (MCU study)
B. Right side grade IV vesicoureteral reflux
C. *Grade I:* VUR does not reach the renal pelvis.
Grade II: VUR extending up to renal pelvis without dilatation of pelvis or calyceal fornices.
Grade III: VUR extending up to kidney with mild dilatation or tortuosity of ureter and renal pelvis and no or minor blunting of calyceal fornices.
Grade IV: Moderate dilatation or tortuosity of the ureter, renal pelvis and fornices with complete obliteration of sharp angles of calyceal fornices.

A-36. A. Osteogenesis Imperfecta
B. Autosomal dominant
C. Fragile bones, blue sclera and deafness
D. Structural/quantitative defect in type I collagen formation
E. Growth hormone (improves bone histology) bisphosphonates (IV pamidronate/oral olpadronate)

A-37. A. Osteopetrosis (marble bone disease)
B. Due to compensatory extramedullary hematopoiesis
C. Narrowing of foramina
D. Bone marrow transplantation, calcitriol, interferon-γ

CHAPTER 23 Statistics

QUESTIONS

Q-1.

A. Define incidence and prevalence.
B. What is the basic difference between 'case control' and 'cohort' study?
C. What is the difference between rate and ratio?
D. Define 'odds.'
E. What is randomized control trial (RCT)?
F. Define 'P' value.
G. Define 1st quartile and 3rd quartile

Q-2.

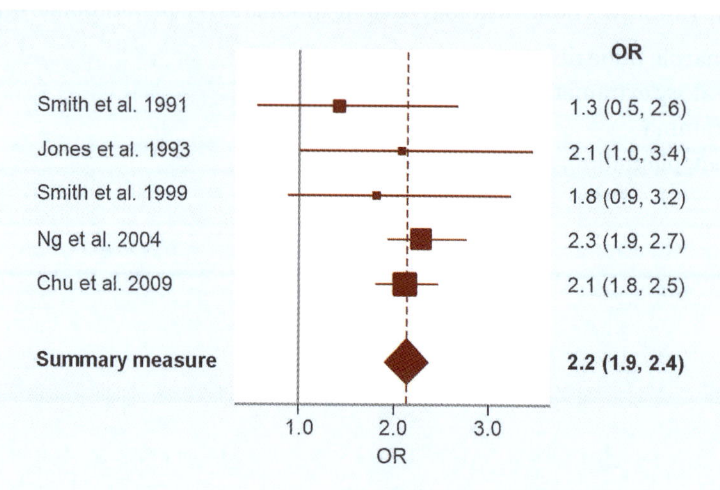

A. What is the name of this plot?
B. What is the another name of this plot?
C. What is the structure of this plot?
D. What is the arrowed figure known as?
E. Where is this plot used in medical research?

Q-3.

A. Define mean, median and mode.
B. When to use each one?

Q-4. The height of 10 children of the same age group is given in centimeters are 101, 98, 98, 99, 102, 101, 100, 98, 101, and 101. Calculate:

A. Mean
B. Median
C. Mode

Q-5.

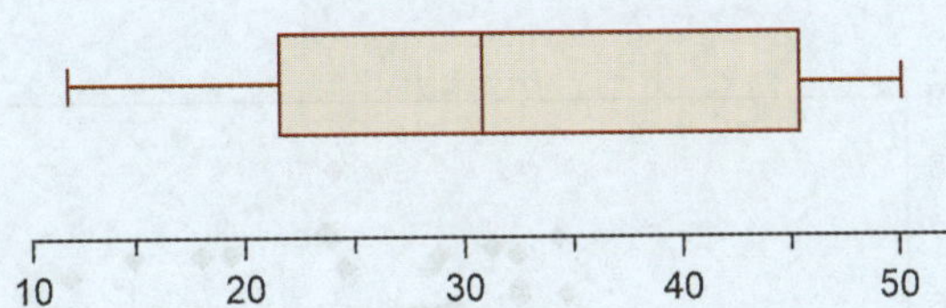

A. What is this plot known as?
B. Describe the plot.
C. What is this plot used for?

Q-6. What is a confidence interval in statistics?

Q-7. What does having a 95% confidence interval mean?

Q-8. Define.

A. Specificity
B. Sensitivity
C. Positive predictive value
D. Negative predictive value

Q-9. State true/false regarding following statements:

A. A case control study is an observational study.
B. A case control study is an analytic study.
C. A case control study cannot be retrospective.
D. A case control study is done to generate hypothesis.
E. A case control study requires a large number of subjects and large number of controls.

Q-10.

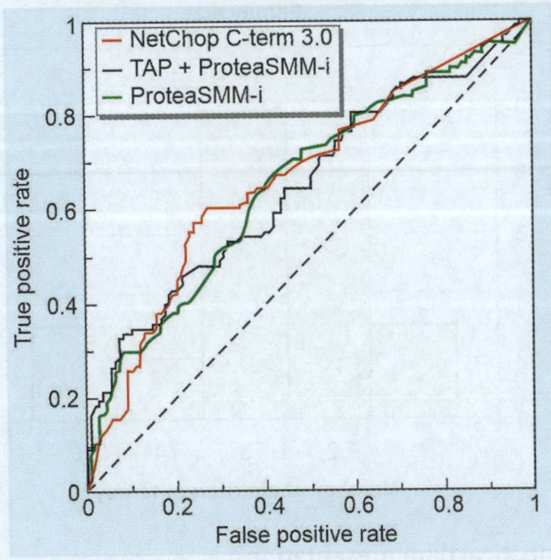

A. What is the name of this curve?
B. What are its uses?
C. What does it represent?

Q-11.

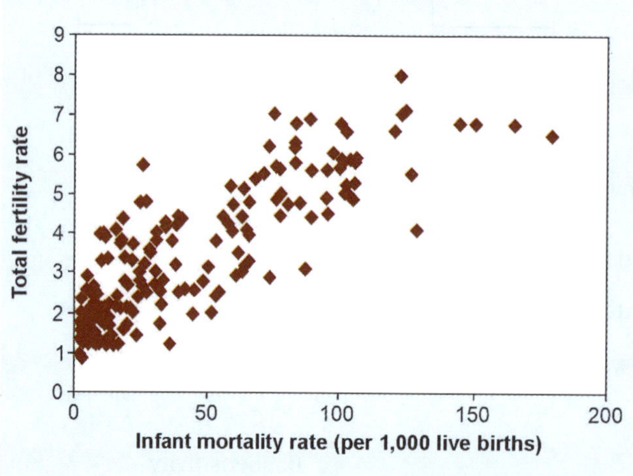

A. What is the name of curve?

B. What are its uses?

Q-12. Write the following journal article in Vancouver style.

Article: Myelin oligodendrocyte glycoprotein antibody associated disorder (MOGA)
Presenting as optic neuritis: A case series.
Author: Shrivastava A, Tandon M, Yadav RK, et al.
Journal: Indian Pediatrics, Year 2024, Volume 61, Page 791–793.

Q-13.

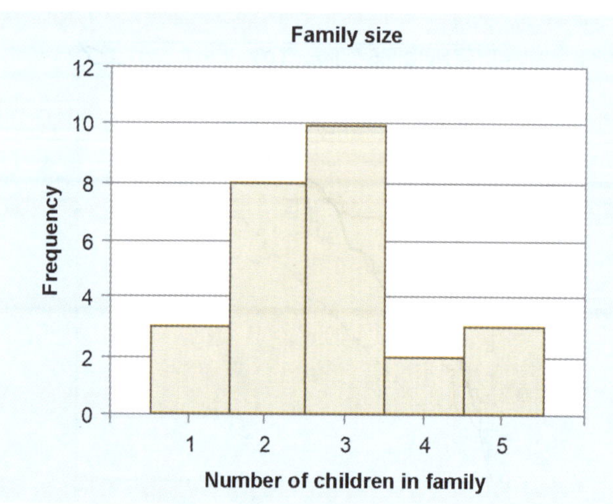

A. What is the name of this statistical data presentation?
B. What are its different visual representation?
C. How does it help in data organization?
D. Give two illustrations for its application in pediatrics.

Q-14.

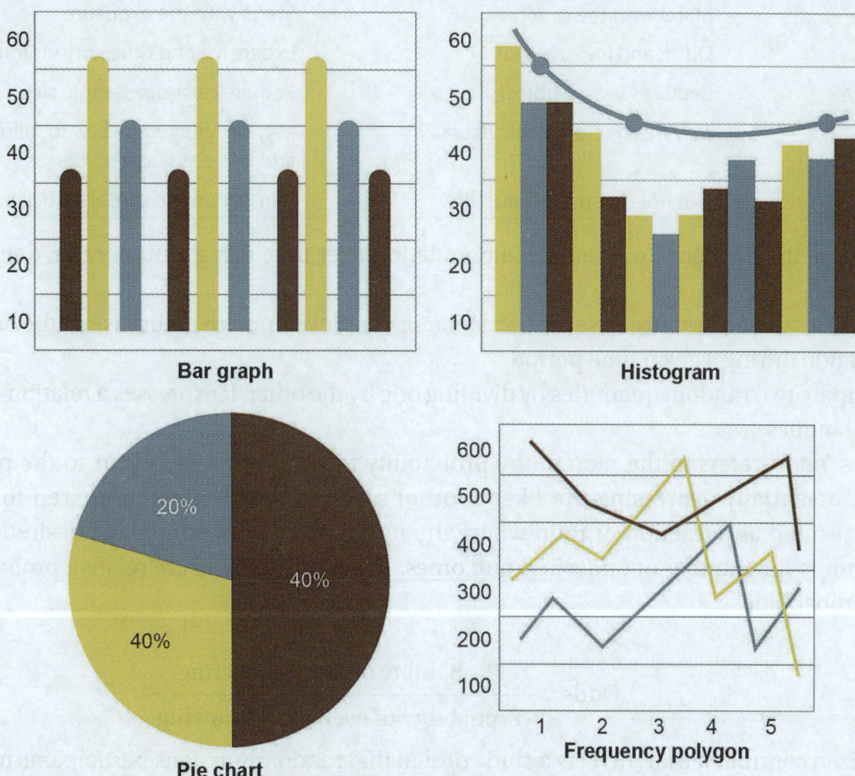

A. What is the name of this statistical data presentation?
B. What are its different visual representations?
C. How does it help in data organization?
D. Give two illustrations for its application in pediatrics.

Q-15. Prepare the frequency distribution table for birth weight among newborns in a hospital.

ANSWERS

A-1. A. *Definition of incidence:* Incidence rate is defined as the number of new cases occurring in a defined population during a specified period of time.

$$\text{Incidence} = \frac{\text{Number of new cases of specific disease during a given time period}}{\text{Population at risk during that period}} \times 1000$$

For example, if there has been 500 new cases of an illness in a population of 30,000 in a year, the incidence would be:

$$500/30000 \times 1000 = 16.7 \text{ per 1000 per year}$$

Definition of prevalence: The term 'disease prevalence' refers to all current cases, old and new, existing at a given point of time, or over a period of time in a given population.

B. Cases control studies and cohort studies both are observational studies. Case-control studies are retrospective, while cohort studies are prospective. The difference between these two studies are as follows:

	Case control study	*Cohort study*
Direction	Starts with the outcome	Starts with the exposure
Time	Quick and inexpensive	Expensive and time consuming
Sample size	Requires fewer subjects	Requires a larger sample size
Bias	May be affected by recall bias	May be affected by loss to follow-up and mis-classification biases
Causality	Can not determine causality	Can determine causal association

C. Rates measure the incidence of events in a population over time using a numerator, denominator and time specification.
A rate measures the occurrence of some particular event (development of disease or the occurrence of death) in a population during a given time period.
Ratios compare two random quantities by dividing one by the other. It expresses a relation in size between two random quantities.

D. In statistics 'odds' refers to the ratio of the probability that an event will occur to the probability that will not occur, essentially expressing the likelihood of an event happening compared to it not happening, often represented as a fraction or ratio where the numerator is the number of desired outcomes and the denominator is the number of undesired outcomes. It is a way to measure relative probabilities rather than absolute probabilities.
Formula:

$$\text{Odds} = \frac{\text{Probability of event occurring}}{\text{Probability of event not occurring}}$$

E. A randomized controlled trial (RCT) is a study design that randomly assigns participants to a treatment group or a control group. RCTs are used to measure the effectiveness of a new treatment or intervention.

F. P-value measures the probability of obtaining the observed results, assuming that the null hypothesis is true. The lower P-value, the greater that statistical significance of the observed difference. P-value of 0.05 or lower is generally considered statistically significant.

G. The observations are arranged in ascending or descending order:
- *Median:* 50% observations are below and 50% are above value.
- *1st Quartile:* 25% observations are below and 75% are above the value.
- *3rd Quartile:* 75% observations are below and 25% are above the value.

A-2. A. Forest plot
B. Blobbogram
C. In this plot, the results of studies used in the review are shown as squares centered on the point estimate of the result of each study. A horizontal line runs through the square to show its confidence interval—usually, a 95% confidence interval.
D. Diamond
E. Meta-analysis

A-3. A. The mean means average. The median is the middle number of a data set from smallest to largest. The mode is the number that occurs the most often.

Mean:
- The average of a set numbers.
- Found by adding the numbers in the set and dividing by the number of values in the set.
- The mean is not usually a value from the original list.

Median:

- The middle value in a set of numbers when ordered from smallest to greatest.
- If there are two middle numbers, the median is the average of those two numbers.
- The letter 'M' is often used to represent the median.

Mode:

- The number that occurs most often in a set of numbers.
- If all the numbers are represented equally, there is no mode.

B.

- The median is often used when data is skewed such as income data.
- The mean is sometimes used when the median and mean are not very different, or when it makes it easier to compare to previous research.

A-4. A. $\text{Mean} = \dfrac{\text{Sum of all}}{\text{Total numbers}} = \dfrac{1000}{10} = 10$

B. $\text{Median} = \text{Middle value in ascending or descending order} = \dfrac{100 + 101}{2} = 100.5$

C. Mode: The value which is the most frequent = 101.

A-5. A. Box and Whisker plot

B.

- The central box represents the values from lower to upper quartile (25–75 percentile).
- The middle line represents the median.
- The horizontal line extends from minimum to maximum value, excluding outside and far out values which are displayed as separate points.

C. Box plots are used to show distribution of numeric data values, especially when you want to compare them between multiple groups.

They display a statistical summary of a variables: median, quartiles, range and extreme values.

A-6. A confidence interval is the mean of your estimate plus and minus the variation in that estimate. This is the range of values you expect. Your estimate to fall between if you redo your test, with a certain level of confidence.

A-7. Confidence in statistics is a way to describe probability. If you construct a confidence interval with a 95% confidence level, you are confident that 95 out of 100 times the estimate will fall between the upper and lower values specified by the confidence interval.

A-8. A. *Specificity:* It is defined as test's ability to correctly reject healthy patients without a condition.

$$\text{Specificity} = \frac{\text{Number of true negatives}}{\text{Number of true negatives + number of false positives}}$$

$$= \frac{\text{Number of true negatives}}{\text{Total number of well individual in population}}$$

= Probability of a negative test given that the patient is well.

- A positive result in a test with high specificity can be useful for 'ruling in' disease, since the test rarely gives positive results in healthy individuals. However, a negative result from a test with high specificity is not necessarily useful for 'ruling out' disease.

B. *Sensitivity:* Sensitivity also called as detection rate in a clinical setting refers to the test ability to correctly detect ill patients out of those who do have the condition.

$$\text{Sensitivity} = \frac{\text{Number of true positives}}{\text{Number of true positives + number of false negatives}}$$

$$= \frac{\text{Number of true positives}}{\text{Total number of sick individual in population}}$$

= Probability of a positive test given that patient has the disease

- A negative result in a test with high sensitivity can be useful for 'ruling out' the disease, since it rarely misdiagnoses those who have the disease.
- A test with 100% sensitivity will recognize all patients with the disease by testing positive. In this case, negative test result would definitively rule out the presence of the disease in the individual. However, a positive result in a test with high sensitivity is not necessarily useful for 'ruling in' disease.

C. Positive Predictive value (PPV) refers to the probability that a patient who tests positive on a diagnostic test actually has the disease being tested for.

A high PPV means that a positive test result is more likely to accurately indicate the presence of the disease.

$$\text{PPV} = \frac{\text{True positives}}{\text{True positives + false positives}}$$

D. Negative predictive value (NPV) refers to the probability that a patient who tests negative for a disease actually does not have the disease.

A high NPV means that a negative test result is very likely to accurately indicate the absence of disease.

$$\text{NPV} = \frac{\text{True negatives}}{\text{True negatives + false negatives}}$$

A-9. A. True. It does not involve any human interventions, only natural occurrence is observed.
B. True
C. False. It is always retrospective.
D. False. It tests already set-up hypothesis.
E. False.

A-10. A. Receiver operating characteristic (ROC) curve
B. ROC curve analysis provides tools to select possibly optimal models and to discard suboptimal ones.
C. It is a graphical representation that plots the sensitivity (true-positive rate) of a diagnostic test against its I – Specificity (false-positive rate) at different cut-off points, allowing for evaluation and comparison of how well a test can be distinguish between diseases and non-diseases individuals across various thresholds; essentially showing the trade of between correctly identifying positive cases and incorrectly identifying negative cases.
A curve closer to the top left corner of the graph indicates better diagnostic accuracy, as it represents high sensitivity with low false positive rate.

A-11. A. Scatter plot chart
B. It is a visual representation that displays the relationship between two numerical variables measured on patients, allowing researchers to see if there is correlation or association between them, e.g., there is any association between total fertility rate and infant mortality rate?

A-12. Shrivastava A, Tandon M, Yadav RK et al. Myelin oligodendrocyte glycoprotein antibody associated disorders (MOGAD) presenting as optic neuritis: A case series. Indian Pediatr. 2024;61:791-3.

Vancouver style: Author's surname initials. Title of Article, Title of journal (Abbreviated). Year of publication, Month and Date, Volume number: Page numbers.

A-13. A. Histogram

B. Histogram is a graphical representation used to visualize the distribution of a continuous variables, like a number of children in family and its frequency to give information on family size.

C. Histogram provides a clear picture how a particular measurement is spread across a population of children, revealing whether the data is normally distributed, skewed to one side or has multiple peaks.

A-14. A. Frequency distribution

B. Frequency distribution is a tool in statistics which can have visual representations in forms of Tables, Histogram, Bar graph, Frequency Polygon and Pie chart.

C. It helps organize large datasets into manageable categories, allowing researchers to easily visualize the distribution of characteristics within a pediatric cohort.

D. Examples of use of frequency distribution in pediatrics:

- Growth monitoring
- Developmental assessment
- Disease prevalence

A-15.
- Recording birth weight of all newborns delivered in a specific period in the hospital. It is called data collection.
- Frequency distribution table can be arranged as follows:

Birth weight (in grams)	***Frequency***
<2500	15
2500–3000	30
3000–3500	45
>3500	20

CHAPTER 24

Drugs and Instruments

QUESTIONS

Q-1.

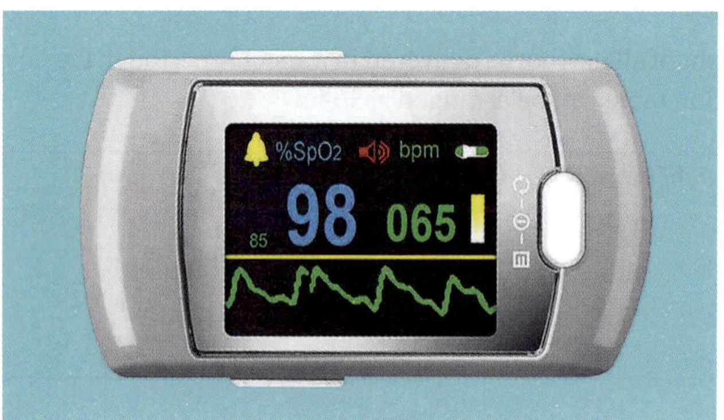

A. Identify the instrument.
B. What does it detect?
C. What level of SpO_2 in room air indicates adequate oxygenation?
D. At what SpO_2 level, it indicates oxygen therapy?
E. At what level of SpO_2, does cyanosis develop clinically?
F. What are limitations of this instrument?

Q-2.

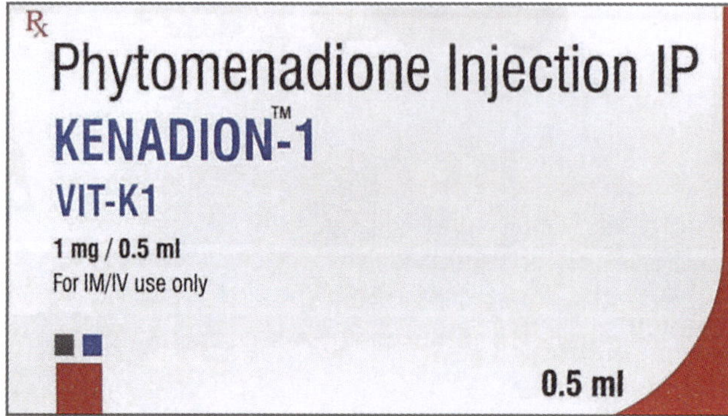

A. Name vitamin K dependent coagulation factors.
B. What are the tests to diagnose deficiency of vitamin K?
C. Define early, classical and late HDN (Hemorrhagic Disease of Newborn).
D. What is the prophylaxis dose of vitamin K in newborns?

Q-3. It is used to evaluate the size of an organ.

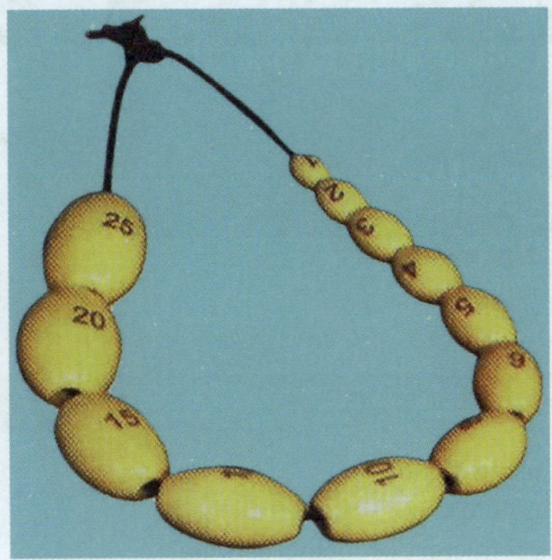

A. Name the instrument.
B. What is the unit of measurement of an organ?
C. What is size of an organ at infantile age, prepubertal age and adult age?

Q-4.

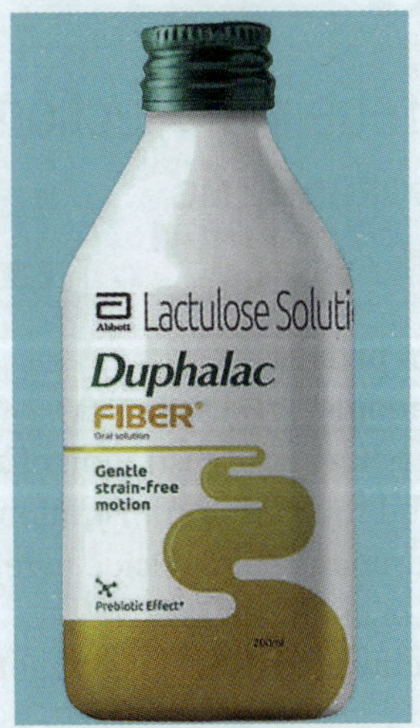

A. What are the indications of using lactulose in children?
B. What is the mechanism of function of lactulose in hepatic failure?
C. What is the dose of lactulose in hepatic encephalopathy?
D. What is dose of lactulose in chronic constipation?

Q-5.

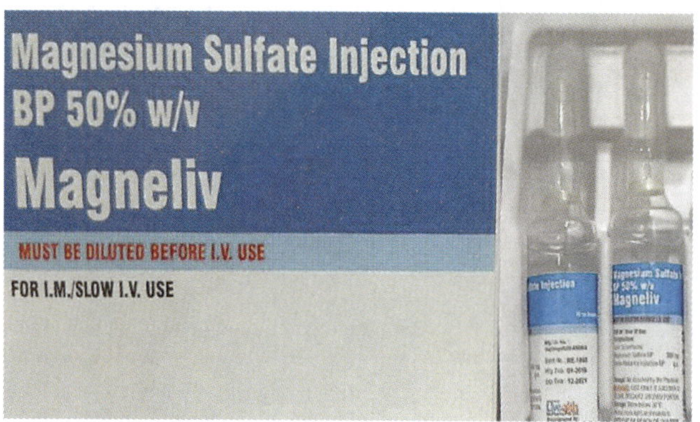

50% Solution
(1 mL = 500 mg)
(4 mEq/mL)

A. What are the indications of using $MgSo_4$?
B. What is the dose of $MgSO_4$ in PEM?
C. What is the dose of $MgSo_4$ in refractory bronchial asthma?
D. What are the manifestations of hypomagnesemia?
E. What are the manifestations of hypermagnesemia?
F. What is the antidote for magnesium sulfate toxicity?

Q-6.

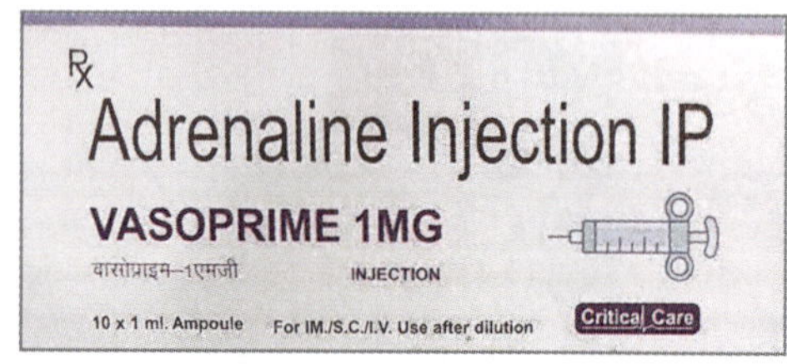

A. What are indications of adrenaline in pediatrics?
B. What is indication of adrenaline in neonatal resuscitation?
C. What precondition must be fulfilled before administration of adrenaline in neonatal resuscitation?
D. What is the concentration, dosage and route of administration of adrenaline in neonatal resuscitation?
E. How will you evaluate after giving adrenaline and decide to repeat the dose in neonatal resuscitation?
F. How will you use adrenaline in case of anaphylaxis?
G. How will you use adrenaline in an acute case of acute laryngotracheobronchitis (croup)?

Q-7.

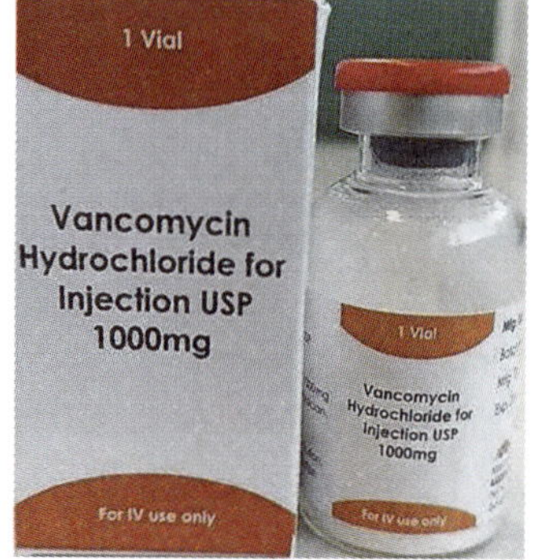

A. What type of drug is it classified in pharmacology?
B. What is the spectrum of activity of this molecule?
C. What are different routes of administration of this drug in specific conditions?
D. What is the dosage?
E. What is the most common side effect of this drug? How can it be prevented?
F. What are other side effects of this drug?

Q-8.

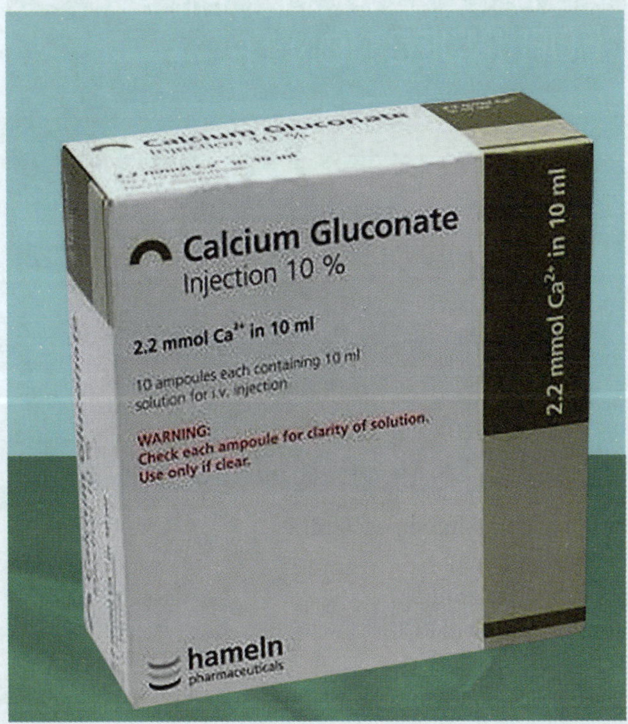

A. What is the concentration of calcium in injection of 10% calcium gluconate?
B. What are the conditions presented as hypocalcemia?
C. How to treat acute symptomatic hypocalcemia?
D. What precautions should be taken while IV calcium therapy?
E. What is the role of IV calcium in a case of severe hyperkalemia?

Q-9.

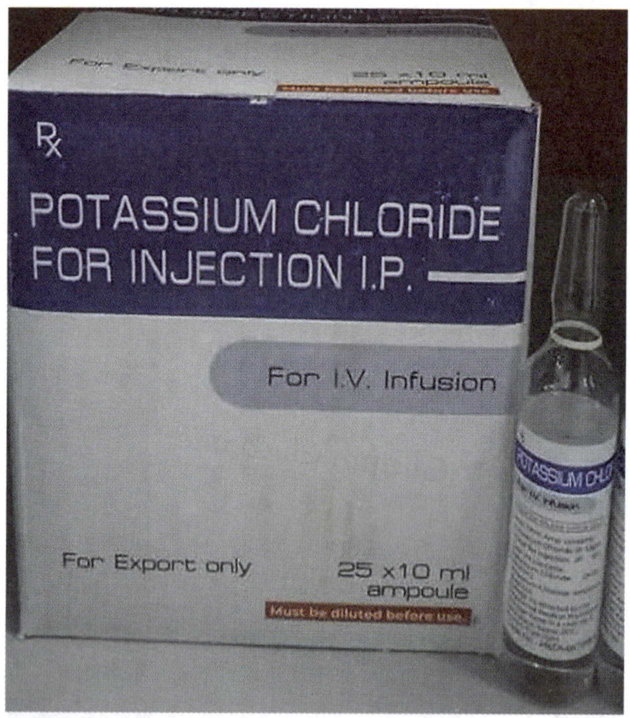

A. What is the concentration of potassium in each mL?
B. What are the causes of hypokalemia?
C. What are ECG changes of hypokalemia?
D. What is the route of administration of KCl?
E. What is the dose of IV KCl?
F. What is the oral preparation for potassium supplementation? What is concentration? What is the oral dose?
G. What precautions are advised for IV and oral potassium therapy?

Q-10.

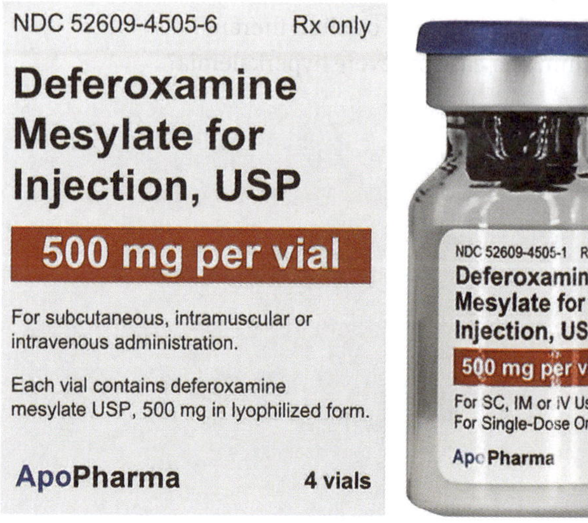

A. What are the indications of this drug in pediatric practice?
B. What are the symptoms of acute iron poisoning?
C. What is the dose of iron causes severe toxicity?
D. What is the dose of deferoxamine in acute severe iron poisoning?
E. What are the indications of deferoxamine in acute iron poisoning?
F. How is it monitored for effective therapy?

Q-11.

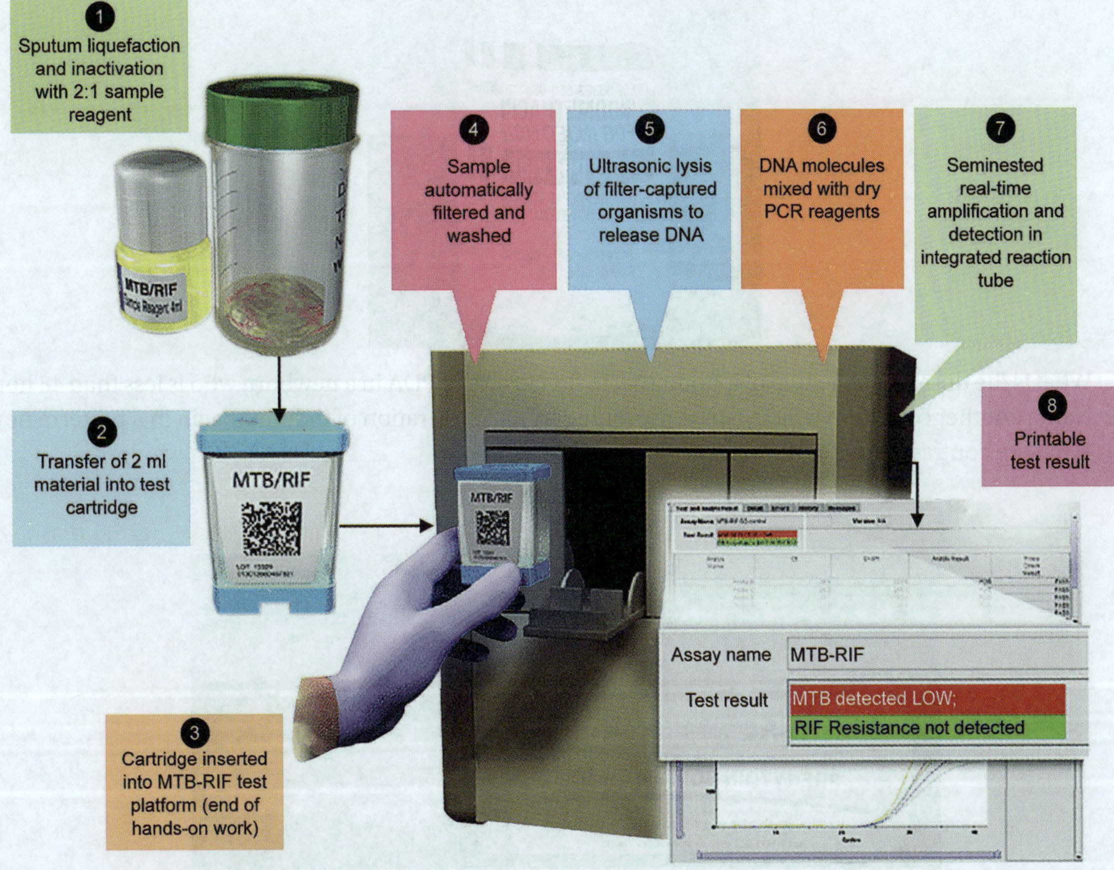

A. For what type of test is the instrument used? For which disease?
B. What is the sensitivity of this test for different specimens used for diagnosis of the condition?
C. What are WHO approved RDTs for this condition?
D. What is the turnaround time for the test by this instrument?

Q-12.

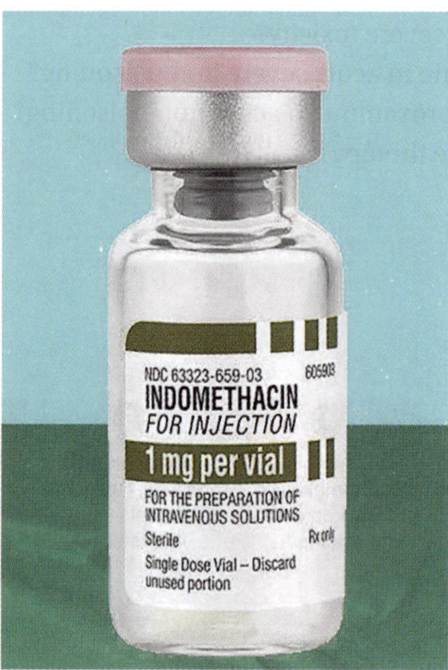

A. What is the dose and schedule of indomethacin for closure of PDA in a newborn who is less than 48 hours old?
B. Name another condition which can be prevented by administration of indomethacin in a preterm newborn.
C. What are contradictions of this drug?

Q-13.

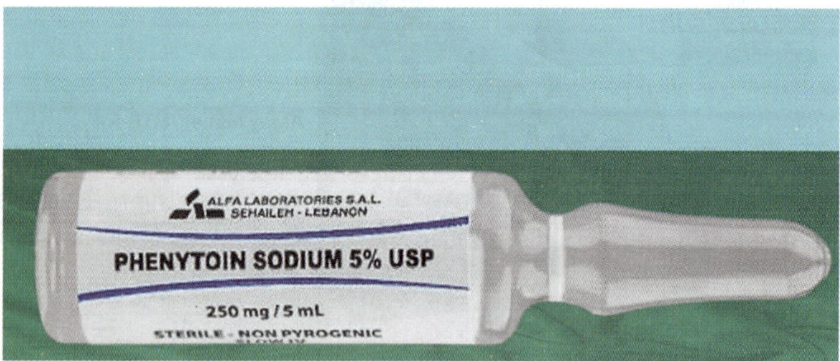

A. What is the loading dose of phenytoin? What is an additional dose?
B. Describe the method of dilution of phenytoin, maximum concentration and rate of administration.
C. What are the adverse effects of phenytoin?
D. How fosphenytoin differs from phenytoin?
E. Why fospherytoin is considered as better alternative to phenytoin?

Q-14.

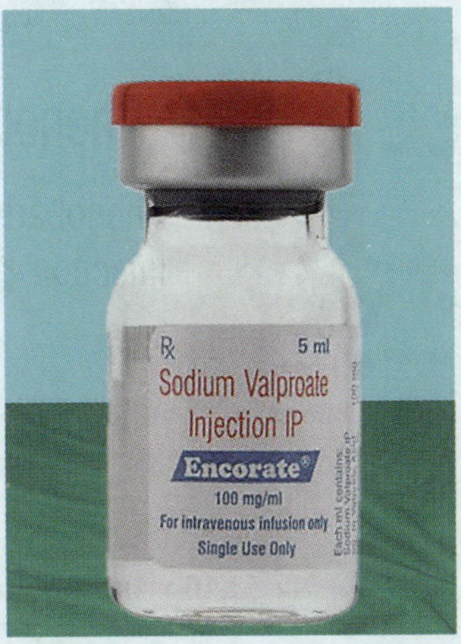

A. What is the dose of sodium valproate by IV route?
B. What are the adverse effects of sodium valproate?
C. What are the indications of sodium valproate in children?

Q-15.

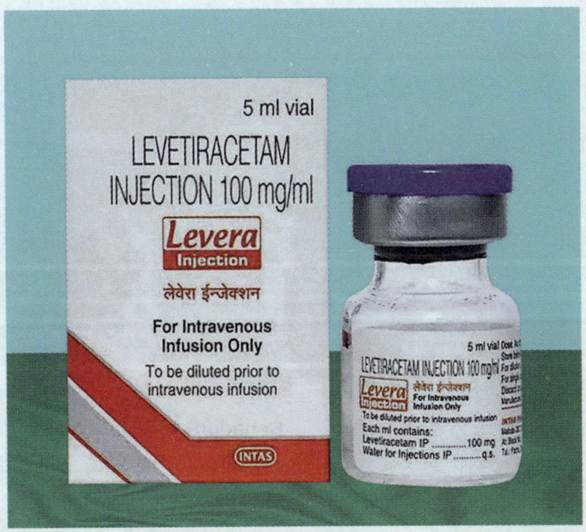

A. What is the intravenous dose of levetiracetam? What is the oral dose?
B. What are the merits of levetiracetam over phenytoin?
C. What are the adverse effects of this drug?

Q-16.

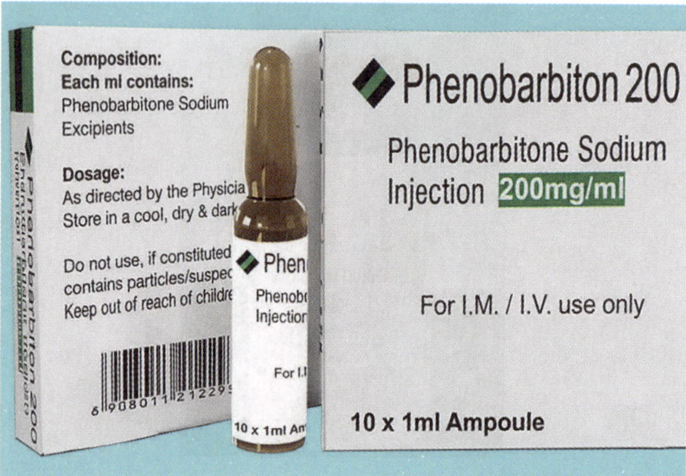

A. What are the indications of this drug?
B. A neonate weighing 2.5 kg presents with generalized seizures. Calculate the loading dose and write in detail of delivering this drug by IV route to control the seizures in this baby.
C. What are contraindications for this drug?

Q-17.

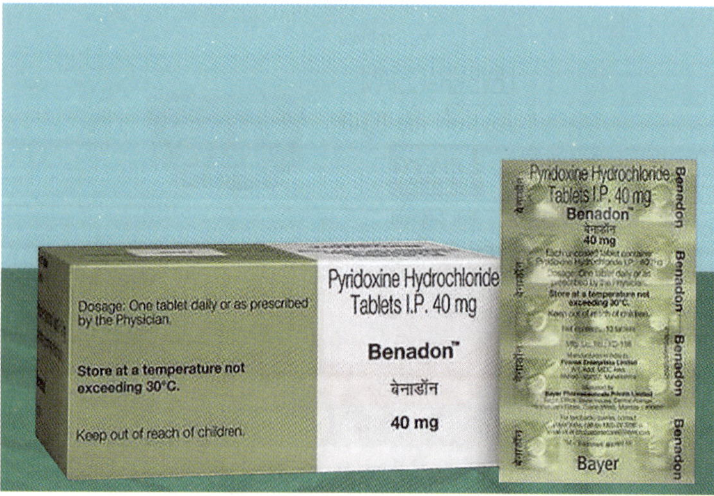

A. Indications of oral pyridoxine.
B. Justification of pyridoxine as supplementation with anti-tuberculous therapy (ATT) in children.
C. What is the dose as supplementation with ATT in children?

Q-18.

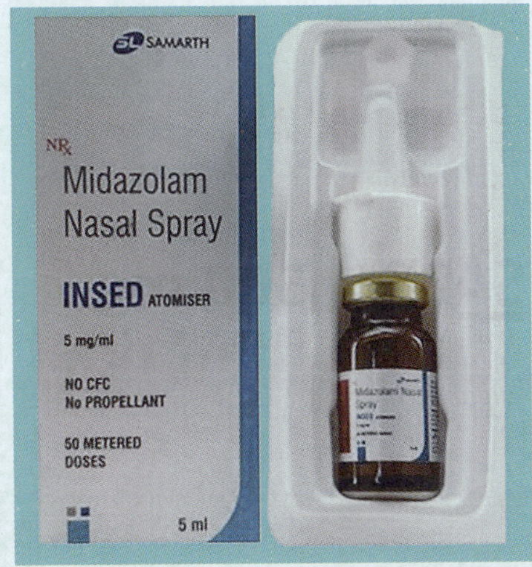

A. Indications of this medicine as nasal spray
B. What is the dose of midazolam as nasal spray?

Q-19.

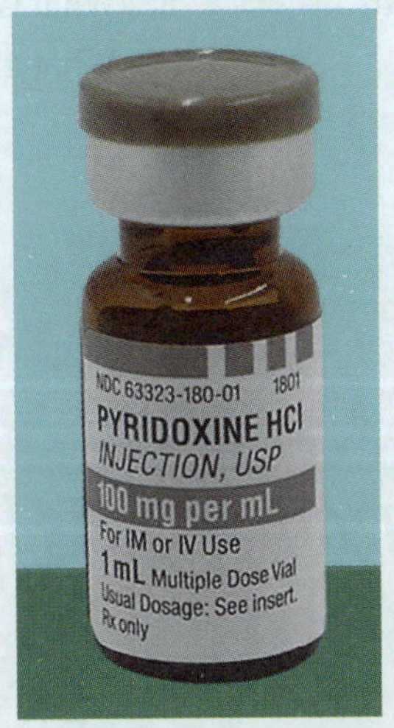

A. What is the indication of parenteral route (IV/IM) of administration of pyridoxine?
B. What is the mechanism of action of pyridoxine in this condition?
C. What is the IV dose of pyridoxine?
D. What are other manifestations or pyridoxine deficiency?
E. What are other indications of pyridoxine?

Q-20.

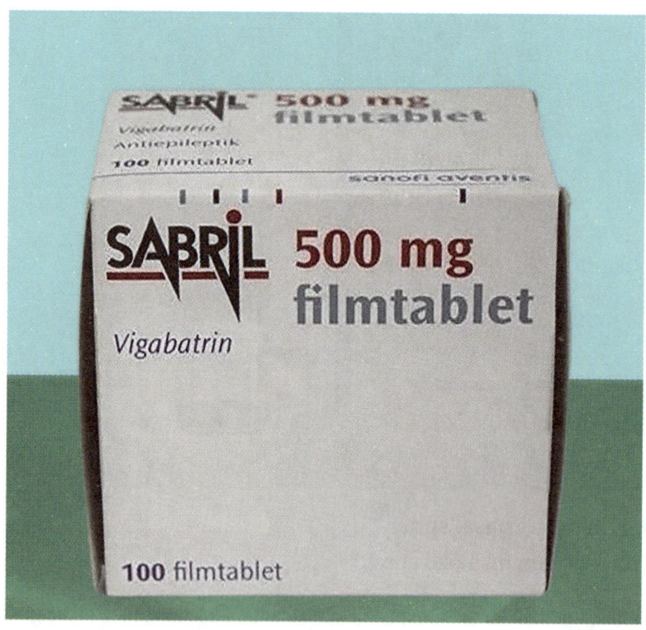

A. What are the indications of vigabatrin?

B. What is the dose of vigabatrin?

C. What is the mechanism of action?

D. What are the adverse effects of it?

Q-21.

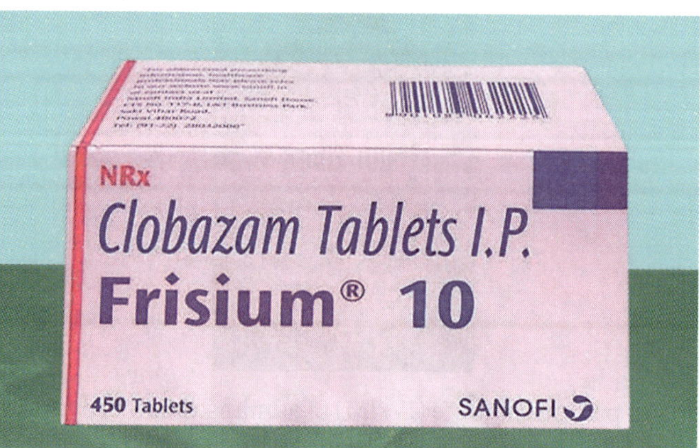

A. What are the indications of clobazam?

B. What is the dose?

C. What is its role as prophylaxis in febrile seizures?

Q-22.

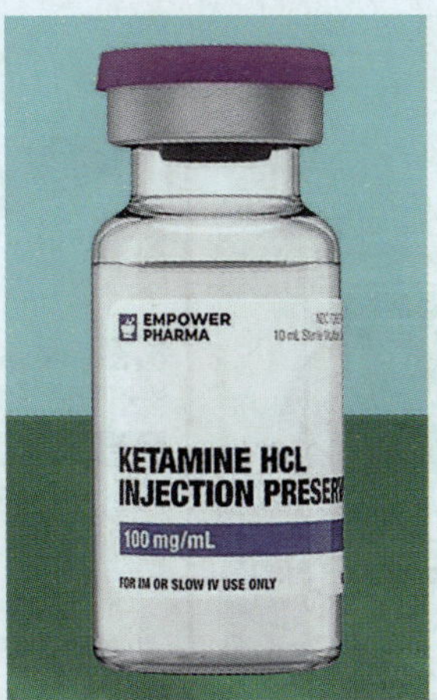

A. What are the indications of ketamine in children?
B. What is the dose of ketamine?
C. What is the duration of anesthesia after IV use?
D. What are the adverse effects of ketamine?
E. What precautions are recommended on use of ketamine?

Q-23.

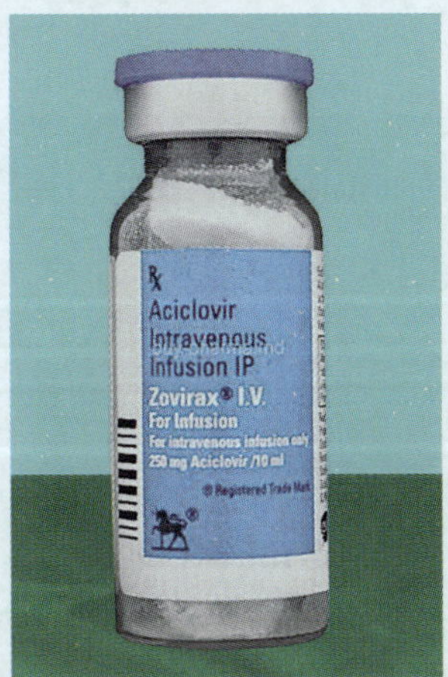

A. What is the pharmacological classification of acyclovir?
B. What is the spectrum of its activity?
C. How can it be prepared for IV route?
D. What is the dose of acyclovir for herpes simplex infection of CNS?
E. What are its adverse effects?

Q-24.

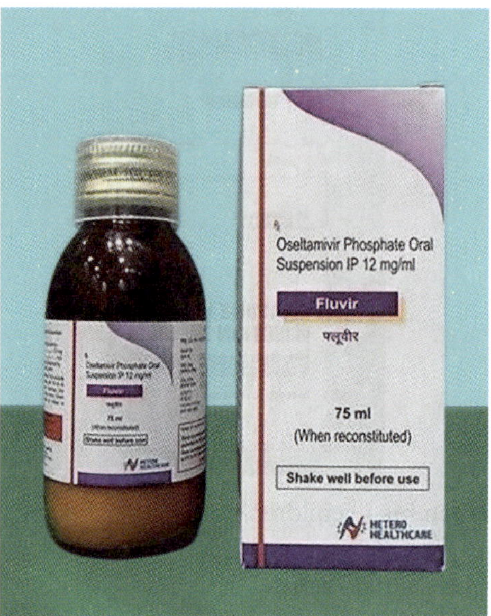

A. What type of drug is it? What is its classification?
B. What are indications of oseltamivir in children?
C. What is dosage of this drug in children?

Q-25.

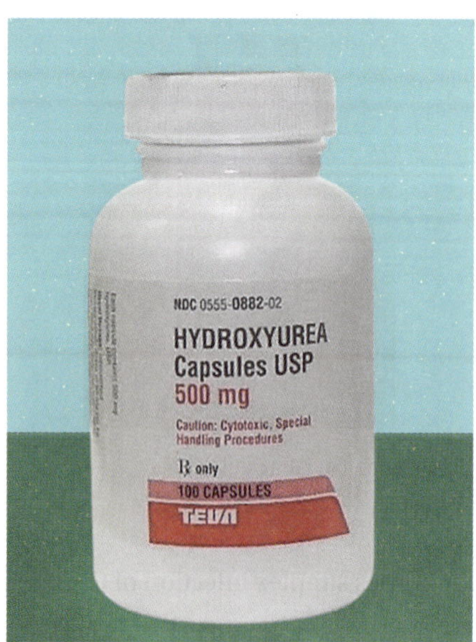

A. How does it help with hemolytic anemia?
B. What are the indications in sickle cell disease?
C. What are the indications in thalassemia?
D. What is dose of this molecule?
E. How should it be monitored for toxicity?

Q-26.

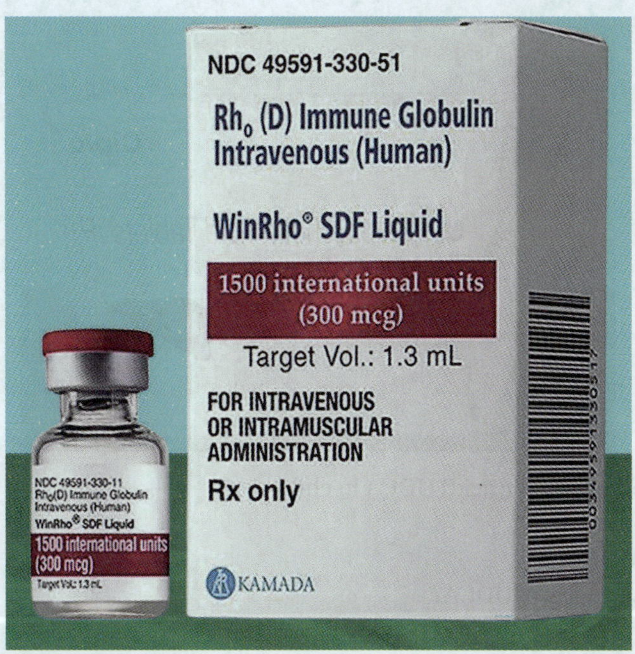

A. What are the indications of IV anti-D?
B. What is the mechanism of its action in said condition?
C. What are the prerequisites for this preparation before using in said condition?
D. What is the dose?
E. What are the adverse effects?
F. What are the merits of IV anti-D above IVIG in ITP?

Q-27.

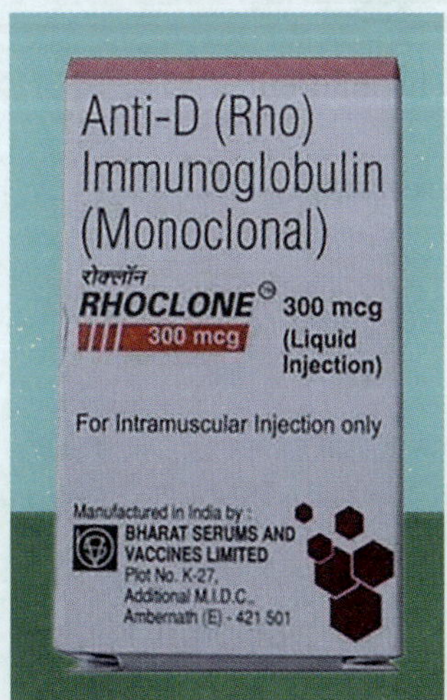

A. Indications of Intramuscular (IM) Anti-D preparation
B. Dosage and schedule of IM Anti-D.
C. How is the dose of this medicine calculated?

Q-28.

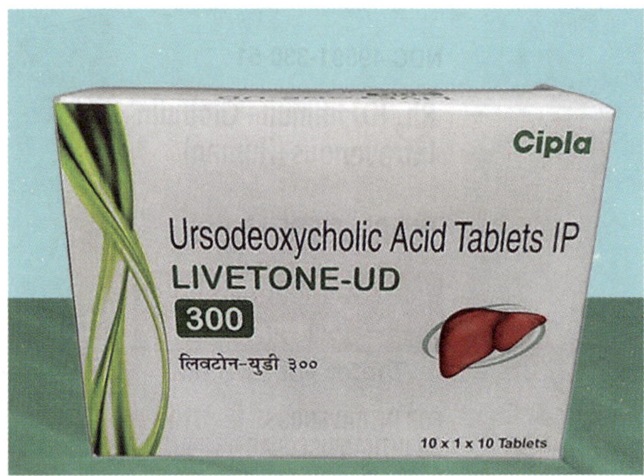

A. Indications of (Ursodeoxycholic acid) UDCA in children.
B. Mechanism of action of UDCA.
C. What is the dose of UDCA?
D. What are the adverse effects of UDCA?

Q-29.

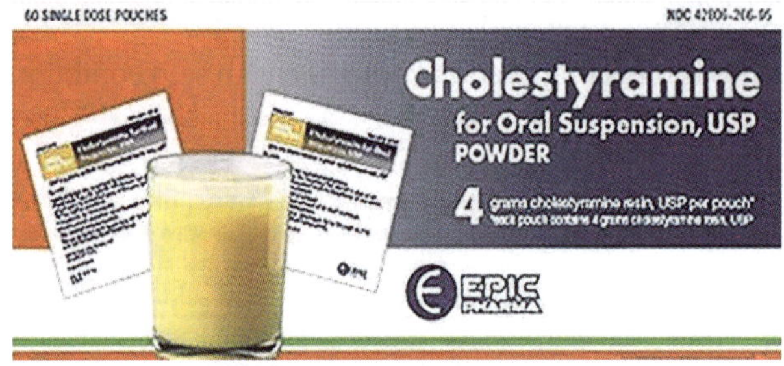

A. Indications of cholestyramine resin in children.
B. What is its mechanism of action?
C. What is the dose of cholestyramine resin?
D. How should it be taken?
E. What are its adverse effects?

Q-30.

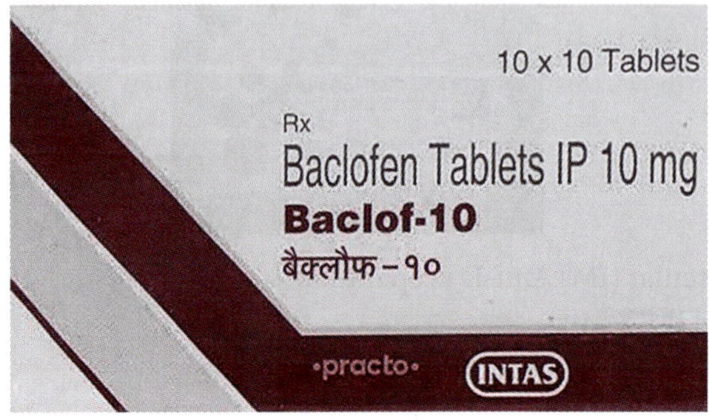

A. What are the indications of baclofen?
B. What is the dose of baclofen?
C. What are the adverse effects?

Q-31.

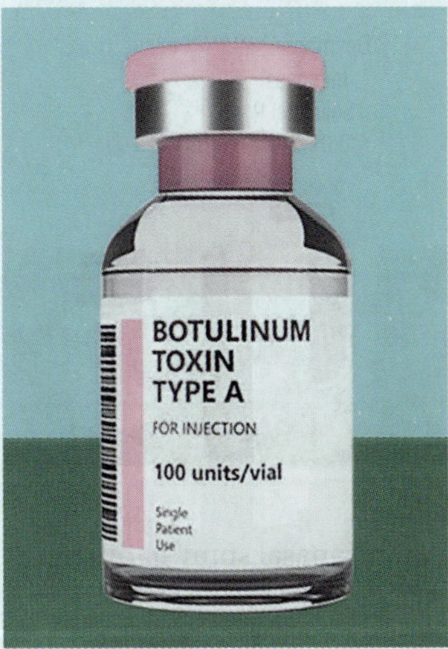

A. What are the indications of botulinum toxin?
B. What is its mechanism of action?
C. What is the dose?

Q-32.

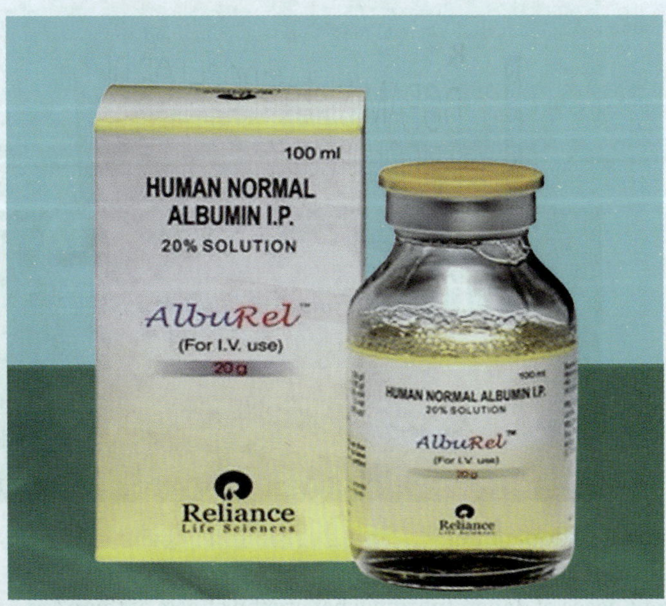

A. What are the indications of albumin therapy in pediatrics?
B. What is the mechanism of its action?
C. What is the dose of albumin?
D. What are the adverse effects?

Q-33.

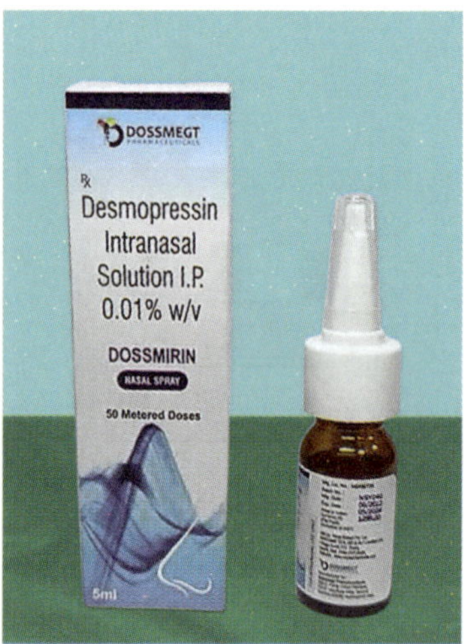

A. Indications of desmopressin in children.
B. What is the dose of desmopressin as intranasal spray in different conditions?
C. What are its known adverse effects?

Q-34. Calculate the dose of dopamine for 10 μg/kg/minute in a patient weighing 20 kg.

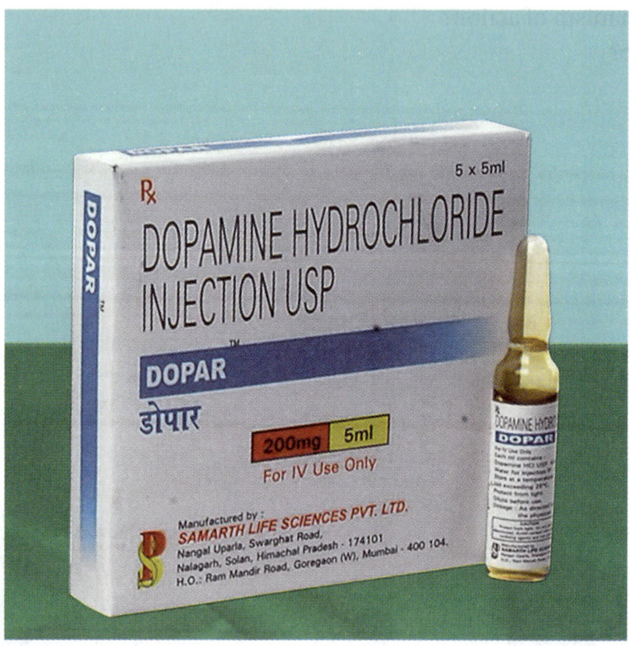

A. What are the indications of dopamine?
B. What is the mechanism of actions?
C. What are the different doses of dopamine and what are the effects of them?
D. What is the formula for calculation of dose of dopamine?
E. What are the adverse effects of dopamine?
F. What are its contraindications?

Q-35.

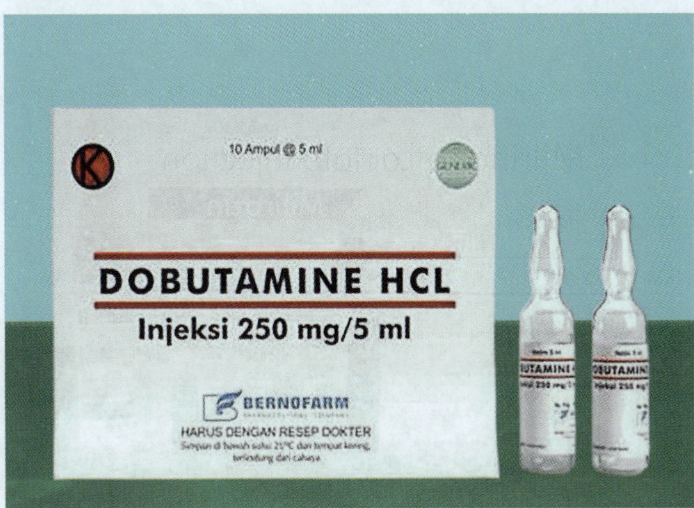

A. What are the indications of dobutamine in pediatrics?
B. What is its mechanism of action?
C. What is the dose of dobutamine?
D. What are its adverse effects?

Q-36.

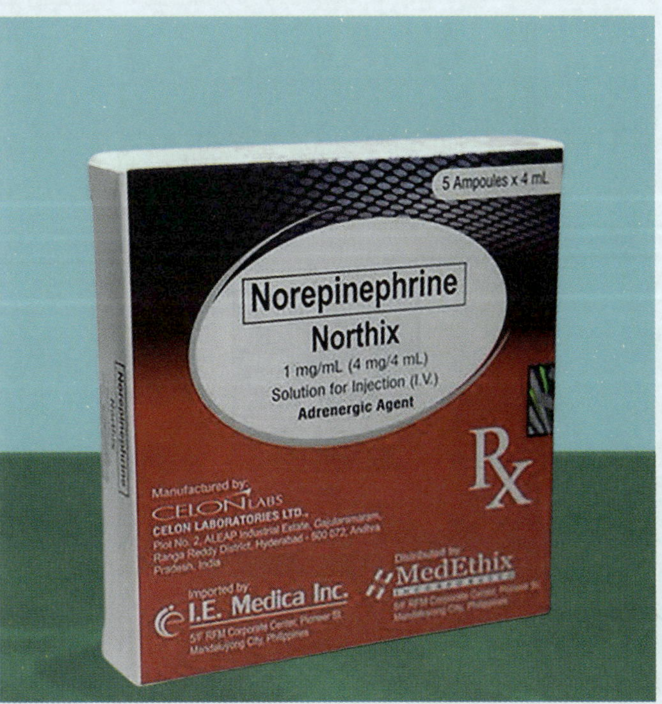

A. What are the indications of norepinephrine?
B. What are mechanisms of action on various organs?
C. What is the dose in shock?
D. What are the adverse effects?

Q-37.

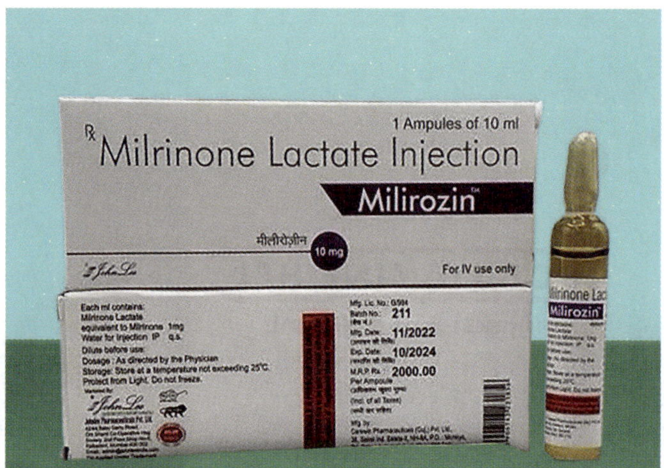

A. Indications of milrinone in pediatrics.
B. What is the mechanism of its action?
C. What is the dose of milrinone?
D. What are its adverse effects?
E. What are the contraindications?

Q-38.

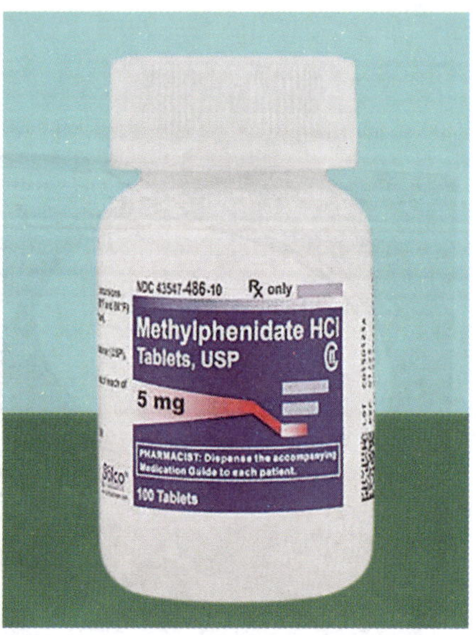

A. What are the indications of methylphenidate?
B. What is the dose?
C. What are the adverse effects?

Q-39.

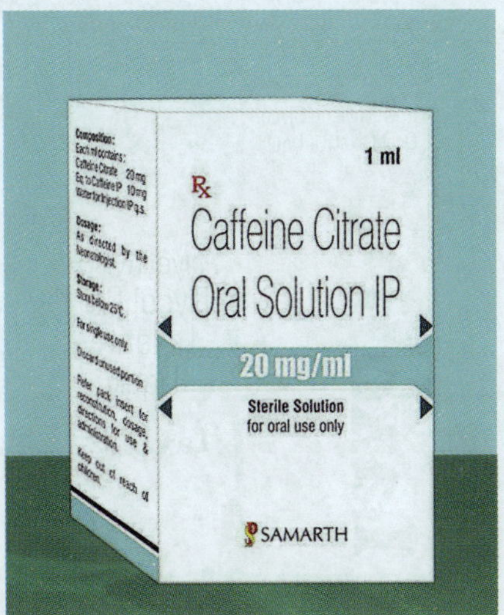

A. What is the indication of caffeine citrate?
B. What is its mechanism of action?
C. What is the dose of caffeine?
D. What are the benefits of caffeine in preterm babies?
E. Any precautions for caffeine in preterms?

Q-40.

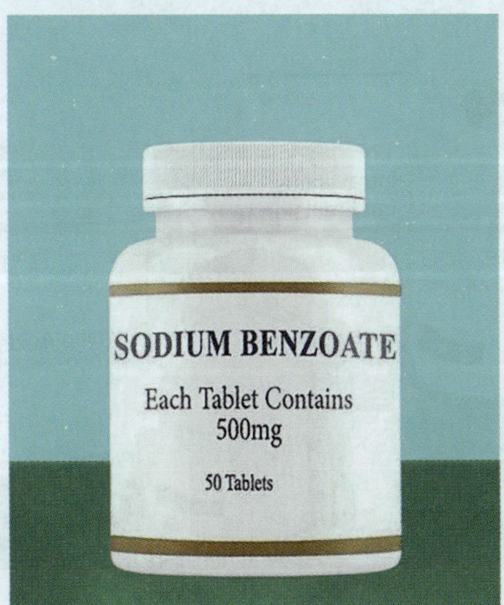

A. Indications of sodium benzoate
B. Dose of sodium benzoate
C. What are its adverse effects?

Q-41.

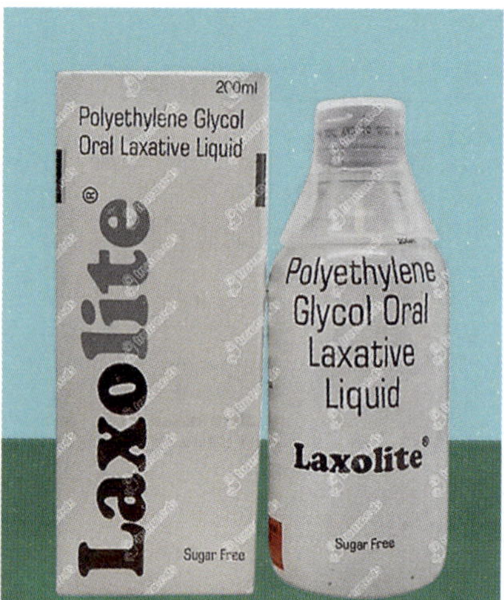

A. What is the indication of polyethylene glycol (PEG) in children?
B. What is the dose of PEG for dis-impaction in a case of constipation?
C. What is the dose of PEG for maintenance therapy in children?
D. What are the adverse effects?

Q-42.

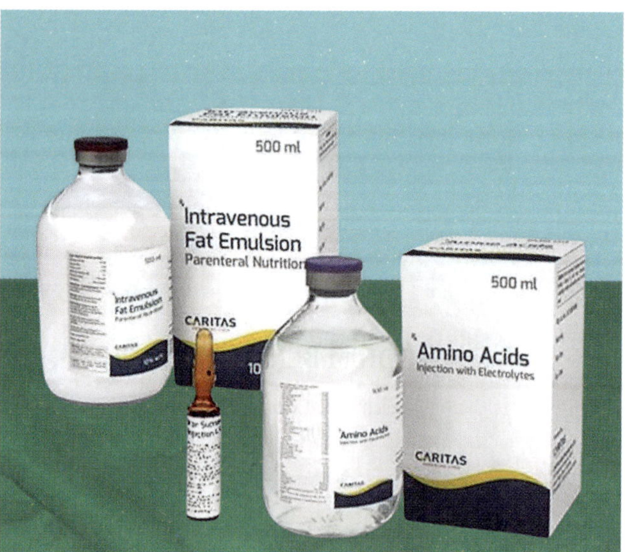

A. Indication for use of this compound
B. What is the dose?
C. What are its indications?
D. What are the side effects of this compound?

Q-43.

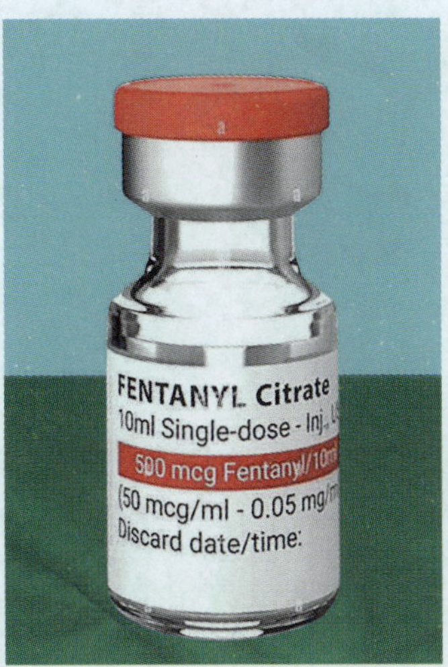

A. What are the indications of fentanyl?
B. What is the mechanism of its action?
C. What is the dose of fentanyl?
D. What are the adverse effects of fentanyl?
E. Which drug can be used to treat the severe respiratory adverse effect?
F. What are other routes of administration of fentanyl?

Q-44.

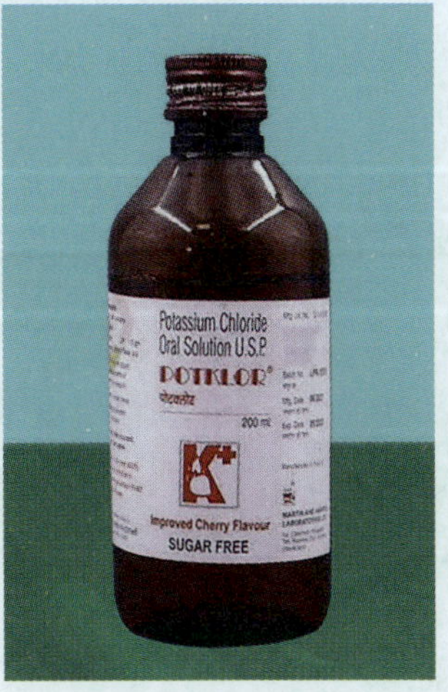

A. What are the causes of hypokalemia in children?
B. What is the concentration of potassium in weight and milliequivalent form in this oral solution?
C. What is the oral dose of potklor?
D. How should it be given orally?

Q-45.

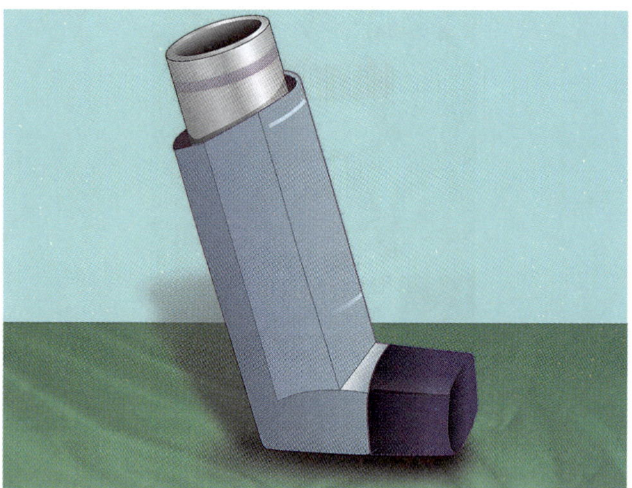

A. Identify the device.
B. What is the indication of its use?
C. What is the mechanism of functioning of this device?
D. How can it be used at different age groups of children?
E. What are the advantages and disadvantages of this device?
F. Which drugs are available in this device?

Q-46.

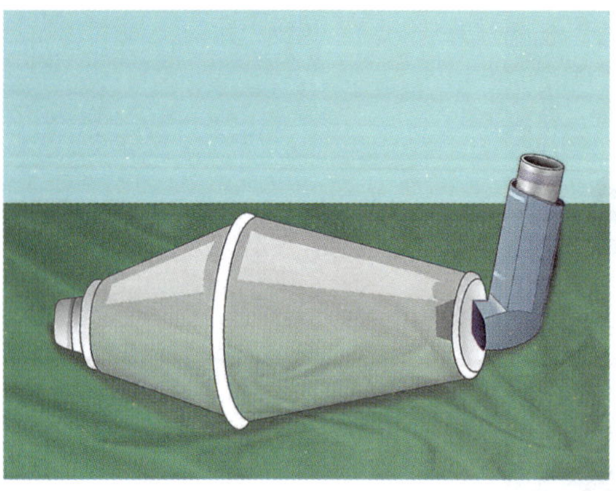

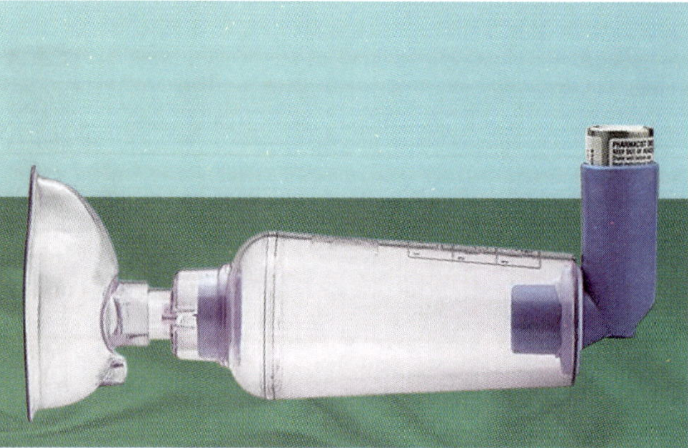

A. Identify the devices.
B. What are the indications of their use?
C. At what different age groups, these devices are used?
D. What are the benefits of these devices?

Q-47.

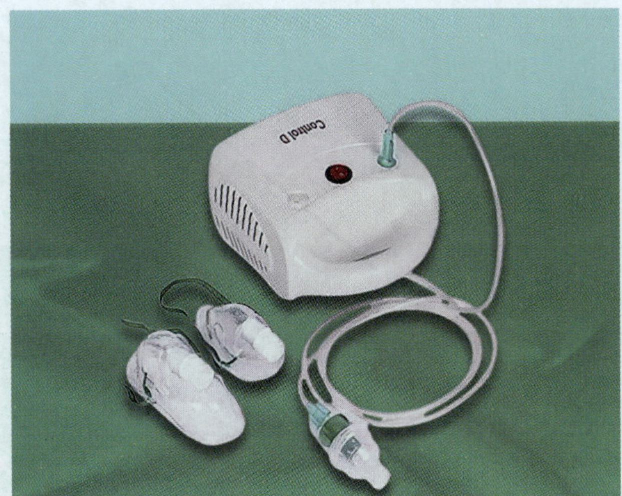

A. Identify the machine.
B. What is the mechanism of its function?
C. Which drugs can be delivered by this device?
D. Advantages of this device.
E. Disadvantages of this device.
F. What different types of the device are available?

Q-48.

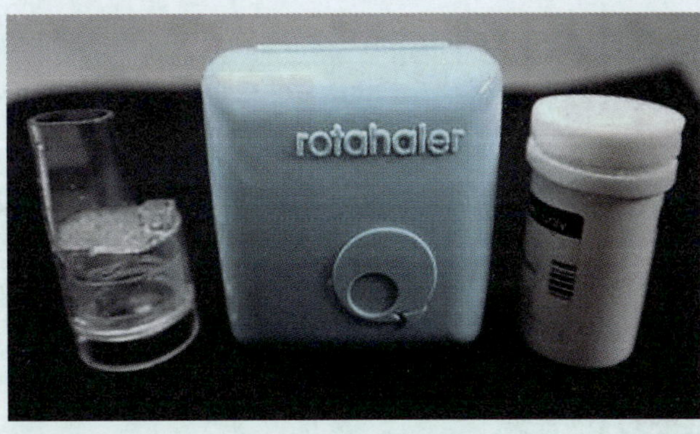

A. Identify the device.
B. Indication for use of this device.
C. Mechanism of its functioning.
D. At what age, can it be used?
E. Advantages and disadvantages of this device.

Q-49.

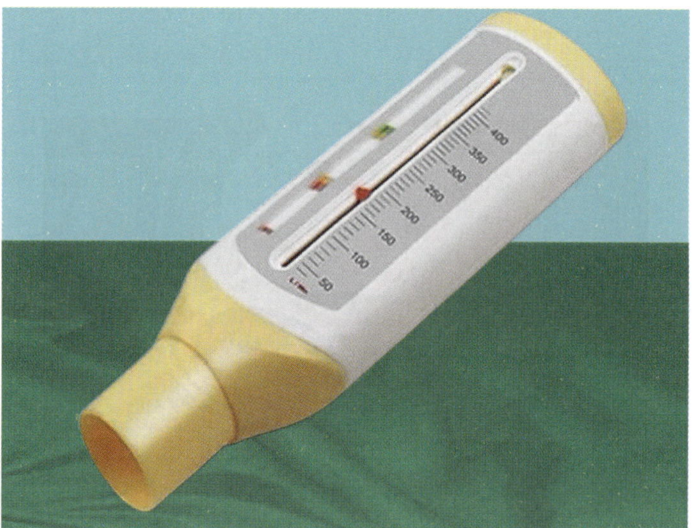

A. Identify the device.
B. What is the technique of using this device?
C. How do you interpret the readings recorded by this device?
D. What is normal peak flow?
E. What are the indications for using this device?

Q-50.

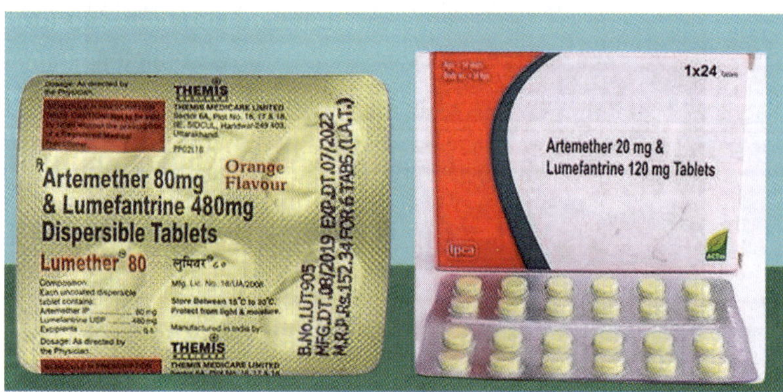

A. What are the indications of using this co-formulated tablet?
B. This co-formulated preparation is called specific therapy. Name it
C. What are the benefits of this co-formulated preparation?
D. What is its dosage?
E. What are other recommended preparations for this condition?

Q-51.

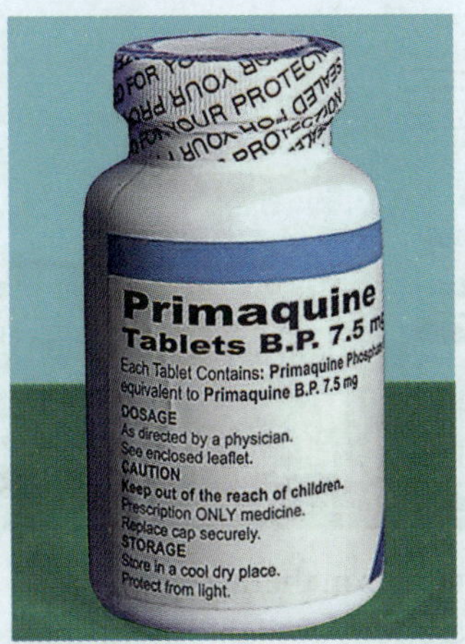

A. What is the role of primaquine in malaria?
B. What is the dosage of primaquine in malaria?
C. For what condition, is it desirable to screen the child before prescribing primaquine?
D. In case of borderline deficiency of said condition, what modification in dosage of primaquine is recommended?

Q-52.

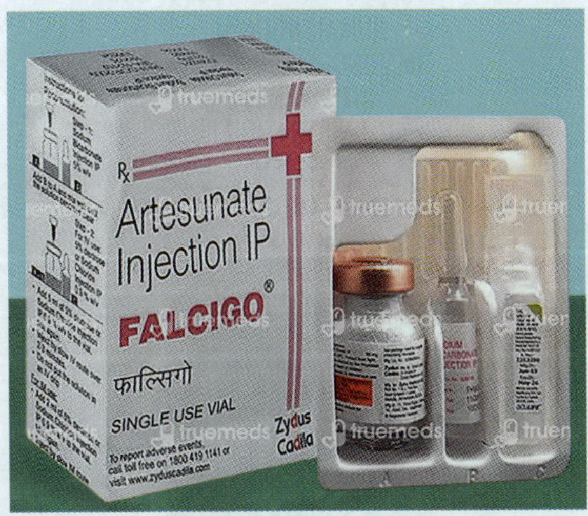

A. Mention the steps of reconstitution of artesunate.
B. Why do we reconstitute artesunate with sodium bicarbonate? What is the concentration of sodium bicarbonate for reconstitution of artesunate?
C. Instead of sodium bicarbonate provided with artesunate, 7.5% sodium bicarbonate can be used?
D. What is the diluent for artesunate injection?
E. What are the routes of administration of artesunate?

Q-53.

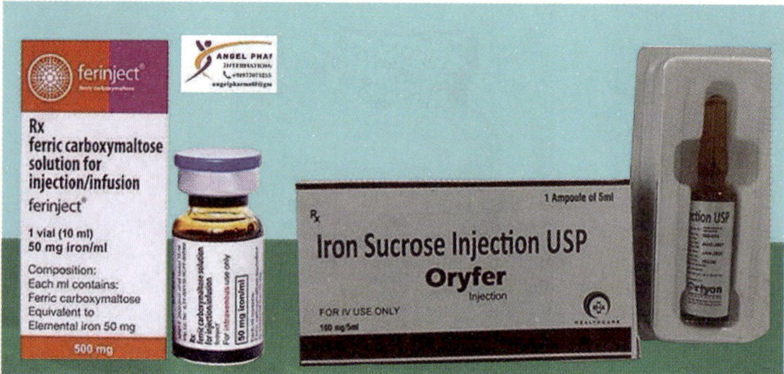

A. What are the indications for parenteral iron therapy?
B. What are safe parenteral iron preparations available in the market?
C. What is formula for dose calculation for parenteral iron therapy?
D. Are there any precautions to be taken during parenteral iron therapy?
E. What is the response to parenteral iron therapy?

Q-54.

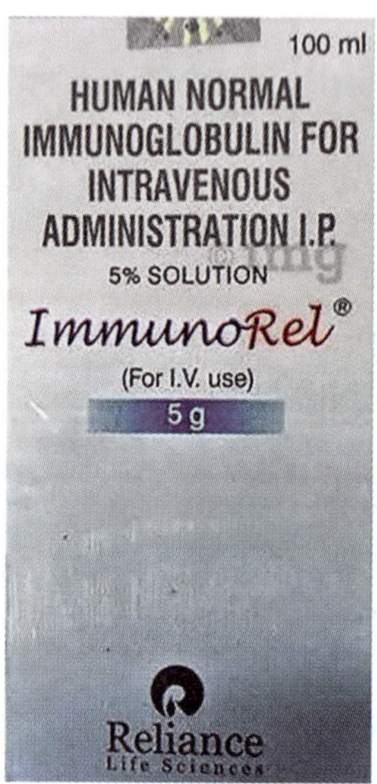

A. What are indications of intravenous immunoglobulin (IVIG) therapy in pediatrics, other than mentioned below?
B. What is the dose in Kawasaki disease?
C. What is the dose in immune thrombocytopenia purpura?
D. What are the infusion-related side effects?

Q-55.

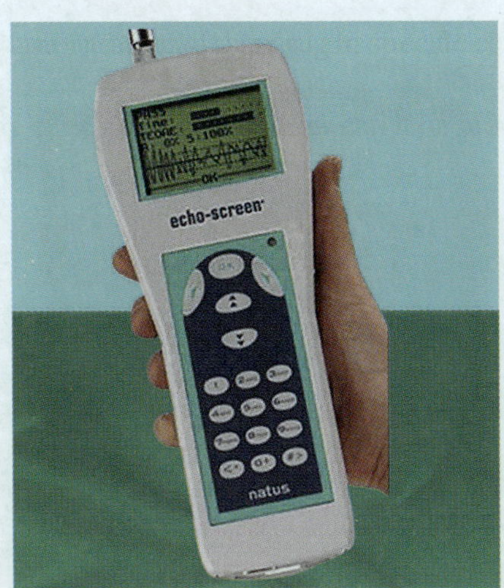

A. Identify the equipment.
B. What is used for?
C. What does it evaluate?
D. What other equipment is used for same purpose? How does it differ from this equipment?
E. What are the current screening recommendations for this parameter in the neonates?
F. What is the recommended sound level in NICU?

Q-56.

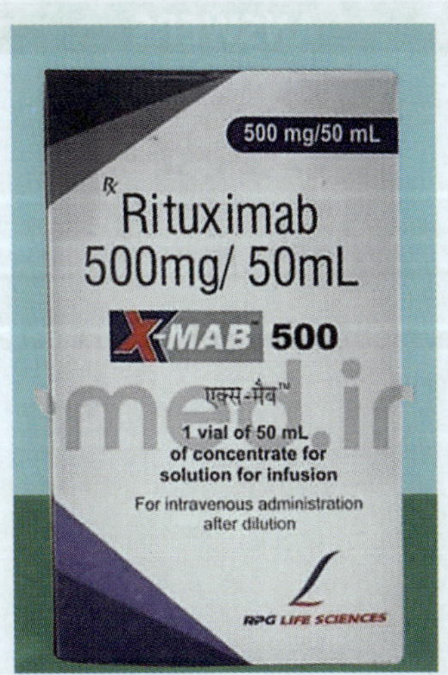

A. What class of drug does rituximab belongs to?
B. What are the mechanisms of action of rituximab?
C. What are the indications of this drug?
D. Describe the process of administration of rituximab.
E. What are its adverse effects?
F. What are the contraindications of this drug?

Q-57.

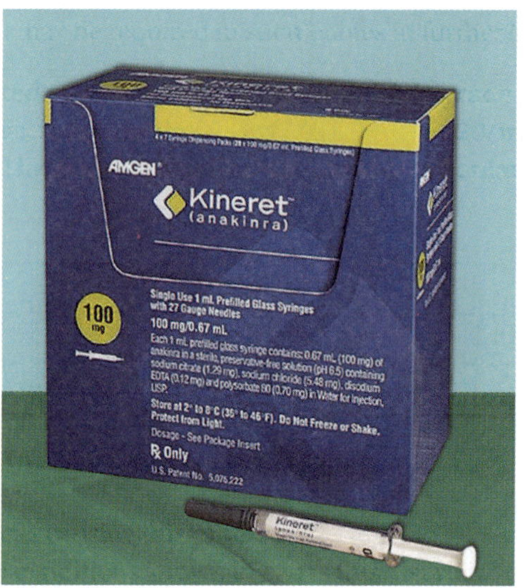

A. What is the mechanism of action of this drug?
B. What are the indications of this molecule?
C. What is the route of its administration?
D. What is the dose of this drug?
E. What are its adverse effects?

ANSWERS

A-1. A. Pulse oximeter
B. Hypoxemia
C. SPO_2 >94%
D. SPO_2 <90%
E. SPO_2 <80%
F. Poor peripheral perfusion, anemia, meth-hemoglobinemia, carboxyhemoglobin

A-2. A. Factors II, VII, IX, X protein C, protein S
B. Increased PT and APTT.
C.
- *Early:* Within 24 hours of life
- *Classical:* Up to 7 days of age
- *Late:* After first week (2–16 weeks)

D. Vitamin K prophylaxis in newborns
IM vitamin K 0.5 mg in less than 1500 G birth weight, 1 mg in more than 1500 G birth weight, single dose

A-3. A. Orchidometer
B. In volume, mL
C. *Infantile:* 2 mL
Prepubertal: 3.5–4 mL
Adult: 17–20 mL

A-4. A.
- Fulminant hepatic failure
- Constipation

B. Lactulose is a nonabsorbable disaccharide. It is metabolized to organic acids by colonic bacteria, and it lowers blood ammonia levels through decreasing microbial ammonia production and through trapping of ammonia in acidic intestinal contents.

C. 1–2 mL/kg/day in 3–4 divided doses. The dose should be titrated sufficient to cause 2–3 watery stools per day.

D. 1–3 mL/kg/day in 2 divided doses

A-5. A.

- Hypomagnesemia in PEM
- Refractory bronchial asthma
- Pre-eclampsia and eclampsia

B. Injection $MgSo_4$ (4 mEq/mL) 2–3 mEq/kg/day (0.5–1 mL/kg/day) 12 hourly IM for 2 days

C. 50 mg/kg in 30 mL glucose solution as IV infusion over 30 minutes.

D.

- Muscular weakness
- Tremors
- Seizures
- Tetany
- Prolonged QT interval
- Arrythmia

E.

- Hypotension
- Hyporeflexia
- Respiratory depression
- Cardiac arrythmia
- Drowsiness, coma and death

F. Calcium gluconate

A-6. A.

- Neonatal resuscitation
- Anaphylaxis
- Croup
- Acute severe bronchial asthma
- Asystole (Pulseless cardiac arrest)

B. If after 30 seconds of PPV with synchronized chest compression, heart rate is <60/minute

C.

- The baby must have adequate ventilation PPV and oxygenation.
- Adrenaline increases oxygen consumption of heart muscles; hence oxygen must be available, otherwise there will be further myocardial damage.

D.

- 1:10,000 concentration
- 0.1–0.3 mL/kg (1:10,000 solution)
- IV through umbilical veins or other veins
- As bolus—rapidly

E.

- Within 30 seconds, if heart rate >60/min continue IPPV till heart rate >100/min and there is spontaneous respiration.
- If heart rate <60/min after 30 seconds, repeat the dose of epinephrine every 3–5 minutes by IV route. Assess other associated conditions like hypovolemia, acidosis etc.

F. Epinephrine (adrenaline) (1:1000 solution) 0.01 mL/kg/dose (maximum 0.5 mL) intramuscular injection on anterolateral aspect of thigh. It can be repeated after 3–5 minutes if required.
G. Adrenaline (1:1000 solution) 0.5 mL/kg (maximum 5 mL) by nebulizer, can be repeated at interval of 2–4 hours, if stridor persists.

A-7. A. Glycopeptide
B. Methicillin sensitive and methicillin resistance *Staphylococcus aureus* (MSSA and MRSA)
C.
- IV route as bactericidal in staphylococcal infections
- Oral route in pseudomembranous colitis

D. 15 mg/kg every 6 hours (60 mg/kg/day)
E.
- "Red man syndrome" is most common side effect. It is infusion rate related.
- Can be prevented by slow infusion.

F.
- Nephrotoxicity
- Ototoxicity
- Neutropenia, thrombocytopenia
- Phlebitis

A-8. A.
- 10% W/V 10 mL ampoule (100 mg/mL of calcium gluconate)
- Elemental calcium, 8.9 mg/ml or 0.45 mEq/mL

B.
- Neonatal hypocalcemia
- Rickets
- Hypoparathyroidism
- Renal failure
- Massive blood transfusion

C. 10% calcium gluconate 1–2 mL/kg IV very slowly over 10 minutes
D.
- Do not given IV calcium to a digitalized patient.
- Monitor for cardiac arrhythmia while giving IV calcium

E. As membrane stabilizing agent to myocardium and protecting from life-threatening complication of hyperkalemia

A-9. A. One mL of 15% KCl (1.5 G/10 mL) = 2 mEq/mL
B.
- Protein energy malnutrition (PEM)
- Acute diarrheal disease
- Diabetes ketoacidosis
- Bartter syndrome
- Gitelman syndrome
- Renal tubular acidosis
- Periodic paralysis
- Diuretic therapy
- Cystic fibrosis

C.
- ST-segment depression
- T-wave flattening
- Prolonged Q–T interval
- Appearance of 'U' waves

D. Injection KCl should be administered by IV infusion and not by IV bolus dose.

E.
- The concentration of K^+ in maintenance IV fluid is 20 mEq/L
- (5 mL of Injection 15% KCl in 500 mL of IV fluid)
- In hypokalemia, it can be increased to 40 mEq/L (10 mL of Injection 15% KCl in 500 mL of IV fluid).
- Maximum concentration of K^+ can be increased to 60 mEq/L in life-threatening hypokalemia.
- ECG monitoring is important while IV infusion of injection KCl.

F.
- Syrup Potklor
- 15 mL of liquid provides 20 mEq of K^+
- 1–2 mEq/kg/day

G.
- It should be given only with good urine flow.
- IV KCl should be given under ECG monitoring.
- Oral potklor should be given diluted to avoid gastric irritation and ulceration.

A-10. A. Chelating agent, used to treat iron and aluminum toxicity.

B.
- Severe vomiting
- Diarrhea
- Abdominal pain
- Dehydration
- Lethargy

C. 60 mg/kg of elemental Iron

D. 10–15 mg/kg/hour IV. Total dose should not exceed 6 G.
100 mg deferoxamine chelates about 8.5 mg of iron

E.
- Clinical features like lethargy, hypotonia, tachypnoea, metabolic acidosis
- Total serum iron >350 μg/dL
- Free serum iron >50 μg/dL

F. *Color of the urine:* Vin rose or red-colored urine indicates presence of free serum iron.

A-11. A.
- Cartridge-based Nucleic Acid Amplification Test (CBNAAT)
- For tuberculosis

B.
- 98% of sputum sample smear positive and 72% in smear negative
- Gastric aspirate 68.8%
- CSF and lymph node aspirates well-sensitive
- Pleural or ascitic fluid yield is poor.

C.
- CBNAAT (Cartridge Based Nucleic Acid Amplification Test)
- CBNAAT ultra
- Truenat
- LPA (Line Probe Assay)
- LAMP (Loop mediated Isothemal Amplification)

D. Around 90 minutes

A-12. A. 200 μg stat → 100 μg at 12 and 24 hours

B. Intracranial hemorrhage

C.

- Poor renal function
- Thrombocytopenia
- Necrotizing enterocolitis (NEC)
- Sepsis

A-13. A.

- Loading dose of phenytoin is 20 mg/kg.
- Additional dose of phenytoin is 10 mg/kg.

B.

- Phenytoin is not compatible with dextrose containing solutions as it gets precipitated. Therefore, infusion of phenytoin should be made only in normal saline.
- Maximum concentration of 10 mg/ml and infused at no more than 1 mg/kg/min in children (up to 50 mg/min in adolescents). Heart rate, blood pressure and ECG should be monitored during infusion.

C.

- Cardiac arrhythmias (attributed mainly due to the solvent propylene glycol)
- Hypotension
- Thrombophlebitis

D.

- Fosphenytoin is a water-soluble phosphate ester of phenytoin. It is a prodrug of phenytoin and has no anticonvulsant effect of its own. It is rapidly converted to phenytoin by non-specific serum phosphates.
- It can be administered three times faster than phenytoin, because of its water solubility and absence of propylene glycol solvent but action of onset is delayed by 15 minutes due to time required for conversion to active form.
- A vial containing 75 mg/mL of fosphenytoin sodium is equivalent to 50 mg/mL phenytoin sodium.

E. Fosphenytoin is considered as better alternative to phenytoin due to following reasons:

- Faster infusion rate.
- Lesser risk of cardiac arrythmias.
- Less local side effects like thrombophlebitis.

A-14. A. 20–40 mg/kg over 5–10 minutes.

B. *Adverse effects of sodium valproate:*

- Hepatotoxicity
- Hyperammonemia
- Pancreatitis
- Encephalopathy

C. *Uses of sodium valproate in children:*

- Epilepsy
- Bipolar disorder
- Migraine
- Sydenham's chorea

A-15. A.

- Loading dose is 20–60 mg/kg at 5 mg/kg/min by IV route.
- Oral dose is 5–10 mg/kg/day divided in 2–3 doses. May be increased weekly by 10 mg/kg. Maximum dose is 60 mg/kg/day or 3000 mg/day.

B. *Merits over phenytoin:*

- It can be administered at a faster rate, 40 mg/kg over 5 minutes as compared to phenytoin, 20 mg/kg over at least 20 minutes.
- Better safety profile.

C.

- Neuropsychiatric adverse events may develop.
- Abrupt withdrawal may precipitate seizures.

A-16. A.

- Neonatal seizures
- Status epilepticus

B.

- 20 mg/kg is loading dose. For the baby with 2.5 kg, total dose is 50 mg.
- Available as an ampoule, containing 200 mg phenobarbitone in each mL.
- 1 mL drug diluted in 9 mL water for injection, each mL contains 20 mg → Take 5 mL (50 mg for baby with 2.5 kg weight) and dilute it in 5 mL and to be given by IV route over 15–20 min, monitoring for respiratory problem.

C.

- Porphyria
- Severe respiratory depression

A-17. A.

- Peripheral neuropathy
- Sideroblastic anemia
- Supplementation with INH therapy
- Dermatitis
- Intractable seizures in neonates

B. Justification for using pyridoxine along with ATT in children:

- Dose of INH has increased to 10–15 mg/kg for children
- High prevalence of malnutrition in children and hence pyridoxine deficiency may be aggravated.
- Clinical diagnosis of peripheral neuropathy is difficult in young children.

C.

- Prophylactic dose of pyridoxine with ATT in children is 10 mg/day.
- Prophylactic dose of pyridoxine with ATT and antiretroviral therapy in children is 50 mg/day.

A-18. A.

- Treatment of acute seizures at home or when parenteral route is not possible.
- As premedication to relieve anxiety before induction of general anesthesia.

B.

- 0.2 mg/kg/dose, maximum 10 mg or 1+1 puffs (one puff in each nostril) per 5 kg weight.

A-19. A. Intractable seizures in neonates.

B. It is pyridoxine dependent seizures, an autosomal recessive disorder. This syndrome results from an inborn abnormality of the enzyme glutamic acid decarboxylase, which results in reduced pyridoxine dependent synthesis of inhibitory neurotransmitter gamma amino butyric acid (GABA). Low concentration of GABA is responsible for intractable seizures.

C. 50-100 mg IV

D. *Clinical manifestations:*

- Intractable neonatal seizures
- Fetal seizures
- Autism
- Breath-holding spell
- Severe mental retardation
- Hepatomegaly, bilious vomiting
- Transient visual agnosia

- Squint
- Severe articulatory apraxia
- Motor dyspraxia
- Microcephaly

E. *Other indications of use of pyridoxine:*
- Pyridoxine deficiency
- Prophylactic with INH therapy
- Severe acute malnutrition
- Sideroblastic anemia
- Homocystinuria

A-20. A. *Indications:*
- Infantile spasms in tuberous sclerosis and Lennox–Gastaut syndrome
- Resistant partial seizures

B. *Dose:* 20–40 mg/kg/day, maintenance dose 100 mg/kg/day in 2 to 3 divided doses.

C. It is Gamma-Aminobutyric acid (GABA) inhibitor. It also has transaminase inhibiting effect.

D. *Adverse effects:*
- Visual field constriction
- Optic atrophy
- Optic neuritis

A-21. A. *Indications:*
- As add on drug in complex partial, generalized tonic–clonic, generalized tonic, absence, myoclonic and Lennox–Gastaut syndrome
- Febrile seizure prophylaxis

B. Dose is 0.3–1 mg/kg/day once a day, preferably at night

C. *For febrile seizures prophylaxis:*
- 0.5 mg/kg/dose 12 hourly for 48 hours
- It should be started on beginning of the fever.

A-22. A. *Indications of ketamine in children:*
- For analgesia of short duration as in bone marrow aspiration
- Induction of anesthesia before ventilation
- Status epilepticus
- Cyanotic spell

B.
- Dose is 0.5–2 mg/kg IV slowly, may administer incremental doses of 0.5–2 mg/kg IV every 15 minutes, if it requires.
- 4–5 mg/kg by Intramuscular route

C. Duration of anesthesia is 5–10 minutes after IV use, very useful for short procedures.

D. *Adverse effects:*
- Hallucination
- Cardiac side effects
- Respiratory depression
- Hypersalivation
- Hypertension
- Increased Intracranial pressure

E. *Precautious while using ketamine:*
- Ketamine should be administered on empty stomach to prevent aspiration of vomitus. Vomiting may occur following administration of ketamine.

- Use of atropine prior to induction of anesthesia by ketamine.
- Administration of overdose or rapid rate may cause respiratory depression.
- Should be administered over a period of 60 seconds.
- Ketamine and phenobarbitone should not be injected from the same syringe because they will form a precipitate.

A-23. A. Antiviral drug

B.

- Herpes simplex virus type 1 and type 2
- Varicella zoster virus
- Epstein–Barr virus
- Cytomegalovirus

C. It is reconstituted in water for injection or normal saline to provide a solution containing 25 mg acyclovir per mL. Intravenous administration should be done as IV infusion over one hour.

D.

- 20 mg/kg 8 hourly IV in infants for 21 days
- 10 mg/kg 8 hourly IV in children for 21 days

E.

- Neutropenia
- Nephrotoxicity
- Neurotoxicity
- Extravasation can cause ulceration and necrosis of surrounding tissues.

A-24. A. Antiviral. It is classified as neuraminidase inhibitor.

B. Treatment of acute, uncomplicated influenza A or B illness in adults and children including neonates older than 2 weeks.

C.

- *Infants 0–8 months:* 3 mg/kg/dose twice a day for 5 days.
- *Infants 9–11 months:* 3.5 mg/kg/dose twice a day for 5 days.
- Children 1–12 years:
  - *<15 kg:* 30 mg twice a day for 5 days.
  - *15 to 23 kg:* 45 mg twice a day for 5 days.
  - *23–40 kg:* 60 mg twice a day for 5 days
  - *>40 kg:* 75 mg twice a day for 5 days.

A-25. A.

- It leads to increase in Fetal Hb (Hb F)
- It also decreases hemolysis by improving hydration of red blood cells in sickle cell disease, thereby, it decreases sickling mechanism which ameliorates the severity of sickle cell disease

B. *Indications in sickle cell disease:*

- Child more than 5 years of age having more than three painful episodes in a year.
- Single episode of acute chest syndrome
- Stroke
- Avascular necrosis of bone

C. It is useful in thalassemia intermedia or non-transfusion dependent thalassemia, but to lesser extent in thalassemia major or transfusion-dependent thalassemia.

D. Starting dose is 15–20 mg/kg with an incremental dose every 8 weeks of 2.5–5 mg/kg if no toxicity occurs, up to a maximum of 35 mg/kg.

E. Hematological toxicity should be monitored by complete blood count and reticulocyte count as it is known to cause bone marrow suppression. It can also cause stomatitis and inflammation of skin.

A-26. A.

- First line therapy for newly diagnosed immune thrombocytopenia purpura (ITP).
- First line therapy for persistent and chronic ITP.

B. The anti-D antibodies coat RBCs and engage macrophage FC receptors. Thus, preferential RBCs destruction takes place in the reticuloendothelial system sparing the platelets.

C. *Prerequisites for IV anti-D in ITP:*

- Patient should be Rh (D) positive
- Hb >10 g/dL
- Patients should not have undergone splenectomy.
- Patients should not have coexisting hemolytic anemia.

D. 50–75 μg/kg

E. *Adverse effects:*

- Headache, nausea, chills, fever
- Some degree of hemolysis is inevitable
- More significant intravascular hemolysis may cause hemoglobinuria and renal failure

F. *Merits of IV anti-D in ITP:*

- Less cost
- Shorter administration time
- Shorter duration of hospitalization

A-27. A. If mother is Rh-negative and the fetus is Rh-positive, Rh-isoimmunization can take place and baby can suffer in the next pregnancy. For prevention of this situation, Anti-D is given to mother as prophylaxis.

B. *Antenatal prophylaxis*

- Prophylactic dose of Anti-D immunoglobulin is given as 300 μg by deep intramuscular route at 28–32 weeks of pregnancy. This will take care of small amount of fetomaternal hemorrhage and prevent isoimmunization. Sometimes, second dose can be repeated.

Postnatal Prophylaxis: Injection Anti-D 300 μg by intramuscular route to the mother within 72 hours to be given.

C.

- During pregnancy small quantity of fetomaternal hemorrhage may take place, maximum may be 10 mL.
- In most of Rh-incompatibility situations, fetomaternal hemorrhage takes place during delivery. Most of times, it is less than 10 mL.
- 10 μg of anti-D is sufficient to prevent sensitization by 1 mL of blood. Therefore, dose of injection Anti-D is calculated 250–300 μg.

A-28. A. *Indications of UDCA:*

- Cholestasis
- Gallstones
- Cystic fibrosis

B.

- UDCA is a hydrophilic substance, replaces the toxic hydrophilic bile-acids from both the bile-acid pool as well as the hepatocellular membrane and improves bile salt dependent bile flow.
- It also stabilizes hepatocellular membranes, protecting against both apoptotic as well as necrotic cell injury.
- It also has immunomodulatory properties.

C. Dose is 10–30 mg/kg/day (maximum 1500 mg/day) in 2–3 divided doses

D. *Adverse effects:*

- Diarrhea
- Rash
- Headache
- Arthralgia
- Elevation of hepatic enzymes

A-29. A. *Indications of cholestyramine resin:*
- Neonatal cholestasis for pruritus
- Obstructive jaundice
- Primary hypercholesterolemia

B. *Mechanisms of action:*
- Removes bile acid from body and helps in pruritus due to cholestasis.
- Reduces LDL cholesterol and useful in primary hypercholesterolemia

C. The dose is 250–500 mg/kg/day.

D. It is available in powder form, mix it with 150–200 mL of fruit juice, water or milk and to be taken one hour before or two hours after the food.

E. *Adverse effects:*
- Malabsorption of fat soluble vitamins
- Constipation
- Steatorrhea
- Metabolic acidosis

A-30. A. *Indications of baclofen:*
- Most useful in spasticity of spinal origin in cerebral palsy
- Spinal cord injury
- Trigeminal neuralgia

B. *Dose of baclofen:*
- *Initial dose:* 2.5 to 5 mg/day
- *Maximum dose:* <7 years 30 mg
  >7 years 60 mg
- *Intrathecal dose:* 25 – 50 mg

C. *Adverse effects of baclofen:*
- Sedation, Hallucination
- Skin rash
- Itching
- Hypotonia, ataxia
- Vertigo
- Increases incidence of omphalocele, if given during pregnancy.

A-31. A. *Indications:*
- To relieve the spasms in a case of spastic cerebral palsy by injecting in the affected muscles.
- Botulinum toxin injected into salivary glands may help to reduce the severity of drooling.

B. *Mechanism of action:*
- Prevents release of acetylcholine from presynaptic terminal and blocks signal transmission at neuromuscular junction
- Reversal of effect is due to preterminal neurite sprouts
- Level of chemical denervation is dependent upon amount of BTX-A injected

C. Dose: 1 unit/kg in each muscle, at interval of 3 months

D. Not to exceed 50 units per injection and not to exceed 400 units in any 3-month period.

A-32. A. *Indications:*
- Acute hypovolemia
- Shock
- Hypoproteinemia (burns, dengue shock syndrome)
- Refractory edema in nephrotic syndrome
- Occasionally, neonatal indirect hyperbilirubinemia

B.
- In case of hypovolemia and shock, it increases osmotic pressure, blood pressure and thereby improves perfusion of cells
- In case of severe hypoproteinemia, albumin is used to replace it as in burns and severe acute malnutrition

C. *Dose of IV albumin:* 0.5–1 G/kg/dose over 2–3 hours

D. *Adverse effects:*
- Fluid overload
- Congestive cardiac failure
- Hypernatremia

A-33. A. *Indications:*
- Diabetes insipidus
- Nocturnal enuresis
- Mild hemophilia

B. *Intranasal dose:*
- *Diabetes insipidus:* 5–30 µg/day in 2 divided doses. >12 years 10–40 µg/day
- *Nocturnal enuresis:* 20 µg at bedtime
- Mild Hemophilia: < 50 kg: 150 µg
  >50 kg: 300 µg

C. *Adverse effects:*
- Facial flushing
- Fluid retention

A-34. A. *Indications of dopamine:*
- Shock—fluid refractory shock
- Shock with myocardial function impairment and hypotension after resuscitation from cardiac arrest
- Shock with low heart rate

B. *Different mechanisms are in action at different doses:*
- At low doses (0.5–2 µg/kg/minute), it acts predominantly on dopaminergic receptors located on the renal, coronary and cerebral vascular beds, causing vasodilatation and increased perfusion.
- At intermediate dose (2–10 µg/kg/minute), it progressively stimulates beta-1 and alpha-1 receptors, causing increased cardiac output and increasing systolic blood pressure.
- At higher dose (10–20 µg/kg/minutes), it causes vasoconstriction and rise in blood pressure.

C.

D. Formula for calculation of dopamine dose:

- $$\frac{\text{Wt. (kg)} \times \text{dose } (\mu\text{g/kg/min}) \times 24 \times 60}{1000 \times 40 \text{ (drug concentration)}}$$

Ml drug → 0.036 × Wt (kg) × dose (µg/kg/min)
Ml dopamine (40 mg/mL) + Normal saline
= 24 mL → 1 mL/hour

- Infusion rate for 20 kg weighing patient for dose of dopamine 10 µg/kg/min
  = 7.2 mL + 16.8 ml NS = 24 mL → Infusion rate 1 mL/hour

$$\frac{20 \times 10 \times 24 \times 60}{1000 \times 40}$$

E. *Adverse effects of dopamine:*
- Tissue necrosis on extravasation
- Cardiac arrhythmias
- Gangrene of peripheral parts of extremities (digits, toes, hands and feet) due to ischemia following severe peripheral vasoconstriction on higher doses (>10 µg/kg/min)

F. *Contraindications of dopamine:*
- Atrial and ventricular tachyarrhythmias
- Drug should be kept away from direct sunlight.
- Calcium and bicarbonate should not be administered in the same line.

A-35. A. *Indications of dobutamine in children:*
- Conditions associated with poor myocardial function
- Conditions associated with low output congestive cardiac failure and normal to moderately decreased blood pressure
- More commonly used in viral myocarditis, cardiomyopathy and myocardial infarct like in Kawasaki disease
- Following corrective or palliative cardiovascular surgery when myocardial dysfunction is suspected or demonstrated
- Children undergoing operation for mitral valve disease

B. *Mechanism of action:*
- Action is on B_1 and B_2 receptors
- More ionotropic than chronotropic effect
- Automaticity of the sinus node
- Enhancement of atrioventricular and intraventricular conduction

C. Dose is 5–20 μg/kg/minute

D. *Adverse effects:*
- Tachycardia
- Hypertension
- Extravasation may cause gangrene.

A-36. A. *Indications of norepinephrine:*
- In children with low blood pressure and a normal or raised cardiac index
- Septic shock—warm shock refractory to volume repletion and dopamine
- Distribute shock

B. *Mechanisms of action of norepinephrine:*
- Stimulation of B_1 receptors
- Potent against alpha-receptor
- Increases systolic and diastolic blood pressure.
- Marked vasoconstriction contributes to marked increased peripheral resistance.

C.
- Available as 1 mg/mL ampoule
- Dose is 0.05 to 0.1 μg/kg/min. IV infusion, not to exceed 2 μg/kg/min
- 0.6 × wt (kg) = mg to mix in 100 mL → 1 mL/hour → 0.1 μg/kg/min

D. *Adverse effects:*
- Cardiac arrhythmias
- Hypertension
- Hyperglycemia

A-37. A. *Indications of milrinone:*
- Septic shock—causing low cardiac output. It is particularly useful in the setting of normal or low cardiac output with increased systemic vascular resistance.
- Congestive cardiac failure
- Use after cardiac surgery

B. *Mechanisms of action of milrinone:* Milrinone causes improvement in cardiac function due to positive ionotropic effect as well as a reduction of afterload and preload secondary to its vasodilator action.

C.
- Available as clear pale-yellow solution 1 mg/mL
- *Dose:* Loading dose 50 μg/kg IV over 15 minutes → followed by continuous infusion 0.5–0.75 μg/kg/min

D. *Adverse effects:*
- Headache
- Ventricular arrhythmia
- Hypokalemia
- Bronchospasm
- Thrombocytopenia

E. *Contraindications:*
- Aortic stenosis
- Pulmonary stenosis
- Myocardial infarction

A-38. A. Attention deficit hyperactive disorder (ADHD) in children above 6 years of age.

B.
- Initial dose 2.5–5 mg orally twice a day, taken 30–45 minutes before the breakfast and lunch.
- *Maintenance dose:* The dose may be increased weekly in increment of 5–10 mg up to a maximum of 60 mg/day in 2 to 3 divided doses. To be used under directions of neurologist or psychiatrist only

C. *Adverse effects:*
- Tachycardia
- Nervousness
- Growth retardation
- Thrombocytopenia

A-39. A. *Indication:* Apnea of prematurity, as a second-line drug after aminophylline.

B. It acts as CNS stimulant, also as ionotropic to myocarditis.

C.
- Injection caffeine citrate available as 20 mg/mL
- 20 mg of caffeine citrate contains 10 mg of caffeine base.
- *Dose:* 10 mg of caffeine base initially followed by 2.5–5 mg/kg/day in 2 divided doses daily.
- Caffeine therapy is usually continued until an infant is free of clinically significant apnea or bradycardia for 5–7 days without positive support or at 34 weeks postmenstrual age.

D. *Benefits of caffeine in preterm babies:*
- Reduces the incidences and severity of apnea of prematurity
- Facilitates successful extubation from mechanical ventilation.
- Reduces the rate of bronchopulmonary dysplasia.
- Improves neurodevelopmental outcomes.

E. *Precautions:*
- Do not use caffeine sodium benzoate in the newborn.
- If theophylline has been administered to the patient within previous 3 days, a modified loading dose, 50–75% of the loading dose, may be given.
- Also caffeine citrate oral solution is available, 20 mg/mL.

A-40. A. *Indications:*
- Hyperammonia in organic acid disorders
- Hyperammonia in urea-cycle disorders

B.
- IV preparation is not available in India.
- Tablet or granules forms are available.
- 250 mg/kg/day in 3–4 divided doses

C. *Adverse effects:*
- Hepatotoxicity
- Abdominal pain
- Blurred vision

A-41. A. *Indications:*

- Functional constipation
- Dis-impaction for rectal impaction
- Maintenance therapy

B.

- *At home:* 1.5–2 G/kg/day in 2 divided doses for 3–6 days, only depending upon the clarity of rectal effluent.
- *In Hospital:*
  - 25 mL/kg/hour oral or by nasogastric tube in young children. Endpoint is clearly effluent.
  - Young children may require IV fluid to maintain hydration.

C. *Maintenance therapy:*

- 0.5–1 g/kg/day >12 months of age

D. *Adverse effects:*

- Dehydration in dis-impaction therapy
- Bloating
- Abdominal pain or cramps
- Loose stools

A-42. A. Parenteral nutrition

B. Dose is 0.5–3.5 G/kg/day

C. When enteral nutrition is insufficient or contraindicated.

D. *Side effects:*

- Dys-electrolytemia
- Cholestasis
- Sepsis—bacterial and fungal
- Thrombosis
- Azotemia
- Thrombocytopenia

A-43. A. *Indications:*

- To produce analgesia during short procedures
- As preanesthetic medicine

B. *Mechanism of action:*

- Classified as opioid analgesia
- It produces analgesia by binding to gamma-receptors in the brain and spinal cord.

C.

- Available as 50 μg/mL for parenteral route.
- *Dose in infants:* 1–4 μg/kg/dose at interval of 1–4 hours by IV route.
- 0.5–5 μg/kg/hour as continuous infusion.
- *Dose in children:*
  - 1–3 μg/kg/dose at 1–4 hours interval by IV route.
  - 1–5 μg/kg/hour as continuous infusion.

D. *Adverse effects of fentanyl:*

- With high dose or rapid administration, it can cause chest rigidity.
- Hypotension
- Respiratory depression
- Bradycardia
- Biliary tract spasm
- Pruritus

E. Chest wall rigidity may develop with dose >5 μg/kg. It can be treated with naloxone or neuromuscular blockade.

F. *Other routes of administration for fentanyl:*
- Oral
- Transdermal (especially for chronic pain)

A-44. A. *Causes of hypokalemia:*
- Severe acute malnutrition (SAM)
- Acute diarrhea disease (ADD)
- Persistent vomiting
- Nasogastric aspiration
- Congenital chloride loosing diarrhea
- Renal tubular acidosis Type I and Type II
- Diuretics-like frusemide
- Salbutamol by nebulizer
- Bartter syndrome
- Cystic fibrosis

B. Concentration of potassium in Potklor oral solution is:
- 1.5 G per 15 mL
- 20 mEq of elemental potassium per 15 mL

C. Oral dose of potassium is 2–4 mEq/kg/day

D. *Oral potassium solution*: Potklor should be mixed with feed to avoid GI irritation. Undiluted potklor can cause gastric mucosal irritation, ulceration and occasionally bleeding.

A-45. A. Meter dose inhaler (MDI), also called pressurized metter dose inhaler (PMDI)

B. Bronchial asthma

C. The drug is suspended in hydrofluoroalkane (HFA) propellant. It delivers a fixed amount of medication in aerosol form each time it is activated.

D.
- ≤4 years → MDI with spacer and mask
- >4 years → MDI with spacer

E.
- *Advantage:* The drug can be effectively delivered on tidal breathing.
- *Disadvantage:* It needs skill and training for proper inhalation in children.

F. *Available drug in MDI device:*
- Salbutamol
- Terbutaline
- Ipratropium
- Budesonide
- Fluticasone
- Salmeterol
- Beclomethasone
- Chromoglycate

A-46. A. I Meter dose inhaler (MDI) with spacer
II MDI with spacer and facemask

B. Bronchial asthma

C. *MDI with spacer and face mask:* <4 years
MDI with spacer: >4 years

D.
- *Benefits of spacer:* Spacers are used as accessories to MDIs. A spacer acts as a temporary reservoir or chamber for the aerosol released from MDI. The child can then inhale from the chamber shortly after the drug is discharged from MDI. They need not coordinate with press and breath.

- *Benefits of mask:* The infants and younger children who cannot inhale through a mouthpiece, a mask is attached to the end of spacer. This eliminates the need for active co-operation of the child.

A-47. A. Nebulizer

B. Nebulizer is a device in which a liquid drug is broken into a small aerosol that can be inhaled.

- *Optimum volume of solution in nebulizer chamber:* 2 to 4 mL
- *Particle size:* 2–5 μm
- *Flow rate:* 4–6 L/minute
- Oxygen driven
- Normal saline should be used as diluent and not distilled water with distilled water, hypo-osmolar solution can lead to reflex vasoconstriction.

C.

- Salbutamol
- Terbutaline
- Ipratropium
- Budesonide
- Tobramycin
- Hypertonic saline (3%)

D. *Advantages of nebulizer:*

- Eliminates need for coordination as required with other devices
- Larger doses of drug can be delivered as may be needed in acute severe asthma.
- Tidal breathing is adequate for inhalation. Therefore, can be given to young children or breathless patients.
- Avoids reflex coughing which may be experienced with other devices.

E. *Disadvantages of nebulizer:*

- Expensive
- Requires regular maintenance
- Infection is possible.
- Takes prolong time (10–15 minutes)

F.

- Ultrasonic nebulizer
- Jet nebulizer

A-48. A. Dried powder inhaler (DPI) or Rotahaler

B. Bronchial asthma

C. DPI is a breath-activated device. It is considered as effective as MDI. In this device, a capsule of powdered drug formulation is inserted into the device and is broken into two halves by rotating the base relative to the mouthpiece. One half of the capsule falls into the Rotahaler, and the patient has to merely inhale through the mouthpiece. It is useful for maintenance therapy or treating mild exacerbations in older children (6 to 12 years).

D. Above 5 years of age

E. *Advantages:*

- Easy to learn, to teach and to use
- Portable (can be kept in the pocket)
- Eliminates the need for coordination between actuation and inhalation.

Disadvantages:

- Younger children (<5 years) cannot use.
- Bad taste due to deposition of drug particles in oral cavity
- Humidity may cause agglutination of particles

A-49. A. Peak flowmeter. There are manual and digital peak flow meters.

B. *Technique of using peak flow meter:*
- Sit or stand up straight
- Confirm that the marker is at the bottom of the meter.
- Take a deep breath, filling your lungs completely and hold it
- Put your mouth around the mouthpiece and close your lips tightly. Make sure your lips form a seal so no air escapes around the outside of the mouthpiece.
- Blow all the air out of your lips as hard and fast a possible in a single exhale.
- Write down the number by the marker on the meter.
- Repeat these steps three times. The highest of these three reading is your daily peak flow.
- Write down your daily peak flow on a sheet of paper, on your calendar, on your smartphone or in your asthma dairy.
- Also record any symptom-like cough, breathlessness, wheezing, medicines taken, etc.

C.
- Peak flow reading depends upon several factors like age, sex, height, etc.
- Healthcare providers generally use a 'traffic-light' system that consists of three zones to determine your peak flow rate
  - *Green:* Asthma is under good control. 80–100% of your personal best
  - *Yellow:* Asthma is not under good control. Peak flow is 50–80% of your personal best.
  - *Red:* Severe asthma. Peak flow is less than 50% of your personal best. Needs emergency care.

D.
- Peak flow is variable according to age, sex and height.
- A normal peak flow in adults is between 400 and 700 L/min. In children, a normal peak flow may range between 150–450 L/min.

E. *Indications for using peak flowmeter:*
- Bronchial asthma
- Chronic lung disease

A-50. A.
- Uncomplicated falciparum malaria
- To switch on this oral preparation once the patient recovers and able to take orally from severe/complicated malaria following parenteral therapy.

B. Artemisinin based combination therapy (ACT)

C. *Benefits of ACT, especially Artemisinin:*
- Artemisinin preparation causes rapid clearance of parasitemia and resolution of symptoms
- Rapid elimination of artemisinin, so that the residual concentration of the drug does not provide a selective filter for the parasites to develop resistance.
- Lack of serious toxic effects
- Gametocidal effect

D.
- Six dose regimens orally twice a day for 3 days
- For 5–14 kg weight 1 tablet at diagnosis, again after 8–12 hours and then twice a day on Day 2 and Day 3.
- For 15–24 kg body weight same schedule with 2 tablets
- For 25–35 kg body weight and above same schedule with 3 and 4 tablets, respectively

E. *Other recommended preparations:*
- Artesunate 4 mg/kg body weight orally once daily for 3 days and a single administration of Sulfadoxine–Pyrimethamine as 25 mg/kg of sulfadoxine and 1.25 mg/kg of pyrimethamine on day one.
- Artesunate as above and mefloquine 25 mg/kg of body weight in two divided doses (15 mg/kg and 10 mg/kg) on Day 2 and Day 3.

Important Points

- Currently, there are insufficient safety and tolerability data on mefloquine in children. Mefloquine shares cross-resistance with quinine which is still an effective drug in our country. Health planners in our country do not advocate use of mefloquine.
- Lumefantrine absorption is enhanced by coadministration with fatty food-like milk.
- Artemether–Lumefantrine is not recommended in children weighing less than 5 kg.

A-51. A.

- Primaquine kills intrahepatic form (hypnozoites) of *Plasmodium vivax* and thereby prevents relapse
- Primaquine also kills gametocytes and thereby prevents transmission of malaria.

B.

- 0.25 mg/kg once daily for 14 days for *P. vivax* to prevent relapse.
- A single dose of primaquine, 0.75 mg/kg for gametocytocidal action.

C. G-6-P-D deficiency test should be performed before primaquine therapy as it can cause hemolysis in this enzyme deficit persons.

D. In cases of borderline G-6-P-D deficiency cases once weekly dose of primaquine 0.6–0.8 mg/kg is given for 6 weeks.

A-52. A. *Reconstitution of artesunate:*

- Inject 5% sodium bicarbonate (1 mL) into the artesunate vial.
- Shake it until dissolved. The solution will be cloudy.
- The reconstituted solution will be clear in about 2 min time. Discard if it is not clear.
- It should be diluted in normal saline or 5% dextrose.
- For IV 1 mL + 5 mL = 6 mL (10 mg/mL). For IM 1 mL + 2 mL = 3 mL (20 mg/mL).
- IV slow bolus over 3–4 mL/minute.
- Prepare a fresh solution for each administration.

B. Artesunate is reconstituted in 5% sodium bicarbonate to form sodium artesunate, the active form of the drug. It is stable in specific pH and therefore reconstituted in 5% sodium bicarbonate. It has poor stability in aqueous solution or neutral pH.

C. To maintain its stability at very specific pH, it is diluted only in 5% sodium bicarbonate. Therefore, 7.5% sodium bicarbonate cannot be used.

D. Diluent is normal saline or 5% dextrose.

E. Artesunate can be given as IV bolus over 3–4 mL/minute and also by intramuscular route.

A-53. A. *Indications for parenteral iron therapy:*

- Poor adherence or intolerability due to gastrointestinal side effects of oral iron.
- Need for rapid replenishment of hemoglobin and iron stores rather than over the course of several months, e.g., in preoperative situations.
- On going blood loss that exceeds the capacity of oral iron to meet needs (heavy uterine bleeding, mucosal telangiectasia)
- Iron malabsorption is due to pre-existing anatomic or physiologic condition, e.g., short bowel syndrome.
- Co-existing inflammatory state that interferes with iron hemostasis.
- Chronic kidney disease.
- Genetic forms refractory to oral iron.

B. Preparations of intravenous iron:

- *Iron sucrose:*
  - Most common form of IV iron used in children.
  - Adverse events including anaphylaxis, are rare, so a test dose or routine pre-medications are not indicated.
  - 1-4 mg/kg elemental iron IV infusion over 1 hour every week with a maximum dose of 200 mg elemental iron per infusion for adolescents and 100 mg of elemental iron per infusion for children.

- *Ferric gluconate:*
  - Approved for children with chronic kidney disease on dialysis and erythropoietin stimulating agents aged > 6 years
  - No test dose or pre-medications are indicated.
  - Maximum dose 125 mg of elemental iron per perfusion
- *Iron dextran:* Low molecular weight iron dextran as single replacement dose, up to 100 mg elemental iron in adults.
- *Ferric carboxy maltose (FCM):*
  - Increasingly used adults
  - Data in pediatric population is limited, but promising
  - Hypophosphatemia is a common complication.
  - 15 mg/kg single rapid over 15 minutes IV infusion without any test dose.

C.

- Hb iron deficit (mg) = Body wt (kg) × (Ideal Hb – desired Hb) × (2.145) + Iron to replenish stores
- Volume product required (mL) = Body wt (kg) × (14-Hb) × 2.145
  Concentration of elemental iron in the product used (mg/mL)

For example, a 6-year-old child weighing 20 kg with Hb 6 g/dL would need 343.2 mg of elemental iron, equivalent to 1.7 mL of iron sucrose injection containing 200 mg/mL of elemental iron

(20 × 8 × 2.145/200)

This child will be given 343.2 mg of elemental iron in four divided weekly doses, 0.43 mL iron sucrose dissolved in 100– 200 mL of normal saline and infused over 1–3 hours every week for 4 weeks.

An intravenous dose of iron for undernourished children should be calculated with present weight, while for obese patients, ideal or lean body weight should be used for calculation.

Lean body weight = BMI 50 × Ht^2

D. Routinely no premedication is indicated. Patients with comorbidity of bronchial asthma, drug allergy and inflammatory arthritis require premedication with 1–2 mg/kg of parenteral methyl prednisolone before IV iron administration.
   - Subjective improvement within a few days
   - Reticulocyte peak at 10 days
   - Symptomatic improvement in 1–2 weeks
   - Complete response may take 4–6 weeks

A-54. A. *Indications for IVIG:*
   - Primary immunodeficiency disorders
   - Immune thrombocytopenic purpura
   - Kawasaki disease
   - Bone marrow transplantation
   - HIV

B. IVIG 2 G/kg in 12 hours duration

C. Single dose of 0.8–1/kg

D. *Infusion-related side effects:*
   - Headache, flushing, chills, myalgia, arthralgia, abdominal pain
   - Uncommon side effects are tightness of chest, hives, anaphylactic reaction.

A-55. A. Oto Acoustic Emission (OAE) machine

B. It is used for hearing screening.

C. It evaluates hearing from middle ear to the outer hair cells in the inner ear, so it is used to screen for sensorineural hearing loss. It cannot detect auditory neuropathy.

D. *Auditory brainstem response (ABR):* It is used to assess auditory pathway from the eighth nerve to the inferior colliculus of the midbrain

E. *Current recommendations:*
- Universal hearing screening of all neonates more than 34 weeks of gestation, at birth, at 72 hours of life by OAE.
- If OAE is abnormal, repeat it at 6 weeks. If it is still abnormal, the ABR should be performed.
- All NICU graduates should undergo ABR.

F. <50 db

A-56. A. Rituximab is classified as monoclonal antibody. It is an anti-CD20 chimeric antibody.

B. Rituximab bonds to CD20 positive cells and causes cell death by antibody dependent cell mediated cytotoxicity (ADCC), complement- mediated cytotoxicity (CDC), antibody dependent phagocytosis (ADP) and direct effect of binding rituximab to CD20.

C. *Indications of rituximab:*
- *Hematological:* HLH, Refractory ITP
- *Neurological:* NMDA encephalitis, NMO spectrum disorders, multiple sclerosis, refractory myasthenia gravis
- *Rheumatological:* SLE and JIA
- *Renal:* Nephrotic syndrome, renal transplant, post-transplant graft versus host disease (GVHD)

D. It is reconstituted with 9% NS or 5% Dextrose and administered as slow IV infusion. No any other drug should be administered in same IV line. Premedication with paracetamol and antihistamine prior to administration rituximab is recommended.

E. *Adverse effects of rituximab:*
- Anaphylactic reaction
- Allergy
- Fever with chills
- Skin rash
- Hypotension
- Cardiac arrhythmias
- Sever bacterial, viral or fungal infections. Reactivation of viruses like herpes, varicella and cytomegalovirus

F. *Contraindications of rituximab:*
- Known hypersensitivity to drug
- Cardiac failure
- Active infection
- Cardiac arrhythmias

A-57. A. Anakinra is an interleukin-1 (IL-1) receptor antagonist. It blocks the biological activity of IL-1 by competitively inhibiting its ability to bind to the IL-1 type 1 receptor (IL-IR1).

B. *Indications of anakinra:*
- Severe active rheumatoid arthritis
- Neonatal onset multisystem inflammatory disease
- Chronic infantile neurological, cutaneous, articular syndrome
- Deficiency of IL-1 receptor antagonist
- COVID-19 pneumonia
- Still's disease
- Macrophage activation syndrome

C. Kineret injection available as 100 mg/0.67 mL prefilled syringe. It is given by subcutaneous route.

D. 100 mg/day in patients of rheumatoid arthritis

E. *Adverse effects of anakinra:*
- Pain, itching, swelling at injection site
- Fever, arthralgia, headache, vomiting, diarrhea
- Flu-like symptoms
- Infections including serious infections.

CHAPTER 25

Counseling

QUESTIONS

Q-1. What is counseling in medical practice?

Q-2. What are key aspects of medical counseling?

Q-3. What are features of active communication?

Q-4. What are aspects of counseling skills?

Q-5. What are steps of facilitate comprehension and understanding the situation?

Q-6. What are nonverbal communication skills?

Q-7. Give examples of closed and open questions?

Q-8. How will you do breaking the bad news?

Q-9. A female child aged 12 months has been diagnosed as a case of simple febrile seizures. Counsel the mother regarding your diagnosis and treatment.

Q-10. A 5-year-old boy is diagnosed as celiac disease. Counsel the parents regarding the diet in details.

Q-11. A 2-year-old girl presents with severe pallor. How will you derive the history in details?

Q-12. A 7-year-old boy has been diagnosed as nephrotic syndrome. He has been started on steroids and has started showing the response and is about to be discharged from hospital. Counsel the parents about the management at home.

Q-13. Explain for urine sample collection by clean catch mid-stream.

Q-14. A newborn is brought to you with meningomyelocele. Parents are anxious for its recurrence in the next pregnancy. Counsel them.

Q-15. A 1-month-old child exclusively breastfed is brought with complaint of frequency of stool 10 to 12 times a day. The baby is otherwise normal, taking breastfeeding well and gaining the weight. Counsel the mother.

Q-16. You are attending to a high-risk delivery of an HIV positive mother. The baby is delivered uneventfully. The baby is normal and hemodynamically stable. How will you counsel regarding the baby?

ANSWERS

A-1. In medical practice, counseling is a collaborative process where a professional helps a patient and his relatives to understand his health condition, cope with emotional distress and develop strategies for managing his health.

A-2. Key aspects of medical counseling

- *Information and education:* Providing clear information about a medical condition, treatment options, potential risks and lifestyle changes.
- *Emotional Support:* Helping patients deal with the psychological and emotional impact of an illness by providing safe space to discuss their feelings and anxieties.
- *Collaborative problem solving:* Working with the patient to find solutions and develop coping mechanisms for managing their health issues.
- *Empowerment:* Encouraging patients to take an active role in their health care, which can lead to better treatment outcomes and adherence.
- *Specific applications:* This includes presurgical counseling, medication counseling, counseling for procedures and counseling how to manage a chronic disease.
- *Professional roles:* While doctors provide counseling, specially trained staff like social workers or dedicated counselors also provide these services, often focusing on the psychosocial and emotional aspects of a patient's health journey.

A-3. Features of active communication

- Nature of disease and its consequences should be explained in simple language, should not be in threating tone.
- We should understand the concerns and difficulties of the patient and family members.
- Relevant information should be provided to them so that they can draw appropriate conclusion.
- All possible treatment options should be explored.
- Suggestions can be given, but no commands.

A-4. Counseling skills

- Comprehension and understanding situation
- Empowerment and support
- Hand holding and monitoring

A-5. Steps of facilitate comprehension and understanding situation

- Ambience and presentation should be appropriate.
- Factual questions should be open
- During communication, you should show interest.
- Empathy with patient should be obvious.
- Do not use judging words.

A-6. Nonverbal communication skills

- Posture is important
- Social distance should be observed
- Eye contact is essential
- They should not feel that you are in hurry
- Barrier should not be there
- Empathetic touch is desirable

A-7. Examples of closed and open questions

Closed questions	***Open questions***
Do you wash hands before collection of blood?	How do you ensure hygiene before collection of blood?
Do you donate blood?	How will you manage for blood?
Can you look after him at home?	Who will look after him at home?

A-8. Breaking the bad news

- Introduce yourself and speak in an empathetic tone
- Check prior information/knowledge
- Come to the point straight and mention the diagnosis/critical condition, etc.
- Give a pause for the parents to respond
- Console/offer water/tissues, if required
- Give only necessary information and offer to meet the parent for further conversations/meetings with the family
- Ask if any questions

A-9.
- Greet the mother. Introduce yourself
- State that from history and physical examination, diagnosis of your child is simple febrile seizures
- Explain that this condition is common in children between the age of 6 months and 5 years
- Explain that the seizure has a tendency to recur in case of fever in the future in 30 to 50% of children.
- Inform that they should consult a doctor at the earliest in case of fever. Oral clobazam (0.5 to 1 mg/kg/day) should be given for 3 days
- Fever should be treated promptly by antipyretics (paracetamol)
- In case of seizure,
  - Keep the child in prone or lateral position with head low position, keeping head on one side to prevent aspiration if he develops vomiting
  - Use midazolam nasal spray to control convulsions
  - Paracetamol suppository may be used by rectal route to control the fever
  - Do not put any object in the mouth of the child. Avoid injury to tongue.
- Reassure the parents that the condition has an excellent prognosis for long-term neurodevelopment
- Ask the parents if they have any query and encourage them to ask the questions
- Wish the parents and offer a telephone number for use in an emergency.

A-10.
- Establish rapport. Introduce yourself.
- Explain that based on history, clinical examination and investigations performed, your son has celiac disease, a condition in which the child is has allergy to wheat and wheat products.
- Explain that the treatment of this condition is to exclude all the wheat products from his diet, in addition to items made from oats and barely for the lifetime.
- Give some examples of wheat containing preparations like *atta, maida, sooji, chapatis, roti,* bread, biscuits, noodles, *halwa, laddu, upma,* etc. If you are not sure regarding the item whether it contains wheat or not, best way is not to consume it.
- State alternative foods like rice, maize, bajra, jowar, sago which can be eaten. All milk products can be taken.
- Suggest that all the family members should adhere to the same diet.
- Explain that with changes in food in a case of celiac disease, improvement in symptoms, gaining weight and height are seen within few months (usually 3 to 6 months)
- Repeat serological tests after 3 months is desirable.
- Ask the parents regarding their doubts and queries
- Wish them and offer your telephone number where they can contact you in case of any query

A-11.
- Establish the rapport. Introduce yourself.
- Ask about onset of pallor whether it was sudden or gradual
- Ask dietary history in detail
- Ask for history of worms infestation.
- Ask regarding the history of any brown, pink or bluish spots on the body.
- Ask for any drug for longer duration, e.g., aspirin in a case of Kawasaki disease
- Ask for associated symptoms like fever, weight loss
- Ask for H/o jaundice
- Ask for H/o blood transfusion
- Ask for history similar problem in family
- Ask for community, consanguinity, geographical and family background

A-12.
- Establish rapport. Introduce yourself.
- Explain that from history, clinical examination and laboratory reports, your child has a kidney disease called nephrotic syndrome in which the protein is lost in the urine.
- Inform that the treatment for the disease has been started and that the swelling over body will gradually decrease and disappear after few days. Explain the need to continue the treatment as per advice and that medicines should not be stopped or modified by their own.
- Explain regarding course of steroids and its toxicity, steroid face, excessive weight gain, increased appetite, hirsutism, etc.
- Explain regarding regular examination of urine for proteinuria (by dipstick or boiling method). Emphasize regarding monitoring the weight, blood pressure and urine output. All the results should be brought during each visit.
- Explain to take normal diet, no extra salt. He can attend the school
- Explain the parents to attend the hospital immediately if he develops pain in abdomen, vomiting, fever, etc.
- Explain regarding immunization. No live vaccines during steroid therapy. Killed vaccines may be given, but effect may be compromised. Ideally, vaccines should be given after 6 weeks of discontinuation of steroids. Pneumococcal, *H. influenzae* B and meningococcal vaccines should be given when he is off the steroids for 6 weeks.
- Ask the parents if they have any query and encourage them to ask the questions
- Wish them and offer your telephone number which can be of use in case of an emergency situation.

A-13.
- Genitalia should be cleaned with soap and water antiseptic washes and forced preputial retraction are not advisable
- Child is asked to squat, retract the prepuce in males and separate the labia in females and then ask to void the urine
- Discard the initial part of urine. Mid part of urine should be collected directly in sterile container
- Plating of the urine specimen within 1 hour of collection. If delay is anticipated, sample should be preserved at 4°C in refrigerator.

A-14.
- Establish the rapport.
- State that based on history, examination and investigations, the diagnosis is meningomyelocele.
- Inform about the possibility of recurrence in the next pregnancy
- Explain that the recurrence can be prevented by use of folic acid
- Advise that folic acid should be started 2 months before conception in the dose of 4 mg once a day and continued for 3 months after conception.
- Ask if mother has any doubts and encourage her to ask the questions
- Wish mother and offer your contact number

A-15.
- Establish the rapport. Introduce yourself.
- Explain the mother that her baby has no diarrhea. Exclusively breastfed baby has least chances of developing infection. Following points should be stressed to convince her
- Baby remains alert and active, takes breastfeeding well
- Passes urine for more than five times a day, indicating there is no dehydration
- Child is gaining the weight. In a case of diarrhea, development of dehydration of weight loss are very common.
- Increased frequency of stool and watery diarrhea in a breastfed baby may be due to,
  - Lack of good sphincter control
  - Gastrocolic reflex
  - More lactose content in breast milk may give rise to watery stool
- Emphasize that it is not diarrhea and there is no need of any medicine. Explain her not to give nut meg and any opium derivative.
- Ask the mother for any doubt.
- Wish the mother and offer your contact number for any query if she has.

A-16.
- Establish the rapport introduce yourself.
- Give the mother options regarding feeding the baby, exclusive breastfeeding, top feeding only and no mixed feeding
- Explain the benefits of breastfeeding for the baby and risk of not giving breastfeeding.
- Inform that breast milk can transmit the virus to the baby.
- Stress the need for hygiene for top feeding and hazards of unhygienic methods. She should know the technique of top feeding and expenses for top milk
- Emphasize that after choosing either of these two, do not change to mixed feeding.
- Ask the parents for their doubt or query. They should be given some time for making the decision.
- Wish them and offer your contact number for clarification of any query if she has.

CHAPTER

26 Preventive and Social Medicine

QUESTIONS ON UNDER-FIVE MORTALITY (U5MR)

Q-1. Define U5MR.

Q-2. What is U5MR of India?

Q-3. What are most common causes of U5MR in India?

Q-4. What is the major contributing factor for U5MR?

ANSWERS

A-1. U5MR is defined as the deaths between birth and 5 years of age per thousand live births

A-2. U5MR of India is 32/1,000 live births [Samples Registration System (SRS), 2020]

A-3.
- 62% deaths are attributed to neonatal deaths
- Others are pneumonia, diarrhea

A-4. Severe acute malnutrition (SAM) is major predisposing factor

QUESTIONS ON CHILD HEALTH INDICATORS

Q-1. Define infant mortality rate (IMR).

Q-2. Define neonatal mortality rate (NMR).

Q-3. Define early neonatal mortality rate (ENMR).

Q-4. Define late neonatal mortality rate (LNMR).

Q-5. Define perinatal mortality rate (PNMR).

Q-6. What is the formula for calculation of IMR?

Q-7. What is current IMR of India?

Q-8. What are most common causes of NMR?

Q-9. What is the formula for calculation of PMR?

Q-10. What is the formular for calculation of NMR?

Q-11. What parameters are considered as indicator of socioeconomic development?

Q-12. What is current NMR of India?

Q-13. What is current PMR of India?

ANSWERS

A-1. *IMR:* Number of infants dying between birth of exactly 1 year of age expressed per 1,000 live births, per year.

A-2. *NMR:* The number of deaths among live births, during first 28 days of life per 1,000 live births per year.

A-3. *ENMR:* The number of child deaths <7 days of life expressed as per 1,000 live births in that reference year.

A-4. *LNMR:* The number of child deaths between 7 and 28 completed days of life expressed as 1,000 live births in that reference year.

A-5. *PNMR:* The number of deaths of fetus after 28 completed weeks of gestation plus the number of early neonatal deaths per 1,000 live births per year.

A-6.

$$\text{IMR} = \frac{\text{Number of deaths in children} <1 \text{ year of age in a year}}{\text{Total number of live births in a year}} \times 1{,}000$$

A-7. Current IMR of India is 28 (SRS 2020).

A-8. Most common causes of NMR are prematurity, low birth weight, congenital malformations, birth asphyxia, sepsis and birth trauma.

A-9.

$$\text{PMR} = \frac{\text{Number of still births} + \text{Deaths during first week of life in a year}}{\text{Total number of live births per year}} \times 1{,}000$$

A-10.

$$NMR = \frac{\text{Number of death in neonates aged <28 days in a year}}{\text{Total number of live births a year}} \times 1,000$$

A-11. Perinatal and neonatal mortality rates can be used as socioeconomic development and for international comparisons

A-12. Current NMR of India is 20 (SRS 20)

A-13. Current PMR of India is 18 (SRS 20).

QUESTIONS ON PREVENTION AND SOCIAL MEDICINE

Q-1. What color bin should be chosen for following items?

A. Metallic implant
B. Scalpels
C. Blood bag
D. Urine bag
E. Soiled diaper
F. Expired polio vaccine

Q-2. Answer the questions pertaining to 'adoption'

A. Define adoption
B. What is the role of a pediatrician in adoption?

Q-3.

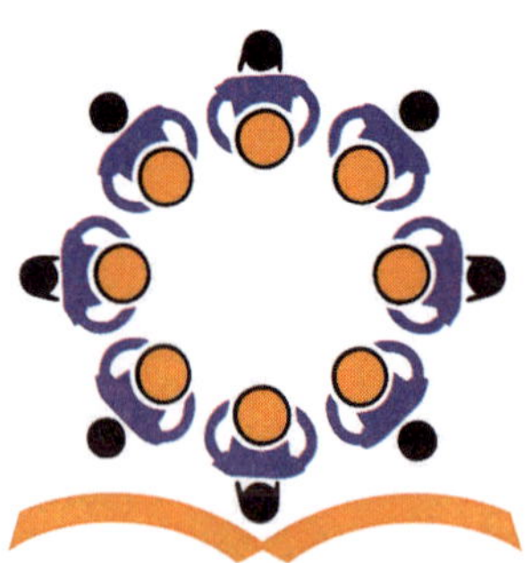

A. Identify the logo.
B. What are the objectives of this program?
C. What are the principles of this program?
D. When was this program launched by Government of India?
E. When was this program renamed? What is renamed program?

Q-4. Answer following questions pertaining to POCSO.

A. What is full form of POCSO?
B. When was it enacted?
C. What is the objective of this act?
D. What is the punishment period as per this act?
E. What is the role of a pediatrician in this act?

Q-5. Answer the questions related to 'DEIC'

A. Full form of DEIC.
B. DEIC comes under which National Program?
C. DEIC supports children under which age group?
D. What is the aim of DEIC?
E. What four DS are targets of DEIC?

Q-6. Answer the questions related to radiation exposure.

A. What is the imaging modality that exposes to maximum radiation in a single procedure?
B. What conditions are associated with exposure to ionizing radiation?
C. What radio pharmaceutical exposure needs discontinuation of breastfeeding?
D. What imaging modalities do not involve ionizing radiation?

Q-7. What are the effects of these chemical substances on children?

A. Tobacco smoke
B. Lead
C. Asbestos

Q-8. A 10-year-old boy was playing in paddy field. After some time, he developed difficulty in speaking, swallowing, lethargy and drooping of eyelids.

A. What is probable diagnosis?
B. What bedside investigation is useful? How will you interpret it?
C. What is the dose of antivenom as per national snake bite protocol?
D. What is the indication to repeat antisnake venom?

Q-9. Answer the questions pertaining to scorpion bite.

A. Describe the gradings of severity of scorpion bite.
B. What are systemic manifestations of scorpion bite?
C. What is initial treatment of scorpion bite?
D. What is the specific treatment of scorpion bite?

ANSWERS

A-1. Color bin for disposal of specific item

A. Blue
B. White
C. Yellow
D. Red
E. Yellow
F. Yellow

A-2. A. Adoption is defined as a legal process of providing a new family for child when birth family desires or unable to parent.
B. A pediatrician should discourage illegal adoption, should perform detailed, comprehensive medical evaluation and support the adopting family.

A-3. A. Mid-Day Meal Scheme
B. Objectives of Mid-Day Meal Program
- To enhance enrollment of children in schools.
- To improve nutritional status of school children

C. Principles of Mid-Day Meal Program
- Should supply one-third of calories and half of the protein required
- It is supplementation and not a substitution

D. 1995
E. Renamed in 2021, as PM POSHAN (Pradhan Mantri Poshan Shakti Nirman)

A-4. A. Protection of Children from Sexual Offences Act
B. 2012
C. To prevent perpetrators and ensuring safe and secured childhood
D. Imprisonment not less than 20 years
E. To examine and to treat the victim, to report to police, to protect privacy of the child

A-5. A. District Early Intervention Center
B. National Health Mission (Rashtriya Bal Swasthya Karyakram)
C. Up to age of 6 years
D. It provides referral support to children detected with health conditions during screening
E.
- Defects at birth
- Deficiencies
- Diseases
- Developmental delays

A-6. A. PET-CT (Position Emission Tomography-Computed Tomography)
B. Conditions associated with exposure to ionizing radiation
- Fanconi syndrome
- Ataxia telangiectasia
- Cokayne syndrome

C. Iodine 131
D. Ultrasonography and MRI have no ionizing radiation

A-7. A. Bronchial asthma
B. Anemia, neurodevelopmental delay and encephalopathy
C. Mesothelioma

A-8. A. Snakebite
B.
- 20 minutes whole blood clotting time is a bedside test in such patients to perform
- Take 2 mL of fresh venous blood in a new, heat-treated glass vial
- Keep it for 20 minutes, undisturbed. If it is not clotted after 20 minutes, it is suggestive of hypofibrinogenemia.

C. 8–10 vials, irrespective of age and weight of the child. It is reconstituted in 5–10 mL/kg of normal saline over 1 hour.
D. Indications to repeat it
- Deteriorating neurotoxicity or CVS signs after 2 hours of ASV dose.
- Delayed clotting screen time after 6 hours of time dose.

A-9. A. *Grade 1:* Isolated pain
Grade 2: Hypertension, sweating, vomiting and priapism
Grade 3: Cardiogenic shock and pulmonary edema
Grade 4: Tachycardia hypotension and pulmonary edema
B. *Systemic manifestations*
- Pulmonary edema
- Acute renal failure
- Liver necrosis
- Pancreatitis

C. Initial management
- *Symptomatic*
  - Paracetamol 15 mg/kg
  - Ice packs and xylocaine
  - Midazolam
- Hemodynamic monitoring

D. Specific management
Prazosin 30 μg/kg/dose. Repeat prazosin after 3 hours of first dose as clinical response.

SECTION 2

Spotters Diagnosis

CHAPTER 27

Down Syndrome

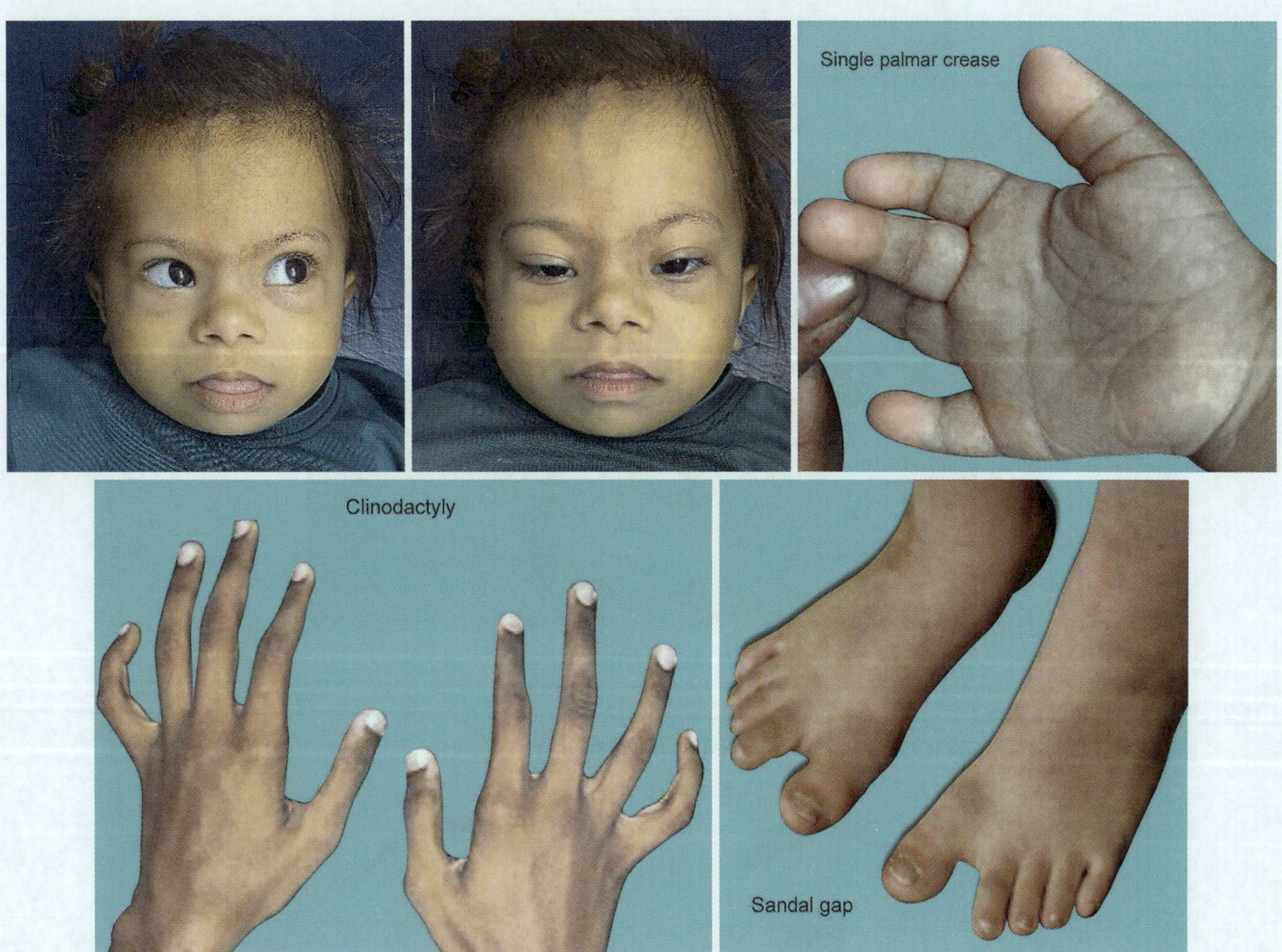

QUESTIONS AND ANSWERS

Q-1. What is hypertelorism?

- Increased distance between two body parts or organs, e.g., eyes, kidneys, nipples. Commonly used for eyes—orbital hypertelorism.
- The distance between two medial canthi measured at the level of posterior lacrimal crest is known as inner canthal distance (ICD).
- The outer canthal distance (OCD) is distance between two lateral canthi.

- The distance between two mid-pupillary regions in the front gaze is called as inter pupillary distance (IPD).
- The Palpebral fissure length (PFL) is the distance between the medial and lateral canthi.
- *Orbital hypertelorism:* Increased ICD, OCD and IPD. Normal PFL **(Figs. 1 and 2)**.

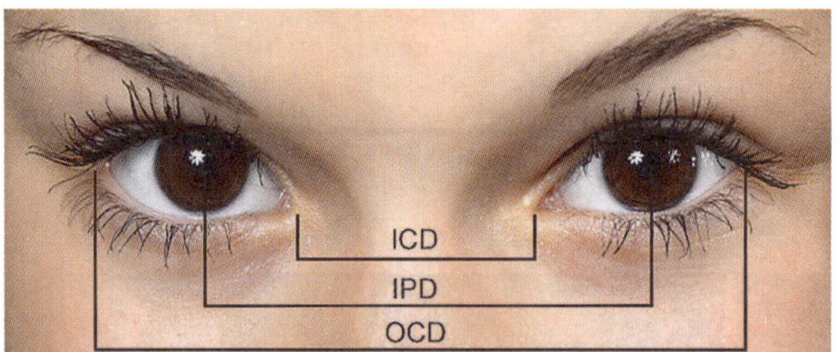

Fig. 1: Measurement of ICD, IPD and OCD.

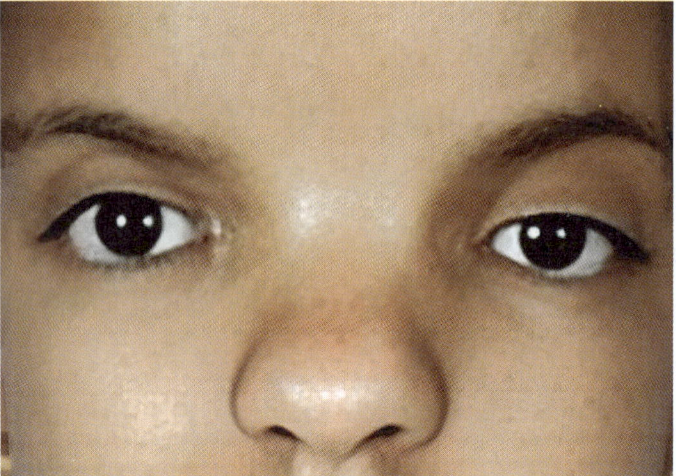

Fig. 2: Hypertelorism.

Q-2. What is telecanthus?

Increased ICD, normal OCD and IPD, but smaller PFD **(Fig. 3)**

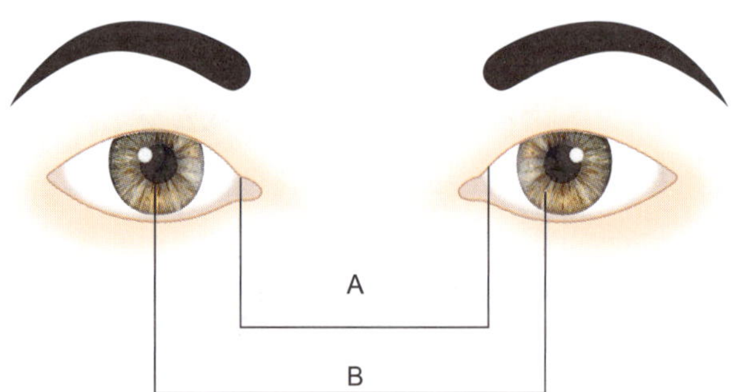

Fig. 3: Telecanthus.

Q-3. What is epicanthal fold?

A skin fold of the upper eyelid covering the inner corner of the eye is called as epicanthal fold **(Fig. 4)**.

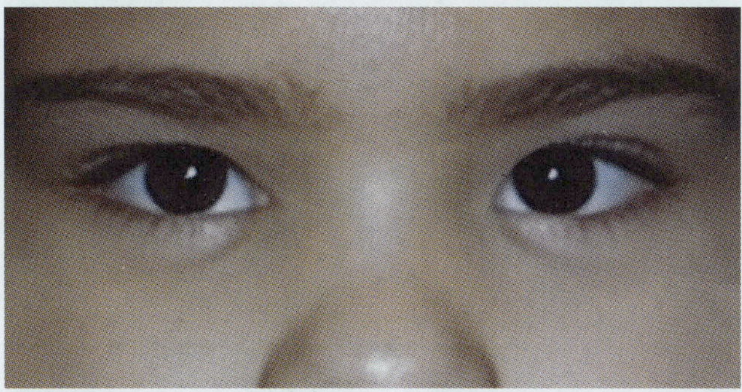

Fig. 4: Epicanthal fold.

Q-4. What is long philtrum?

- Length of philtrum >13 mm in a female.
- Length of philtrum >15 mm in a male **(Fig. 5)**

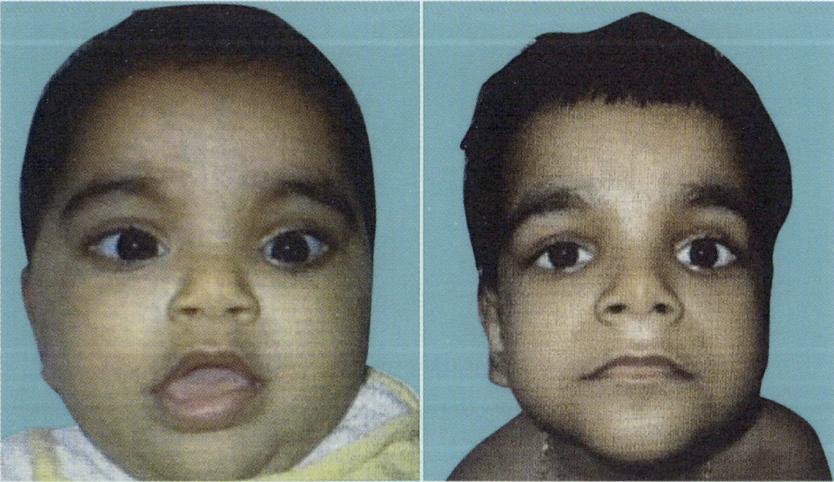

Fig. 5: Long philtrum.

Q-5. What is slanting of eyes?

- A line drawn from the inner corners to the outer corners determines the slant of eyes.
- *Upward slanting of eyes:* Down syndrome **(Fig. 6)**
- *Downward slanting of eyes:* Soto syndrome.

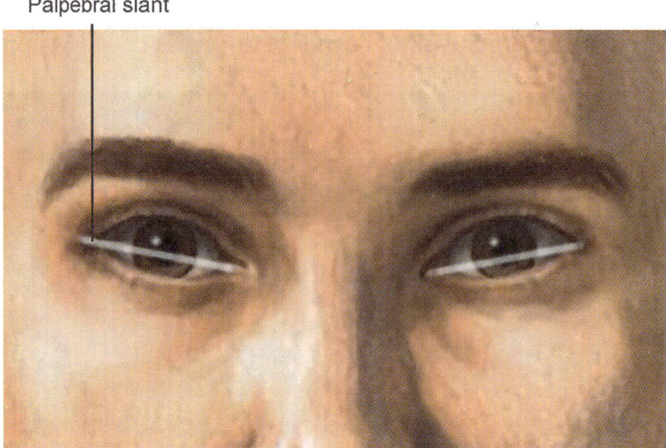

Fig. 6: Upward slanting of eyes.

Q-6. What is low set ears?

The ear is low set when the helix of ear meets the cranium at the level below a horizontal plane through both inner canthi **(Fig. 7)**.

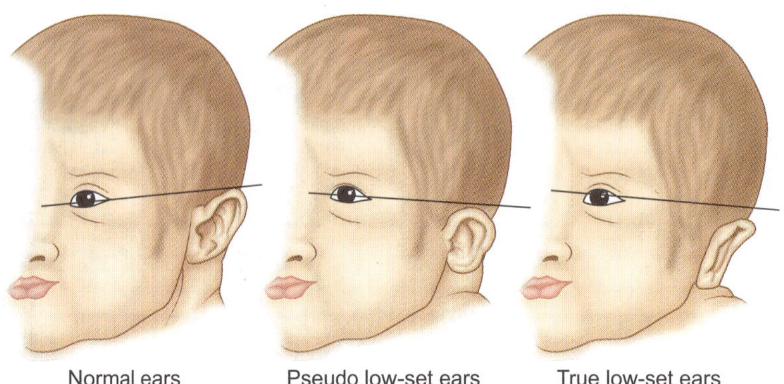

Fig. 7: Low set ears.

Q-7. What is cephalic Index?

$$\frac{\text{Maximum breath}}{\text{Maximum length}} \times 100$$

- <76 → Dolichocephaly (scaphocephaly)
- 7–80 → Mesocephaly
- >80 → Brachycephaly

Q-8. What is Mongolism?

- Mongolism and Mongoloid are other terms used for Down syndrome.
- Mongolian is for specific race. Chinese, Japanese and Korean are mongoloids.
- Now, Mongolism and Mongoloid like terms are not used for Down syndrome.

Q-9. What is the relation between maternal age and Down syndrome?

Down syndrome is classically associated with increased maternal age. However, Down syndrome due to fusion of 21st and 22nd chromosome is associated with increased paternal age also.

Maternal age (years)	*Risk of Down syndrome*
30	1:1,000
35	1:350
40	1:100
45	1:50

Q-10. What is nondisjunction?

- Nondisjunction is characterized by an extra chromosome from faulty cell division during meiosis.
- 75% maternal origin.
- 25% paternal origin.

Q-11. What is translocation?

Transfer of all or a segment of a chromosome from one chromosome to another nonhomologous chromosome.

- *Balanced translocation:* A full complement of genetic material is transferred. No loss or gain of genetic material. No abnormalities in the carrier. Offspring may inherit an unbalanced translocation.
- *Unbalanced translocation:* Full complement of genetic material not present, only acrocentric chromosome involved. Leads to translocation Down syndrome, spontaneous abortions, etc.

Q-12. What is mosaic Down syndrome?

- Seen in <1% Down syndrome.
- Cells with trisomy 21 and normal karyotype are seen.
- Milder clinical features.

Q-13. What are the mechanisms of Down syndrome?

- 95% due to meiotic nondisjunction.
- 4% due to Robertsonian translocation—the extra chromosome is not free but translocated to chromosome 14 and rarely to 22/21.
- 1% due to mosaicism.

Q-14. Is Down syndrome inherited?

No, Down syndrome is chromosomal disorder and not inherited. But, yes, if parents are translocation carrier.

Q-15. What are Hall's criteria for diagnosis of Down syndrome?

In 1996, Hall described the clinical criteria which helps to diagnose Down syndrome in neonates. At least 4 of these abnormalities may be seen in all neonates with Down syndrome and 6 or more in 90% of them.

- Flat facies 90%
- Sluggish Moro reflex 85%
- Hyperextensible joints 80%
- Excess skin folds in nape of neck 80%
- Hypotonia 80%
- Upward slant of eyes 80%
- Dysplastic pelvis 70%
- Clinodactyly 60%
- Ear anomalies 60%
- Simian crease 50%

Q-16. What are gastrointestinal manifestations of Down syndrome?

- Esophageal atresia
- Duodenal atresia

- Annular pancreas
- Hirschsprung's disease
- Imperforate anus
- Meckel's diverticulum

Q-17. In which chromosomal anomaly is Meckel's diverticulum seen?

Down syndrome.

Q-18. What cardiac anomalies are known in Down syndrome?

- Endocardial cushion defect
- VSD
- PDA
- Auricular ASD
- Aberrant subclavian artery
- MVP, TVP, AR are seen after the age of 20 years.

Q-19. What are the neurological features of Down syndrome?

- Intellectual disability
- Hypotonia
- Alzheimer's disease after 30 years
- Reactive depression in adolescents and young adults.
- Autistic behavior.

Q-20. What are the manifestations of Down syndrome in the extremities?

- Short broad hands and fingers
- Simian crease
- Clinodactyly (Siegert sign)
- Large ATD angle (due to distal position of palmar axial tri radius).
- Ulnar loops in all digits.
- Sandle sign (Goldstein sign)—increased gap between first and second toe.
- Kennedy crease (deep vertical crease between first and second toes).

Q-21. What are the effects on dentition in a child with Down syndrome?

- Hypoplasia
- Irregular placement
- Dental carries

Q.22. What causes are possible for prolonged jaundice in Down syndrome?

- Annular pancreas
- Hypothyroidism
- Constipation (increased enterohepatic circulation)

Q-23. What are the hematological manifestations of Down syndrome?

- Acute leukemia (AML and ALL)
- Juvenile chronic myeloid leukemia
- Myeloproliferative disorders
- Congenital thrombocytopenia

Q-24. What are endocranial manifestations of Down syndrome?

- Hypothyroidism (TSH should be done at birth, yearly for 3 years and at puberty).
- Girls may menstruate and may be fertile.
- Boys are sterile.

Q-25. What are the ocular manifestations of Down syndrome?

- Small—almond-shaped eyes
- Upward slanting of eyes (mongoloid slant).
- Myopia
- Squint
- Cataract
- Brush field spots
- Glaucoma
- Refractive errors

Q-26. What is the importance of atlanto-occipital dislocation in Down syndrome?

- *Incidence:* 10 to 30%
- Due to laxity of ligaments around C_1 and C_2
- Features of spinal cord compression.
- Take lateral neck X-ray every 3–5 years
- Atlantodens interval >5 mm is significant.

Q-27. What is the risk of recurrence of Down syndrome?

- Advanced maternal age (>35 years)
- If parents have a child with Down syndrome
- If one of the parents is a translocation carrier.
- Rarely, normal parents may have two or more children affected with trisomy 21. In such cases, gonadal mosaicism should be suspected as the cause for recurrence of the disease in the family.

Q-28. Is there any fertility issue with Down syndrome?

- Girls menstruate, fertility is reported.
- Males are always sterile.

Q-29. What are the indications of prenatal diagnosis of Down syndrome?

- Maternal age >35 years.
- Previous child with Down syndrome.
- Translocation carrier status of parents.

Q-30. What are the advantages of chorionic villus sampling (CVS) over amniocentesis?

- In CVS, chorionic villi are aspirated via transcervical catheter or transabdominal needle under USG guidance.
- Done at 10–12 weeks of gestation (16 weeks amniocentesis). Hence, gives sufficient time to terminate pregnancy, if indicated.
- Amniotic fluid AFP cannot be performed.

Q-31. What are the indications for amniocentesis?

- Advanced maternal age (>35 years).
- Previous child with cytogenic abnormality
- First degree relative with neural tube defect.

The optimum time for amniocentesis is 16–18 weeks of gestation. Diseases like Down syndrome, fragile X syndrome or any chromosomal abnormality can be predetermined by this method. The risk of fetal loss is 1–1.5%.

Q-32. What is PUBS?

- PUBS → Percutaneous umbilical cord blood sampling (cordocentesis).

- The site for needle insertion into the placenta is determined by USG and the needle-guided through the mother's abdomen and uterine wall into the fetal vein of the umbilical cord, where fetal blood sample is obtained.
- Demerits of PUBS
  - Can be done at 18 weeks of pregnancy or later.
  - More invasive.
  - May cause complications like bleeding at the site of puncture, infection and premature rupture of membrane.
  - Higher rate of fetal loss than amniocentesis.

Q-33. What are the first trimester screening tests for Down syndrome?

- Biochemical markers
  - Free β-hCG
  - Pregnancy associated plasma protein A (PAPPA) (2.5 times lower in DS pregnancies).
- *Fetal ultrasound marker:* Nuchal translucency thickness measured in the sagittal plane between 10 and 13 gestational weeks. It is 2 times more than normal.

Q-34. What are the biochemical markers of Down syndrome?

Alpha fetoprotein	Decreased
Human chorionic gonadotropin	Increased
Unconjugated estriol	Decreased
Inhibin A	Increased
PAPPA	Decreased
Uman placental lactogen	Increased

Q-35. What are the new biochemical markers for Down syndrome?

- ADAM-12 (a disintegrin and metalloprotease): Reduced.
- Pregnancy-specific beta 1 glycoprotein.
- Invasive trophoblastic antigen (ITA).
- Highly glycosylated form of hCG.

Q-36. What are the sonographic features associated with fetal Down syndrome?

Major anomalies	***Markers***
• Cardiac defects • Duodenal atresia • Ventriculomegaly • Hydrops	• Nuchal thickening • Hyperechoic bowel • Echogenic focus in heart • Pyelectasia • Choroid plexus cysts • Short frontal bone • Clinodactyly • Short limbs • Hypoplastic/absent nasal bone • Widened Sandal gap

Q-37. What is triple test?

- Also known as Bart test or Kettering test.
- Maternal markers done at 16 weeks.
- Low alpha-fetoprotein.

- Low unconjugated estriol.
- High hCG.
  It helps to detect 60% of all Down syndrome pregnancies.

Q.38. What is quadruple test?

- Triple test + inhibin A
- Inhibin A is increased
- It help to detect 75% of Down syndrome

Q-39. What is integrated test?

- Assessment of serum PAPP-A and nuchal translucency in the first trimester.
  and
  Measurement of serum alpha-fetoprotein, unconjugated estriol, hCG and Inhibin A in the second trimester.
- Integrated test has a detection rate of 80–85%.
- False-positive rate of 5%.

Q-40. What are important aspects of management of a child with Down syndrome?

- Neurodevelopmental patterning
- Special schooling
- Vocational rehabilitation
- Friendly-fond of music and dance
- Management of cardiac problems
- Screening for hypothyroidism, celiac disease, leukemia
- Atlanto-occipital dislocation.

Q-41. What is natural history of Down syndrome?

- Muscle tone tends to improve with the age.
- Rate of development slows down with age.
- Social performance is better compared to other milestones.
- They are good babies, happy children, enjoy mimicry, music and dance.
- *Cause of mortality:* CHD, LRTI
- Life expectancy may be 50 to 60 years
- May be carrier for hepatitis B surface antigen.

Q-42. When World Down Syndrome Day is celebrated?

- On 21st March since 2012.
- 21st March is selected as there is trisomy of 21 chromosome in Down syndrome (triplication of 21 → 21/3).

CHAPTER 28

Hydrocephalus

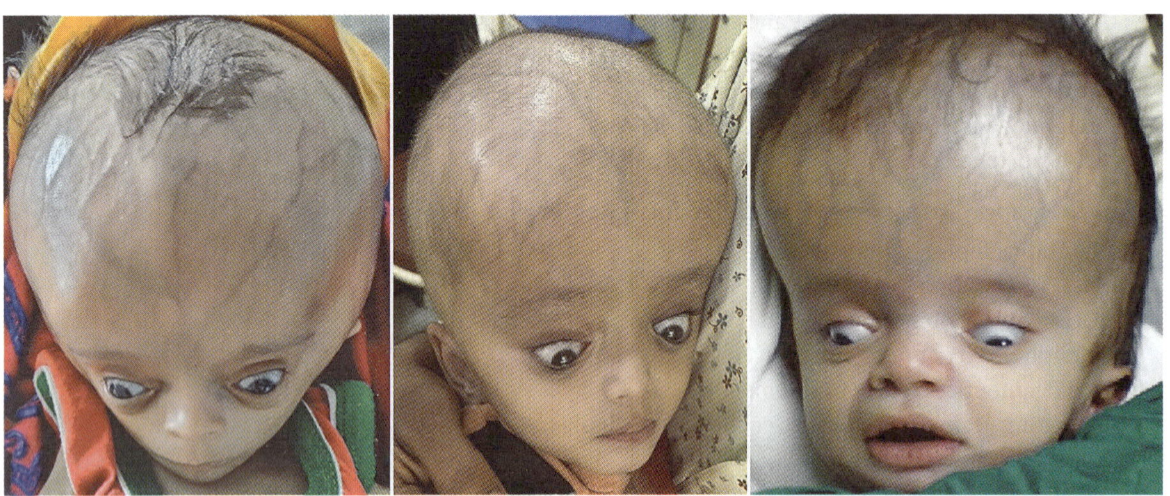

QUESTIONS AND ANSWERS

Q-1. What is your spot diagnosis?

Hydrocephalus.

Q-2. What points are favoring for hydrocephalus?

- Large head
- Failure of upward gaze
- Sunsetting sign
- Dilated scalp veins
- Tense anterior fontanelle

Q-3. What is the definition of hydrocephalus?

Abnormal excessive accumulation of CSF in the brain, leading to raised intracranial pressure and pathological dilatation of cerebral ventricles.

Q-4. What is the classification of hydrocephalus?

- Congenital/acquired
- Obstructive (noncommunicating)/nonobstructive (communicating)

Q-5. Anatomical and physiological points on CSF and cerebral ventricular system.

- Normal CSF production is 20 mL/h (0.35 mL/min)
- Total CSF volume is 150 mL in adults and 50 mL in infants
- Capacity of lateral and third ventricle is 20 mL

- Length of Aqueduct of Sylvius is 8–12 mm (3 mm long and 2 mm in diameter in a child)
- CSF is produced by choroid plexus in the ventricles. CSF flows from the lateral ventricles through the foramen of Monro to the third ventricle, then through aqueduct of Sylvius to the fourth ventricle. From the fourth ventricle, CSF exits through the median aperture—foramen of Megendie and lateral aperture—foramina of Luschka into the subarachnoid space, which surrounds brain and spinal cord.

Q-6. What are the causes of hydrocephalus?

Congenital hydrocephalus	*Acquired hydrocephalus*
• Aqueductal stenosis • Arnold Chiari malformation • Dandy-Walker syndrome • Vein of Galen malformation • Intrauterine infections • Benign intracranial cyst • Hydranencephaly • Achondroplasia	• Meningitis • TBM with defective absorption of CSF • Posterior fossa tumors • Intracranial hemorrhage • Head injury • Choroid plexus papilloma • Inflammation (sarcoidosis) • Third ventricular cyst • Pineal tumor • Arachnoid cyst

Q-7. What are the clinical features of hydrocephalus?

	History	*Examination*
Infants	• Projectile vomiting without nausea and salivation • Irritability/lethargy/drowsiness • Altered sensorium • Poor feeding • Failure to thrive • Progressive increase in head size • Impairment of eye movements • Seizures	• Abnormal excessive head circumference • Failure of upward gaze • Sun setting sign • Dilated scalp veins • Bulging of anterior fontanelle • Hypertonia
Children after AF closure	• Headache • Vomiting • Irritability • Drowsiness • Blurred vision • Double vision • Loss of bladder control • Changes in personality and memory	• Cranial nerves palsy • VI nerve palsy (False localizing sign) • Failure of upward gaze • Bradycardia • Apnea • Papilledema • Unsteady gait and difficulty in walking?

Q-8. What are the clinical manifestations of acute hydrocephalus?

- Headache
- Vomiting
- Papilledema
- Respiratory difficulties (Cheyne-stoke breathing)
- Full, wide, tense anterior fontanelle
- Irritability, lack of interest
- Decerebration and decortication
- Altered sensorium—loss of consciousness

Q-9. What are the clinical manifestations of chronic hydrocephalus?

- Enlarged head
- Cracked pot sound (McEwan sign)
- Restricted upward gaze
- Visible scalp veins
- Sutural diastasis
- Impaired mentation
- Seizures
- False localizing sign (6th nerve palsy)
- Bradycardia
- Hypertension
- Cardiac arrhythmias

Q-10. What is the mechanism of sun-setting sign?

There is dilatation of supra pineal recess in a case of hydrocephalus. Dilated supra pineal recess compresses the quadrigeminal plate which is the nucleus for upward gaze. Due to compression over quadrigeminal plate there is loss of upward gaze resulting in sun setting sign.

Q-11. Why the scalp veins become prominent and visible in hydrocephalus?

The scalp veins become dilated due to raised intracranial pressure. Also the scalp becomes thin and shining in hydrocephalus. Dilated scalp veins become prominent and visible through thin scalp.

Q-12. Why is there unsteady gait and difficulty in walking in older children with hydrocephalus?

There is limb spasticity and difficulty in walking with unsteady gait due to stretching of pyramidal and periventricular tract fibers. On examination, there may be hypertonia, exaggerated deep tendon reflexes and extensor planter reflex.

Q-13. What conditions may have loss of upward gaze?

- Hydrocephalus
- Tumor in the pineal region
- Damage to dorsal midbrain
- Trauma
- Niemann-Pick disease

Q-14. Common causes of large head

- Familial macrocephaly
- Hydrocephalus
- Rickets
- Hemolytic anemia
- Subdural effusion
- Megalencephaly
- Hydranencephaly
- Achondroplasia

Q-15. At what age cracked-pot sign (Macewen sign) can be elicited as reliable sign of raised intracranial pressure?

- Between 2 and 18 years of age
- Less than 2 years, AF and sutures are open, therefore cracked pot sign can be present normally.
- Up to 18 years of age, there is fibrous closure of the sutures, can open up due to raised intracranial pressure and cracked-pot sign is positive. There is osseous closure of the sutures at the age of 18 years and therefore, cannot open up in spite of raised intracranial pressure.

Therefore, presence of cracked-pot sign (Macewen sign) between 2 and 18 years of age is suggesting raised intracranial pressure.

Q-16. Why is there bradycardia in hydrocephalus?

Due to raised intracranial pressure in a case of hydrocephalus, there is stretching of vagus nerve, causing vagal stimulation and bradycardia.

Q-17. What is the pathophysiology of posthemorrhagic hydrocephalus in preterm babies?

There is fibrosing arachnoiditis, meningeal fibrosis and subependymal gliosis as sequelae of intraventricular and germinal matrix hemorrhage. These changes result in impaired absorption and physiology of CSF flow, resulting in hydrocephalus.

Q-18. What clinical parameter should be monitored on follow-up of high-risk neonates and infants for early detection of hydrocephalus?

- Accurate serial measuring and recording head circumference is essential for early detection of hydrocephalus in this group.
- Normal rate of growth of head circumference in infants:
  - *At birth:* 33–35 cm
  - Head circumference increases 2 cm per month for first 3 months, 1 cm per month between 3 and 6 months, 0.5 cm per month from 6 to 12 months of age.
- If head circumference increases, >1 cm every fortnight in first 3 months of age, suspect hydrocephalus.
- Persistent widening of squamoparietal sutures after 15 days of life, should be considered unusual and be vigilant for hydrocephalus.

Q-19. What is pathophysiology of communicating (nonobstructive) hydrocephalus?

There is no obvious block in the CSF pathway and it is mainly because of impairment of absorption by subarachnoid villi. It is common following subarachnoid hemorrhage and meningitis due to blunting of villi as a sequelae of inflammation. Blunting of subarachnoid villi results in impairment of CSF absorption.

Q-20. What investigations should be performed in a case of hydrocephalus?

- *X-ray skull:* Limited value. Suture widening, erosion of posterior clinoid, silver beaten appearance and ballooning of sella turcica can be the evidences of chronic raised ICP.
- *Ultrasonography (USG):* USG through anterior fontanelle can demonstrate ventricular enlargement in infants. It is the procedure of choice for imaging fetal brain. It is not the best modality to identify lesions in the posterior fossa. It can easily identify hemorrhage and serve as a tool for serial monitoring of the ventricular dimensions.
- *CT head:* It provides adequate information about etiology and type of hydrocephalus. In obstructive hydrocephalus, both lateral and third ventricles are dilated. In communicating hydrocephalus, there is generalized enlargement of ventricles. In addition, there will be presence of CSF in subarachnoid spaces, as there is defective absorption of CSF. The normal bifrontal width of lateral ventricle is on average of 30% of brain width at this level. When this ratio (Evans ratio) is >30%, it is suggestive of hydrocephalus.
- *MRI brain:* MRI brain is considered as gold standard in the diagnosis and surgical planning of the hydrocephalus. It shows the extent of dilatation of ventricle site and nature of block. MRI brain gives better details of the posterior fossa lesion when compared to a CT scan. MRI brain can reveal dilated lateral and third ventricle among those with aqueduct stenosis.

Q-21. What is the medical treatment of hydrocephalus?

- Acetazolamide (Diamox), a carbonic anhydrase inhibitor reduces the CSF production. The dose is 25 mg/kg/day in divided doses, can be increased up to 100 mg/kg/day with strict watch on electrolytes and ABG.
- Frusemide 0.5 mg/kg.

- Mannitol 0.25 to 0.5 G/kg 6 hourly
- Dexamethasone 0.15 mg/kg 6 hourly can be used for a short time in postinfective hydrocephalus.
- Hypertonic saline (3% Nacl) 3 to 5 mL/kg
- *Oral glycerol:* 1.5 g/kg every 6 hourly.

Q-22. What is surgical treatment of hydrocephalus?

- *Lumbar drainage:* Tapping of CSF from spinal subarachnoid space can help in reducing intracranial pressure in communicating hydrocephalus. Post- tapping headache and tonsillar herniation are known complications of this procedure.
- *Ventriculoperitoneal shunt (VP shunt):* Most accepted procedure in treatment of hydrocephalus is ventriculoperitoneal shunt. The peritoneal end can be inserted in peritoneal cavity. The most commonly used VP shunts are Chhabra, Upadhyay and currently flow regulated shunt devices that sense flow through a magnetic strip. The CSF from the ventricle is drained via a silicon tube into abdomen. A subcutaneous tunnel carries the shunt from the ventricle to peritoneum. The known complications associated with VP shunt are infection, shunt obstruction, migration, bleeding, ascites and subdural effusion. The success rate of VP shunt is 70–90%.
- *Ventriculoatrial shunt (VA shunt):* Ventriculoatrial shunt is performed in the children with abdominal disease. VA shunt can lead to glomerulonephritis and endocarditis.
- *Endoscopic third ventriculostomy (ETV):* Endoscopic third ventriculostomy is an excellent minimally invasive procedure for hydrocephalus in which internal shunting is done within ventricular system. An osteotomy is made along the floor of third ventricle which drains CSF in prepontine cistern, by passing aqueduct of Sylvius obstruction. The success rate is 70–90% depending upon the cause of hydrocephalus. Rescue ETV is indicated in repeated shunt failure. The complication rate is 8–10%. The fatal complications are rate but can happen with rupture of basilar artery or its branch. Damage to fornix, thalamus, septal and thalamostriate vein can result during surgery and may cause neurological deficit.

Q-23. What are other types of hydrocephalus?

- *External hydrocephalus—Benign Hydrocephalus (BEH):* BEH is a condition in infants characterized by a rapid increase in head circumference, often associated with enlarged subarachnoid spaces on neuroimaging. There may be normal or mildly enlarged ventricles.
  Most children with BEH experience normal development with the condition typically resolving or stabilizing withing first few years of life.
- *Normal pressure hydrocephalus (NPH):* NPH is a rare condition with excess CSF builds up in the ventricles of the brain, disrupting brain function. The fluid pressure is usually normal. It can cause problems with walking, bladder control, thinking and reasoning. It can worsen, if left untreated.
- *Arrested hydrocephalus (static or chronic hydrocephalus):* Arrested hydrocephalus occurs when the progression of hydrocephalus is halted and the condition of the child stabilizes. It can happen spontaneously or after treatment, with a new balance achieved between CSF production and absorption, normal intracranial pressure and minimal neurological issues.
- *Hydrocephalus ex vacuo:* It is unilateral dilatation of lateral ventricle due to cortical atrophy. It occurs following brain damage often from stroke, injury or neurodegenerative diseases. There is shrinkage of brain tissues, leading to an apparent enlargement of the ventricle. This is not truly hydrocephalus, but rather a compensatory change where the shrinking brain tissue creates more space that is occupied by CSF.
- *Hydranencephaly:* It is a condition in which the hemisphere of brain are absent to a great degree and the cranial cavity is filled up with CSF.

Q-24. What is pathophysiology of papilledema development in hydrocephalus?

CSF is absorbed by optic nerve roots which causes enlargement of optic nerve sheaths, resulting in development of papilledema.

Q-25. What is Omaya reservoir and its utility in hydrocephalus?

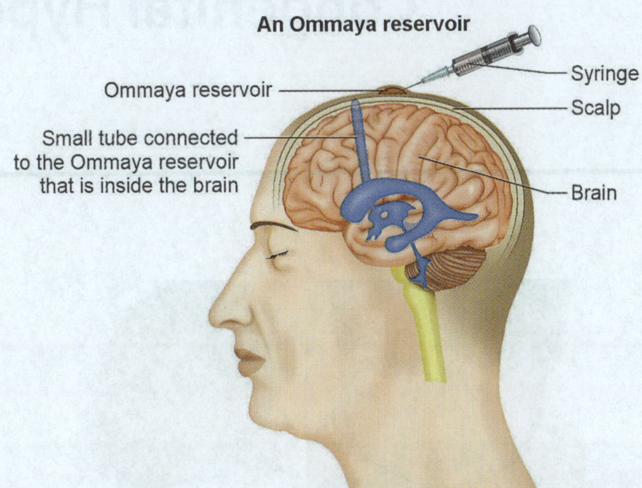

Ommaya reservoir is a ventricular access device with an intraventricular catheter system for the purpose of chronic access to the intrathecal space. Ommaya reservoir is a highly effective implant that provides long term access to the CSF and has simplified administration of antibiotics, antifungals, antineoplastic drugs directly into the brain. This device is named after its inventor, a Pakistani neurosurgeon Ayub Khan Ommaya in 1963.

Indications

- Administration of intrathecal chemotherapeutic agents for intracranial neoplasms as well as hematological conditions with CNS involvement as in ALL.
- Administration of Intrathecal antibiotics, for chronic relapsing meningitis and MDR CNS infections
- Chronic drainage of CSF for infants with intraventricular hemorrhage.
- Chronic aspiration of fluid from tumor cysts not amenable to treatment such as craniopharyngiomas.
- Aspiration of subdural hematoma or effusion.

Contraindications

- Scalp infection
- Brain abscess

Complications

- Infection
- Suboptimal position
- Subdural hematoma or subdural hygroma
- Mechanical failure of device

CHAPTER

29 Congenital Hypothyroidism

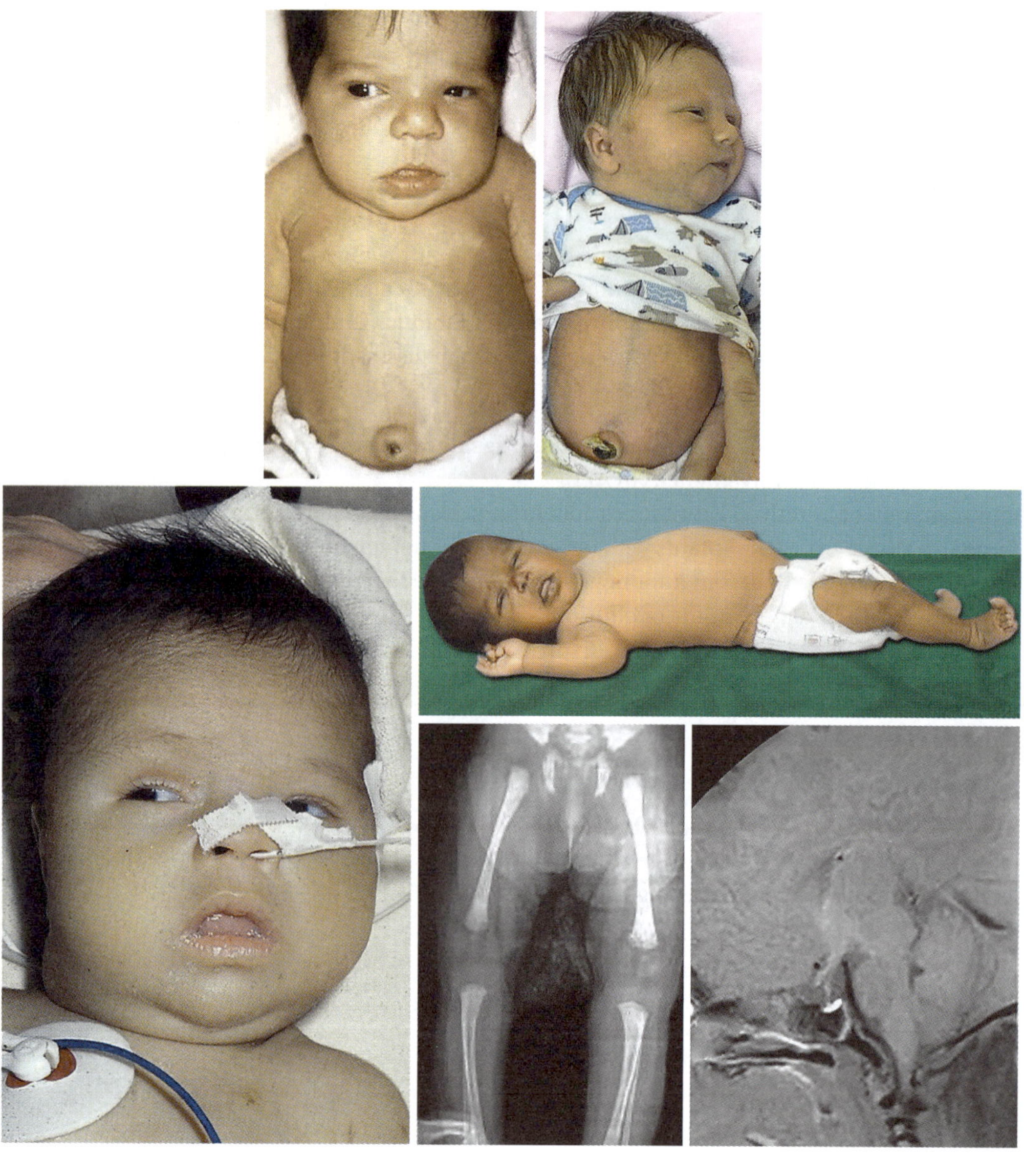

QUESTIONS AND ANSWERS

Q-1. What is the spot diagnosis?

Congenital hypothyroidism (CH) (Cretinism)

Q-2. What are the causes of congenital hypothyroidism?

- *Dysgenesis*
  - Agenesis of thyroid
  - Hypoplastic thyroid
  - Ectopic thyroid
- *Dysmorphogenesis*
  - Organification defect
  - Iodide trapping defect
  - TSH unresponsiveness
  - Defective thyroglobulin synthesis
  - Iodotyrosine deiodinase deficiency
- *Central hypothyroidism*
  - Panhypopituitarism
  - Hypothalamic-pituitary anomalies
  - Isolated TSH deficiency
- *Drug-induced*
  - Antithyroid drugs
  - Iodine
  - Maternal antibody-induced

Q-3. What are the clinical features of congenital hypothyroidism?

- Large for date
- Postmaturity
- Edematous face
- Wide fontanels
- Persistent open posterior fontanelle
- Rough, dry skin
- Large abdomen
- Umbilical hernia
- Constipation
- Large tongue
- Feeding/Sucking/Difficulty/Chocking spells
- Pallor
- Hypothermia
- Prolonged physiological jaundice (UDGT activity is diminished due to paucity of thyroxine)
- Hoarse cry
- Hypotonia
- Excessive sleepiness
- Delayed development
- Associated congenital anomalies
  - Congenital heart disease
  - Chromosomal disorder

- Microcephaly
- Club foot
- Subluxation of the hip

Q-4. What maternal factors can cause transient hypothyroidism in the infant?

- Iodine deficiency in the mother
- If mother is hypothyroid, the infant may have severe hypothyroidism at birth as the placental transfer of thyroxine is minimal in this situation

Q-5. What are normal thyroid hormone values in the newborn period? What will be thyroid hormone status in CH?

Age	TSH (ICMA) mIU/L	T_4 (RIA) µg/dL
Preterm (28–36 weeks of gestation) First week of life	0.7–27	4–17.4
Cord blood (≥37 weeks of gestation)	2.3–13.2	5.9–15
Birth to 4 days	1–38.9	14–28.4
2–20 weeks	1.7–9.1	8.1–15.7
21 weeks–20 years	0.7–6.4	5.6–14.9

- Newborn physiological TSH surge occurs half an hour after birth and lasts about 2 to 4 days.
- Thyroid function tests should be interpreted specifically for the age of the child and should include either serum free T_4 or total T_4 and TSH.
- T_3 estimation is not useful as it may often be normal in CH.
- Low serum total or free T_4 concentration with markedly elevated serum TSH level are seen in nearly all cases of CH except central hypothyroidism, where in low serum total or free T_4 are seen along with low or normal serum TSH. It will need to be distinguished from thyroxine binding globulin (TBG) deficiency.

Q-6. What radiographs will be useful in diagnosis of CH?

Radiographs of both knees will show absence or small size of lower femoral and/or upper tibial epiphyses.

Q-7. What is the role of thyroid nuclear imaging in diagnosis of CH?

Thyroid nuclear imaging is useful to decipher the etiology of CH and helps in convincing the parents regarding the permanent nature of the condition and the need for lifelong therapy. CT scan provides anatomical details of the thyroid. When nuclear scan is not available readily, therapy with thyroxine should never be delayed.

Q-8. Is there any role of ultrasonography in diagnosis of CH?

Thyroid ultrasonography is useful to delineate the presence of the thyroid when it is not demonstrate on nuclear scan because of poor tracer uptake caused by maternal thyroid antibodies or antithyroid drug therapy.

Q-9. What is the treatment of CH?

- Levothyroxine tablet in dose of 10–15 µg/kg/day once daily for newborns.
- The tablet is crushed and mixed with a small quantity of water or expressed breast milk and administered with a spoon or dropper ensuring all the particles are given entirely, preferably on an empty stomach.
- Thyroxine is unstable in suspension form.
- The parents should be educated for daily regular therapy for life long. Dosage adjustment will be required on follow-up.
- Repeat thyroid function tests a month after commencing the therapy and subsequently once in 3–6 months.
- Monitoring the growth and development at regular interval is essential.

- Ectopic thyroid should never be removed.
- If thyroxine had been commenced on purely clinical grounds without confirming the cause, thyroxine may be stopped after 4–6 weeks after the age of 3 years to establish the permanent nature of hypothyroidism.

Q-10. What is the prognosis of CH?

Early initiation of thyroxine therapy for permanent hypothyroidism will lead to acquisition of normal academic skills and these children will compare well with their unaffected peers.

Q-11. What is newborn screening for hypothyroidism?

Screening is defined as identification of unrecognized disease or defects by rapidly applied tests in apparently healthy individuals on a large scale. Newborn screening (NBS) is the practice of screening newborn shortly after birth for potentially fatal disorders that are treatable, but difficult or impossible to detect clinically. Newborn screening is available for few disorders like CH that are important public health problems with facilities for diagnosis available. It has a latent period for disease manifestation that bears long term consequences on growth and development, and an effective treatment is available that improves survival of the affected babies.

Newborns screening is offered to all babies at birth through simple tests conducted on cord blood or a drop of blood collected from heel-prick of the baby on a filter paper. The filter paper requires special equipment for measurement of the analytes. NBS for CH is available in few state government programs in India.

Q-12. What is the interpretation of NBS for CH?

- A TSH surge occurs in all babies after birth, hence TSH levels are elevated in first 24–48 hours. Therefore, the ideal time to obtain the blood spot is from placental end of umbilical cord, immediately after birth or in the postnatal period after 48–72 hours of birth to minimize the chances of false-positive TSH surge.
- An elevated TSH on cord blood or blood spot needs to be confirmed on a venous sample before informing the family of a confirmed diagnosis of CH.
- In babies with TSH >80 mIU/mL, the diagnosis of CH is almost confirmed. In such babies, thyroxine should be started immediately without waiting for confirmatory venous sample.

Chapter 30 Acquired Hypothyroidism

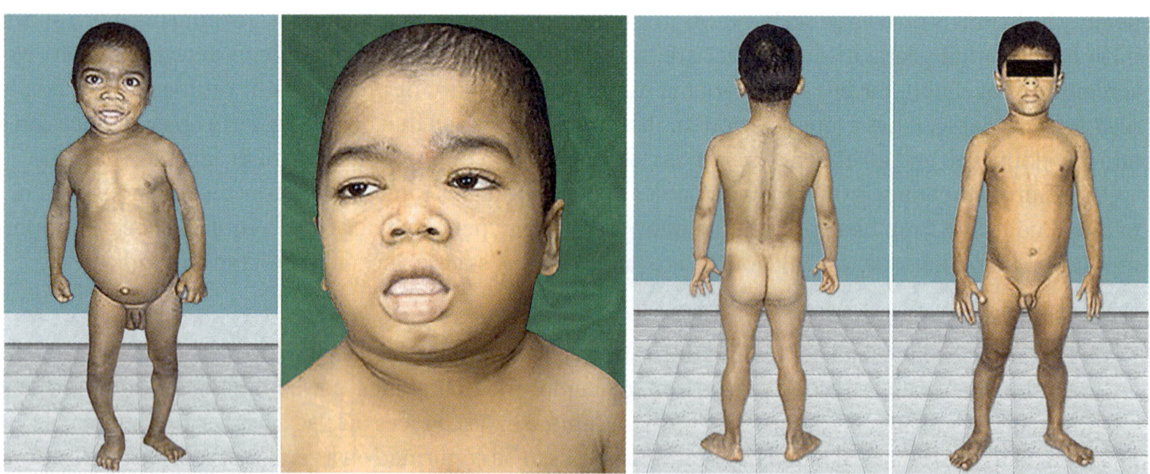

QUESTIONS AND ANSWERS

Q-1. What is acquired hypothyroidism?

Childhood hypothyroidism with onset after 6 months of age is also known as acquired hypothyroidism and may be primary (at level of thyroid gland), secondary (at pituitary level) or tertiary (at level of hypothalamus)

Q-2. What are the causes of acquired hypothyroidism in children?

- *Primary hypothyroidism*
  - Hashimoto thyroiditis (chronic lymphocytic)
  - Chromosomal and other disorders associated with autoimmune thyroiditis
  - Late onset CH
    - Thyroid dysgenesis
    - Thyroid dyshormonogenesis
  - Drugs
    - Anticonvulsants
    - Lithium
    - Antithyroid drugs
  - Infection
  - Infiltration
  - Iodine deficiency
- *Secondary/tertiary hypothyroidism*
  - Craniopharyngioma
  - Tumors compressing pituitary/hypothalamus

- Neurosurgery
- Cranial irradiation
- Head trauma
- *Thyroid hormone resistance*

Q-3. What conditions are associated with autoimmune thyroid disease?

- Down syndrome
- Turner syndrome
- Noonan syndrome
- Klinefelter syndrome
- Celiac disease
- Addison disease
- Type I diabetes mellitus
- SLE
- Polyglandular disorder
- Vitiligo
- Alopecia
- Juvenile idiopathic arthritis autoimmune

Q-4. What are the clinical features of acquired hypothyroidism?

Symptoms	*Signs*
• Lethargy, somnolence • Decreased physical activity • Poor school performance • Increasing weight gain • Dry skin • Cold intolerance • Constipation • Delayed puberty • Family history of thyroid or autoimmune disorders	• Short stature • Pallor • Myxedematous face • Coarse facial features • Goiter • Bradycardia • Cold extremities • Brittle hairs • Proximal myopathy • Pseudohypertrophy • Delayed relaxation of ankle jerk (Hung up ankle reflex) • Pseudotumor cerebri • Delayed dentition • Delayed puberty • Delayed skeletal age • Absorption and metabolism of vitamin B_{12} and folic acid are affected leading to megaloblastic anemia • Conversion of carotene into vitamin A requires thyroxine. Deficiency of thyroxine leads to accumulation of fat-soluble carotene into skin imparting yellowish color of the skin. Sclera is not yellow

Q-5. What laboratory tests are recommended for diagnosis of hypothyroidism?

- *Thyroid function tests:* Estimation of serum T_3, T_4, TSH.
  - Low T_3, T_4 and raised TSH indicates primary hypothyroidism. Serum T_3 estimation is not useful as it may be normal in hypothyroidism.
  - Low T_4 or free T_4 levels with normal or low serum TSH suggests secondary hypothyroidism. In this situation, TBG deficiency should be ruled out.
  - TRH stimulation test will help distinction between secondary and tertiary hypothyroidism. In secondary hypothyroidism, TRH will not elicit TSH response, but in tertiary hypothyroidism, increased TSH response will be seen.

- In chronic Lymphocytic thyroiditis, antithyroid globulin antithyroid peroxidase (anti-TPO) antibody titers are increased.
- Ultrasonography, thyroid nuclear scan and fine-needle aspiration cytology are indicated in the presence of thyroid nodule.
- Children with predisposing factors like Type I diabetes mellitus, Down syndrome, celiac disease, etc. should be monitored with annual thyroid function tests.
- Histopathological examination of thyroid tissues in autoimmune thyroiditis.

Q-6. What radiological changes are seen in a case of hypothyroidism?

- The distal femoral and proximal tibial epiphyses, normally present at birth, are absent in congenital hypothyroidism in a newborn.
- Retardation of skeletal age.
- Epiphyseal dysgenesis (multiple foci of ossification)
- Beaking of lower thoracic and upper lumbar (12th thoracic and 1st and 2nd lumbar) vertebrae
- Skull changes
  - Large fontanels
  - Wide sutures
  - Wormian (inter sutural) bones
  - Enlarged sell turcica, rarely erosion and thinning of posterior clinoid process
- Delayed eruption of teeth
- Cardiac enlargement and pericardial effusion

Q-7. What is the management of acquired hypothyroidism?

- Thyroxine replacement therapy using levothyroxine is the main stay of treatment in hypothyroidism, regular and continuous therapy.
- The dose of levothyroxine for different age groups

Age	***Dose of thyroxine (µg/kg/day)***
6–12 months	5–8
1–3 years	4–6
3–10 years	3–5
10–18 years	2–4

- A dose of 100 µg/M^2/day is alternate way for calculation of dose of thyroxine
- The goal is to keep serum free T_4 in the mid normal range and TSH in the normal range.
- Almost 20% of patients with Hashimoto thyroiditis recover, become euthyroid and do not require lifelong thyroxine therapy. After attaining puberty, a 6-month trial of discontinuation thyroxine may be considered with serial measurements of free T_4 and TSH every 3 months.

Q-8. What is the prognosis in a case of hypothyroidism?

- Prognosis is good with early diagnosis and regular treatment for recommended duration.
- If it is late diagnosed, physical stature may not be attainable.
- Permanent intellectual or neurological deficits are less likely if age at diagnosis is beyond 3 years.
- Children with acquired hypothyroidism who have received thyroxine at least 5 years before the onset of puberty may attain their genetic potential for final adult height.

Q-9. What is subclinical hypothyroidism?

Subclinical hypothyroidism is defined as a normal serum total or free T_4 and mildly evaluated TSH. It is considered due to several reasons like minor developmental abnormalities, obesity, mild autoimmune thyroiditis and mutation in the gene for TSH receptors. Since few cases of subclinical hypothyroidism progress to overt hypothyroidism, treatment may be deferred periodic follow-up testing undertaken. Elevated thyroid antibodies or presence of goiter are considered risk factors for the development of eventual overt hypothyroidism. If over a period of 2 years, the thyroid profile remains stable without increase in serum TSH, further periodic monitoring is not required.

Q-10. What is sick euthyroid syndrome?

In nonthyroidal conditions like acute or chronic severe illness, surgery, trauma, fasting, malnutrition and certain drugs, the classical findings of low T_4 and free T_4, low T_3 with a low or normal TSH are called as sick euthyroid syndrome. There is no need of thyroid replacement in these conditions.

CHAPTER 31

Duchenne Muscular Dystrophy

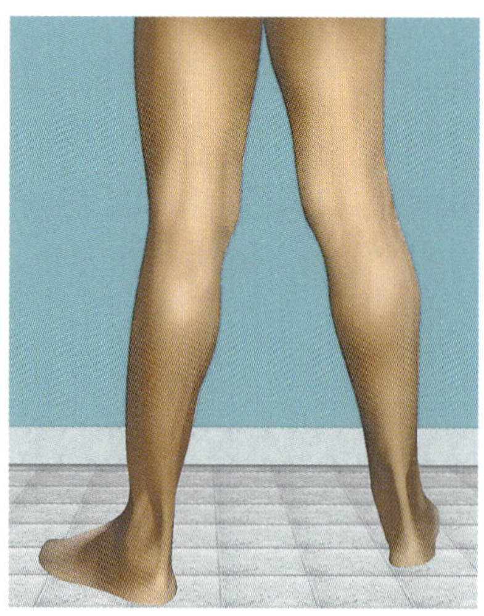

QUESTIONS AND ANSWERS

Q-1. What is the spot diagnosis?

Duchenne muscular dystrophy (DMD) or pseudohypertrophic muscular dystrophy

Q-2. What are the diagnostic clinical features in this boy?

- Hypertrophy of bilateral calf muscles
- Gower sign is present

Q-3. What type of genetic inheritance occurs in this disorder?

- X-linked recessive disorder. Males are affected and females are carriers.
- 30% of cases are new mutations where mother is not a carrier

Q-4. Can DMD affect the females?

Yes, it can happen rarely, but possible following situations:

- The girl is subject of Turner syndrome
- The carrier girl's normal X-chromosome is inactivated by Lyon hypothesis
- Affected females have milder disease manifestations

Q-5. What do you mean muscular dystrophy?

A group of genetically determined disorders where the skeletal muscles show progressive degeneration without any involvement of central or peripheral nervous system

Q-6. What are essential criteria for muscular dystrophy?

- Primary myopathy
- Genetic in origin
- Progressive in nature
- As the disease advances, there is degeneration and death of muscles

Q-7. Name the muscular dystrophies with mode of inheritance

- Duchenne muscular dystrophy—X-inked recessive
- Becker muscular dystrophy—X-linked recessive
- Limb girdle type of muscular dystrophy—autosomal recessive or autosomal dominant
- Congenital muscular dystrophy—autosomal recessive
- Myotonic dystrophy—autosomal dominant
- Fascio—scapulohumeral or scapula peroneal muscular dystrophy—X-linked recessive

Q-8. What is the difference between DMD and Becker type of muscular dystrophy?

- Both are pseudohypertrophic muscular dystrophy
- Both are X-linked recessive
- Both have same genetic defect at the same gene locus (*Xp Z1*)
- DMD presents early and is severe form of disease, where as Becker type is milder form of disease and presents later age group
- DMD shows manifestations by 2 to 4 years, where as Becker type starts manifesting between 5 to 25 years
- DMD may progress to nonambulatory stage in the first decade or early second decade. The death in DMD cases is usually in second decade.
- The patients of Becker type muscular dystrophy, remain ambulatory in adolescence or adulthood, death occurs in third decade, some cases may live around 40 years.

Q-9. Why is it called pseudohypertrophic muscular dystrophy?

Some muscle look bulky, hypertrophic. But the muscles are weak. It is not true hypertrophy. There is hypertrophy of some muscle fibers, infiltration of fat in the muscle groups and proliferation of collagen fibers, resulting in bulky in appearance, but are weak. Therefore, it is called as pseudo hypertrophic muscular dystrophy.

Q-10. What is the pathogenesis of DMD?

- Dystrophin is located subsarcolemmally and is a cytoskeletal protein
- Absence of dystrophin leads to delocalization of dystrophin associated proteins from the membrane, disruption of the cytoskeleton with resultant membrane instability and increased susceptibility to mechanical stress.
- In addition, altered membrane permeability and abnormal calcium homeostasis are thought to play a role.
- The absence of nitric oxide synthetase, delocalized from the subsarcolemmal membrane, may contribute to dystrophic features, in direct ways.

Q-11. What are the clinical features of DMD?

- Motor delay or an abnormal gait are most frequent presenting symptoms
- Difficulty in getting up from the ground.
- Frequent falls.
- Toe-walking.
- Most present between 3 and 5 years
- Less frequent problems are language or global developmental delay
- Raised SOGT or SGPT are found when these investigations are performed for other reasons
- Gower's sign present

- Hypertrophy of calf muscles
- By the age of 6 to 7 years, weakness becomes more evident. Due to weakness of paraspinal muscles, lordosis and protuberant abdomen become obvious
- Weakness of gluteal muscles, particularly gluteus medius, waddling gait develops
- Due to weakness of quadriceps, there is knee buckling and falls which are spontaneous or result from pushes and on uneven surface.
- As the condition advances, extensors of the knee and hip joints become further weak and children find it more difficult to stand on their own and gradually take to the wheel chair. This stage is reached between 9 and 12 years of age.
- Contractures of muscles in tendo Achilles and ilio-tibia bands
- Kyphoscoliosis
- Respiratory difficulty

Q-12. What are notable points on physical examination of DMD patients?

- Muscle hypertrophy is most prominent and evident in the calf muscles, but other muscles like deltoids, brachioradialis, infraspinatus, glutei, temporalis and tongue are enlarged in size. As the disease advances, hypertrophy may become less evident, but gastrocnemius and deltoid muscles often remain prominent. Occasionally, there may be no hypertrophy of muscles.
- Weakness of muscles in initially involves the lower limbs. It begins in the quadriceps and gluteal muscles and then tibialis anterior is weakened, resulting in foot-drop. At this stage, they walk on toes. The ocular, facial, bulbar and hand muscles are usually spared. Because of simultaneous hypertrophy of deltoid superolaterally, infraspinatus interomedally and wasting of posterior axillary fold, the appearance looks like valley (valley sign). It is best seen while arms are abducted at 90° and hand upward, examiner observing the posterior shoulder girdle.
- Deep tendon reflexes are depressed in weak muscles and ankle reflex continues to be elicited till very late in the disease.
- Cardiac involvement starts early and subclinical disease is seen in under 6 years of age. Overt cardiac symptoms begin after 10 years of age. One-third patients are symptomatic by 14 years and it is present in all patients over 18 years of age. Cardiac conduction defects are less commonly seen.
- Restrictive lung disease is common in DMD. Obstructive sleep apnea is seen in DMD children as early as the first decade.
- The average intelligence of DMD tends to be lower.
- Scoliosis, long bone fractures due to fall and osteoporosis are common orthopedic problems in DMD.
- There is increased risk of malignant hyperthermia following exposed to halothane or succinylcholine.

Q-13. What investigations should be performed for diagnosis of DMD?

- Raised SGOT, SGPT and CPK levels
- Nerve conduction and electromyography
- Muscle biopsy.
- Molecular genetic testing is important for accurate diagnosis, genetic counseling and prenatal diagnosis.
- Multiplex ligation dependent probe amplification (MLPA) is a more sensitive technique for detecting deletions.
- CPK levels are raised in many carriers.
- MLPA can detect the carrier status.

Q-14. Explain the mechanism of waddling gait.

Gluteus medius spans from iliac crest to the greater trochanter. In normal individuals, when one leg is raised off the ground, opposite gluteus medius contracts, keeping both anterior superior iliac spines at same level. With a weakness medius, pelvis tilts to the side of the raised, this alternates as child walks, resulting in waddle.

Q-15. What are managements options available for DMD?

- *General management and surveillance:* Nutrition, physiotherapy
- Corticosteroid therapy
  - *Proposed mechanism:* Alteration of regulation of genes in muscle fibers , slowing the rate of skeletal muscle breakdown, reducing cytotoxic T cells, lowering cytosolic calcium concentrations and increasing myogenic repair.
  - *Optimum dose:* Prednisolone 0.75 mg/kg/day lower dose 0.3 mg/kg/day result in lesser degree of benefit and higher dose 1.5 mg/kg/day do not result in additional benefits.
  - *Dosing regimens:* 1.25 mg/kg and 2.5 mg/kg alternate day doses; 10 days on and 10 days off; 10 days on and 20 days off; followed by 5 mg/kg/day is another option.

  It is generally believed that corticosteroid treatment should be started early, optimal duration is not defined. Improvement in muscle strength is seen in 10 days, which is maximum at 3 months and is maintained up to 10 months.
- Gene therapy.
- Stem cell therapy.

Q-16. What are the common causes of death in DMD?

- Pulmonary infections
- Respiratory failure
- Cardiac decompensation

Q-17. What are preventive measures for DMD?

- Genetic counselling
- Detection and counselling of female carrier
- Parental diagnosis

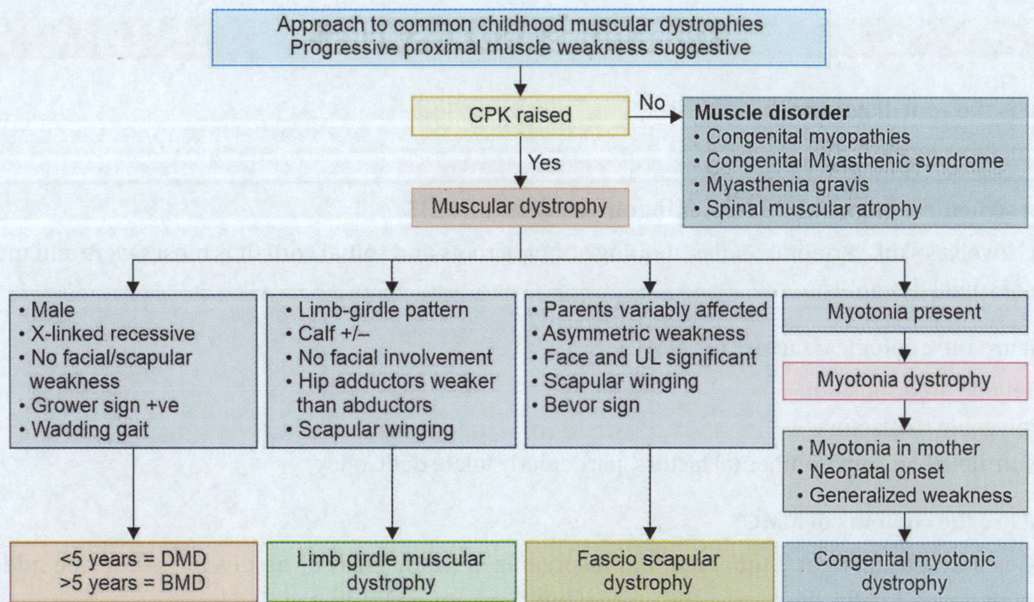

CHAPTER 32 Meningomyelocele and Neural Tube Defects

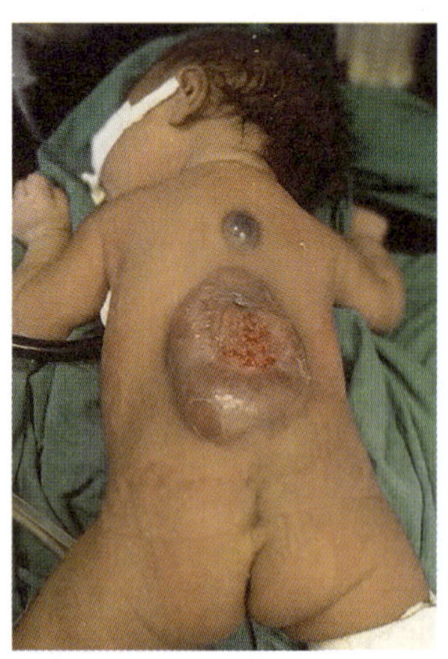

QUESTIONS AND ANSWERS

Q-1. What is the spot diagnosis?

Meningomyelocele.

Q-2. What structures are involved in meningomyelocele (MMC)?

MMC involves skin, vertebral bodies, meninges, nerve roots and spinal cord. It is most severe and most complex form of spinal dysraphism.

Q-3. What are the etiological factors for MMC?

- Genetic predisposition
- Polygenic risk factors
- Nutritional and environmental factors, particularly folate deficiency

Q-4. What are the contents of MMC?

MMC is a dysplastic neural tube, red, flat disorganized flashy mass of tissues located in the midline of CSF containing sac. Usually, the sac may be present but may rupture leading to CSF leak.

Q-5. What is the most common site?

- Most common location is lumbosacral region (75%) but may be variable. Thoracic defects are more complex and have more complications.
- MMC in cervical region are more protuberant.

Q-6. What are the clinical manifestations of MMC?

- Weakness or paralysis of the lower limbs
- Urinary bladder and bowel sphincter dysfunction
- Complications like infection
- Hydrocephalus is frequently present
- MMC is a very often associated with developmental dysplasia of hip (DDH) and congenital talipes equinovarus (CTEV) or club foot
- Sensory loss and trophic ulcers
- Although intelligence is normal in the majority, cognitive and language difficulties may be present

Q-7. What are common urinary tract and bowel dysfunction in this condition?

- Overflow incontinence
- Loss of sacral tone
- Loss of sacral and rectal sensations
- Loss of detrusor muscle activity
- Normal bladder control may be in 10% of patients
- Fecal incontinence
- Constipation

Q-8. What are the complications of MMC?

- Tethering of cord or restriction of growth of spinal cord
- Arnold-Chiari malformation
- Hydrocephalus (75–80%), 90% with thoracolumbar MMC and 95% in patients with associated Arnold-Chiari malformation
- Renal failure

Q-9. What are various neural tube defects (NTDs) and spinal cord malformations?

- Spina bifida occulta
- Meningocele
- Meningomyelocele
- Anencephaly
- Encephalocele
- Dermal sinus
- Lipoma involving conus medullaris or filum terminale
- Tethered cord
- Syringomyelia
- Diastematomyelia
- Caudal regression syndrome

Q-10. What is the incidence of NTDs and what is the risk of recurrence of it?

- Incidence of NTDs is 1.5 to 2.5 per 1,000 live births
- 4.1 per 1000 live births in India. NTDs in North India is 3.9 to 9 per 1,000 births and 11.4 per 1,000 births in some pockets of South India.
- Risk of recurrence in the next pregnancy is 4% which increases to 10% and 25% with subsequent pregnancies.

Q-11. What are etiological factors for NTDs?

- Inheritance
- Multifactorial

- Environmental
- Folic acid deficiency
- Vitamin B_{12} deficiency
- Maternal malnutrition
- Exposure to radiation and alcohol
- Trisomy 13 and 15
- Maternal drugs
  - Valproate
  - Carbamazepine
  - Trimethoprim
  - Oral contraceptives
  - Clomiphene during pregnancy
  - Retinoic acid

Q-12. What are cranial disruption?

- Anencephaly
- Encephalocele
- Craniorachischisis
- Iniencephaly

Q-13. What is spina bifida occulta?

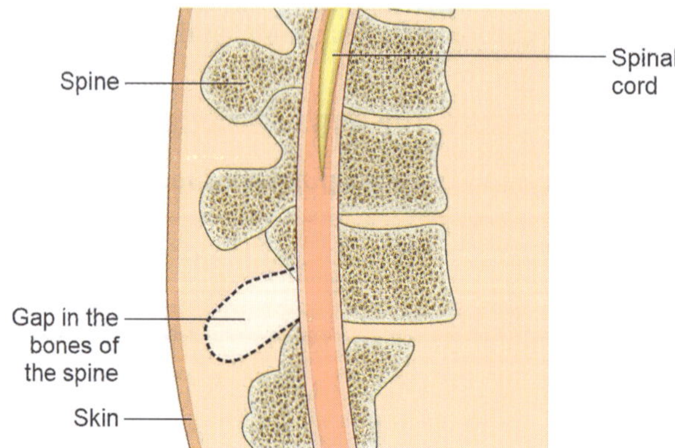

- It is midline defect of vertebral bodies without involvement of spinal cord or meninges
- Common NTD (5% of population)
- Common in lower lumbar region (L5-S1)
- No neurological symptoms and signs
- Detected incidentally on radiographic study
- No treatment is required
- In 10% of patients, there may be cutaneous markers like tuft of hairs, midline lipoma or angioma, pit, lump or dermal sinus over the back
- May be associated with syringomyelia, diastematomyelia or a tethered cord
- USG is helpful in diagnosis
- Every patient of spina bifida occulta must be investigated with MRI to detect other known anomalies

Q-14. What is dermal sinus?

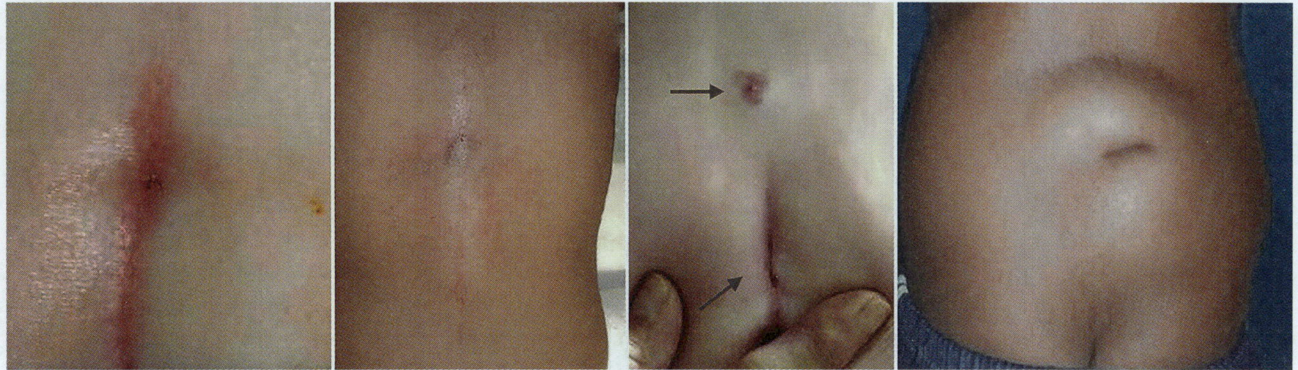

- Dermal sinus is a small opening on the skin
- Most common sites are lumbosacral and occipital regions
- The sinus leads into a narrow passage which may lead to a dead end or pass through the dura and act as midline cutaneous marker over the location of meningocele or encephalocele
- May cause recurrent meningitis
- Look for other associated conditions like diastematomyelia and tethered cord which may require surgical interventions

Q-15. What is tethered cord?

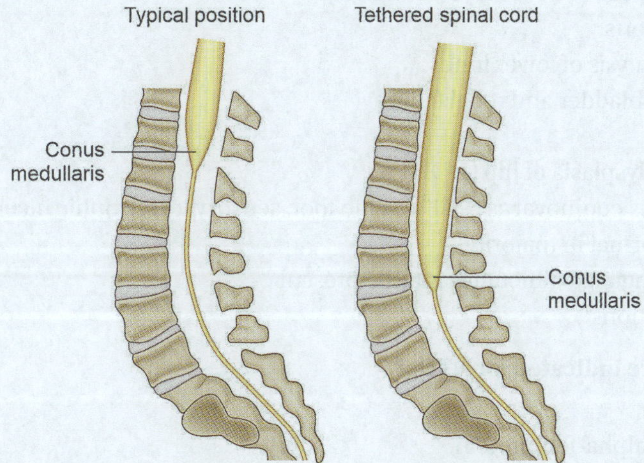

- The developing cord initially extends till the sacrum and gradually ascends to its final level of L_2 vertebra, due to differential growth of the cord and vertebral bodies
- In case of tethering, the cord is forcibly fixed at upper sacral vertebrae and its upward migration is prevented
- It leads to severe traction and neurological damages
- The traction-induced damage progressively worsens with the growth of the vertebral column and spinal movement
- The tethering may be due to fibrous band, bony or cartilaginous spur or the stalk of lipoma
- *Clinical manifestations:* Lower limb paresis, bladder symptoms like UTI, neurogenic bladder and constipation
- Surgical treatment is the remedy.

Q-16. What is diastematomyelia?

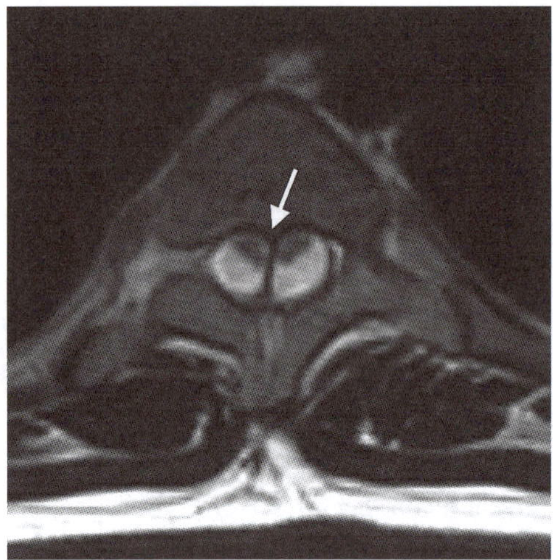

- Spitting of the cord into two halves, each with a separate dural covering.
- Spitting of the cord is due to septum which is ordinarily a bony or cartilaginous spur attached anteriorly to the vertebral body.
- It may have variable length with the hemicords merging into a single entity distal to the spur
- One-half of the cord may show hypoplasia or dysplasia
- The dividing spur needs to be removed surgically
- Clinical manifestations
  - Weakness or paralysis of lower limbs
  - UTI, neurogenic bladder and renal failure
  - Hydrocephalus
  - Developmental dysplasia of hip (DDH)
  - Congenital talipes equinovarus (CTEV), club foot, sensory loss, trophic ulcers
  - Intelligence is normal in majority
  - Cognitive and language difficulties may be present
  - Chiari malformations

Q-17. What investigations are indicated for NTDs?

- Antenatal diagnosis
  - Maternal serum alpha-fetoprotein
  - Fetal ultrasonography
  - Acetylcholinesterase (ACh) in amniotic fluid
- Investigations after birth
  - X-ray chest and spine
  - USG for NTD, head and abdomen
  - CT scan/MRI of brain and spine
  - Karyotyping and cytogenetic analysis
  - Evaluation of genitourinary system
  - Urine culture
  - Renal scans
  - Urodynamic study
  - Vesicocystourethrogram

Q-18. What are preventive measures for NTDs?

- Antenatal screening for NTD
- Medical termination of pregnancy, if indicated
- Folic acid supplementation (70% reduction)
- Vitamin B_{12}, zinc, vitamin A and other nutrients

Q-19. What is periconceptional folic acid supplementation?

- *All prospective mothers:* Folic acid 0.4 mg/day, 2 months prior to conception to 3 months after conception.
- *Prospective mothers with previous child NTD:* 4 mg/day, 2 months prior to conception to 3 months after conception.

CHAPTER 33 Tuberous Sclerosis and Neurocutaneous Disorders

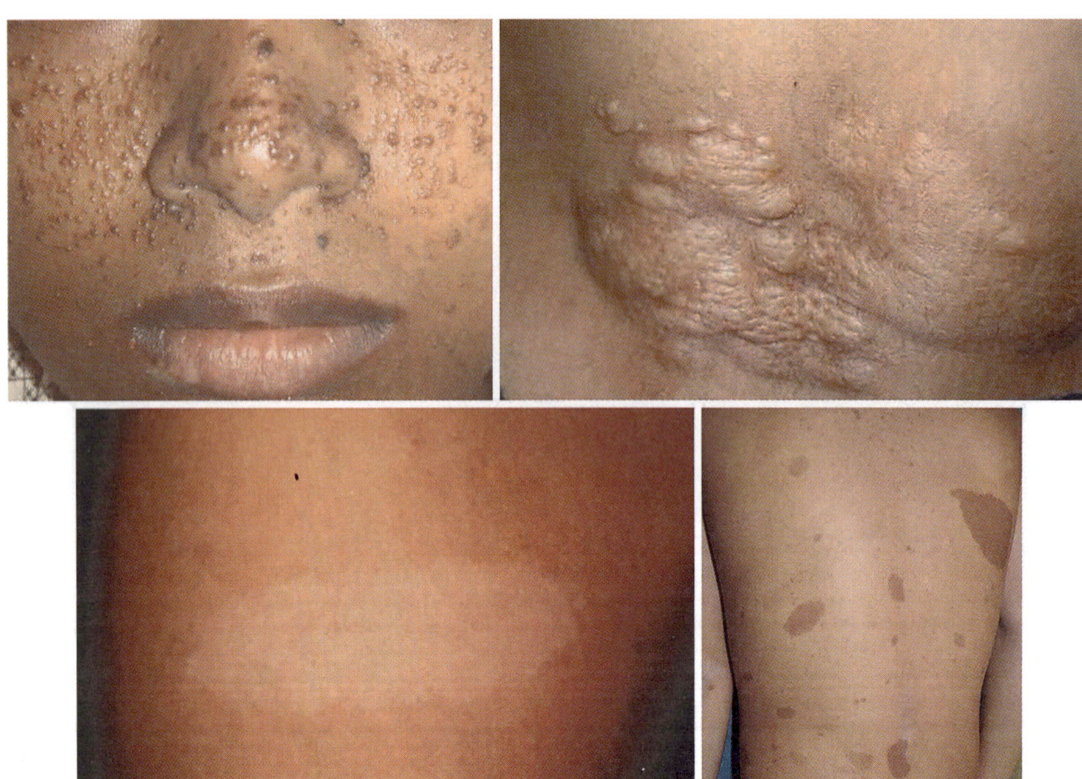

QUESTIONS AND ANSWERS

Q-1. What is spot diagnosis?

Tuberous sclerosis (Bourneville disease).

Q-2. What is the incidence of tuberous sclerosis (TS)?

1:5,800 live births.

Q-3. What is the type of genetic inheritance of TS?

Autosomal dominant (AD).

Q-4. What is the etiology of this disease?

- One-third of cases are inherited, rest are sporadic due to spontaneous mutation.
- Current molecular diagnostic methods detect mutation in either *TSC1* or *TSC2* gene in 85% of tuberous sclerosis complex (TSC) patients, both inherited and sporadic cases.

Q-5. What are clinical features of TSC?

The clinical features of TSC depend on the location of the tubers which are predominantly located in the brain, skin, eyes, heart, kidneys and lungs.

- Cutaneous manifestations
  - In 96% patients
  - Facial angiofibroma (adenoma sebaceum), pink or red papules, butterfly distribution over nose and cheeks.
  - Ash leaf macules (hypomelanotic macules)
  - Gingival fibromas
  - Shagreen patch
- Neurological manifestations
  - Seizures
  - Most common, 85% of patients
  - Onset in first year of life
  - Infantile spasm or focal seizures
  - Poor response to antiepileptic drugs
  - Unfavorable factors include onset of seizures in infancy, multiple seizures types, specific EEG changes
  - Cortical tubers act as epileptic foci
  - Neuropsychiatric disorders
  - Profound cognitive impairment
  - Behavioral disorders
  - ADHD
  - Autistic spectrum disorders
  - Memory and attention deficits
  - Hydrocephalus and increased intracranial pressure
- Renal manifestations
  - Angiomyolipomas (80%)
  - Renal cyst
  - Polycystic kidney disease
  - Renal cell carcinoma
- Cardiac manifestations
  - Rhabdomyomas (50–60%), can cause outflow obstruction, interference with valvular function and arrhythmias
- Ophthalmic manifestations
  - Retinal hamartomas (50%)
  - Visual impairment
- Pulmonary manifestations
  - Pulmonary cysts
  - Lymphangiomyomatosis

Q-6. What are diagnostic criteria for tuberous sclerosis?

- Genetic diagnostic criteria
  - *TSC1* or *TSC2* pathogenic mutation in DNA from normal tissues
  - Normal result does not exclude TSC
- Clinical diagnostic criteria
  - Major features
    - Hypomelanotic macule (≥3 at least 5 mm diameter)
    - Angiofibromas or fibrous cephalic plaque

- Ungual fibromas
- Shagreen patch
- Multiple retinal hamartomas
- Cortical dysplasia
- Subependymal nodules
- Subependymal giant cell astrocytoma
- Cardiac rhabdomyoma
- Lymphangioleiomyomatosis
- Angiomyolipomas
- Minor features
  - Confetti skin lesions
  - Dental enamel pits
  - Intraoral fibromas
  - Retinal achromic patch
  - Multiple renal cysts
  - Non renal hamartomas
- *Definitive diagnosis:* Two major features or one major feature with more than or equal to two minor features
- *Possible diagnosis:* Either one major feature or more than or equal to two minor features

Q-7. What investigations should be performed in TSC?

- Neuroimaging
- Ophthalmic examination
- Echocardiogram
- Renal USG study
- EEG
- Chest CT scan

Q-8. What is the treatment of TSC?

- *Antiepileptic medicines:* Vigabatrin/ACTP
- Neuropsychological evaluation and appropriate treatment
- Cortical tubers and subependymal nodules
  - Asymptomatic may not require active treatment
  - Surgical intervention for large and growing nodules causing ventricular enlargement
- Rapidly changing or disfiguring skin lesions may be considered for excision, laser or topical application of medicine.
- Retinal lesions are left alone and follow-up on any symptom
- Angiomyolipoma
  - Embolization followed by corticosteroids for presenting with acute hemorrhage
  - Nephrectomy is avoided
- Lymphoangioleiomyomatosis (LAM)
  - mTOR inhibitors
  - Lung transplantation

Q-9. What are neurocutaneous disorders?

- Tuberous sclerosis complex
- Neurofibromatosis type 1
- Neurofibromatosis type 2
- Sturge-Weber syndrome

- Von Hippel–Lindan syndrome
- Ataxia telangiectasia
- Incontinentia pigmenti
- Epidermal nervous syndrome

Q-10. What is neurofibromatosis type 1 (NF1)?

- Also known as Recklinghausen's disease
- Most common, 1:3,000 individuals
- Autosomal dominant
- Clinical features
  - After the skin, bone and peripheral nervous system involvement is common.
  - Café-au-lait spots
  - Skin fold freckling (85%) noticeable in axillae, groins, base of neck, upper eyelids and under the breast
  - Neurofibromas—benign tumors arise from Schwann cells, increase in number after puberty
  - Iris lisch nodules—highly specific to NFI, require slit lamp examination
  - Optic gliomas
  - Skeletal dysplasia

Q-11. What are the complications of NFI?

- Neurological complications
  - Aqueductal stenosis
  - Chiari malformation
  - Gliomas
  - Optic pathway glioma
  - Cognitive impairment
  - Epilepsy
  - Multiple sclerosis
  - Neuropathy
- Glaucoma
- Skeletal complications
  - Scoliosis
  - Osteoporosis
  - Skeletal dysplasia
  - Congenital heart disease
  - Restrictive lung defect
  - Pheochromocytoma
  - Rhabdomyosarcoma
  - Breast carcinoma

Q-12. What are diagnostic criteria of NFI?

- Six or more café-au-lait spots measuring at least 5 mm before puberty or 15 mm after puberty
- Skin fold freckling
- Two or more neurofibromas or one plexiform neurofibroma
- Two or more iris lisch nodules
- Optic glioma
- Characteristic skeletal dysplasia
- Affecting first degree relative diagnosis ≥2 criteria

Q-13. What is neurofibromatosis type 2 (NF2)?

- Autosomal dominant
- 1:60,000
- Clinical features
  - Usually present in early adulthood
  - Visual disturbances, more frequent in children
  - Vestibular schwannomas in adults
  - Meningioma
  - Neuropathy
  - Posterior subcapsular cataract
  - Intracutaneous plaque

Q-14. What are diagnostic criteria for NF2?

Bilateral vestibular schwannomas (VS) of family history of NF2 plus.

1. Unilateral VS or
2. Any two of meningioma, glioma, neurofibroma, schwannoma, posterior lenticular opacities

Additional criteria: Unilateral VS plus any two of maningioma, glioma, neurofibroma, schwannoma and posterior lenticular opacities

Or

Multiple meningiomas (≥2) plus unilateral VS or any two of glioma, neurofibroma, schwannoma or cataract.

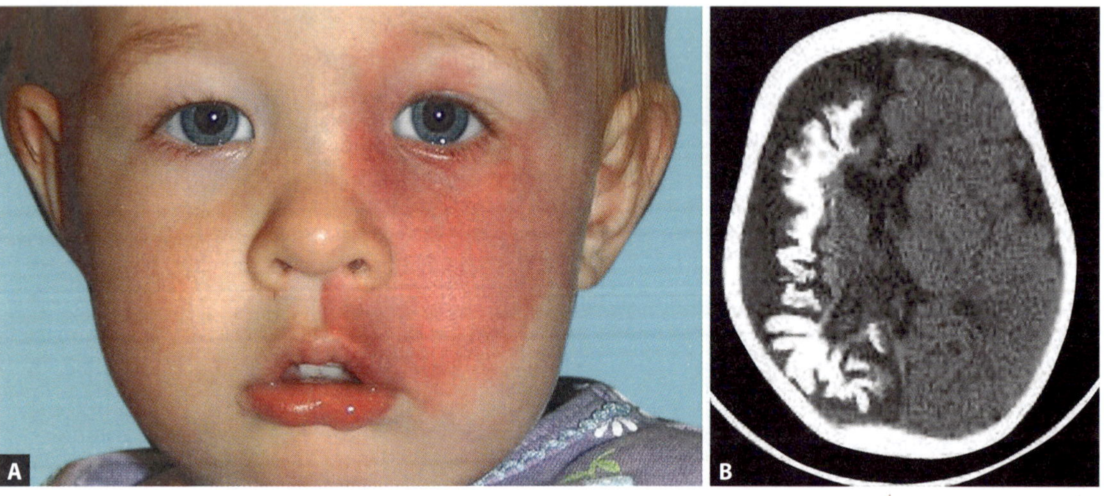

The child shown in **Figure A** presented with seizures and focal neurological deficit (left side weakness). His CT scan finding was as shown in **Figure B**.

Q-15. What is your diagnosis?

Sturge-Weber syndrome, also called as encephalofacial angiomatosis.

Q-16. What are the clinical manifestations of Sturge-Weber syndrome?

- Portwine stain over ophthalmic distribution of the trigeminal nerve
- Vascular glaucoma and vascular malformation of the eye
- Neurological manifestations
  - Epilepsy (75–85%)
  - Focal neurological deficit (hemiplegia)
  - Psychomotor delay
  - Headache and migraine

- Ocular involvement
  - Eyelid hemangioma
  - Glaucoma
  - Conjunctival and episcleral hemangioma
  - Diffuse choroidal hemangioma

17. What investigations should be performed in this case?

- *MRI brain:* Leptomeningeal angioma, ipsilateral cerebral volume reduction
- *CT scan brain:* Superior to MRI for demonstration of characteristic calcifications, double lined gyri form pattern of calcification parallelling cerebral convolutions (railroad track sign)

CHAPTER 34

Turner Syndrome

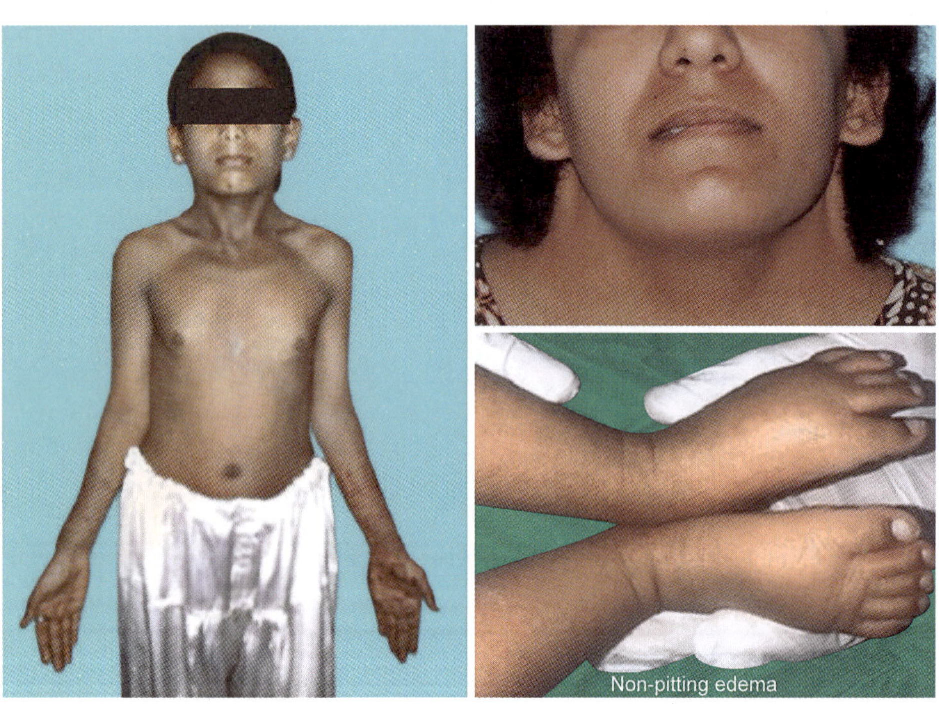

QUESTIONS AND ANSWERS

Q-1. What is the spot diagnosis?

Turner syndrome.

Q-2. What is the type of disorder it?

Turner syndrome is a chromosomal disorder caused due to loss of one 'X' chromosome.

Q-3. What is the incidence of Turner syndrome?

- 1 in 2,500 live born females
- A 45,X karyotype is observed in 1–2% of conceptions, 10% of miscarriages and 1% of stillbirths

Q-4. What is the mechanism of Turner syndrome?

- The most common type of Turner syndrome is due to errors in meiotic segregation of chromosomes, leading to one gamete with two X chromosomes and another with no X chromosome. This type of abnormality is seen in about 45% of patients and karyotype is 45,X.
- The other mechanisms of Turner syndrome include isochromosome X9 (15–18%), mosaic 45,X/46,XX (7–16%), ring X chromosome or partial deletion of XP or X9.

Q-5. What are the clinical features of Turner syndrome?

- Short stature
- Characteristic facies—drooping of eyes
- Small mandible
- Low set ears
- Low hair line
- Nuchal folds
- Shield chest
- Wide spaced nipples
- Cubitus valgus
- Hypoplastic nails
- Hyperconvex nails
- Nonpitting edema of hands and feet, pretibial edema is very characteristic in newborns
- High arched palate
- Pigmented nevi
- Short fourth metacarpal
- Left-sided cardiac anomalies (30%) like coarctation of aorta (30%), aortic stenosis, bicuspid aortic valve (50%)
- Renal anomalies like horse shoe kidneys
- Ovarian failure
- Intellectual disability
- May have learning disability
- Hearing impairment
- Delayed or absent puberty
- Infertility
- Autoimmune diseases like hypothyroidism and celiac disease
- Inflammatory bowel disease (IBD) are common
- Skeletal deformities like scoliosis, sternal malformations

Q-6. What is confirmatory test for diagnosis of Turner syndrome?

- Chromosomal analysis is indicated in any female with short stature
- Karyotyping
- Cytogenetic analysis of chromosomes
- FISH or PCR-based methods

Q-7. What is the management of Turner syndrome?

- Cardiac assessment—clinical, echo and MR angiography to detect cardiac anomalies.
- Renal assessment for detection of anomalies like horseshoe kidney, double collecting system, UTI, hypertension.
- Free T4 and TSH should be performed annually, hypothyroidism occurs in 10–30% of individuals with Turner syndrome.
- Hearing and visual assessment
- Screening test (TTGA) to detect celiac disease as they have high risk for it.
- Growth hormone (GH) therapy should be considered in all girls with Turner syndrome whose height is below the 5th centile for Turner syndrome and are not exhibiting significant catch up on disease specific charts by 3–4 years of age. GH therapy accelerates growth in patients with Turner syndrome and final height increments range from 5 to 15 cm. GH therapy also contributes to achievement of peak bone mass in combination with estrogen.
- Hormonal replacement (estrogen) therapy under supervision of pediatric endocrinologist.

Cleft Lip and Cleft Palate

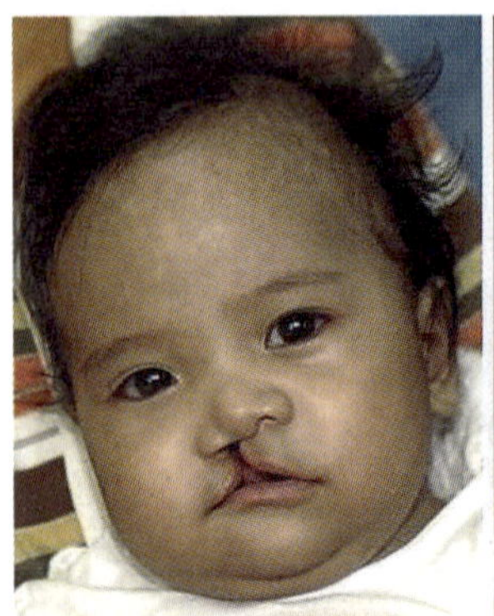

Unilateral cleft lip

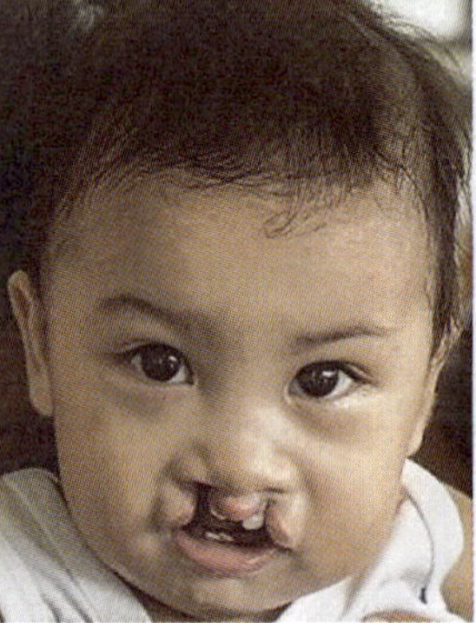

Bilateral cleft lip

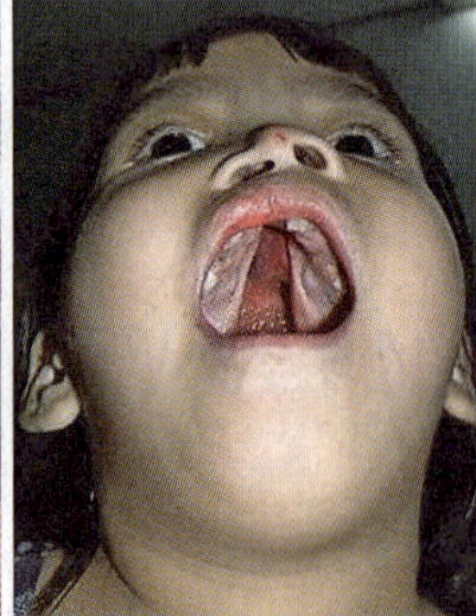

Cleft palate

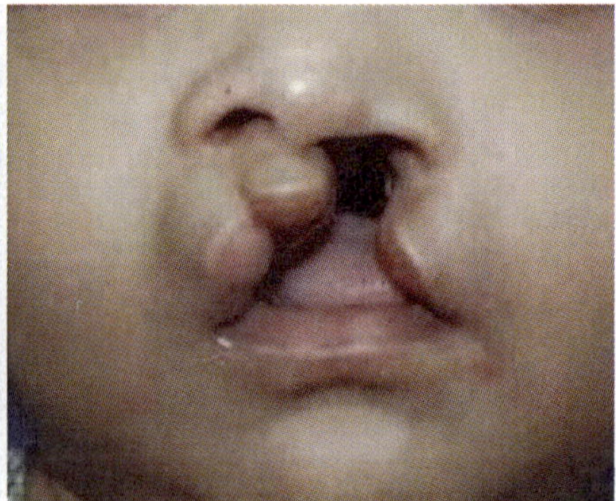

QUESTIONS AND ANSWERS

Q-1. What is the spot diagnosis?

Cleft lip and cleft palate.

Q-2. What is the genesis of cleft lip (CL) and cleft palate (CP)?

- Cleft lip develops because of hypoplasia of the mesenchymal layer, resulting in a failure of medial nasal and maxillary processes to join.
- Cleft palate results from failure of palatal shelves to approximate or fuse.

Q-3. What factors are playing the role for development of cleft lip and palate?

- Clefts of lips are more common in males
- Cleft palate is seen more common in females
- Maternal drug exposure
- Syndromic conditions—approximately 400 syndromes are associated with cleft lip and palate.
- Presence of susceptible genes.
- Cleft lip may be associated with craniofacial anomalies.
- Cleft palate may be associated with central nervous system anomalies.

Q-4. What is the risk of cleft lip and cleft palate in next sibling getting affected?

- Normal parents with one cleft child 4% risk for the next child to have CL/CP.
- Normal parents with two kids with CL/CL 9% risk for the next sibling.
- One parent affected with CL/CL, no affected kid 4% risk for the next child.
- One parent and one child with CL/CP 17% risk for the next child.

Q-5. What are clinical manifestations?

- Cleft lip can vary from a small notch in the vermilion border to a complete separation involving skin, muscles, mucosa, tooth and the bone.
- Clefts of lip may be unilateral (more on the left side) or bilateral and can involve the alveolar ridges.
- Isolated cleft palate occurs in midline and might involve only the uvula or can extend into or through the soft and hard palates to the incisive foramen.
- When cleft palate is associated with cleft lip, the defect can involve the midline of the soft palate and extend into hard palate on one or both sides, exposing one or both nasal cavities as a unilateral or bilateral cleft palate.
- The palate can also have a submucosal cleft indicated by a bifid uvula, partial separation of muscle with intact mucosa, or a palpable notch at the posterior of the pate.
- 75% clefts are unilateral and 25% bilateral.

Q-6. What is the classification of CL/CP?

- Isolated CL/CP, unilateral/bilateral, complete/incomplete
- Combined CL and CP, unilateral/bilateral, complete/incomplete
- Syndromic

Q-7. What are the clinical problems of this malformation?

- Feeding problems
- Nasal regurgitation and aspiration
- Middle ear infection
- Speech problems
- Psychosocial problems
- Dental problems

Q-8. Can it be diagnosed by antenatal ultrasonography?

Craniofacial clefts can be diagnosed by antenatal ultrasonography, as early as 18–20 weeks of gestation.

Q-9. How can be feeding managed of this baby, till the malformation is repaired?

- Normal feeding requires the creation of suction by velopharyngeal closure and compression by orbicularis oris muscle and tongue. Babies with CL/CP cannot create a negative pressure for suction or compression. So they may be given expressed breast-milk using special feeding devices or breastfed using feeding obturators. The teat should be kept on the uncleft side and gently squeezed after every 3 to 4 sucks. Feeding should not exceed 20–30 minutes, since longer feeds are energy consuming leading to poor weight gain.
- If bottle fed, the baby should be kept upright to prevent nasal regurgitation.
- Special teat or bottle which can be squeezed while the baby is sucking is now available. This will push the milk into the babby's mouth and will compensate for suction.

Q-10. What is the surgical treatment schedule of this malformation?

- *Birth:* Initial assessment, presurgical evaluation and orthodontics
- *3–6 months:* Primary lip repair
- *9–12 months:* Palate repair (before speech develops)
- *2 years:* Speech assessment
- *3–5 years:* Lip revisions
- *8–9 years:* Initial intervention orthodontics
- *10 years:* Alveolar bone grafting
- *16 years:* Nasal revision
- *17–20 years:* Orthognathic surgery

CHAPTER 36

Achondroplasia

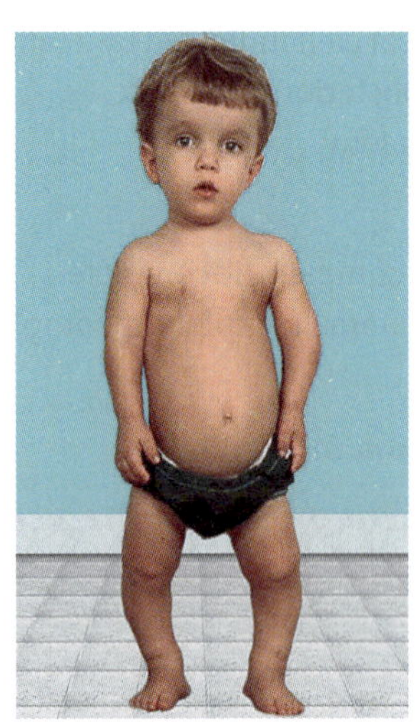

QUESTIONS AND ANSWERS

Q-1. What is the spot diagnosis?

Achondroplasia.

Q-2. What diseases are associated with advanced paternal age?

- Achondroplasia
- Apert syndrome
- Crouzon syndrome
- Marfan syndrome
- Autism spectrum disorder

Q-3. What are the clinical features of achondroplasia?

- Short limb dwarf
- Rhizomelic short limbs
- Large head
- Frontal bossing
- Hypoplasia of the midface
- Trident configuration of hands
- Hyperextensibility of joints
- Mild to moderate hypotonia
- Motor milestones may be delayed
- Intelligence is normal
- Hydrocephalus

Q-4. What is the mechanism for development of hydrocephalus?

Hydrocephalus develops due to disparity of skull and brain. Hydrocephalus results from increased intracranial venous pressure due to stenosis of the sigmoid sinus at the level of the narrowed jugular foramina. USG cranium should be done at birth and 2 months and 4 months.

Q-5. What is the management of achondroplasia?

- Measurement of growth and head circumference using growth charts standardized for achondroplasia.
- Neurological examination—CT/MRI brain.
- Surgical enlargement of foramen magnum in case of severe stenosis.
- Management of middle ear infections and dental crowding.
- Control of obesity.
- Growth hormone.
- Limb lengthening and deformity correction.

Q-6. What is the prognosis of achondroplasia?

- The risk of sudden unexpected death in infants with achondroplasia is high in first year attributable to abnormalities of craniocervical junction causing cervical compression.
- Overall mortality between ages 20 years and 35 years is 10 times more than in general population.
- Increased incidence of obesity.
- Average life expectancy is decreased by 10 years.

CHAPTER 37

Craniosynostosis

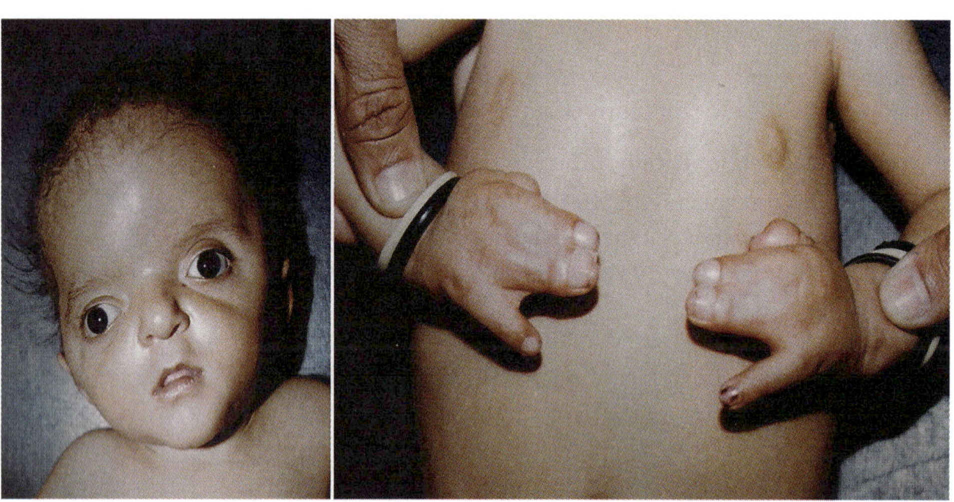

QUESTIONS AND ANSWERS

Q-1. What is craniosynostosis?

Craniosynostosis refers to premature closure of one or more sutures of the skull. It may be syndromic or isolated. The bone is unable to grow in a direction perpendicular to the fused sutures and therefore disproportionate growth occurs in a parallel direction leading to characteristic appearance of the head.

Q-2. What are common syndromes associated with craniosynostosis?

- Apert syndrome
- Crouzon syndrome
- Carpenter syndrome
- Jackson-Weiss syndrome
- Muenke syndrome
- Pfeiffer syndrome
- Loeys-Dietz syndrome
- Saethre-Chotzen syndrome
- Shprintzen-Goldberg syndrome

Q-3. What are the types of craniosynostosis?

- *Primary:* It is part of abnormality of skull development.
- *Secondary:* Results from failure of brain growth and expansion
  - Microcephaly
  - Following insertion of ventriculoperitoneal shunt
  - Medications during pregnancy like valproate or metabolic disorders

Q-4. What are the features of Apert syndrome?

- Usually sporadic condition
- It is associated with advanced paternal age
- Autosomal dominant inheritance
- Premature fusion of multiple sutures, especially the two coronal sutures
- Symmetric complex syndactyly of the hands and feet
- Severe acne during puberty
- Developmental delay in most patients

Q-5. What are the features of Crouzen syndrome?

- Autosomal dominant
- Brachycephaly resulting from closure of bilateral coronal sutures
- Pan synostosis is also common
- Orbits are underdeveloped and ocular proptosis is prominent
- Hypoplasia of maxilla and orbital hypertelorism are typical facial features
- Beaked nose
- High arch palate
- Dental abnormalities
- Acanthosis nigricans

Q-6. What are the features of Carpenter syndrome?

- Craniosynostosis
- Broad forehead
- Hypertelorism
- Syndactyly
- Polydactyly
- Congenital heart defects
- Kyphoscoliosis
- Genu valgum

Q-7. What is the treatment of craniosynostosis?

- Minimally invasive surgery (endoscopic)
- Open surgery
- The goal of surgery is to relieve pressure on the brain and allow it to grow properly and reshaping the skull

CHAPTER 38

Mucopolysaccharidosis

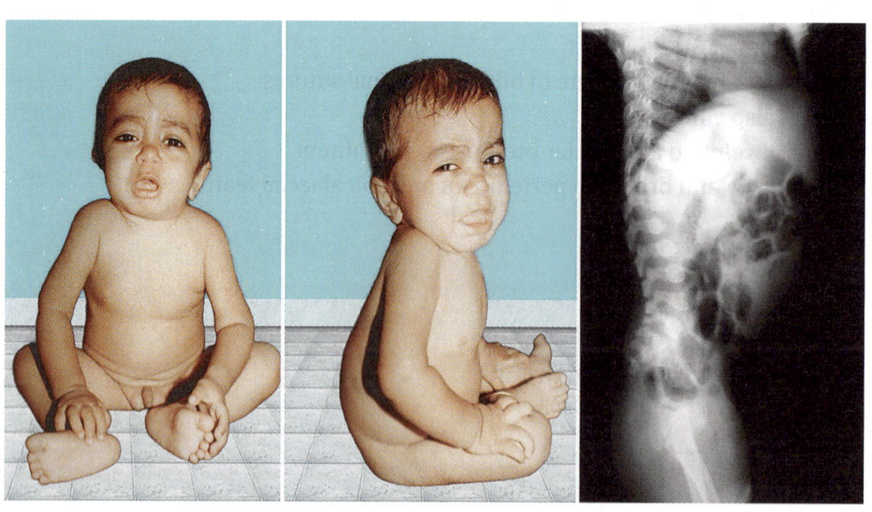

QUESTIONS AND ANSWERS

Q-1. What is spot diagnosis?

Mucopolysaccharidosis.

Q-2. What are types of mucopolysaccharidosis (MPS)?

Type	*Name*
MPS I – H	Hurler syndrome
MPS I – HS	Hurler–Scheie syndrome
MPS I – S	Scheie syndrome
MPS II	Hunter syndrome
MPS III – A	Sanfilippo syndrome A
MPS III – B	Sanfilippo syndrome B
MPS III – C	Sanfilippo syndrome C
MPS III – D	Sanfilippo syndrome D
MPS IV – A	Morquio syndrome A
MPS IV – B	Morquio syndrome B
MPS VI	Maroteaux–Lamy syndrome
MPS VII	Sly syndrome
MPS IX	Natowicz syndrome

Q-3. What are the clinical features of MPS?

- Mucopolysaccharidoses are clinically distinct group of disorders with variable degree of growth failure, intellectual disability, coarse facial features, joint contractures, organomegaly, corneal clouding, glycosaminoglycans and dysostosis multiplex with onset in infancy and childhood.
- Hurler syndrome is prototype for clinical features of MPSs presenting with three phenotypes of different severity. Similar features are shared by Hunter syndrome and Sly syndrome though Sly syndrome can present with hydrops fetalis.
- *Coarse facial features:* Large head with prominent forehead, flat nasal bridge, hirsutism, thick lips, large tongue and broad nasal tip.
- Skeletal changes include restricted joint mobility (contractures), dysostosis multiplex and short stature.
- Dysostosis multiplex refers to the skeletal changes like thick skull bones, widened sell turcica, broad oar-shaped tibs, bullet-shaped phalanges and metacarpals, irregular epiphyses and metaphysis, beaked or ovoid vertebral bodies and broad diaphysis. Tapering of lower iliac wing is often evident and is a very useful radiological sign.
- Variable degree of intellectual disability is seen and is progressive.
- Loss of vision (pigmentary retinopathy)
- Hearing loss.
- Otitis media.
- Obstructive sleep apnea.
- Recurrent respiratory tract infections.
- Hepatomegaly
- Splenomegaly
- Umbilical hernia.
- Inguinal hernia.
- Widely spaced teeth.
- Cardiomyopathy, regurgitation across the valves, arrhythmias
- Hydrocephalus.
- Spinal cord compression.
- Subcutaneous nodules (pebble-like) in MPS II are seen over back, neck and chest.
- Patients with severe forms of the disease usually succumb in the first or second decade of life.
- Milder variants have a later age of onset and intellectual functioning is better preserved MPS I–S has almost normal intelligence.
- MPS III has more severe cognitive and neurological impairment than the somatic manifestations and that may be very mild. Behavioral problems, development delay, dementia, poor social and communication skill are the predominant symptoms.
- MPS IV is unique in terms of skeletal involvement with pronounced spondyloepiphyseal dysplasia, anterior-middle beaking of vertebral bodies, short ulna forming 'V' shaped angle with lower end of radius and proximal pointing of metacarpals, joint laxity, genu vulgus, pectus carinatum and atlantoaxial instability. Intellect is well preserved. Corneal clouding is always seen.
- MPS VI has somatic manifestations similar to MPS I, II and VII, but differ in terms of preserved intellectual function.

Q-4. What is approach to diagnosis in a case of MPS?

- Documentation of clinical features.
- Three generation pedigree.
- Skeletal survey.
- Slit lamp examination of eye.
- Urinary glycosaminoglycans (GAG).
- Enzyme analysis on leucocytes or cultured fibroblasts
- Genetic testing

Q-5. What is the management of MPS?

- Multidisciplinary approach—clinical genetics, genetic counseling, biochemistry, orthopedics, cardiology, neurology, ophthalmology, otorhinolaryngology.
- Hematopoietic stem cell transplantation.
- Enzyme replacement for MPS I, II and VI.

Q-6. What are preventive steps for MPS?

- Early diagnosis and multidisciplinary approach for management.
- Prenatal diagnosis.
- Genetic counseling.
- Newborn screening.

CHAPTER 39

Spinal Muscular Atrophy

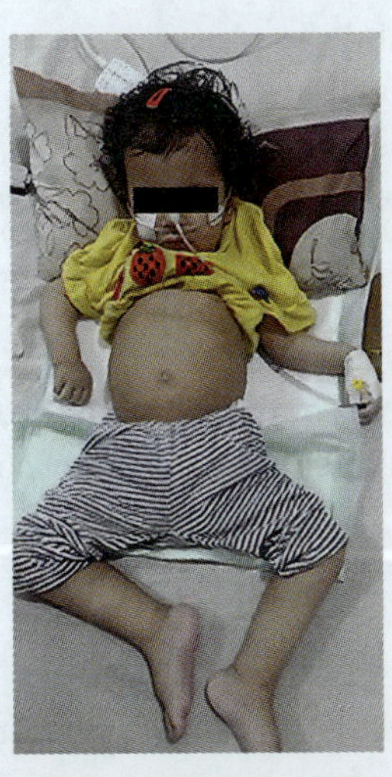

QUESTIONS AND ANSWERS

Q-1. What is your spot diagnosis?

Floppy infant—probably spinal muscular atrophy (SMA)

Q-2. What type of neurological disorder is it?

It is neuromuscular disorder due to degeneration of anterior horn cells of spinal cord with or without bulbar motor neurons involvement.

Q-3. What are clinical subtypes of SMA?

SMA type	*Genetics*	*Age of onset*	*Clinical features*	*Maximum function achieved*	*Prognosis*
0–Prenatal	SMN gene *AR*	Intrauterine	• Reduced fetal movements • RD at birth	Requires ventilatory support at birth	Fatal at birth
1–Infantile SMA (Werdnig–Hoffmann)	SMN gene *AR*	0–6 months	• Floppy infant • Bulbar + respiratory involvement	Sits with support	Death by 2 years of age
2–Intermediate SMA (Dubowitz disease)	SMN gene *AR*	6–18 months	Delayed motor milestones	• Sit without support • Unable to walk	Variable
3–Juvenile SMA	SMN gene *AR*	After 18 months	Pseudomyopathic	Able to walk with assistance	Variable
4–Adult SMA	SMN gene *AR*	Usually after 30 years (above 5 years)	Pseudomyopathic/ neuropathic pattern	Able to walk independently	• Slow progression • Normal life span

Q-4. What are the clinical features of SMA subtypes?

- SMA type 0
  - Decreased fetal movements
  - Proximal muscle weakness
  - Hypotonia
  - Areflexia
  - No arthrogryposis
  - Respiratory muscle weakness—asphyxia + encephalopathy
- SMA type 1 (Werdnig-Hoffman disease)
  - Most common—50% of all SMA subtypes
  - Presents in the neonatal period or within 6 months of life
  - Never attain the ability to sit independently
  - Severe generalized hypotonia, proximal more than distal weakness and areflexia. Severe head lag
  - Frog-like position
  - Fasciculations often present
  - Extraocular movements are always normal
  - Intercostal muscles are severely weak, but diaphragm involvement occurs in the disease
  - Respiratory distress and aspiration pneumonia are very common due to intercostal muscle weakness
  - Contractures may develop
  - Usually die before 2 years of age
- SMA type 2
  - Normal at birth
  - Presents to clinician as delayed motor milestones with normal language and social milestones
  - Onset is between 6 and 18 months of age
  - Able to sit without support with variable bulbar and respiratory involvement
  - May acquire standing position, but they never achieve independent walking
  - They have prominent hip and knee contractures, kyphoscoliosis and club feet
  - Eventually they become wheelchair confined
- SMA type 3 (Kugelberg-Welander disease)
  - Normal at birth
  - Manifest motor weakness after 18 months of age
  - Attain independent walking, they have difficulty in climbing stairs, getting up from squatting position and use Gower's maneuver to do so
  - Waddling gait with excessive lumbar lordosis and protuberant abdomen
  - Pseudohypertrophy of calf muscles occurs due to relative preservation of calf muscles compared to thigh muscles
  - Fasciculation is very common
- SMA type 4 (Adult onset, pseudomyopathic type)
  - Usually occurs after the age of 30 years
  - Clinical features are similar to intermediate type.
  - Bulbar, respiratory involvement and bony deformities are rare.
  - Majority have a normal lifespan.

Q-5. What are diagnostic tests for SMA?

- Molecular diagnosis
- Nerve conduction study—may be normal
- EMG shows features of denervation like fibrillation potentials, positive waves and fasciculations
- Muscle biopsy

Q-6. What is the management of SMA?

- Family education and counseling
- Genetic counseling
- Pulmonary care

Q-7. Consensus statement for standard care in SMA.

Complications	*Monitor*	*Management*
Respiratory failure	• ABG • Chest X-ray • Oxygen saturation	• Noninvasive ventilation • Invasive ventilation, if required
Impaired cough		• Manual assisted coughing • Cough assist devices
Pooling of secretions		• Frequent suctions, • Chest physiotherapy • Prevention of aspiration
Aspiration pneumonia	• Total count • Chest X-ray	Antibiotics
Prevention of respiratory infections		• Influenza vaccine • Pneumococcal vaccine
Nutritional support and hydration		• Feeding tube • Adequate diet • Gastrostomy/jejunostomy
Speech	Speech assessment	Speech therapy
Neurorehabilitation		• Physical therapy • Occupational therapy • Prevention of contractures • Prevention of osteopenia and fractures
Scoliosis		• Corrected surgery • Spinal brace
Orthoses		• Walkers • Limb orthoses

Q-8. What are new therapeutic strategies for SMA?

- Neuroprotective strategies
  - *Riluzole:* A glutamate antagonist, creatine to improve metabolism
  - *Albuterol:* Anabolic substance
- Antisense oligonucleotides
- Histone deacetylase inhibitors
- Gene therapy
- Stem cell therapy

SECTION 3

Viva

CHAPTER 40

Nutrition

BREASTFEEDING

- **Breast Milk**
  - Ideal food for infants from birth to 6 months.
- **Initiation of Breastfeeding**
  - Within 1 hour of birth irrespective of type of delivery.
- **Exclusive Breastfeeding**
  - Only breast milk for first 6 months of life
  - Nothing else, not even the water
  - Except vitamin drops or any medication, if indicated.
- **NFHS - 5 (2019–2020) data**
  - BF initiation within 1 hour: 41.8%
  - Exclusive BF: 64%.

Benefits of Breast Milk

- **Nutritionally superior**
  - Breast milk contains all the nutrients in the proportion that a neonate needs for optimum growth and development.
  - Digestibility
  - *Nutritive value:* 67 kcal/100 mL
- **Carbohydrates**
  - 6–7 g/dL
  - Majority of carbohydrate is lactose.
  - Lactose promotes calcium and magnesium absorption.
  - Galactocerebroside (Galacto-oligosaccharide) helps in myelination and brain growth
- **Proteins**
  - 0.9 to 1.1 g/dL
  - Quality of protein is superior: Whey protein.
  - Lactalbumin and lactoglobulin.
  - Taurine and cysteine, necessary for brain growth.

Breast milk	*Cow's milk*
Whey protein predominant	Casein predominant
Ratio of whey: Casein is 60:40	Ratio of whey: Casein is 20:80
Whey protein is easily digestible	• Casein is poorly digestible • Casein causes constipation

- **Fats**
  - 3.5–4 g/dL
  - Rich in polyunsaturated fatty acids, necessary for myelination of the neural tissues.

- Contains omega-2 and omega-6 fatty acids, helps in synthesis of prostaglandins and cholesterol for steroid hormones.
- Long chain polyunsaturated fats (LCP) promote brain growth and reduces dyslexia and hyperactivity.

- **Human milk oligosaccharides**
  - Nondigestible carbohydrate
  - Acts as prebiotics
  - Helps in developing healthy microbiome
- **Vitamins and minerals**
  - Quantity and bioavailability of vitamins and minerals good
- **Water and electrolytes**
  - Water content 88%
  - Baby does not require additional water even during summer
  - Low solute load—less burden to kidneys
- **Immunological components**
  - Breastfed neonate is 14 times less likely to die of diarrhea and 4 times less likely to die of pneumonia.
  - It supplies enzymes which increase digestibility also act as defence against microbes.
    - Amylase
    - Lipoprotein lipase
    - Bile salt stimulated lipase—kills amoeba and giardia
    - Oxidases
    - Lactoperoxidases
    - Leucocyte myeloperoxidase
  - Lactalbumin—rich in tryptophan—precursor of serotonin that plays an important role as neurotransmitter.
  - Lactoferrin—ensures absorption of iron and zinc, also bacteriostatic. It binds iron and makes it unavailable to the bacteria. It inhibits *E.coli.*
  - Levels of Para Amino Benzoic Acid (PABA) offer protection against malaria.
- Bifidus factor—promotes colonization of lactobacilli and bifidobacterium.
- Macrophages
- Lysozymes
- Complements
- Secretory IgA
- **Other benefits**
  - Breast milk contains several growth factors, enzymes and hormones.
  - Epidermal growth factor—enhances maturation of the intestinal cells.
  - Reduces risk of allergy
  - Lipase—increases digestion of fat.
- **Protection from other illnesses**
  - Diabetes mellitus
  - Cardiac diseases
  - Cancer
  - Allergy
  - Infections
- **Mental growth**
  - Good maternal bonding
  - Higher IQ
- **Benefits to mother**
  - Helps in uterine involution and reduces the risk of postpartum hemorrhage
  - Lactation amenorrhea provides effective contraception

- BF is convenient and time saving
- Reduces risk of breast cancer to mother
- Prevents DM type II

Prolactin Reflex (Milk Secretion Reflex)

- The anterior pituitary produces prolactin, which mediates milk production by the alveolar epithelial cells.

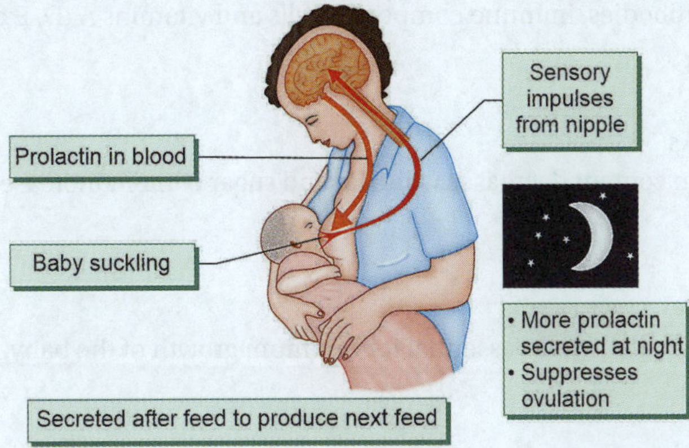

Fig. 1: Prolactin reflex.

- When the neonate sucks, the nerve ending in the nipple caries the impulse to the anterior pituitary which releases prolactin.
- The more neonate sucks at the breast, the greater milk production.
- Earlier the initiation, the sooner the reflex. The greater the demand more is the production. Therefore, mothers should initiate feeding early, do it frequently and allow complete emptying of the breast at each session.
- There is a higher production of prolactin during night, therefore, night feeding helps to maintain the reflex.

Oxytocin Reflex (Milk Ejection Reflex)

- The posterior pituitary produces oxytocin, which is responsible for ejection of milk from the milk glands to the lactiferous sinuses.
- A baby's thought, sight or sound stimulates this reflex.
- The mother's positive emotions and relaxed, confident attitude help the milk ejection reflex. On the contrary, tension, lack of confidence, pain and lack of sleep hinder the milk flow.

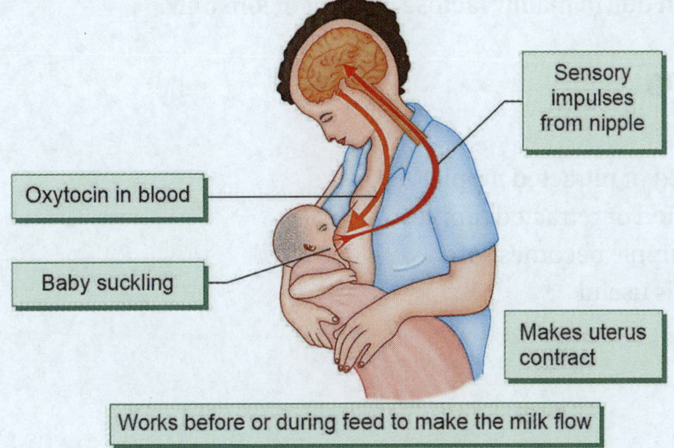

Fig. 2: Oxytocin reflex.

Composition of Breast Milk

Human milk is not only species—specific, but also specific for an individual.

Colostrum

- Initial 3–4 days of delivery.
- Small in quantity (10 to 40 mL/day), yellow and thick.
- Contains large amount of antibodies, immune competent cells and vitamins A, D, E and K.

Transitional Milk

- From 3 to 4 days until 2 weeks.
- Immunoglobulin and protein content decreases while fat and sugar content increases.

Mature Milk

- Follows transitional milk.
- Thinner and watery, contains all nutrients essential for optimum growth of the baby.

Preterm Milk

- Contains more protein, sodium, iron and immunoglobulins and calories to meet the requirement of preterm baby.
- May require fortification with additional nutrients to meet high calories, protein and mineral requirements for very preterm babies.

Fore Milk

- Milk secreted at the start of feed.
- Watery and high in protein, sugar, vitamins and minerals.
- It quenches the baby's thirst.

Hind Milk

- Richer in fat, providing more energy.
- Provides sense of satiety.

Fore Milk Syndrome

If mother feeds only fore milk without ensuring the hind milk, baby may develop diarrhea with perianal excoriation, failure to thrive and colicky pain due to mainly lactose content of fore milk.

Problems of Breastfeeding

Inverted Nipples

- Flat or small nipples inverted or retracted nipples.
- Latching is difficult in inverted or retracted nipples.
- Neonate sucks nipple and nipple becomes sore.
- Inverted syringe technique is useful.

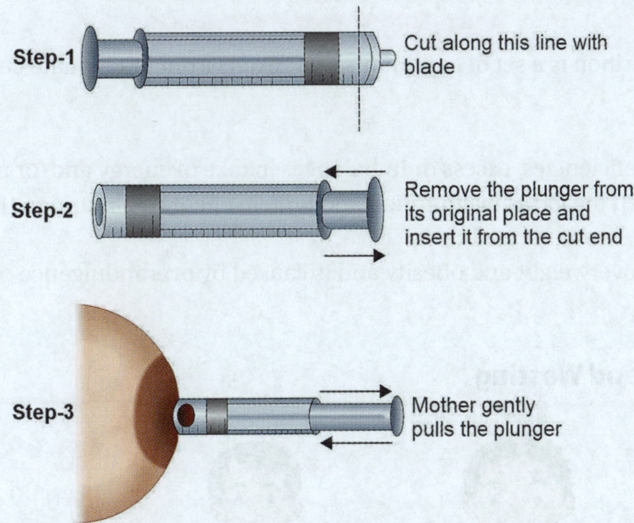

Fig. 3: Inverted syringe technique.

Sore Nipples

- Baby sucks nipple rather than areola, due to incorrect technique or retracted nipple, nipple becomes sore.
- Frequent washing with soap and water can also make nipple sore.
- Correct positioning and latching is the remedy.

Breast Engorgement

- Milk production accelerates from the second to third day of delivery and if feeding is delayed, it may result in engorgement of breast.
- Breast becomes hard, warm and tender with shiny skin.
- Early and frequent feeding in correct breastfeeding technique can prevent breast engorgement.
- Treatment consists of hot fomentation, massage and frequent feeding or expression of milk. Paracetamol can be given to relieve the pain.
- Development of breast abscess may require incision and drainage.

Criteria Indicating Enough Secretion of Breast Milk

- Baby is satisfied and sleeps for 2 to 3 hours after breastfeeding.
- Passing urine at least 6–8 times in 24 hours.
- Gaining the weight.

Storage of Expressed Breast Milk (EBM)

- Room temperature: Up to 4 hours.
- Refrigerator: Up to 24 hours.
- Freezer (-20. C): Up to 3 months.

Contraindications to Breastfeeding

- Congenital lactose intolerance.
- Galactosemia.
- Intake of antimalignant drugs, anti thyroid drugs and antipsychiatric drugs like lithium and radiotherapy to mother.

UNDERNUTRITION

- **Undernutrition:** Undernutrition is a set of conditions that results from inadequate consumption, poor accretion or excessive loss of nutrients.
- **Malnutrition:**
  - Malnutrition refers to deficiencies, excess or imbalances in take of energy and/or nutrients.
  - In practice, however, often the terms malnutrition and protein energy malnutrition (PEM) are used interchangeably with undernutrition.
- **Overnutrition:** It includes overweight and obesity and is caused by over indulgence or excessive intake of nutrients or pathological conditions.

Under Weight, Stunting and Wasting

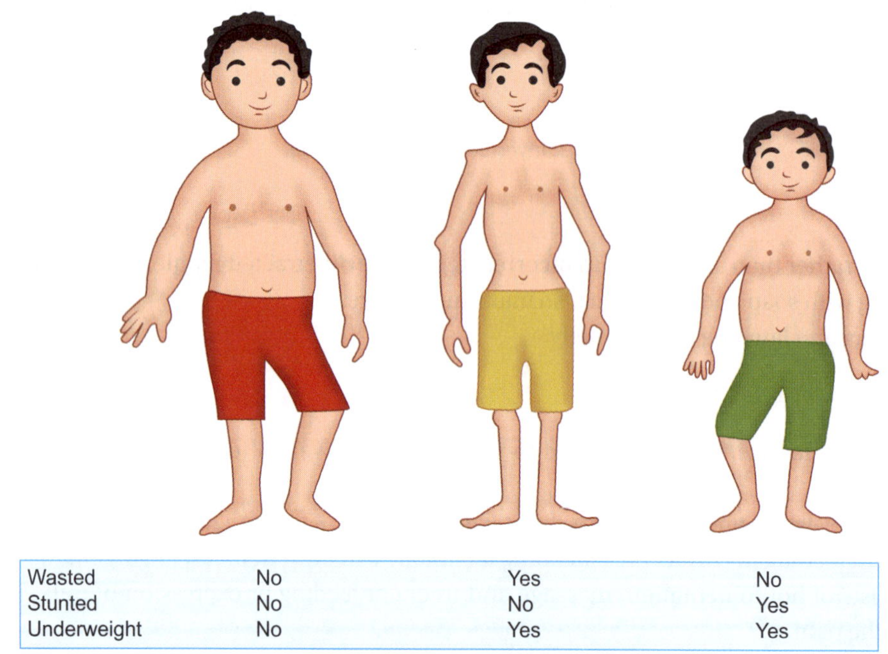

Wasted	No	Yes	No
Stunted	No	No	Yes
Underweight	No	Yes	Yes

Fig. 4: Underweight, stunting and wasting.

Underweight

An underweight child has low weight for age. The weight of the child is less than minus 2 standard deviation scores (-2 SDS) on the WHO Growth standard for her/his age. An underweight child could be wasted or stunted or both.

- **Stunting:**
  - Stunting denotes low height for age. The height or length of the stunted child is below minus 2 standard deviation scores (< -2 SDS) at her/his age. A stunted child is short for her/his age.
  - Stunting indicates chronic malnutrition.
- **Wasting:**
  - Wasting means low weight for height. A child whose weight for her/his actual height is less than minus 2 standard deviation scores (< -2 SDS) at her/his age on the WHO Growth Standard has wasting.
  - Thin appearance.
  - Indicates acute malnutrition as a result of recent acute illness like diarrhea, measles, etc.

Classification of Undernutrition

Indicator	< -2 Z score	-2 to -3 Z score	< -3 Z score
Weight for age	Underweight	Moderate underweight	Severe underweight
Height for age	Stunting	Moderate stunting	Severe stunting
Weight for height	Wasting	Moderate wasting	Severe wasting

Micronutrients

- **Type I:**
  - Iron
  - Calcium
  - Iodine
  - Vitamin A
  - Thiamine
  - Riboflavin
  - Vitamin B_{12}
  - Folate
  - Selenium
- **Type II:**
  - Body does not store, needs to be supplemented
  - Essential amino acids
  - Potassium
  - Magnesium
  - Zinc
  - Phosphorus

Marasmus

- Severe form of wasting
- Greek word—marasmus means wasting
- *Most common age:* 0 to 3 years
- Energy deficit
- *Clinical features:*
  - Looking alert
  - Irritable
  - Hungry
  - Appears very thin skin and bones and has no fat
  - Sunken eyes
  - Depressed anterior fontanelle
  - Baggy pant appearance—loose skin of buttocks hanging down due to loss of fat
  - Monkey facies following loss of buccal pad of fat
  - Sparse—hypopigmented hairs
  - No edema

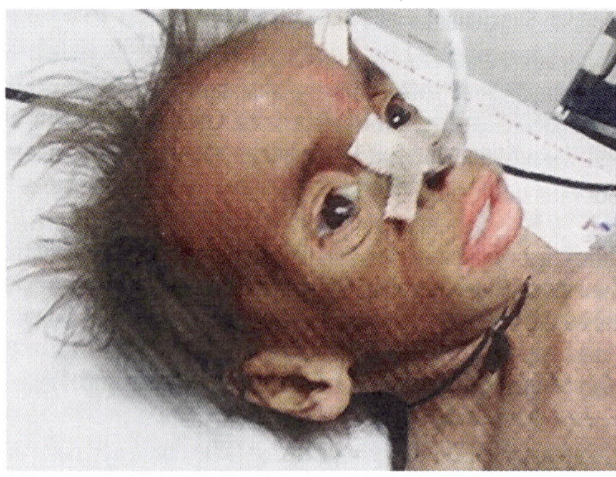

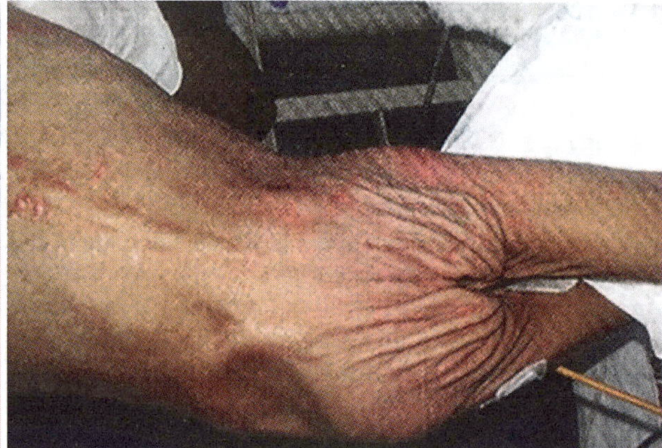

Grades of Marasmus

- *Grade I:* Loss of fat from axillae and groins
- *Grade II:* Loss of fat from axillae, groins, thighs and buttocks
- *Grade III:* Wasting at axillae, groins, thighs, buttocks, chest and abdomen
- *Grade IV:* Last loss of buccal pad of fat

Kwashiorkor

- Coined the name by Cicely Williams in 1933.
- From 'Ghana' language, meaning 'red boy'.

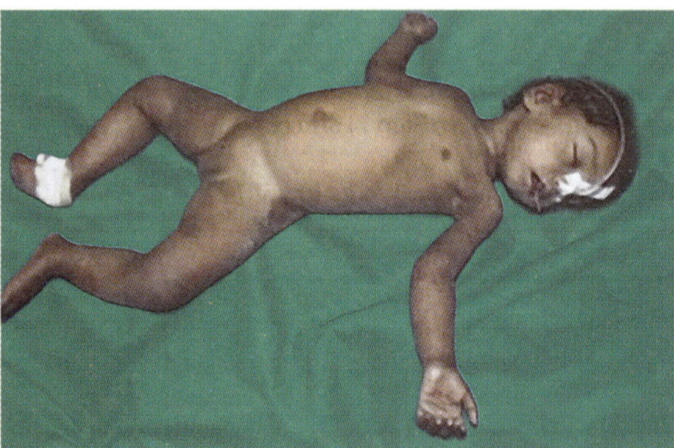

- Also called 'Sugar baby'
- Most common age 1 to 4 years
- Uncommon in India, now
- *Essential (cardinal) features:*
  - Edema
  - Growth retardation
  - Apathetic (psychomotor changes)
  - Muscle wasting
- *Edema:*
  - Hypoalbuminemia
  - Retention of fluid and water due to increased capillary permeability
  - Free radical induced damage to cell membrane included by infection
  - Edema starts from legs and face and becomes generalized.

- Ascites is rare unless there is a coexistent cause of tuberculosis.
- *Psychomotor changes:* Lethargic, listless, apathetic
- Loss of appetite
- *Dermatosis:*
    - Dry and scaly skin with cracking
    - Flaky paint (hypopigmented or reddish skin, peeling plaques of dermatosis)
    - Pavement dermatosis (jet black patches over flexures and pressure sites, especially of extremities)
    - Buttocks, perineum and thighs are common sites
    - Multiple, punctate pinkish areas over legs
    - Perioral lesions due to riboflavin and zinc deficiency
    - Deep and indolent ulcerations and fissures in flexures or over pressure points
- *Hair changes:*
    - Hypopigmented, lusterless, thin, easily pluckable
    - Flag sign of hairs
    - Pallor
    - Deficiency of vitamins, zinc, niacin, tyrosine

Grading of Kwashiorkar

- *Grade I:* Bilateral pedal edema
- *Grade II:* Pedal and facial edema
- *Grade III:* Pedal, facial, paraspinal and chest edema
- *Grade IV:* Generalized edema with ascites

Indicators of Dehydration in Malnutrition

- It is difficult to assess for dehydration in children with malnutrition due to overlapping of several clinical features.
- Specific indicators of dehydration are:
    - Dry oral mucosa
    - Excessive thirst
    - Oliguria
    - Weak pulse
    - Hypothermia

Severe Acute Malnutrition (SAM)

- Special classification recommended by WHO for identifying and managing children with life threatening undernutrition in public health program settings.
- Children with SAM have a mixture of features of marasmus and kwashiorkor.
- 6 to 59 months.
- Diagnostic criteria of SAM
    - Weight for heigh < -3 STD on the WHO growth standard.

      Or
    - Bilateral pedal edema

      Or
    - Mid upper arm circumference <11.5 cms.

Management of Moderate Acute Malnutrition (MAM)

- >80% of malnutrition associated deaths are due to MAM.
- Vital to intervene in children with MAM at the community level before they develop complications.

- Definition of MAM
  Weight for height between -2 and -3 SDS and/or MUAC between 11.5 and 12.5 cm. without edema.
- *Management:*
  - Nutritious home food
  - Frequent feeding (up to 7 times a day)
  - Use of fat to increase the energy
  - Milk and eggs are excellent animal origin foods
  - Combination of cereals and legumes
  - Protein 3 g/kg/day
  - Vitamins
  - Minerals
- Weight gain is best measure of the efficacy of treatment.

Severe Acute Malnutrition

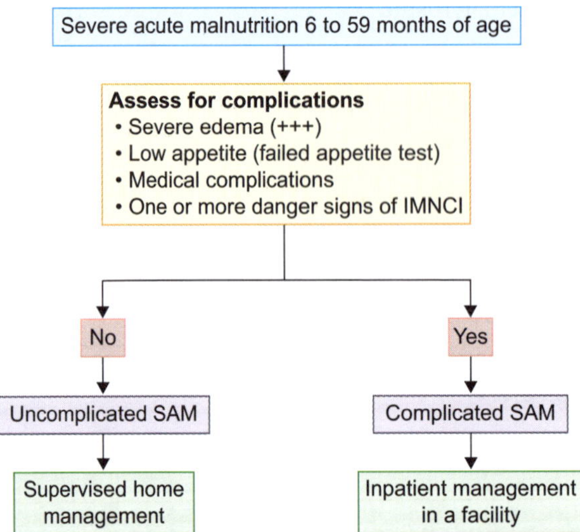

- Medical complications like severe anemia, pneumonia, diarrhea, dehydration, tuberculous, HIV, Heart disease, Cerebral palsy etc.

Supervised Home Management of a Child with Uncomplicated SAM

- **Nutrition therapy:**
  - Initially catch up diets → home foods → Continue breastfeeding. 175 kcal/kg/day.
  - Should be fed 6–8 times a day.
  - Should be fed lovingly, actively, ensuring hygiene.
- **Other treatments:**
  - Oral amoxicillin for 5 days
  - Vitamin A
  - Albendazole - single dose
  - Vaccination
- **Sensory stimulation**
- **Supervision and support:**
  - Home visits by health workers, initially daily, later twice a week
  - Involve a peer counselor

- **Monitoring by health workers (ASHA/AWW/ANM):**
  - Assess intake, solve feeding issues
  - Treat or refer for medical problems
  - Assess growth weekly

Management of Complicated SAM

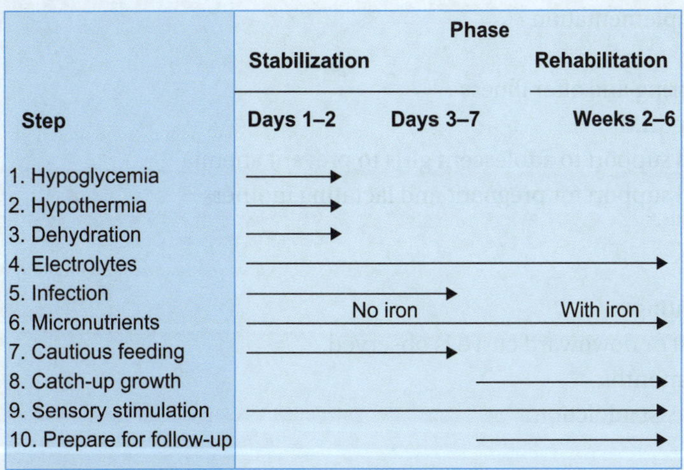

Indications for Hospital Management in SAM

- Age <6 months
- Presence of any emergency signs
- Hypothermia (Axillary temp <35°C)
- Fever (Axillary temp >39°C)
- Edema
- Persistent vomiting
- Diarrhea and dehydration
- Severe anemia
- Very weak, apathetic
- Fast breathing, chest indrawing
- Evidence of systemic infections or complications
- Extensive skin lesions, eye lesions
- Purpura/bleeding tendency

Ten Reasons for High Mortality in SAM

1. Inability to distinguish between acute and rehabilitation phases
2. Excessive use of IV Fluids
3. Fluid overload due to lack of monitoring during rehydration
4. Use of diuretics for edema
5. Use of albumin for edema
6. Not keeping child warm and euglycemic
7. Low index of suspicion of infection
8. Early use of diet high in protein and sodium
9. Failure to monitor food intake
10. Early treatment of anemia with oral iron

Ten Key Interventions for Prevention of Malnutrition

1. Breastfeeding within 1 hour of birth
2. Exclusive breastfeeding for first 6 months of life
3. Age appropriate food from 6 months to 2 years
4. Hygienic, complementary feeding practices
5. Immunization
6. Biannual vitamin A supplementation
7. Deworming
8. Appropriate feeding during and after illness
9. Therapeutic feeding for SAM
10. Adequate nutrition and support to adolescent girls to prevent anemia
11. Adequate nutrition and support for pregnant and lactating mothers

Invisible PEM

- Not overt wasting or stunting.
- Growth chart shows a flat or downward curve is observed.
- Most common age 6–24 months.
- Often associated with breast addiction.

Appetite Test

- **Procedure**
  Ask the mother to offer energy dense therapeutic food to the child in a quiet area gently. Child is allowed to drink water while feeding.
- **Interpretation**
  - *Passed test:* If child eats early.
  - *Failed test:* If refuses therapeutic food even after persistent encouragement.

Amount of Ready to Use Therapeutic Food (RUTF)

Weight (kg)	*Amount of RUTF (g/day)*
3–4.9	105–130
5–6.9	200–260
7– 9.9	260–400
10–14.9	400–460

Vitamin A

Vitamin A Deficiency

- Leading cause of blindness in preschool children in India
- Follicular hyperkeratosis of skin
- Toad skin
- Night blindness
- Xerophthalmia
- Bitot's spots
- Keratomalacia
- High risk of contacting severe systemic infections especially measles

WHO Classification of Xerophthalmia

Primary Signs

- *XIA:* Conjunctival xerosis
- *XIB:* Bitot spots
- *X2:* Corneal xerosis
- *X3A:* Corneal ulceration (<1/3 of cornea)
- *X3B:* Corneal ulceration (>1/3 of cornea)

Secondary Signs

- *XN:* Night blindness
- *XF:* Fundal changes
- *XS:* Corneal scarring

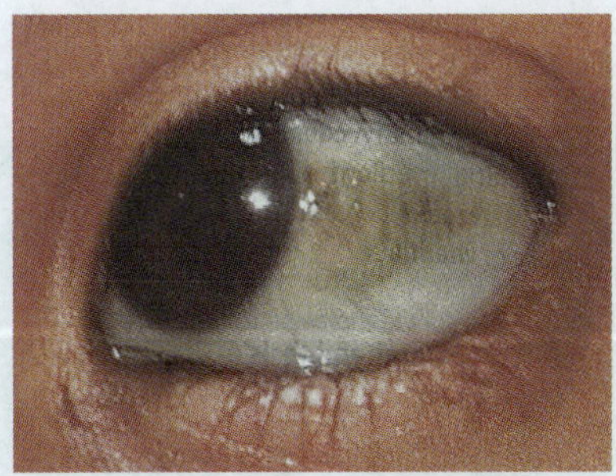

Treatment of Vitamin A Deficiency

Age	*Dose in IU*
<6 months	50,000
6–12 months	1 lakh
>1 year	2 lakhs

Three Doses

- First day
- Next day
- 4 weeks later

Prophylaxis Program against Nutritional Blindness (1970)

- 6–59 months
- Vitamin A 1,00,000 units 9 months with measles vaccine
- 2,00,000 units at 15–18 months with DPT booster
- Then 6 monthly till the age of 5 years (total 9 doses)

Any Child with Measles or SAM

- *<1 year:* 1,00,000 units
- *Older children:* 2,00,000 units
- Consecutive 2 days

NUTRITIONAL RICKETS

Rickets is Defined as Failure of Mineralization of Growing Bones

Clinical Features:

- Wide open AF
- Large head
- Frontal, parietal and occipital bossing (Hot cross bun appearance) (caput quadratum)
- Craniotabes (sign of active rickets)
- Pigeon chest
- Rachitic rosaries
- Pectus carinatum
- Harrison's sulcus
- Knock knee
- Widening of wrist
- Double malleoli

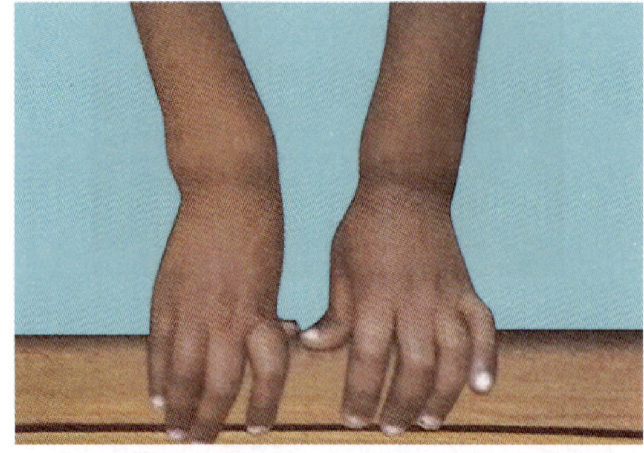

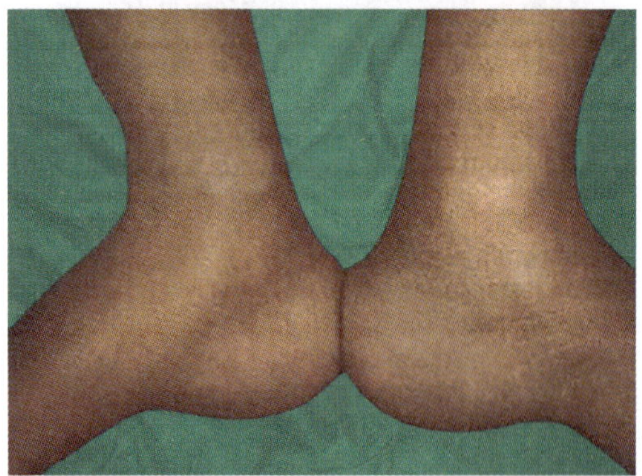

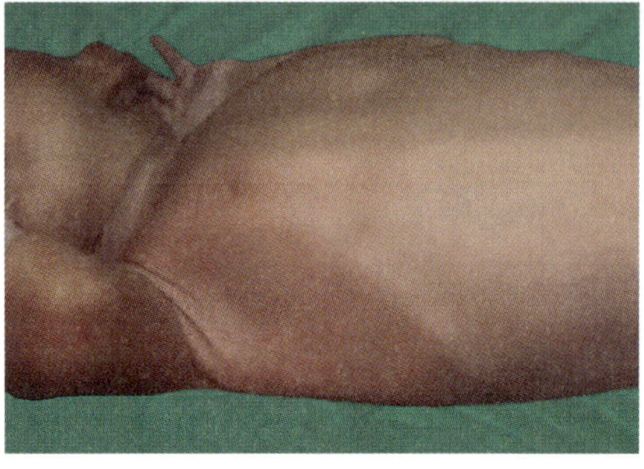

Treatment Guidelines for Nutritional Rickets

Age	*Daily dose of vitamin D for 12 weeks*	*Alternative intermittent dose regimen*
<6 months	2,000 IU	Not recommended
6–12 months	2,000 IU	Equivalent of 2,000 IU/day may be given on a weekly or monthly basis
>12 months	2,000 IU	60,000 IU every 2 weeks for 5 doses

Rickets

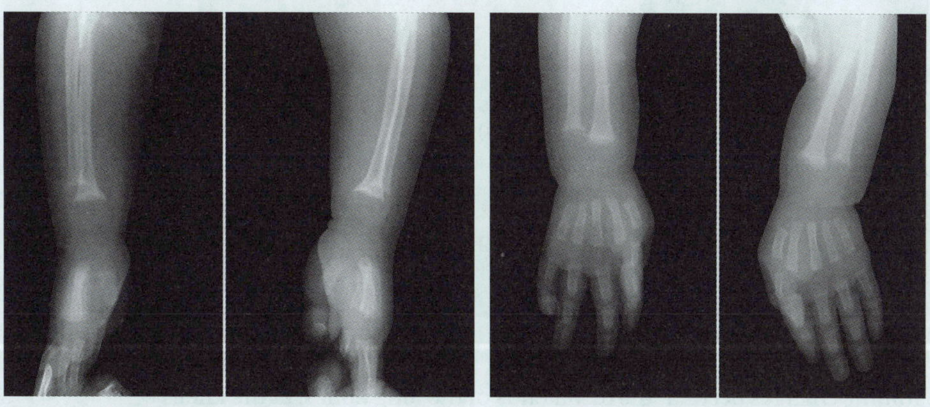

Radiological Features of Rickets

- Nonmineralization of growing bones is called rickets
- Rapidly growing bones of the body are commonly affected (wrists and knees)
- Loss of zone of provisional calcification (Increased distance between the epiphysis and the metaphysis)
- Fraying (Blurring of metaphyseal margin) (If cloth frays, some of the threads at the end start to come apart)
- Apparent increase in width of growth plate
- Splaying (Widening of metaphysis) (Splay means to spread out or become wide apart at the end)
- Cupping of metaphysis (Depression of metaphysis)
- Osteoporosis (decrease in bone density)
- Deformities (bow legs, coxa vara, lumbar lordosis, kyphoscoliosis)
- Rachitic rosary (beaded enlargement of anterior metaphysis of ribs)
- Pathological fractures (Green stick fracture)

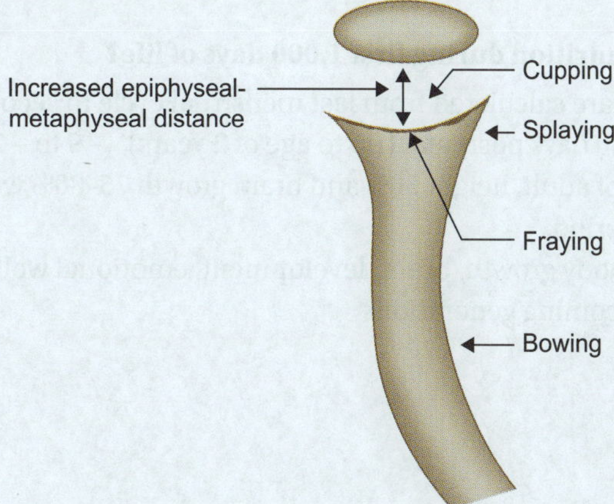

Scurvy

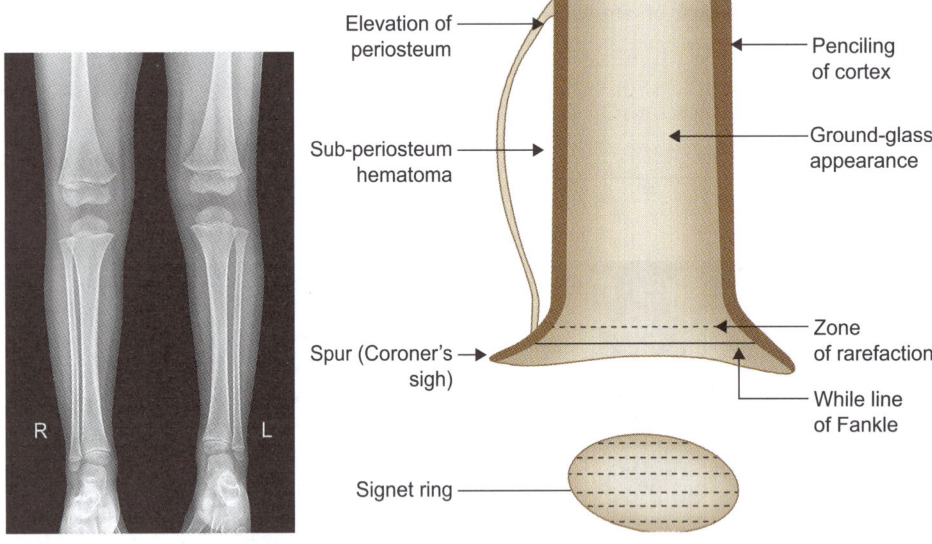

Radiological Changes of Scurvy

- Typical radiographic changes occur at the distal ends of the long bones, at the knees
- Ground-glass appearance
- Pencilling of cortex (Thinned out cortex)
- Wimberger's sign (Signet ring) (Hallo sign of Wimberger) (Epiphysis is out lined as a rim standing out against a rarified body with pencilling)
- Corner sign (Pelken spurs) (projection of calcified matrix beyond the usual limits of shaft forming spurs)
- Zone of rarefaction
- Frankel's sign (Dense white line at the end of long bones)
- Extremely severe may have subluxation of epiphyses
- Fissuring and fractures above calcified cartilage in the metaphysis
- Subperiosteal hematoma
- Subluxation of ribs (step like) at the costochondral junction (clinically scorbutic rosary)

QUESTIONS AND ANSWERS

Q-1. What is the importance of nutrition during first 1,000 days of life?

- The first 1,000 days of life are calculated from last menstrual cycle to second birth day
- Intrauterine 270 days + 730 days postnatal (up to age of 2 years), (– 9 to + 24 months)
- Body growth occurs 20% of adult, height 50% and brain growth 75–80% with responsive social and emotional expressions during this period.
- It is very crucial time for body growth, brain development, emotional well being, immunity and future health of the individual and the coming generations

Q-2. What is Global Strategy for IYCF feeding during first 1000 days of life?

- Initiation of breastfeeding as soon as possible
- Exclusive breast feeding during first 6 months of life
- Introduction of optimal complementary feeds at 6 months
- Age appropriate feeding from 6 months to 2 years
- Hygienic complementary feeding practices
- Breastfeeding to be continued minimum for 2 years and beyond
- Responsive feeding
- Monitor on Growth Charts
- Immunization + Vitamin A supplementation + Deworming
- Appropriate feeding during and after illness
- Therapeutic feeding for children with SAM
- Adequate nutrition and support for adolescent girls to prevent anemia and for pregnant and lactating mothers

Q-3. What is Iron Folic Acid (IFA) supplementation Government of India program for women?

- 60 mg iron + 500 μg (0.5 mg) folic acid per day from 14th week of pregnancy and continued throughout pregnancy for 180 days and to be continued for 180 days, post partum
- Women of child bearing age (nonpregnant and nonlactating) and adolescents: IFA (60 mg iron + 0.5 mg FA) per week

Q-4. What are different methods for assessment of malnutrition in children?

- Anthropometric assessment (Gold standard)
- Dietary assessment, including feeding practices (24 Hours recall method)
- Clinical assessment
- Biochemical tests
- Epidemiological and ecological
- Functional assessment for organ and its morphology
- Radio-imaging

Q-5. How to perform anthropometry in children?

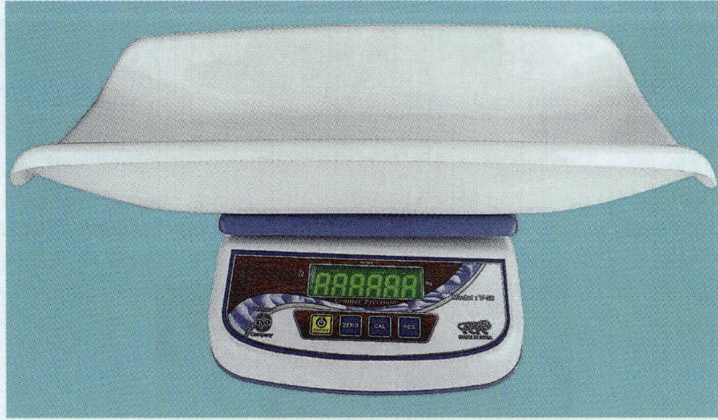

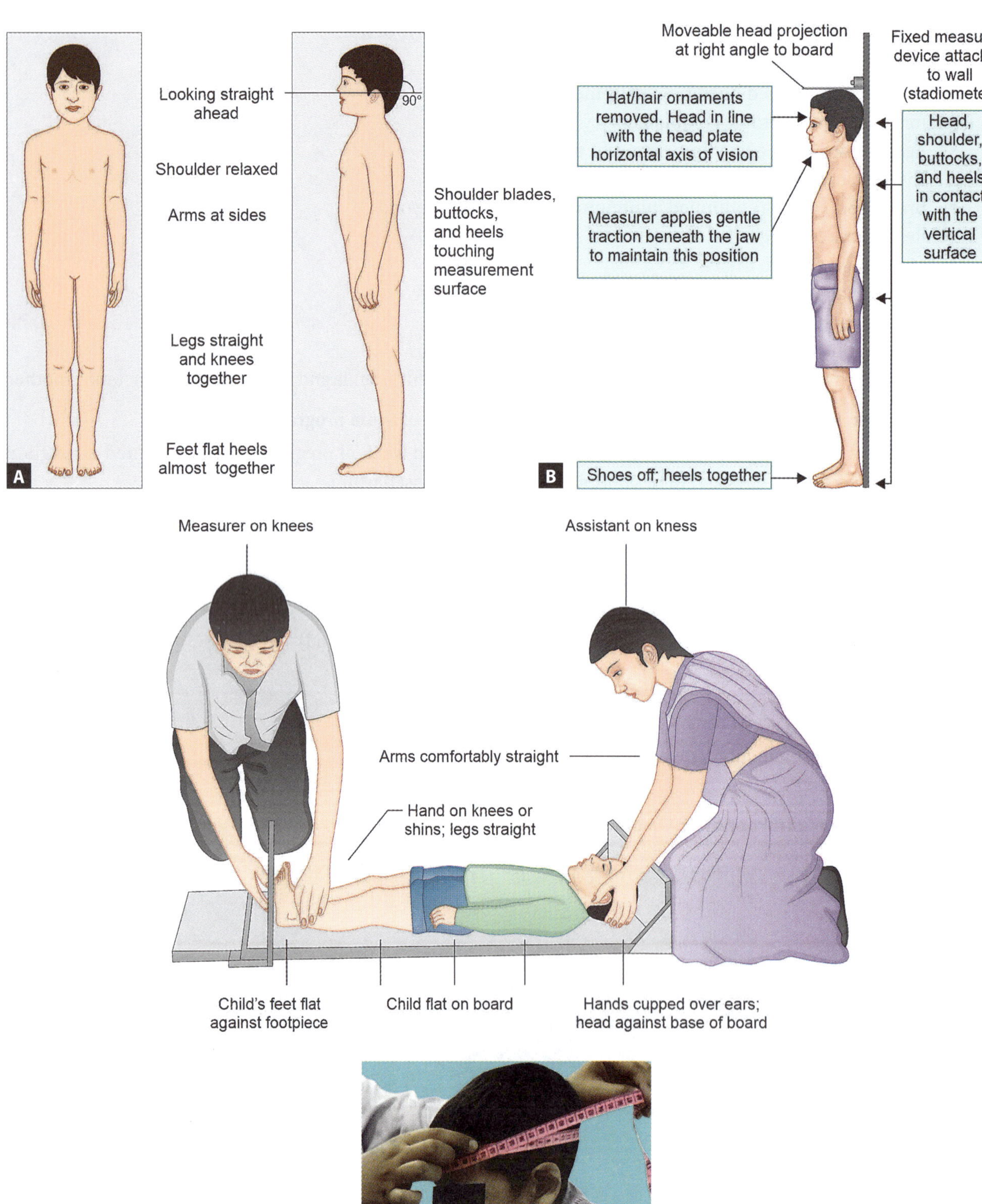
Looking straight ahead
90°
Shoulder relaxed
Arms at sides
Legs straight and knees together
Feet flat heels almost together
Shoulder blades, buttocks, and heels touching measurement surface
A
Moveable head projection at right angle to board
Fixed measuring device attached to wall (stadiometer)
Hat/hair ornaments removed. Head in line with the head plate horizontal axis of vision
Head, shoulder, buttocks, and heels in contact with the vertical surface
Measurer applies gentle traction beneath the jaw to maintain this position
B
Shoes off; heels together
Measurer on knees
Assistant on kness
Arms comfortably straight
Hand on knees or shins; legs straight
Child's feet flat against footpiece
Child flat on board
Hands cupped over ears; head against base of board

Q-6. How to measure mid upper arm circumference?

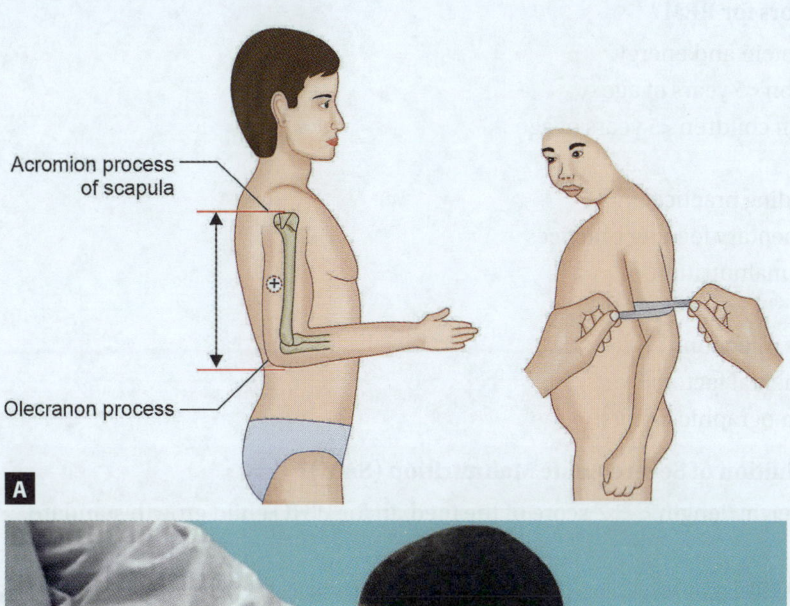

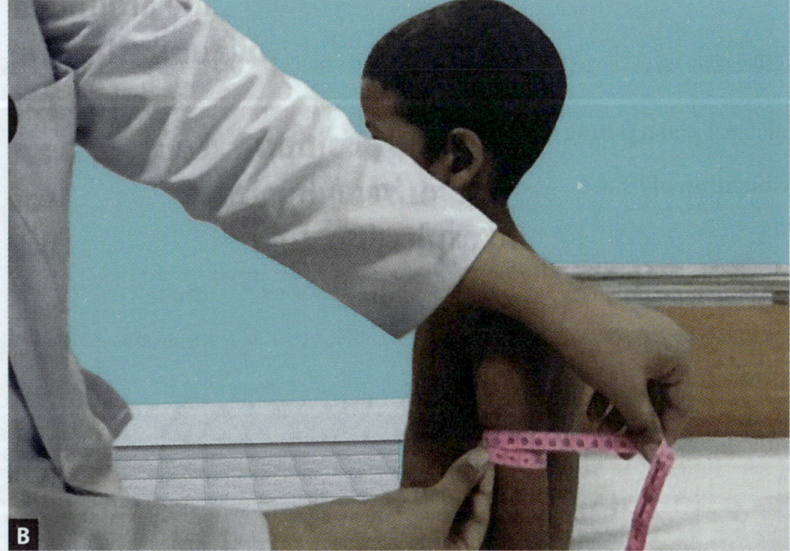

Q-7. What are interpretations of MUAC in children?

- ≥12.5 cm → Normal
- 11.5 to 12.4 → Moderate Acute Malnutrition (Wasted)
- <11.5 → SAM (severely wasted)

The Bangle Test

- Internal diameter 4 cm
- If it crosses elbow, child is malnourished

The Shakir's Tape

- *Green:* >13.5 cm
- *Yellow:* 12.5 to 13.5 cm
- *Red:* <12.5 cm

Q-8. What is protein energy malnutrition (PEM)? What is prevalence of PEM in India? What are common etiological factors for PEM?

- Deficit of protein and energy
- Most common <5 years of age
- 65% of Indian children <5 years of age
- *Etiology:*
  - Breastfeeding practice
  - Complementary feeding practices
  - Maternal malnutrition
  - LBW
  - Recurrent infections
  - Environmental factors
  - Socio-demographic factors

Q-9. What is the definition of Severe Acute Malnutrition (SAM)?

- Weight for height/length <-3 Z score of the median for WHO child growth standard
  and/or
- MUAC <11.5 cm
  and/or
- Presence of bilateral pedal pitting edema

Q-10. What is IAP classification of PEM?

IAP Classification

% of expected weight for age	*Grade*
>80%	Normal
71–80%	I
61–70%	II
51–60%	III
<50%	IV

Q-11. What is Gomez classification of PEM?

Weight for age (%) of expected	*Nutritional status*
>90	Normal
75–90	I
60–75	II
<60	III

Q-12. What is Grading of Marasmus?

- *Grade I:* Loss of fat from axillae and groin
- *Grade II:* Loss of fat from axillae, groin, thighs and buttocks
- *Grade III:* Wasting at axillae, groin, thighs, buttocks, chest and abdomen
- *Grade IV:* Last loss of buccal pad of fat

Q-13. What is appetite test?

- The appetite test in SAM management is a method to assess a child's ability to consume Ready to Use Therapeutic Food (RUTF). It helps to determine whether a child with SAM can be treated as an out patient with RUTF or needs to be admitted for inpatient care due to poor appetite.
- Appetite test should be carried out in quiet, comfortable environment.
- Mother/care giver should wash his/her hands.
- Allow the child to sit comfortably on lap and offer RUTF.
- Encourage the child to finish the food
- If the child is able to finish the amount recommended for weight, child can be shifted to outpatient management.

Q-14. What are criteria for passing appetite test?

Body weight (kg)	*Minimum amount needed to be consumed to pass the appetite test*
<4	15 mL
4–6.9	25 mL
7–9.9	35 mL
10–14.9	50 mL

Q-15. What are indicating for hospitalization in SAM?

- Age <6 months
- Any emergency signs
- Hypothermia (axillary temp <35ºC)
- Fever (axillary temp >39ºC)
- Edema
- Diarrhea and dehydration
- Severe anemia
- Persistent vomiting
- Apathetic
- Fast breathing, chest indrawing
- Extensive skin lesions
- Eye lesions
- Purpura (bleeding tendency)
- Infection

CHAPTER 41

Nutritional Anemia

QUESTIONS AND ANSWERS

Q-1. What is the prevalence of nutritional anemia?

- Nutritional anemia is the most common type of anemia clinically encountered in children
- The deficiency of main micronutrients required for the synthesis of hemoglobin like iron, folic acid and vitamin B_{12} are grouped under nutritional anemias
- Iron deficiency anemia (IDA) is the most widespread micronutrient deficiency
- It is estimated to affect one third of world population out of which 90% cases are from developing countries
- Infants, preschool children, adolescents and women of child-bearing age groups are at the greatest risk of developing IDA

Q-2. What are important facts to know concerned with IDA?

- A full term new born infant contains about 0.5 g (75 mg/kg) of iron, compare to 5 g of iron in adults
- Infants and young children should continue to absorb 1 mg of iron daily to reach the adult level of stores of 5 g
- 1 mg of iron should be absorbed daily to maintain positive iron balance in childhood. Because less than 10% of dietary iron is usually absorbed, a dietary intake of 8-10 mg of iron daily is necessary
- IDA is common despite abundance of iron in the Earth's crust because of factors like poor dietary intake, impaired iron absorption, blood loss leading to insufficient iron for RBC production
- *Rich sources of dietary iron:*
  - Meat, eggs
  - Dates
  - Jaggery
  - Millet, Ragi
  - Green leafy vegetables
  - Sprouts
- Though breast milk contains small quantity of iron, the bioavailability of this iron (lactoferrin) is about 50–70% and hence it is adequate for the first 6 months of life
- Delayed clamping of umbilical cord (one minute) can improve iron status of the baby and reduce the risk of IDA
- *Factors retarding absorption of iron:*
  - Alkaline pH
  - Phosphates
  - Phytates
  - Bran
  - Calcium
  - Tannins
  - Antacids
  - Cobalt, lead

Q-3. What are common causes of iron deficiency anemia (IDA)?

- *Decreased iron stores:*
  - Preterm babies
  - SFD babies
  - Twins
- *Decreased intake:*
  - Lack of breast milk
  - Delayed introduction of complementary feeds
  - Iron poor diet
- *Top milk/Cow's milk:*
  - Lower bioavailability of iron
  - Bovine milk is rich in calcium that retards iron absorption
  - Cow's milk allergy can cause GI blood loss
  - Predominant milk diet
- *Increased requirements:*
  - Preterm babies
  - SFD babies
  - Adolescent growth spurt
  - Pregnancy
  - Lactation
- *Malabsorption:*
  - Celiac disease
  - Chronic diarrhea
  - Giardiasis
  - Cow's milk allergy
  - Chronic infectious like HIV, TB
  - GI surgery
- *Losses:*
  - Repeated blood sampling
  - GI bleeding like portal hypertension, drugs like NSAIDs, hook worm infestation, CMPA, Polyp, Meckel's diverticulum, menstruating women
  - Malaria
  - Peptic ulcer
  - Bleeding diathesis
  - Hemangioma
  - IBD

Q-4. What are clinical manifestations of IDA?

- Peak incidence occurs between 6 months and 3 years followed by adolescents 11–17 years and pregnant and lactating mothers
- Pallor (most common)
- Hypoperfusion, hypoxemia, oedema in nephrotic syndrome, hypothyroidism like conditions also present with apparent pallor, which should be excluded
- Look for pallor at lips, tongue, conjunctiva, palms and nails
- *Degree of pallor:*
  - *No pallor:* No anemia
  - *Palmar pallor:* Some anemia
  - *Palmar creases pallor:* Severe anemia

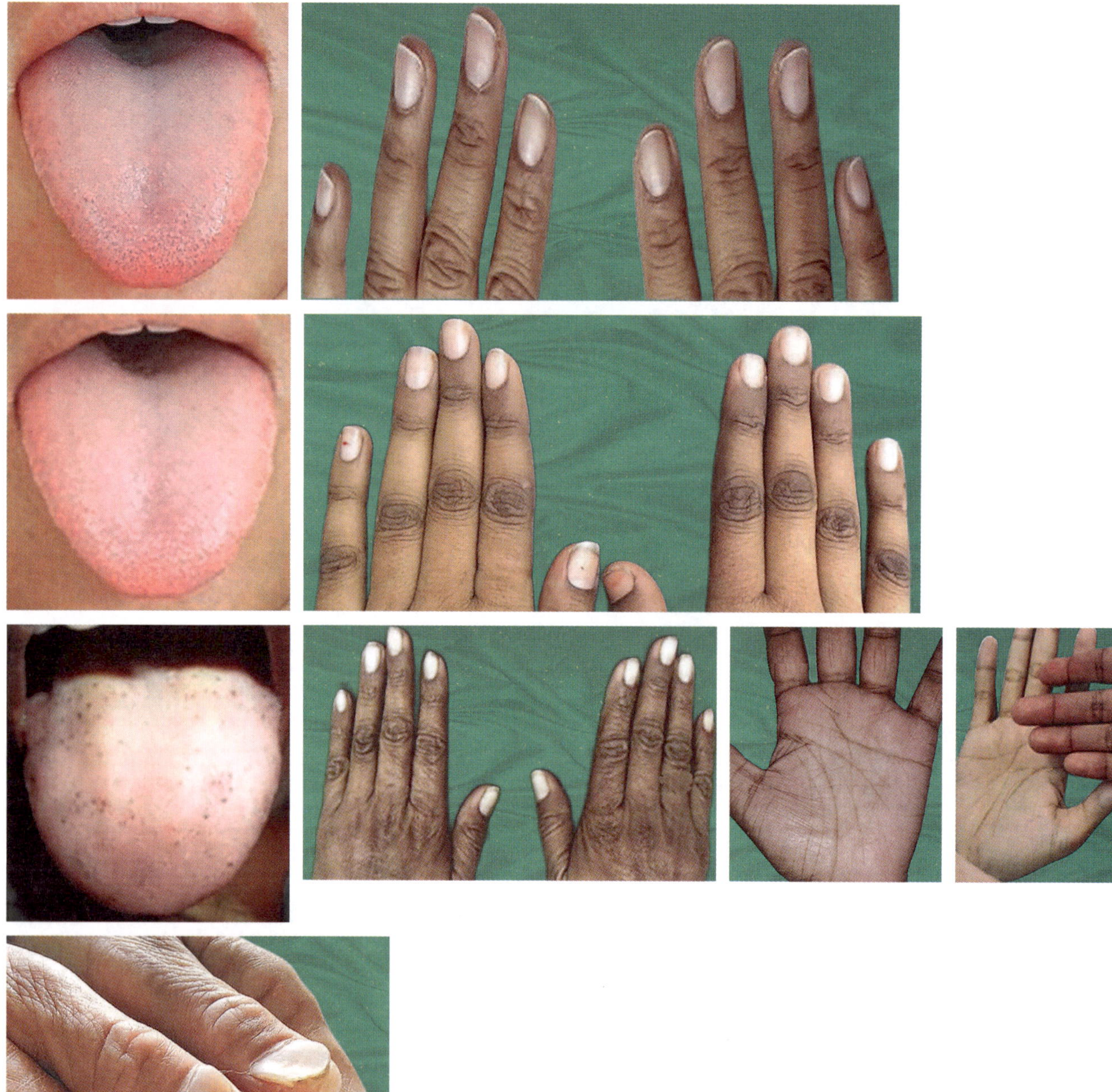

- Pica (Geophagia, Pagophagia, Amylophagia, etc.)
- Platynychia, Koilonychia
- Mild splenomegaly and frontoparietal bossing (caput quadratum) may be present in long standing IDA.
- Increased susceptibility to infection (due to reduced immunity)
- Signs of congestive heart failure
- Easy fatigability
- Anorexia
- Irritability

- Cognitive dysfunction
- Short attention span, impaired mental and motor development (scholastic performance affected)
- Glossitis, stomatitis
- Dysphagia (due to esophageal webs)
- Plummer–Vinson or Paterson Kelly syndrome

Q-5. What are the causes of IDA with clubbing?

- Celiac disease
- Inflammatory bowel disease (IBD)
- Bacterial endocarditis
- A–V fistula

Q-6. What conditions have IDA as the risk factor?

- Breath-holding spell
- Febrile seizures
- Stroke

Q-7. What investigations should be performed in a case of IDA?

- **Complete hemogram**
  - Hemoglobin is reduced
  - Total RBC count is reduced
  - MCV (<80 fL) and MCHC (<32%) are reduced
  - Red cell distribution width (RDW) is increased (>14.5%)
  - WBC within normal limits
  - Platelets count normal or increased
  - Peripheral smear microcytic and hypochromic RBCs with anisocytosis and poikilocytosis
  - Reticulocyte count is normal unless iron therapy
- Serum Iron reduced (<75 mg/dL) and TIBC raised (>350 µg/dL)
- Transferrin saturation <16%
- Serum Ferritin reduced (<15 ng/mL)
- Depletion of stainable iron from bone marrow
- Normal serum iron level varies considerably, diurnal variation with a peak in the morning and trough in the evening. Dietary intake also can alter the iron levels in the plasma. May also be affected by chronic infections, malignancies and chemotherapy as well as iron medication. Serum Iron is not a reliable test.
- Factors affecting serum iron concentration do not alter values of TIBC, Gold standard test, highly specific and adequately sensitive test, sensitive laboratory index of iron status.
- *S. Ferritin increases in:*
  - Inflammatory conditions (collagen disorders)
  - Chronic infections
  - Malignancies
  - Chronic liver diseases

  In these conditions, S. ferritin is raised as an inflammatory markers and therefore IDA is missed.
- If CRP and serum ferritin both are raised, consider them as inflammatory markers and ferritin level is not reliable to assess iron status.

Q-8. What are differential diagnosis of IDA?

Parameters	*Iron deficiency anemia*	*Anemia of chronic disease*	*Thalassemia trait*
MCV	Decreased	Normal or decreased	Markedly decreased
RDW	Increased	Increased or normal	Increased or normal
Red cell morphology	Microcytic, hypochromic anisopoikilocytosis	Normocytic, normochromic	Microcytic, hypochromic, polychromasia
RBC count	Decreased	Decreased	Normal
Serum iron	Decreased	Decreased	Normal
TIBC	Increased	Decreased	Normal
Transferrin Saturation	Decreased	Decreased or normal	Normal or increased
S. Ferritin	Decreased	Increased or normal	Normal
Hb electrophoresis	Normal	Normal	Hb A2 > 3.5%
Marrow hemosiderin	Low or absent	Normal or increased	Normal

Q-9. What is the treatment of IDA?

Medicinal Iron Therapy

- Oral iron therapy is the ideal treatment
- 3 to 6 mg/kg/day of elemental iron, 3 to 4 mg/kg/day is sufficient for optimal response
- Hb level is usually reached in 3 months, it should be continued for another 2 to 3 months to build up iron stores
- Ferrous compounds are better absorbed than ferric iron:
  - Ferrous sulfate (20% elemental iron)
  - Ferrous gluconate (30% elemental iron)
  - Ferrous fumarate (33% elemental iron)
  - Ferric ammonium citrate (18% elemental iron), it is most commonly used ferric salt
- Iron polymaltose complex (IPC) is a novel iron preparation, which contains nonionic iron and polymaltose in a stable complex. Not as efficacious as other preparations
- Carboxyl iron is a small particle preparation of highly purified metallic iron, safe and lesser side effects, much less toxic than other ionized forms of iron
- Colloidal iron is a readily available iron preparation, hardly any data is available
- Iron in the form of Hb is not useful. Large volumes need to be taken
- Enteric coated tablets are more expensive and may not disintegrate in the stomach and hence absorption may not be adequate
- Slow releasing preparations improves absorption and lesser side effects
- Sprinkles are devised by UNICEF
- Iron should be taken as empty stomach in single dose or two divided doses
- Phytates, calcium and tea retard the absorption of iron
- Vitamin B_{12} and Folic acid may be given with iron
- *Side effects of iron:*
  - Nausea and vomiting
  - Diarrhea
  - Constipation
  - Abdominal discomfort
  - Ferrous salts—high incidence of GI side effect (23%)
- Iron absorption is maximum during initial phase of therapy. It declines from 14% in the first week to 7% in the 4th week and 2% after 4 months

Parenteral Iron Therapy

- **Indications**
  - Severe intolerance to oral iron
  - GI bleeding aggravated by oral iron
  - Preoperative in urgent surgery
  - Malabsorption syndromes
- **Total dose**

$$\text{Iron (mg)} = \frac{\text{Wt (kg)} \times \text{Hb deficit (g/dL)} \times 80}{100 \times 3.4 \times 1.5}$$

OR

$$\text{Wt (kg)} \times \text{Hb deficit (g/dL)} \times 4$$

- **Preparations available**
  - Iron dextran complex (No longer preferred)
  - Iron sucrose
  - Sodium iron gluconate
  - Ferumoxytol
  - Ferric carboxymaltose (not approved for use in children)
- **Side effects**
  - Skin rash
  - Arthralgia
  - Myalgia
  - Anaphylaxis (rare)
- **Indications for hospitalization**
  - Severe anemia (Hb <5 g/dL)
  - CCF
- **Indications for PCV transfusion**
  - Rarely needed
  - Severe anemia with CCF
  - Hb <4 g/dL
  - Ongoing blood loss

Q-10. How will you monitor response to iron therapy?

- *12 to 24 hours:*
  - Replacement of intracellular iron enzymes
  - Subjective improvement
  - Decreased irritability
  - Increased appetite
  - Increased serum iron
- *36 to 48 hours:*
  - Initial bone marrow response
  - Erythroid hyperplasia
- *48–72 hours:*
  - Reticulocytosis, peaking 5–7 days
- *4–30 days*
  - Increase in the Hb level (0.1 g/dL/day)

  - Increase in MCV
  - Increase in ferritin
- *1–3 months*
  - Replacement of stores

An increase in Hb >1 g/dL after 1 month of iron therapy is usually the most practical means to establish the diagnosis of IDA.

Q-11. What are the preventive measures for IDA?

- Exclusive BF for 6 months
- Timely introduction of complementary feeds at 6 months of age.
- Iron supplementation for preterm and LBW infants from 2 months of age.
- Restrict cow's milk (bovine milk) consumption
- Intake of dates, jaggery, millet and green leafy vegetables

Q-12. What is the dosage and duration of Iron Folic Acid Supplementation at various age group in Government Health Program?

S. No.	*Age group*	*Dose*	*Regime*	*Service delivery*
1.	6–60 months	1 mL IFA syrup containing: • 20 mg elemental iron and • 100 µg folic acid	• Biweekly throughout the period 6–60 months of age and • De-worming for children 12 months and above	Through ASHA Inclusion in MCP card for entry by ASHA
2.	5–10 years	*Tablets:* • 45 mg elemental iron 400 µg folic acid	• Weekly throughout the period 5–10 years of age and • Biannual de-worming	• In school through teachers • For out-of-school children: through Anganwadi Centre (AWC) + Mobilization by ASHA
3.	10–19 years	*Tablets:* • 100 mg elemental iron • 500 µg folic acid	• Weekly throughout 10–19 years of age • Biannual de-worming	• In school through teachers • For out-of-school: through Anganwadi centre (AWC) + Mobilization by ASHA
4.	Pregnant and lactating women	*Tablets:* • 100 mg elemental iron • 500 µg folic acid	• 1 tablet daily for 100 days starting after first trimester • To be Repeated for 100 days postpartum	ANC/ANM/ASHA Inclusion in MCP card
5.	Women in reproductive age (WRA)	*Tablets:* • 100 mg elemental iron • 500 µg folic acid	Weekly throughout the reproductive period	Through ASHA during house visit for contraceptive distribution

Q-13. What is refractory IDA?

- Refractory IDA is a frequently encountered problem in practice
- Refractory IDA is defined as failure to respond to therapeutic dose of iron (3 to 6 mg/kg/day) administered for at least 4–6 weeks.

Q-14. What will you check before evaluation of refractory IDA?

- **Compliance**
  - Most common reason for poor response to iron therapy
  - GI intolerance in <10% of patients with standard doses of iron
  - Dose and frequency can be reduced (once a day), may be administered with food.
  - Intermittent administration (weekly thrice) can be tried (Inferior to daily iron therapy).

- **Dose**
  Therapeutic dose of oral iron is 3 to 6 mg/kg/day, may be given 3 mg/kg/day
- **Formulation**
  - Check the formulation—elemental iron per mL, per 5 mL, strength of tablet, etc.
  - Ferrous salts have better bioavailability than ferric salts (20% elemental iron).
  - Ferrous fumarate and ferrous gluconate can also be used.
- **Diet modification**
  - Less milk
  - *Iron rich food:* Dates, millet, jaggary, green leafy vegetables

CHAPTER 42

Chronic Hemolytic Anemia: Thalassemia

QUESTIONS AND ANSWERS

Q-1. What is the definition of anemia?

Anemia is defined as reduction in oxygen carrying capacity of blood, due to reduced hemoglobin, concentration and red cell mass leading to tissue hypoxia.

Q-2. What other causes of pallor can be mistaken for anemia?

- Congestive cardiac failure (due to decreased perfusion)
- Nephrotic syndrome (due to edema and waxy skin)
- Hypothyroidism
- Vasovagal syncope
- Hypoproteinemia
- Poor perfusion (due to peripheral vasoconstriction)

Q-3. What are WHO cut-off values for diagnosis of anemia at different age groups?

Age/Sex	*Hb (g/dL)*
Newborn	<14
At 3 months	<9
6 months to 6 years	<11
6-14 years	<12
Adult male	<13
Adult female	<12
Pregnant woman	<11

Q-4. What are the gradings of anemia?

- Mild: Hb < 10 g/dL
- Moderate: Hb 7-10 g/dL
- Severe: Hb 7-5 g/dL
- Very severe: Hb < 5 g/dL.

Q-5. What are the pointers of chronic anemia?

- Growth retardation
- Exercise intolerance, tiredness, easy fatigability
- Behavioral changes
  - Irritability—excessive crying
  - Breath holding spell
  - Temper tantrum
  - Reduced attention span
  - Deteriorating school performance

- Poor academic achievement
- Decreased cognition
- Altered immunity (cell-mediated and humoral)

Q-6. What are the features of chronic hemolytic anemia?

- History of progressive pallor
- History of recurrent blood transfusions
- Firm hepatosplenomegaly
- No significant lymphadenopathy
- No bleeding manifestations like petechiae and purpuric spots (except hypersplenism)

Q-7. What is the most common hemolytic anemia in India?

Thalassemia.

Q-8. What are other names of thalassemia?

- Mediterranean anemia
- Cooley's anemia

Q-9. When Thalassemia was reported in World and in India?

- It was first reported in 1920-1925 by Cooley.
- First case of Thalassemia in India was reported by Dr Mukharjee from Kolkata in 1938.

Q-10. In which communities in India prevalence of thalassemia is more?

- Sindhi
- Punjabi
- Khatris
- Gujarati
- Lohanas
- Mohars

Q-11. What is the primary defect in thalassemia?

- The defect lies in the globin chain gene. It is in the form of deletion, nucleotide substitution or insertion. If the defect involves β-chain gene, the problem is β-thalassemia and if the defect is in α-chain gene, the problem is α-thalassemia. Commonest form is β-thalassemia.
- The pattern of inheritance is autosomal recessive. If it is heterozygeous, the problem is β-thalassemia trait or carrier. If it is homozygous, the disease is β-thalassemia disease. Depending on genetic expression, β-thalassemia homozygous can be β^0 or β^+, no β-chain is formed and β^+ some β-chain is formed. β^0 homozygous thalassemia is called thalassemia major. β^+ homozygous thalassemia is called thalassemia intermedia.
- Most defects are due to mutations and more than 200 mutations are responsible for β-thalassemia worldwide.
- Thalassemia major : $\beta^0\beta^0$
- Thalassemia intermedia: $\beta^+\beta^+$ or $\beta^0\beta^+$

Q-12. What is ∈ β-thalassemia?

Thalassemia β-chain gene (β^0 or β^+) can occur together with other β-chain structural variant, most commonly Hb ∈ gene causing a disease expression like homozygous β-thalassemia. The disease is called ∈ β-thalassemia. The clinical picture is like thalassemia major or intermedia depending pon β^0 or β^+.

Q-13. What is the genesis of anemia in β-thalassemia major?

- The principle cause is ineffective erythropoiesis. There is deficiency of β chain leading to imbalance between α-chain and β-chain, results in relatively excess α-chain form aggregation which gets deposited in the inner

wall of RBCs. The cell wall integrity of the developing RBCs is lost at the haemopoietic site and thus there is premature destruction of RBCs. α-chain is also utilized for synthesis of HbF (2 α 2 γ).
- The life span of circulating RBCs containing HbF is less and there is hemolysis.

Q-14. What are common presenting features of β-thalassemia major?

- Common presenting symptoms
  - Progressive pallor
  - Growth failure
  - Enlargement of abdomen due to hepatosplenomegaly
  - Diminished activity, tiredness, generalized weakness
  - Breathlessness with severe anemia
- Common presenting signs
  - Hemolytic facies
  - Anemia—moderate to severe
  - Hepatosplenomegaly
  - Sometimes, mild icteric tinge
  - Skin discoloration due to pallor, hemosiderosis and occasionally icteric tinge.

Describe thalassaemic facies.

- Frontal and parietal bossing
- Large head
- Maxillary overgrowth and prominent zygoma
- Malar prominence
- Hypertelorism, depressed nasal bridge
- Prominent epicanthic folds
- Dental malocclusion
- Sallow complexion

Q-15. What is the cause for specific thalassaemic facies?

In response to microcytic hypochromic anemia, there is increased erythropoietin production, which leads to hyperplasia of bone marrow. It occurs specially in diploic spaces in skull, specifically spongy bones. It causes expansion of skull bones causing facial disfiguration, thalassaemic facies.

Q-16. Why is there hepatosplenomegaly in thalassemia major?

- Extramedullary erythropoiesis is the major cause
- Hemolysis and hemosiderosis are aggravating the size of organs

Q-17. What is the consistency of liver and spleen?

Firm consistency.

Q-18. What are the clinical differentials of severe anemia and hepatosplenomegaly in early infancy (3-6 months of age)?

- Thalassemia major
- Diamond-Blackfan syndrome
- Malaria
- Osteopetrosis
- Parvovirus infection
- Physiological anemia of infancy (rare)

Q-19. What are the causes of jaundice in β-thalassemia major?

As such β-thalassemia major does not have frank jaundice, at the most may have icteric tinge. Jaundice in thalassemia may be due to,

- Transfusion transmitted infections like hepatitis B, hepatitis C, CMV etc.
- In chronic cases, there may be hemosiderosis, leading to cirrhosis of liver and hepatocellular failure.
- Immune hemolysis due to repeated transfusions.

Q-20. What is the age of presentation of thalassemia?

- Most patients of β-thalassemia major present after the age of 6 months, usually before the age of 2 years.
- β-thalassemia intermedia usually presents at the age of 5 to 7 years (>2 years)

Q-21. What is β-thalassemia trait or carrier?

- They are heterozygous subjects carrying one gene for β-chain defect in one chromosome.
- Most of β^0 minor ($\beta\beta^0$) or β^+ minor ($\beta\beta^+$) carriers are mildly anaemic.
- Hematological picture is microcytic, hypochromic anemia, almost similar to iron deficiency anemia.
- MCV and MCH are reduced. MCHC and RDW are usually normal. RBC count is increased. In iron deficiency anemia, RBC count is decreased and RDW increased.
- Thalassemia trait have increased HbA2, 3.5% to 7%, also mild increased HbF.
- Rarely, carrier may be silent showing no clinical or hematological abnormality and HbA2 level is normal.

Q-22. What are the differentiating points for β-thalassemia major, intermedia and trait?

- Thalassemia Major
  - Manifestations are present in first year of life, latest by 2 years of ag.
  - Pallor, FTT, growth retardation common
  - Hemolytic facies
  - Hepatosplenomegaly
  - Transfusion dependent
  - Pigmentary changes of skin are present in children who received multiple transfusion, it is due to hemosiderin deposition in skin
  - If thalassemia major remains undiagnosed or untreated, does not survive beyond the age of 3 to 4 years.
  - If aggressive transfusion is done without iron chelators, they die in adolescent age or early adulthood.
- Thalassemia intermedia
  - Mild anemia
  - Growth retardation
  - Mild to moderate jaundice
  - Hemolytic facies
  - Hepatosplenomegaly
- Thalassemia trait/minor/carrier
  - Asymptomatic
  - Mild anemia, microcytic, hypochromic like IDA
  - May be drop of Hb during stress or pregnancy
  - Hb A2 > 3.5%.

Q-23. What investigations should be performed in a case of clinically diagnosed homozygous thalassemia?

- Hb : Low
- Peripheral blood smear examination.
  - *RBC morphology:* Microcytic, hypochromic RBCs, anisocytosis, poikilocytosis, presence of target cells, nucleated RBCs, basophilic stippling, polychromasia, reticulocytosis
  - Apparently, reticulocytosis should be decided with reference to corrected reticulocyte count (CRC). CRC is low because of ineffective erythropoiesis.

- Red cell indices
  - MCV ↓
  - MCH ↓
  - MCHC ↓
  - RDW may be normal
- *HbF:* >90% in thalassemia major and 60-80% in thalassemia intermedia
- *Hemoglobin electrophoresis:* Big HbF band and small HbA bands are found in thalassemia major, while in thalassemia intemedia big HbF, small HbA band and HbA_2 band are found.
- Radiological evaluation
  - *Skull:* Hair on end appearance
  - *Hand:* Increased translucency due to diminished bone density and thinning of cortex of the metacarpal bones.
- Unconjugated serum, bilirubin may be mildly raised.
- Serum ferritin : raised.

Q-24. How to confirm the thalassemia trait?

Hb electrophoresis by HPLC (High performance liquid chromatography): HbA2 is increased, 3.5 to 7% HbA_2 band may exceed 3.4% in megaloblastic anemia secondary to vitamin B_{12} and folic acid deficiency. Hence, raised HbA_2 level should be evaluated with peripheral blood picture to confirm thalassemia trait.

Q-25. In which conditions HbA2 may be raised, besides thalassemia trait?

- β-thalassemia "silent carriers"
- Concomitant iron deficiency anemia

Q-26. What are screening tests for thalassemia trait in the community?

- *MCV and MCH estimation of RBCs:* Both are low.
- *NESTROFT (Naked Eye Single Tube Red Cell Osmotic Fragility Test):* The fragility is reduced. It is best method for screening in the community.
- Both tests are sensitive and specific.

Q-27. When should be screening for thalassemia trait be done?

It must be done before marriage, may be done earlier also. If it is done after marriage and both the parents are carriers, the antenatal diagnosis is the option.

Q-28. How antenatal diagnosis of thalassemia is done?

- Samples for diagnostic study
  - Chorionic villous sampling (CVS) at 10-12 weeks of gestation.
  - Fetal blood collection by cordocentesis at 18-20 weeks of gestation.
- DNA analysis and PCR molecular tests
  - Finding out gene deletion
  - Detection of mutation in DNA

Q-29. What are the complications of β-thalassemia major?

The complications are due to severe anemia, haemosiderosis and hypersplenism. The major complications are:

- Cardiac complications
  - Congestive cardiac failure due to severe anemia.
  - *Due to hemosiderosis:* Pericarditis, pericardial effusion, restrictive cardiomyopathy, cardiomegaly, CCF, cardiac arrhythmias, valvular regurgitation.
  - Refractory heart failure due to anemia and hemosiderosis.

- Cirrhosis of liver following hemosiderosis.
- Diabetes mellitus due to hemosiderosis of pancreas affecting islet cells.
- *Pituitary hemosiderosis:* Hypogonadism, delayed puberty, growth hormone deficiency.
- Hypersplenism can lead to pancytopenia.
- *Bone:* Pathological fracture due to osteoporosis and osteopenia.

Q-30. What is formula for calculation of corrected reticulocyte count (CRC)?

$$\text{CRC} = \frac{\text{Actual RC x PCV}}{45}$$

Q-31. What is reticulocyte?

- Reticulocytes are immature red cells, they have lack of nucleus.
- Reticular mesh like network of ribosomal RNA is seen in the cell, hence they are called as reticulocytes.
- They circulate in blood for a day and then mature into an RBC.
- 2 to 6% in infants.
- 0.5 to 2% in adults.

Q-32. What are the differences between thalassemia minor/trait and iron deficiency anemia?

	Thalassemia trait	***Iron deficiency anemia (IDA)***
Anemia	Mild	Mild to moderate
Hemoglobin	Slightly low	Low, depends upon degree of IDA
RBC	Raised for Hb level	Decreased with Hb level
MCV	Low	Low
MCh	Low	Low
RDW	Normal	High
Serum Iron and Ferritin	Normal	Low
TIBC	Normal	High
HbA_2 level	>3.5%	<3.5%

Q-33. What is Mentzer's index:

- Mentzer's Index : $\frac{\text{MCV}}{\text{RBC count}}$
- <13: Thalassemia trait
- >13: Iron deficiency anemia
- It is only for patients with mild anemia

Q-34. What are the principles of treatment of β-thalassemia?

- To maintain Hb level in a physiological range by adequate PCV therapy. It will minimize bony deformity, hepatosplenomegaly, iron absorption from the gut and maintain a good quality of life.
- Iron chelation therapy to prevent hemosiderosis and its complications.
- Splenectomy.
- Definitive and curative treatment
  - Bone marrow transplantation
  - Stem cell transplantation
  - Gene therapy

Q-35. What are the goals of transfusion therapy in thalassemia?

- To obviate the ill effects of hypoxia
- To suppress endogenous erythropoiesis
- To promote normal growth and development and good quality of life
- To prevent complications of under transfusion like hemolytic facies
- To prevent hepatosplenomegaly
- To ensure safe blood transfusion practices
- To provide transfusion services most suited to patient

Q-36. What are the transfusion regimen in thalassemia?

Transfusion regimen	*Pretransfusion Hb level (g/dL)*
Palliative	8
Moderate	9.5 to 10.5
Hypertransfusion	10-12
Supertransfusion	>12

Q-37. What is fresh blood?

4 to 5 days old.

Q-38. Who should not donate the blood for transfusion to these children?

Parents and first degree relative.

Q-39. Among all the four types of transfusion therapy, which one is preferred?

Hypertransfusion.

Q-40. What are the problems of supertransfusion?

Supertransfusion increases iron load and vascular complications due to high viscosity of blood when Hb is more than 16 g/dL.

Q-41. How much blood should be transfused?

Usually 10-15 mL/kg PCV is transfused over 2 to 3 hours regularly at 15-20 days interval.

- In a normal child may be transfused 3-4 mL/kg/h, while in patients with cardiac decompensated it should be given 1-2 mL/kg/h.

Q-42. What measures should be taken to prevent transfusion reactions?

- Ideally triple saline washed RBCs should be used.
- Leukocyte filters should be used. The filters actively filter out WBCs and platelets from transfused cells. CMV can also be filtered out.
- Elimination of leukocyte will prevent transfusion reactions and allo-immunization to HLA antigens, which is important considering future bone marrow transplantation.

Q-43. What infection risks ae known in patients of thalassemia?

- Transfusion transmitted infections: Hepatitis B and C, HIV, CMV, Malaria, etc.
- Leucopenia due to hypersplenism can lead to infection.
- Yersinia enterocolitis.
- Listeria monocytogens
- Mucormycosis

Q-44. Which vitamin supplementation is advised in patients of thalassemia?

- Folic acid—requirement is increased due to erythroid hyperplasia.
- Vitamin E.

Q-45. What is the indication of starting chelation therapy in thalassemia?

- After approximately 10 transfusions.
- Serum ferritin level exceeds 1000 ng/mL.

Q-46. Why is there iron overload in thalassemia?

- Transfused exogenous iron.
- Hemolysis due to disease.
- Excessive absorption of iron from gut.

Q-47. What iron chelating agents are available?

- Desferrioxamine or Deferoxamine
- Deferiprone
- Defersirox

Q-48. What are the doses, route of administrations and side effects of different iron chelators?

	Deferoxamine	***Deferiprone***	***Deferasirox***
Route of administration	• By subcutaneous route by infusion pump • May be given IV	Oral route	Oral route
Dosage	Continuous infusion for 8-10 hours/day for 5 days a week, plasma half life is only 20 minutes	Daily, divided in 3 doses	Once a day long plasma half life of 10-15 hours
Efficacy	• Best chelating agent • Best for hepatic iron chelation • Prevents cardiac haemosiderosis	Less efficacious than deferoxamine but more effective in removing cardiac iron load	• Can be started in children above 2 years. • Good efficacy in removing hepatic iron load
Cost	Costly	Less costly	Moderately costly
Side effects	• Ototoxicity • Ocular toxicity • Impaired bone growth • Local skin reaction	Agranulocytosis Arthritis Arthralgia GI disturbances	• Can raise SGPT and SGOT • Proteinuria • Skin rash • GI disturbances

Q-49. What is the best method to know iron burden in thalassemia?

- Liver biopsy
  - Chemical measurement of non-hem iron.
  - Histochemical study of iron deposition in liver cells.
- The assessment of liver iron concentration can be done noninvasively by quantitative MRI of liver.
- Myocardial iron concentration can also be assessed by quantitative MRI.
- Serum ferritin level: Indirect method, less reliable, but more feasible.

Q-50. What are the indications of splenectomy in thalassemia?

- Hypersplenism
  - Frequency transfusions are required, more than 200 mL/kg/year.
  - Annual PCV transfusion 1.5 times of basal requirements.
  - Difficult to maintain Hb > 10g/dL.
  - Pancytopenia
- Mass effect of hugely enlarged spleen.

Q-51. How does splenectomy help?

It decreases the requirement of blood transfusion. It cannot cure thalassemia.

Q-52. How does bone marrow transplantation help in thalassemia?

It cures thalassemia, no further blood transfusion or chelation therapy is required. The child lives normal life. Success rate is 65-98%. However, genetic transmission of thalassemia from the subject can not be prevented.

Q-53. What is alternative of marrow transplantation in thalassemia?

Cord blood stem cell transplantation can be done.

Q-54. What is minimum age for bone marrow transplantation in thalassemia?

2 to 3 years is optimal, but can be done at any age.

Q-55. Who can be donor for bone marrow or cord blood stems cell transplantation?

HLA matched subject, usually a sibling. For bone marrow transplantation, both HLA and blood group matching is required. For cord blood stem cell transplantation only HLA compatibility is required.

Q-56. What is time schedule for development of complications in poorly chelated thalassemic children?

- Increase in serum ferritin: 15-20 transfusions
- Hepatic fibrosis: 3-5 years
- Liver cirrhosis: 10-15 years
- Sub clinical cardiac dysfunction: 10-12 years
- Cardiac disease: 12-15 years
- Cardiac failure: >15 years
- Endocrinal dysfunctions: 15-20 years

Q-57. What are MRI interpretations for hepatic and cardiac iron overload?

Iron overload	*Liver iron hepatic T_2 (ms)*	*Cardiac iron cardiac T_2 (ms)*
None	>6.3	>20
Mild	2.7 to 6.3	12-20
Moderate	1.4 to 2.7	8-12
Severe	<1.4	<8

Q-58. How will you monitor children with thalassemia?

- Each visit
  - CBC
  - Weight, height on growth charts
  - Size of liver and spleen
  - Adverse reaction of blood transfusion, if any
- Three monthly
  - Urine analysis
  - Liver and renal function tests
  - Serum ferritin
- Yearly
  - Annual blood transfusion requirement

  - Hepatic serology (HbsAg, anti-HCV, HIV tests)
  - T2 MRI for cardiac iron overload
- After 10 years (yearly)
  - ECG, Echocardiography
  - Endocrine tests for thyroid, hypoparathyroid, diabetes mellitus
  - Bone mineral density
  - 25 hydroxy vitamin D3 level
- Sexual development (LH, FSH, Testosterone, Tanner staging)

CHAPTER 43

Development

QUESTIONS AND ANSWERS

Q-1. What is the timeline for development of human brain?

- 25% of its adult size in newborn
- 80% by age 3
- 90% by age 5.
- 95% by age 6.

Q-2. What are the principles of development?

- Development always proceeds in cephalocaudal manner, from head to toe
- Rate of development may vary, but the sequence is same, e.g. head control always precedes sitting, however, the age of acquisition of these milestones may vary
- Generalized mass activity is replaced by specific individual response
- Primitive reflexes to be lost before voluntary functions are acquired
- Persistence of a primitive reflex, beyond the age at which it should have disappeared, indicates and predicts abnormal development

Q-3. What are common causes of abnormal development?

- Intrauterine infections
- Perinatal asphyxia
- Postnatal insults in a growing brain (first 5 years of life)
  - Trauma
  - Meningitis
  - Intra cranial hemorrhage
  - Kernicterus
  - Hypoglycemia

Q-4. What are the domains of development?

- **Motor development**
  - *Gross motor:* Pertaining to development of locomotion
  - *Fine motor:* Pertaining to development of finer limb movements and co-ordination, e.g. grasping, transferring objects
- **Cognition/problem solving:** Refers to mental abilities, e.g. imitation, simple problem solving, drawing, reading, writing
- **Personal and social:** Reaction to other persons and his adjustments to domestic life, social groups and community conventions e.g. social behavior, feeding, play activity, dressing
- **Language and speech:**
  - Ability to communicate
  - Receptive language
  - Expression of language including speech, gestures, signs

Q-5. What is the age for development of different gross motor milestones?

Age	Milestone
3 months	Neck holding
5 months	Rolls over
6 months	Sitting with support
8 months	Sitting without support
9 months	Stands with support
12 months	Creeps well, stands without support, walks but falls
15 months	Walks alone
18 months	Runs, explores drawers
2 years	Walks up and downstairs (2 feet/step), Jumps
3 years	Rides tricycle, Alternate feet climbing upstairs
4 years	Hops on one foot, Alternate feet going downstairs
5 years	Skips

Q-6. What is the age for development of important gross motor milestones?

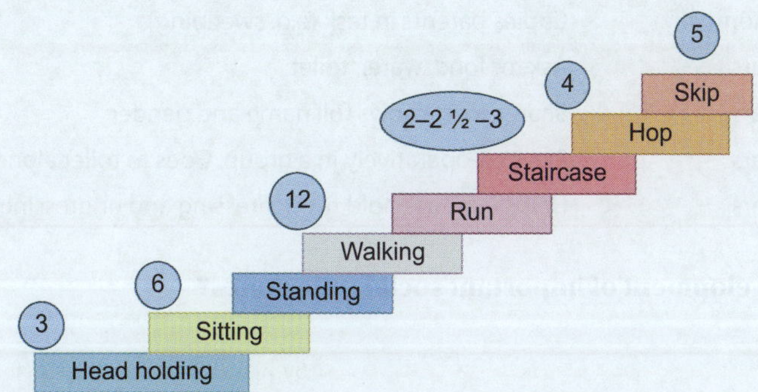

Q-7. What are the key Fine Motor Milestones?

Age	Milestone
4 months	Bidextrons reach (reaching out for objects with both hands)
6 months	Unidextrons reach, transfers objects
9 months	Immature pincer grasp
12 months	Mature pincer grasp
15 months	Imitates scrubbing, tower of 2 blocks
18 months	Scribbles, tower of 3 blocks
2 years	Tower of 6 blocks, vertical and circular stroke
3 years	Tower of 9 blocks, copies circle
4 years	Copies cross
5 years	Copies triangle

Q-8. What is the age for development of important fine motor milestones?

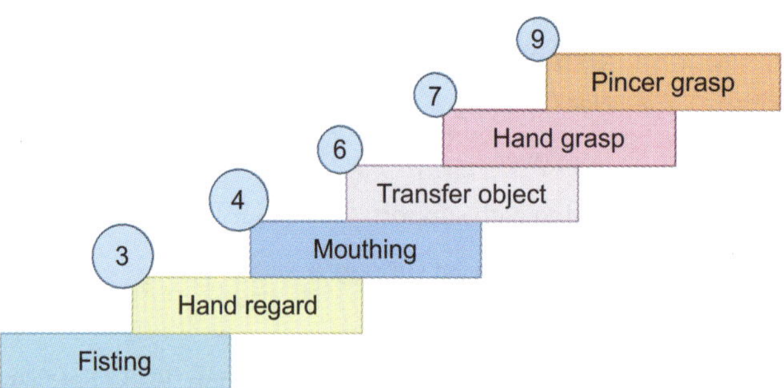

Q-9. What are key social and adaptive milestones?

Age	Milestone
2 months	Social smile (Smile after being talked to)
3 months	Recognizes mother
6 months	Recognizes stranger, stranger anxiety
9 months	Waves "bye bye"
12 months	Comes when called
15 months	Jargon
18 months	Copies parents in task (e.g. sweeping)
2 years	Ask for food, water, toilet
3 years	Shares toys, knows full name and gender
4 years	Plays co-operatively in a group, Goes to toilet alone
5 years	Helps in house hold tasks, dressing and undressing

Q-10. What is the age for development of important social milestones?

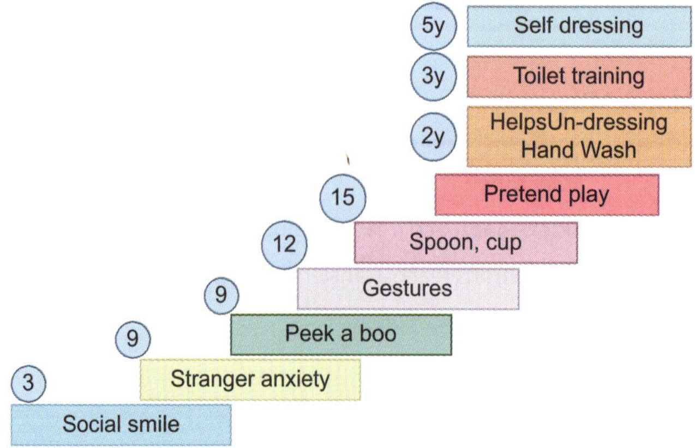

Q-11. What are key language milestones?

Age	Milestone
1 month	Alerts to Sound
3 months	Cooing (musical vowel sounds)
4 months	Laugh loud
6 months	Mono syllables (ba, da, pa) ah – goo sounds
9 months	Bi syllables (baba, mama, dada)
12 months	1-2 words with meaning
18 months	8-10 words vocabulary
2 years	2-3 words sentences, uses pronouns "I", "Me", "You"
3 years	Ask questions, Knows full name and gender
4 years	Says song or poem, tells stories
5 years	Asks meaning of words

Q-12. What is the age for development of important receptive milestones?

Milestone	Age
Turns to voice	3-6 months
Responds to name	4-9 months
Understands "NO"	9-18 months
Follows 1 step command	12-20 months
Points body parts	12-24 months
Follows two-step command	22-30 months

Q-13. What is the age for development of different expressive milestones?

Milestone	Age
Cooing	3 months
Laugh	3-6 months
Babbling	5-9 months
Dada/Mama	9-14 months
5 words	1 years
50 words	2 years
250 words	3 years

Q-14. What are the different tests to assess vision in children?

- Can fixate and follow a moving person or dangling ring at birth
- Following dangling ring held 8–10 inches away
  - Up to range of 45 at birth
  - Up to range of 90 by 4 weeks
  - Up to range of 180 by 12 weeks
- Can fixate to mother as she talks to her at one month
- Binocular vision begins at 6 weeks and established by 4 months

- Fixates intently on an object shown to him at 3–4 months
- Adjusts his position to follow objects by 6 months of age
- Follows rapidly moving objects by 1 year of age

Q-15. What are different tests to assess hearing in children?

- New born responds to sounds by startling, blinking, crying, quieting or changing activity
- Make a sound of a bell kept 1.5 feet away and out of the field of vision to test hearing
  - Turns his head towards the sound by 3 to 4 months.
  - Child turns head to the side and then downward to the sound produced below the ear level by 5 to 6 months of age
  - Can make out sound produced above the level of ears by 7 months
- Looks at source of sound diagonally by 10 months

Q-16. What are the risk factors for impairment of hearing?

- **Less than 28 days**
  - Severe jaundice
  - VLBW
  - Low Apgar
  - Meningitis
  - Ventilation
  - Ototoxic drugs
  - Stigmata of syndromes:
- **1 month to 2 years**
  - Parental concern
  - Recurrent otitis
  - Severe head trauma
  - Mumps, Meningitis
  - Neurodegenerative

Q-17. What are the prerequisites for assessment of development in a child?

- **Prerequisites**
  - Place should be comfortable and free from distractions
  - Child should not be hungry, tired, ill or irritated
  - Child should be in a playful mood with mother
  - Developmental assessment in a sick child can be deferred until he recovers well

Q-18. What are the contents of development kit?

- A red ring (diameter 6–7 cm tied to a string)
- Nine red cubes
- Paper pellets
- Spoon
- Cup with handle
- A book with thick pages
- Picture book
- Red pencil, paper
- Doll and mirror
- Red ball
- Red wool
- A bell

Q-19. What risk factors can be identified in history for developmental delay?

- **Prenatal factors**
  - Genetic
  - Maternal factors
    - Maternal nutrition
    - Exposure to drugs and toxins
    - Maternal diseases and infections
- **Neonatal risk factors**
  - IUGR
  - Prematurity
  - Perinatal asphyxia
- **Postnatal factors**
  - Nutrition
  - Iron deficiency
  - Iodine deficiency
  - Infectious disease
- Environmental factors
- Psychosocial factors
- Protective factors
  - Breastfeeding
  - Optimum nutrition
  - KMC
  - Nurturing family
  - Stimulating environment
  - Absence of illness

Q-20. What are identifiable risk factors on physical examination for developmental delay?

- Anthropometry—serial measurements especially head circumference
- Nutrition
- Abnormal growth—FTT, microcephaly
- Major congenital anomalies like spina bifida or midline defects
- Dysmorphism
- Neurocutaneous skin lesions like café-au-lait spots, neurofibromatosis
- Abnormal findings on eye examination like poor vision, cataract
- Abnormal findings on ear examination like low set ears, abnormal shape of ears, recurrent OM
- Hepatosplenomegaly
- Skeletal abnormalities
- Neurologic abnormalities like hypertonia, hypotonia, brisk DTR, etc.
- Features of intrauterine infections
- Signs of hypothyroidism

Q-21. What are warning signs for developmental delay?

- Shrill/high pitched cry
- Excessive sleepiness/irritability
- Opisthotonus/Frog like posture
- Seizures
- Abnormal movements
- Microcephaly
- Large head

- Poor eye following
- Poor response to sound
- Asymmetrical/Absent/Persistent neonatal reflexes
- Hypotonia/Hypertonia/Dystonia
- Delayed developmental milestones

Q-22. What are different development screening test?

- Screening is a brief assessment procedure designed to identify children requiring detailed assessment
- **Phatak's Baroda screening test**
  - Meant to be used by child psychologists rather than physicians
  - Indian adaptation of the Bayley developmental scale
  - Applied to children up to 30 months
- **Ages and stages questionnaire (ASQ – 3)**
  - Age based parent completed questionaries
  - One month to 5.5 years of age
  - Takes 10–15 minutes for parents to complete
  - Takes 2–3 minutes to score
  - Communication, gross motor, fine motor, problem solving and personal social assessed
- **Denver-II (DDST)**
  - Revised in 1992
  - Assesses child for gross motor, fine motor, adaptive, language and personal social behavior
- **Trivandrum Development Screening Chart (TDSC)**
  - Consists of 51 items
  - For 0–6 years
  - For use in community to identify children with developmental delay
- **Clinical Adaptive Test and Clinical Linguistic and Auditory Milestone Scale**
  - Assesses child's cognitive and language skills
  - From birth to 36 months
  - Uses parental reports and direct testing the children
- **Goodenough-Harris drawing test**
  - The child draws a man in the best possible manner and the detail of the drawing determined the score of the child
  - Note the mature grip of pen
  - One can determine the mental age by comparing scores obtained with a normative sample
- **Definitive tests**
  - Indicated once screening tests or clinical assessment is abnormal

Q-23. What points should be taken for consideration before interpretation of developmental assessment?

Points for consideration while interpreting developmental assessment

Use corrected age for developmental status till 2 years of age in preterm born children., e.g. a child born at 32 weeks of gestation (Gestational age 32 weeks) seen at 12 weeks (postnatal age) should be considered a 4-week-old (corrected age)

- Single assessment or isolated examination findings should not be basis for the diagnosis of retardation
- Considerable factors,
  - Recent illness
  - SAM
  - Emotional deprivation
  - Sensory deficits
  - Neuromuscular disorders

Q-24. What is the upper limit age for attainment of different milestones?

Age	Milestone
2 months	Visual fixation or following
6 months	Vocalization
10 months	Sitting without support
12 months	Standing with assistance
14 months	Hands and knees crawling
17 months	Standing alone
18 months	Walking alone
18 months	Single word
3 years	Imaginative play

Q-25. What are the windows of achievement of six major milestones?

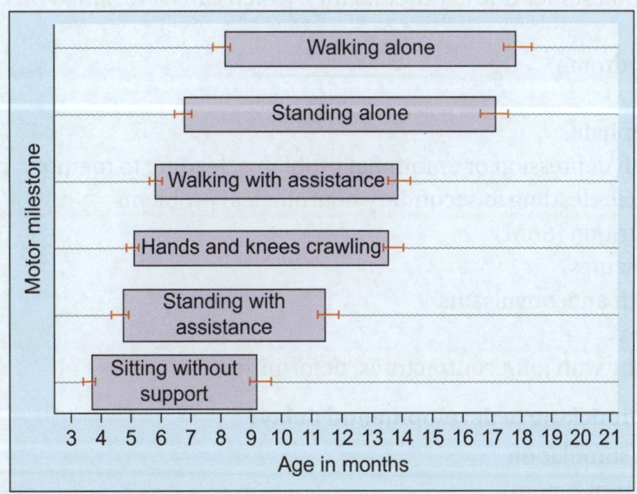

Q-26. What is definition of developmental delay?

- Development in one domain may not necessarily run parallel to that in other spheres
- Rate of development differs in different domains
- In a child with SAM, gross motor milestones may be more affected than language and personal social
- In a child with autism, language and personal social spheres are grossly delayed but may have a normal gross motor development
- **Definition:**
  Developmental delay is refers to significant delay in the acquisition of milestones in one or more developmental domains as compared to the peers. It is defined as a performance two stand deviations or more below (-2 SD) on age appropriate, standardized norm referred testing in one or more of the domains of development.
- **Developmental Quotient**
  - $\frac{\text{Developmental age}}{\text{Chronological age}} \times 100$
  - <70 is labeled as delay
  - DQ should be estimated separately for each area of development

Q-27. What is the definition of global developmental delay?

- Defined as significant delay in two or more of the developmental delays
- Usually, children with global developmental delay have delay across all domains
- Global developmental delay term is reserved for children <5 years of age
- Intellectual disability is the term used for children >5 years of age. Formal IQ testing is done

Q-28. What is developmental deviance?

- Nonsequential, unevenness in the achievement of milestones within one or more streams of development
- May be physiological, normal variant. Some infants never attain creeping, still walking will be achieved within physiological range
- Most of the times, it is pathological

Q-29. What is developmental regression?

- Loss of previously acquired skills ore milestones
- Most common in brain degenerative disorders

Q-30. What is developmental pseudoregression?

Transient loss of some milestones due to other factors, which can be regained on correction of basic cause

- Hypothyroidism
- Infantile Tremor syndrome
- HIV
- Progressive hydrocephalus
- Disable children with depression or emotional problems, leading to memory, mood and behavior changes
- Nutritional deficiencies leading to secondary neurological problems
- Severe acute malnutrition (SAM)
- Poorly controlled seizures
- Over medication with anticonvulsants
- Intercurrent illnesses
- Static encephalopathy with joint contractures, deformities, etc.

Q-31. What conditions are mimicking to developmental delay?

- Less environmental stimulation
- Vision and hearing impairment
- Autism
- Epilepsy
- Transient tone abnormalities
- Child with chronic illness
- Severe Acute Malnutrition (SAM)
- Muscular Disorders (DMD)
- Space occupying lesions (SOL) of brain
- Hydrocephalus
- Metabolic disorders
- Genetic syndrome

Q-32. What are the markers of cerebral palsy of infancy?

- Preference of hand before 1 year
- Cross midline to pick up toy
- Persistent fisting (>4 months of age)
- Long roll rather than segmental roll
- Leg scissoring
- Persistent primitive reflexes

Q-33. What are the causes of global developmental delay?

- **Prenatal**
  - Genetic, chromosomal
  - Acquired like nutritional deficiencies, maternal infections, fetal alcohol syndrome, maternal substance use
- **Perinatal**
  - Hypoxic ischemic encephalopathy (HIE)
  - Infections
  - Stroke
  - Hypoglycemia
  - Metabolic disturbances
- **Postnatal**
  - CNS infections (Bacterial meningitis, encephalitis)
  - Intracranial hemorrhage
  - Kernicterus
  - Stroke
  - Trauma
  - Severe malnutrition

CHAPTER 44

Neonatal Resuscitation

INTRODUCTION

- Around 6 lakh newborns die every year in India. Approximately 19% of these deaths are attributed to birth asphyxia.
- The term birth asphyxia connotes the inability of the newlyborn baby to establish optimum respiration after birth. Birth asphyxia leads to progressive hypoxia, hypercapnia, hypoperfusion and acidosis. It affects all major organ systems like central nervous system (CNS), heart, lungs, gastrointestinal tract (GIT) and kidneys. It leads to multiorgan failure. Hypoxic ischemic encephalopathy (HIE) resulting from asphyxia may lead to long-term neuromotor and other sequelae.
- Approximately 85% of all neonates born at term gestation not require resuscitation.
- The American Heart Association (AHA) and the American Academy of Pediatrics (AAP) have recently updated resuscitation guidelines. Around 10% of neonates require initial steps of drying and stimulation and approximately 5% require positive pressure ventilation at birth.

PATHOPHYSIOLOGY OF BIRTH ASPHYXIA

- When a fetus does not receive enough oxygen, it leads to a brief period of rapid breathing and still the asphyxia continues, the respiratory movements cease and develops primary apnea. During primary apnea, the heart rate begins to fall, the neuromuscular tone gradually diminishes, but the blood pressure is preserved. In most cases, during this phase, tactile stimulation will restart respiration.
- If the asphyxia continues, the infant develops deep gasping respiration, the heart rate continues to fall, blood pressure also starts to fall and the baby becomes flaccid. The breathing becomes weaker till the infant takes the last gasp and results a secondary apnea. The infant is now unresponsive to stimulation and does not resume respiratory efforts unless resuscitation in the form of positive pressure ventilation (PPV) is initiated.
- As a result of fetal hypoxia, the infant may go through primary and secondary apnea stages before birth. Hence, apnea at birth may be either primary or secondary apnea. These two situations are clinically indistinguishable, the infant is not breathing in both conditions, the heart rate may be below 100 per minute. Therefore, when the baby is delivered with an apnea, assume that the baby has secondary apnea and institute full resuscitation without wasting much time in tactile stimulation.

PREPARING FOR RESUSCITATION

- Even with knowledge of risk factors, one can predict birth asphyxia only in 50% of the cases. In rest of cases, birth asphyxia and need of resuscitation would be a surprise. Therefore, the team must view each delivery as an emergency and be ready to provide resuscitation and to manage the situation.

PREPARATION FOR DELIVERY

- At least one person should be available, who is solely responsible for the neonate and is capable of undertaking full resuscitation. In an anticipated need for resuscitation, more than one person may be needed. Coordinated team efforts are required to ensure effective resuscitation.

- Check list
  - Inquire about antepartum and intrapartum risk factors
  - Anticipate emergencies and plan accordingly.
  - Assemble a team
  - Use effective communication
  - Check the equipment
  - Ask for additional help, if required

ROLE OF APGAR SCORES IN RESUSCITATION

The Apgar score is an objective method for evaluation of the baby's condition. It is usually performed at 1 minute and again at 5 minutes after birth. However, resuscitation must be started before 1 minute score is assigned. Therefore, the Apgar score is not used to guide the resuscitation.

Apar score does not help to decide whether the baby needs resuscitation, but the serial scores help in knowing how well the neonate responds to resuscitative efforts. Extended Apgar scores should be obtained every 5 minutes for up to 20 minutes if the 5-minute Apgar score is less than 7.

NEONATAL RESUSCITATION SUPPLIES AND EQUIPMENT

Suction Equipment

- Mechanical suction
- Suction catheters 10,12 or 14 F
- Meconium aspirator

Bag and Mask Equipment

- Neonatal resuscitation bags (self-inflating)
- Face masks (For both term and preterm babies)
- Oxygen with flow meter and tubing

Intubation Equipment

- Laryngoscope with straight blades No. 0 (preterm), No. 1 (term)
- Extra bulbs and batteries (for laryngoscope)
- Endotracheal tubes (internal diameter of 2.5, 3, 3.5 and 4 mm)

Medicines

- Epinephrine
- Normal saline or Ringer's lactate
- Naloxone hydrochloride

Miscellaneous

- Linen, shoulder roll, gauze
- Radiant warmer
- Stethoscope
- Syringes 1, 2, 5, 10, 20, 50 mL
- Feeding tube 6 F
- Umbilical catheters 3.5 and 5 F
- Three-way stopcocks
- Gloves

NEONATAL RESUSCITATION ALGORITHM

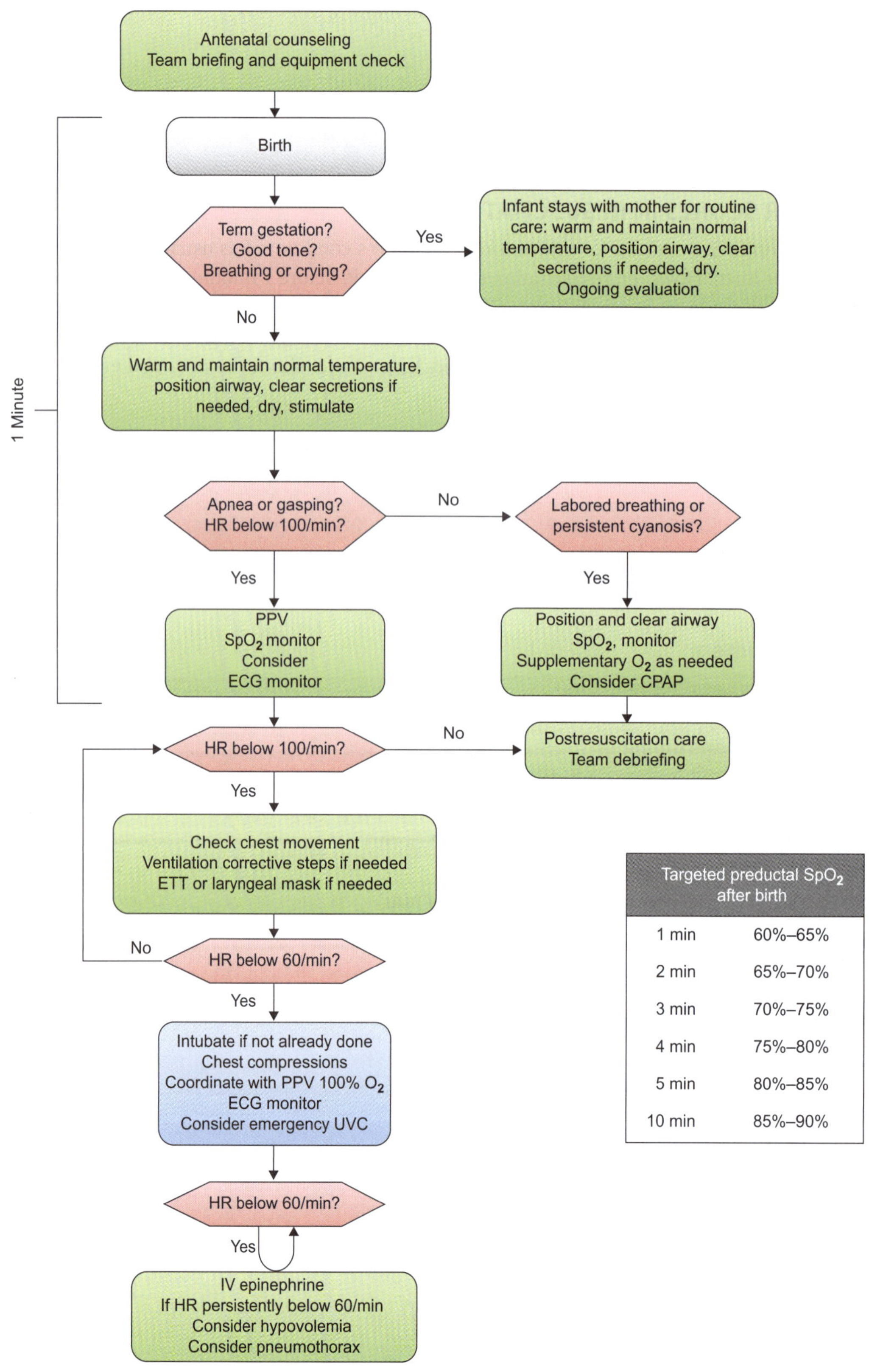

Targeted preductal SpO_2 after birth	
1 min	60%–65%
2 min	65%–70%
3 min	70%–75%
4 min	75%–80%
5 min	80%–85%
10 min	85%–90%

Once the baby is delivered, one should ask three questions about the newborn:

1. Term gestation?
2. Good muscle tone?
   Flexed posture and active movements of the neonate indicates good tone.
3. Breathing or actively crying?
   If the answers to all three questions are 'yes,' the infant stays with the mother and receives routine care.

Routine Care

- *Warmth:* Provided by putting the neonate directly on the mother's abdomen and chest in skin-to-skin contact.
- *Clearing of airway if required:* Position the neonate and wipe the baby's mouth and nose using a clean cloth, no need to suction routinely.
- Dry the neonate using a dry and warm cloth. Remove wet linen and cover the baby.
- *Ongoing evaluation for vital parameters:* Helping mother in breastfeeding will facilitate an easy transition to an extrauterine environment.

Delayed Cord Clamping (DCC)

- In all neonates, preterm and term, those who do not require resuscitation, cord clamping must be delayed for 30–60 seconds, delayed cord clamping.
- There is no enough evidence to recommended DCC in neonates needing resuscitation. In such babies, clamp and cut the cord immediately and initiate resuscitation without delay. If the answer to any of these three questions is 'no,' the baby needs resuscitation. After cutting the cord, start the 'initial steps.'

Initial Steps

Warmth

Place the neonate under the source of heat, preferably a radiant warmer. Do not cover the neonate with blankets or towels to endure visualization and let the radiant heat reach to the baby.

Dry and Stimulate

- Dry the neonate properly with prewarmed linen to prevent heat loss. Wet linen should be removed.
- Suctioning and drying may be enough stimulation to initiate breathing.
- If the baby continues to have poor breathing, additional tactile stimulation can be provided by gently rubbing the trunk, back and extremities. However, do not take much time for tactile stimulation.

Positioning

- Place the neonate on her back or side with the neck slightly extended, sniffing position. It keeps the airway open and facilitates breathing. Hyperextension or flexion of the neck should be avoided as they may interfere with respiration.
- To maintain the correct position, one may place a rolled blanket or towel under the shoulders of the infant, elevating her by 2 to 2.5 cm off the mattress. The shoulder roll is particularly helpful, if the infant has a prominent occiput, resulting from molding, edema, IUGR or prematurity. Airway should be cleared, if it requires.
- If secretions are there, remove from the airway by wiping the nose and mouth with a clean cloth or suctioning with a bulb syringe or a suction catheter.
- Mouth suction should be done before nose to prevent aspiration, when the infant makes a breathing effort on suctioning nose.
- If the infant has copious secretions from the mouth, turn the head to one side to allow secretions to collect in side of the mouth, where it can be easily removed.
- For suctioning, the catheter size should be 12 to 14 Fr. Keep the suction pressure around 80 mm Hg (100 cm of water) and not more than 100 mm Hg (130 cm of water)

- Do not insert the catheter too deep in the mouth or nose as the stimulation of the posterior pharynx can cause vagal response resulting in bradycardia or apnea.

BABY BORN THROUGH MECONIUM-STAINED LIQUOR (MSL)

A neonate born through MSL may aspirate the meconium into the trachea and lungs. Recent evidences have shown that procedures of intrapartum suctioning of the mouth and nose before delivery of the shoulders and postnatal tracheal suctioning of nonvigorous neonates—feeble breathing or hypotonia—are not beneficial. The new guideline does not recommend these procedures anymore.

Evaluation

- After the initial steps, the neonate should be evaluated by checking respiration, heart rate (HR) and color or oxygen saturation by pulse oximetry.
- Observe the chest movement for evaluation of respiration
- Auscultate the heart or palpate the umbilical cord pulsations for 6 seconds. Multiply the number of heart beats or pulsations in 6 seconds × 10 to get heart rate per minute. For example, a count of 14 in 6 seconds is 140 HR/min.
- Look for the tongue, mucous membrane and trunk to evaluate the color. A bluish lip, tongue and central trunk suggests central cyanosis. The presence of cyanosis in extremities (acrocyanosis) does not have any significance.
- *Good breathing efforts, HR ≥ 100/min and no cyanosis:* No additional intervention is indicated. Monitor the baby frequently.
- *Labored breathing or persistent central cyanosis:* Provide CPAP in preterm neonates and supplemental oxygen in term neonate. Monitor oxygen saturation and titrate supplemental oxygen to achieve the targeted saturations.
- *Apnea, gasping breathing or HR less than 100/min:* Provide positive pressure ventilation (PPV)

Supplemental Oxygen

- Provide oxygen by oxygen mask or oxygen tube held in a cupped hand over the baby's face or by a flow inflating bag and mask.
- Do not give oxygen using a self-inflating bag.
- The flow of oxygen should be minimum 5 L/min.

Positive Pressure Ventilation (PPV)

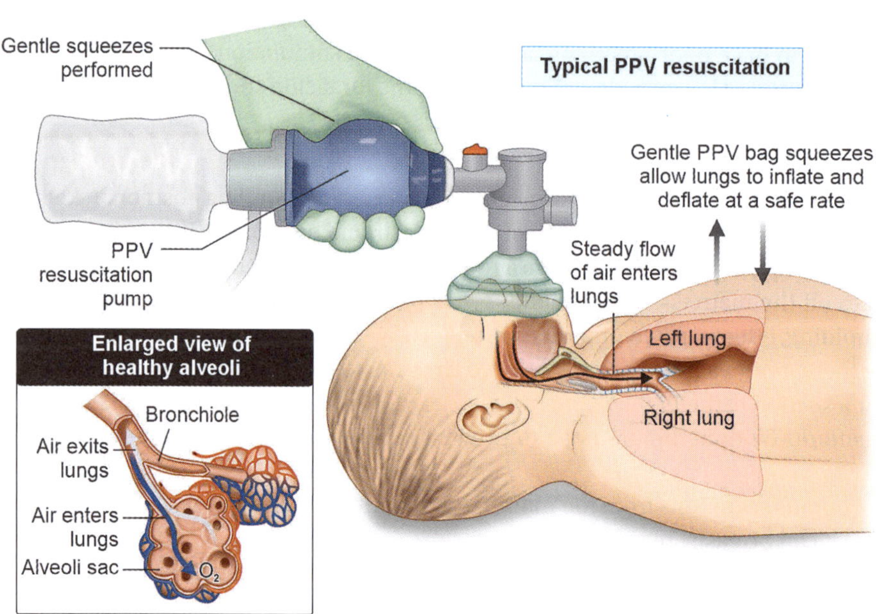

- PPV should be provided with a self-inflating bag (bag and mask ventilation). The resuscitation bag should have a capacity of 250–750 mL. Connect the bag to a source of oxygen and air and a blender that provides the desired concentration of supplemental oxygen.
- *Indications of PPV:*
  - Apnea or Gasping baby
  - Heart rate <100 beats/min
- *Contraindication for PPV:* A confirmed or suspected case of congenital diaphragmatic hernia is a contraindication for using bag and mask resuscitation.
- Oxygen should be used as a drug, appropriate concentration, appropriate flow rate and appropriate duration.

The most preterm neonates need supplemental oxygen during resuscitation. In preterm neonates less than 35 weeks of gestation, 21–30% oxygen concentration should be started, followed by titrating its concentration as per pulse oximetry readings. Starting with a low oxygen concentration prevents the complications of hyperoxia such as retinopathy of prematurity, bronchopulmonary dysplasia, etc.

Room air should be used in neonates of 35 weeks or more to initiate resuscitation. Oxygen saturation should be monitored by pulse oximetry and oxygen concentration should be titrated to maintain oxygen concentration in the targeted range.

Procedure of PPV

- The PPV is the single most effective step in neonatal resuscitation, especially in those babies who do not breathe at birth. Therefore, confirming adequacy of PPV is an important step for successful resuscitation of these babies.
- Usually, neonates respond to PPV after birth with immediate increase in their heart rates. If a neonate is not responding by a rapid increase in heart rate after 15 seconds of PPV, assess whether the baby's chest is moving with PPV and auscultate for breath sounds. If the chest is not rising and there are no audible breath sounds, take ventilation corrective steps (MR SOPA).
- What are three important questions about new born at the time of birth deciding need of neonatal resuscitation?
- What is delayed cord clamping?
- What is the change in intrapartum action for an infant born through meconium-stained liquor (MSL).
- Indications for endotracheal intubation during neonatal resuscitation
- Endotracheal tube size according to gestational age and weight of the baby in neonatal resuscitation
- Drugs used in neonatal resuscitation
- Once the effective chest rise is observed, perform PPV at a rate of 40–60 breaths per minute, following a squeeze, two, three, sequence. Ensure the chest is rising as if the neonate is taking easy breaths. Avoid giving too deep breaths (too much tidal volume). Do not deliver PPV at a high rate.
  After 30 seconds of PPV, evaluate the heart rate and take necessary action.
- Improving the infant's condition is judged by increasing heart rate, spontaneous respiration and improving the color. If the infant fails to improve, check for chest rise. If the chest rise is inadequate, take ventilation corrective measures.
- PPV may cause abdominal distention as the air escapes into the stomach through the esophagus. Distended stomach presses on the diaphragm and compromise ventilation. Therefore, if the ventilation is confirmed for more than 2 minutes, an orogastric tube should be inserted and left open to decompress the abdomen.

ENDOTRACHEAL INTUBATION (ET)

Endotracheal intubation (ET) is required only in few asphyxiated babies. It requires consistent practice to main the skill for ET.

Indications of ET Intubation During Resuscitation

- Neonate's heart rate <100 per minute despite 30 seconds of effective PPV
- When prolonged bag and mask ventilation is required
- When bag and mask ventilation is ineffective

- When chest compression is needed
- When congenital diaphragmatic hernia is suspected
- When the airway is blocked with thick secretions
- ET intubation may be considered for administration of epinephrine

Endotracheal Tube (ET)

- ET should be of uniform diameter throughout the tube length
- Vocal cord guide should be there at tip centimeter markings should be there on tube
- ET tube size depends on the weight or gestation of the baby

Approximate Endotracheal Tube Size

Gestational age (weeks)	*Weight (g)*	*Inner diameter of the tube (mm)*
<28	<1000	2.5
28–34	1000–2000	3
34–38	2000–3000	3.5
>38	>3000	4

- The insertion depth of the endotracheal tube is calculated as:

  Nasotragal length (NTL) + 1 cm

- The ET has a black line near the tube's tip called a vocal cord guide. It helps in deciding position of ET above the bifurcation of the trachea.
- A neonatal laryngoscope with straight blades of size '0' for preterm babies and '1' for term babies is required for intubation. Before intubating, the appropriate blade is attached to the laryngoscope handle, and the light is turned on.

Procedure of ET Intubation

- The infant's head should be in the midline and the neck slightly extended.
- The laryngoscope is held in the left hand between the thumb and the first three fingers, with the blade pointing away from oneself.
- Standing at the head end of the infant, the blade is introduced in the mouth and advanced to just beyond the base of the tongue so that its tip rests in the vallecula.
- The blade is lifted and landmarks looked for the epiglottis and glottis should come into view. Vocal cords on the side surround the glottic opening. Once glottis is visible, the ET is introduced from the right side of the mouth, and its tip is inserted into the glottis until the vocal cord guide is at the glottis level. Thus, it positions it halfway between the vocal cords and the carina.

Chest Compression

Chest compression helps mechanically pump blood to vital organs of the body. Chest compression consists of rhythmic sternum compression that compresses the heart against the spine, increases intrathoracic pressure, and circulates blood to the body's vital organs. Bag and mask ventilation must always accompany chest compression so only oxygenated blood is circulated during chest compression.

Chest compression is indicated if heart rate is <60/min, even after 30 seconds of PPV. Once the heart rate is 60/min or more, chest compression should be discontinued.

- **Procedure**

  Chest compression is performed by the two-thumb technique. The two thumbs are used to depress the sternum, with the hands encircling the torso and the fingers supporting the back.

  - The earlier used two finger technique for chest compression is now not recommended

- When chest compression is performed on a neonate, pressure is applied at the lower third of the sternum. Avoid using force on the xiphoid. To locate the area, slide the fingers on the lower edge of the thoracic cage to find the xiphisternum. The lower third of the sternum is just above it. The thumbs should be remain in contact with the chest during compression and release
- Complications known with chest compression procedure are fracture of ribs, lacerations of liver and pneumothorax.

- **Rate**
  - A positive breath should follow every third chest compression: 90 chest compression and 30 positive-pressure ventilation in one minute.
  - The chest compression should be performed three times over 1.5 seconds, leaving out ½ second for ventilation in a 2-minute cycle.
  - Check femoral or carotid pulsations periodically to determine the efficacy of chest compression

Evaluation

- After 60 seconds of chest compression, check the heart rate.
- *Heart rate <60:* Continue chest compression along with positive pressure ventilation. In addition, epinephrine may be considered
- *Heart rate ≥60:* Discontinue chest compression. Positive pressure ventilation should be continued until the heart rate is above 100 beats per minute and the infant breathes spontaneously.

Medications

- Medicines used in resuscitation are epinephrine and volume expanders
- There is no role of atropine, dexamethasone, calcium, mannitol, dextrose and naloxone for newborn resuscitation in the delivery room.
- Medications are preferably delivered through the umbilical vein. There is no role for intracardiac injection.
- For umbilical vein access, insert a 3.5 Fr or 5 Fr umbilical catheter into the umbilical vein just deep enough to get a free blood flow
- In an emergency, epinephrine can be delivered through the trachea, If the newborn is intubated. Absorption is erratic in the tracheobronchial tree, and it should be used only, if venous access is not possible.
- The drug is injected by a syringe or a feeding tube into the endotracheal tube and dispersed into the lungs by positive-pressure ventilation
- Indications
  - Use of adrenaline is indicated, if heart rate remains below 60 despite adequate ventilation of 30 seconds and 60 seconds of effective ventilation and chest compressions. The dose of epinephrine is 0.2 mL/kg (0.1 to 0.3 mL/kg) of 1:10,000 dilution (1 mg in 10 mL of saline). It should be flushed 3 mL of bolus normal saline.
  - Volume expander in the form of normal saline or Ringer's lactate is indicated when there is a history of blood loss or signs of shock in the neonate

Medications to be Used in the Delivery Room

Medication (concentration)	*Indication*	*Effects*	*Concentration administered*	*Dose of prepared solution*	*Route*
Epinephrine (1:1000)	HR < 60/min after 60 seconds of PPV and chest compression	• Ionotropic • Chronotropic • Peripheral vaso constriction	1:10,000	0.2 mL/kg a repeat dose can be given 3–5 minutes	IV: through umbilical vein (if not umbilical vein, endotracheal route
• Normal saline • Ringer's lactaria	Acute bleeding with hypovolemia	Increased intravascular volume and improves perfusion		10 mL/kg over 5–10 minutes	Umbilical vein

Ventilation Corrective Steps (MR SOPA)

Action	***Condition***
Inadequate seal	Re-apply mask
Blocked airway	Reposition of the infant's head
Blocked airway	Clear secretion by suction
Blocked airway	Ventilate with mouth slightly open
Inadequate pressure	Increase pressure slightly
Consider alternate airway	Blocked airway (endotracheal tube)

CHAPTER 45

Tuberculosis

QUESTIONS AND ANSWERS

Q-1. What is natural history of tuberculosis (TB) infection in children?

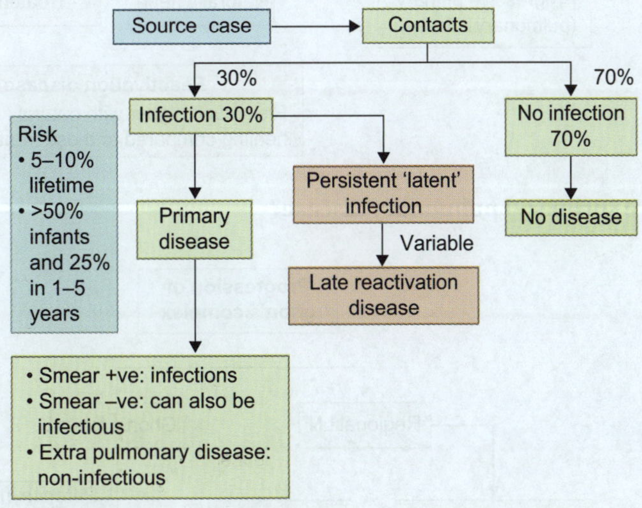

Q-2. What is Wallgren Time Table of TB disease in children

Time	*Manifestations*
3–8 weeks (average 6 weeks)	Incubation period
Early manifestations	Evidence of primary lesion and phenomena accompanying primary infection (erythema nodosum, phlyctenular conjunctivitis)
Usually within 3 months	Miliary TB, TB meningitis
Usually 1 year	Pleural effusion
Usually 3 years	Bone and Joint lesions
Usually within 5 years	Progressive pulmonary disease
After 5 years	• Renal tuberculosis (urogenital) • Skin TB

Q-3. What is the fate of primary complex in childhood TB?

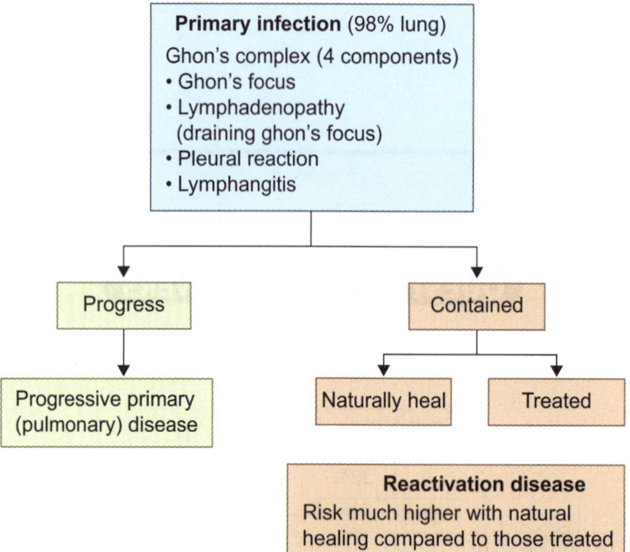

Q-4. What is progressive (primary) pulmonary disease?

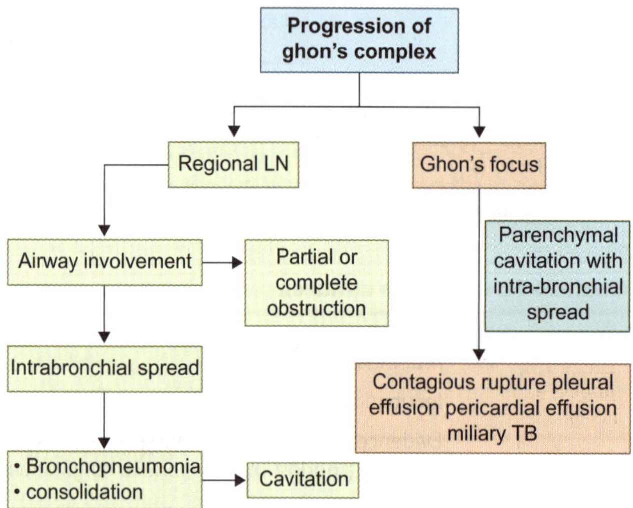

Q-5. What is reactivation or postprimary TB?

- Disease of adolescence and adulthood
- 50% to 90% of TB cases result from reactivation of previously dormant primary infection
- Apical or posterior segments of upper lobes or superior segment of lower lobes
- It usually appears as focal or patchy heterogenous consolidation, consolidation with cavitation or pleural extension
- Tuberculomas are rare

Q-6. What are different skin tests are available for diagnosis of TB?

- Tuberculin skin testing (Mantoux test)
- C-TB

Q-7. Describe Mantoux test (MT) in details.

- 1TU PPD RT 23 Tween 80 is used for Mantoux test. If 1TU PPD is not available, 2 TU PPD fluid may be used. Use of 10 TU fluid is not justified.
- PPD fluid should be preserved at 2 to 8°C
- Mantoux test is performed by intradermal route on volar aspect of forearm, about 2 to 4 inches below the cubital fossa. It will produce 6 mm wheal. The site of test should not be washed or rubbed.
- It should be interpreted between 48 and 72 hours by measuring by transparent ruler or scale. 'O' of the ruler should be place on left edge of the induration and ruler line should be read on the right edge of the induration. Measurement should be recorded in millimeters across the horizontal axis only. Induration should be considered for measurement and not the erythema. It may be read up to 7 days, if the test is positive.
- Test is considered as positive, if induration is >10 mm. It is considered as positive with 5 mm induration in a case of HIV.
- Prior BCG has minimal influence on PPD reaction.
- Positive MT indicates TB infection, not necessarily disease.
- Negative MT does not rule out TB infection.

Q-8. What are the causes of false positive and false-negative Mantoux test?

- Causes of false-positive MT
  - Incorrect technique of interpretation
  - BCG vaccination
  - Infection with *Mycobacterium* other than TB
- Causes of false-negative MT
  - Incorrect technique
  - Improper storage of PPD fluid
  - Immune deficiency—primary or secondary like HIV, severe acute malnutrition, immunosuppressive drugs like steroids
  - Infections like measles, pertussis
  - Vaccinated with live viral vaccine within 6 weeks in neonates
  - Severe form of TB

Q-9. What is C-TB test?

- The C- TB test is a modern TB skin test that uses ESAT- and CF -10 proteins, which are specific to *Mycobacterium tuberculosis*.
- It is tuberculin skin testing (TST) with higher specificity, not affected by BCG vaccination.
- The antigen is injected by intradermal route and is read 48–72 hours later by measuring induration
- It is useful for diagnosis of latent TB.
- Not available in India at present.

Q-10. What is Interferon Gamma Release Assays (IGRA)?

- IGRA measures production of interferon gamma by peripheral mononuclear cells.
- Early Secreted Antigen Target 6 (ESAT 6) and Culture Filtrate Protein 10 (CFP 10) antigens are used.
- These two antigens are present only in M-TB and not other mycobacteria or BCG vaccine strain.
- Principle is similar to skin test
- Does not differentiate TB infection from disease
- Used in low prevalence disease countries to detect latent TB infection.
- Utility of this test in high burden disease situation is not clear
- Currently there is no role of IGRA in clinical practice for the diagnosis of TB

Q-11. What are advantages and disadvantages of IGRA test?

Advantages

- Single visit
- Result is available in 24 hours
- No skill is required in administration
- Prior BCG does not interfere
- Prior tests do not booster subsequent testing

Disadvantages

- Samples need to be processed within few hours of collection
- Nonstandardized labs, failure to run controls, decreased accuracy
- Limited data in children <5 years of age, those recently exposed and immune compromised
- No data on semi repeated testing
- Test is expensive

Q-12. Which radiological lesions are considered as highly suggesting tuberculosis on chest X-ray in children?

- Miliary pattern
- Hilar and/or paratracheal lymphadenopathy with or without parenchymal involvement
- Fibrocavitary lesions

Q-13. What is the utility of ultrasonography in diagnosis of TB?

- To assess pleural fluid collection
- It is useful to differentiate thymus and anterior lymph nodes
- Identifying best place for aspiration or FNAC or biopsy in a peripheral lesion

Q-14. What is the utility of CT scan in diagnosis of TB?

CT scan is sometimes necessary but is costly and gives significant radiation. It should be used judicially.

- Persistent pneumonia
- Certain CT patterns can be highly suggestive of TB although not diagnostic like necrotic mediastinal lymphadenopathy, centrilobular nodules with tree in bud pattern and cavities with surrounding consolidations.
- Chest CT scan, also, may offer an opportunity for CT guided biopsy for tissue diagnosis.

Q-15. Bacteriological diagnosis is the only confirmatory method of diagnosis of TB. What are the tests for bacteriological diagnosis?

- Microbiological diagnosis
  - Ziehl-Neelsen stain of smear
  - Culture for AFB
- Molecular diagnosis
  - CBNAAT (Cartridge-based nucleic acid amplification test)
  - CBNAAT ultra
  - True Nat
  - Line Probe Assay (LPA)
  - LAMP (Loop Mediated Isothermal Amplification)

Q-16. Sputum examination is an important test for diagnosis of TB. What is good sputum sample? How should it be preserved and transported?

- A good sputum sample consists of recently discharged material from the bronchial tree with minimum amount of oral or nasopharyngeal material, presence of mucoid or mucopurulent material and should be 2–5 mL in volume. It should be collected in a sterile container after rinsing the oral cavity with clean water.

- The collected specimens should be transported to the laboratory as soon as possible after collection. If delay is unavoidable, the specimen should be refrigerated up to one week to inhibit the growth of unwanted microorganisms.

Q-17. Describe the steps for gastric aspirate collection procedure.

- Explain the procedure and take consent from the parent or guardian.
- Patient should be fasting for 4–6 hours prior to collection procedure. In an admitted child it may be done early in the morning, while the child is still asleep and in bed.
- Place the patient in supine position and restrain using the long-folded sheets
- The infant feeding tube, Ryle's tube needs to be placed in the body of stomach through mouth can be ascertained by measuring the distance from tip of the nose to the tragus and then from tragus to the midpoint between xiphisternum and umbilicus.
- Apply lubricant jelly to the tube.
- Gently insert the tube through the nose in the direction perpendicular to the face up to the measured length. This can often be assisted by asking the patient to swallow.
- Fix it to the nose with an adhesive tape.
- It is important to confirm that the tube is correctly positioned in the stomach. This can be ascertained by pushing some air with a syringe into the tube and simultaneously auscultating for the gush of air over the epigastrium with a stethoscope. In case, the patient starts choking or coughing while inserting the tube then the tube should be withdrawn and reinserted after the patient has settled.
- Once the Ryle's tube has been inserted into the stomach, its position can be checked by hearing gush of air over the epigastrium. One can also aspirate the stomach contents to confirm the position.
- Gently aspirate from the tube keeping the patient in the supine position.
- If there is no aspirate or the quantity is inadequate, try re-aspiration after shifting the patient in the left and right lateral positions.
- If one still does not get adequate specimen in both supine as well as lateral positions, further aspiration can be retried by shifting the tube a little in or out, in an effort to hit the stomach contents. The repeat aspiration should be done while rotating the patient through supine and lateral positions.
- In case, direct aspiration fails to provide adequate specimen, one should instill about 10 mL normal saline through the tube slowly. Align it to gravitate on its own.
- After instilling, reaspirate rotating the patient through supine as well as left and right lateral positions.
- Repeat these steps till gastric aspirate is obtained.
- Collect the aspirate in the sterile container. A specimen is considered adequate if it contains about 10–15 mL of stomach contents.
- After collection of gastric aspirate, gently remove the tube by closing its cap or pinching the tube.

Q-18. Describe the steps for procedure for induced sputum sample collection.

- Patient should be nil by mouth for 2–3 hours prior to the procedure.
- Explain the procedure and take consent from the parent or guardian.
- Procedure should be performed in a well-ventilated room having an exhaust fan. Wearing a N95 face mask is must.
- Baseline values of respiratory rate, pulse rate, chest retractions, wheeze and oxygen saturation should be taken prior to the procedure.
- Priming with salbutamol should be done either through MDI or nebulizer.
- Nebulize with 5 mL of 3% saline.
- While the child is nebulized, give a container to the child to collect expectorated sputum.
- Child may start expectorating while being nebulized with 3% saline. If the sample is adequate, the procedure may be stopped and expectoration should be sent to the laboratory for further processing.

- If required, chest percussion can be performed. The percussion will bring the secretions from the peripheral to central airways, from where the child can expectorate the sputum. The palms of hands while percussion should be made into a cup shape formed by fingers and thumb, instead of flat hand. One should cover all areas of chest in sitting, supine and prone positions.
- The sputum should be collected in sterile container and should be sent to the laboratory immediately.
- The patient should be monitored for 30 minutes after the procedure for respiratory rate, pulse rate, chest retractions, wheeze, etc.

Q-19. What is the utility of smear microscopic examination for diagnosis of TB?

- Special AFB staining with Ziehl-Neelsen (ZN) stain has been used to visualize AFB in the sputum or tissue samples for more than 100 years.
- It needs a high bacterial load of approximately 5×10^3 to 10^4 bacilli per mL of sputum.
- LED (Light Emitting Diode) fluorescence microscopy increases the sensitivity by 10%, however, need of dark rooms and trained personnel pose some operational issues.
- Sensitivity of smear microscopy is 10% low compared to culture.

Q-20. What is CBNAAT? Mention regarding the procedure, its sensitivity and specificity in various body specimens, advantages and limitations.

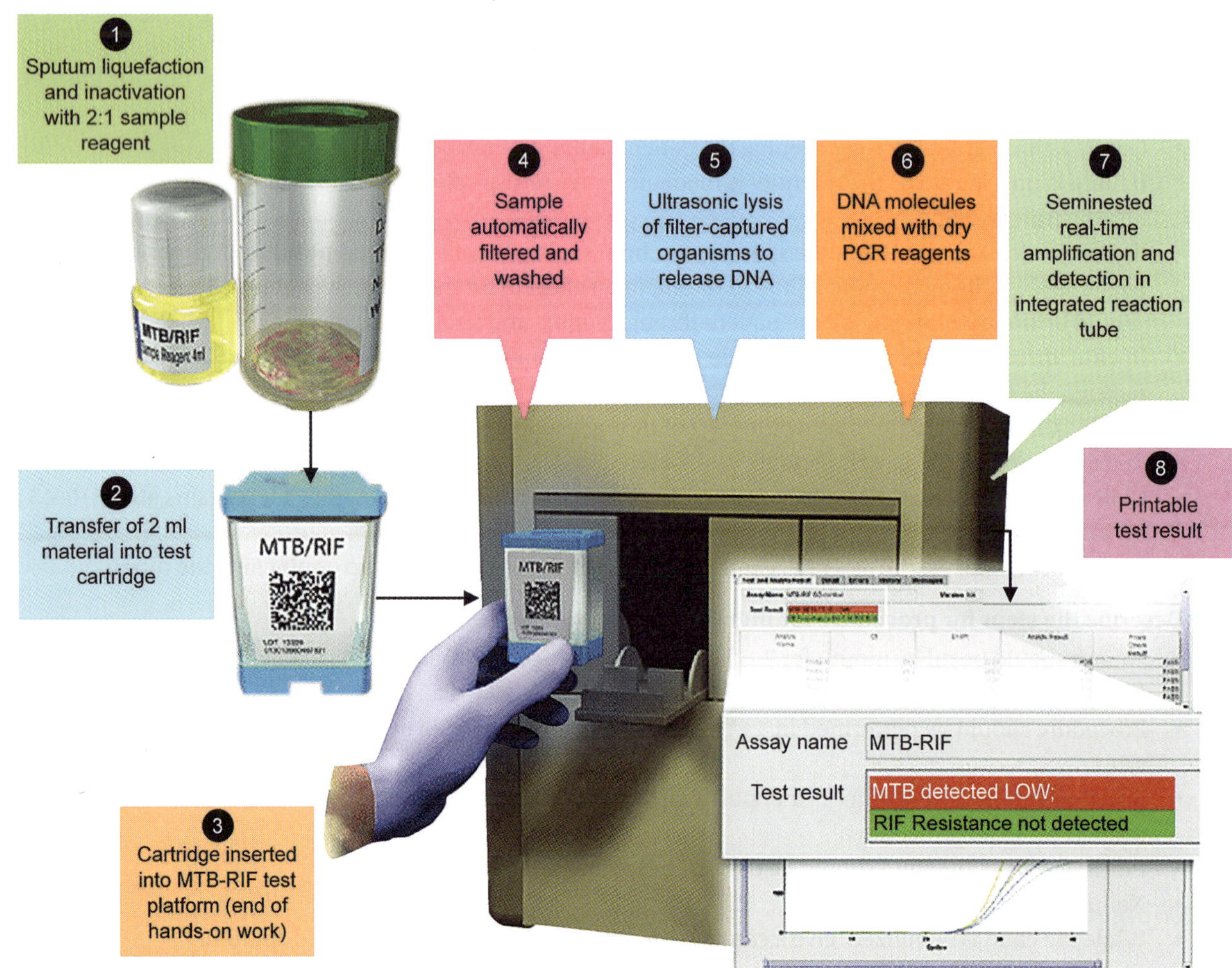

- CBNAAT (Cartridge-based nucleic acid amplification test) is a real time PCR rapid technique for diagnosis of TB and detection of rifampicin resistance conferring mutations within 2 hours.
- Steps for testing the specimen in CBNAAT machine:
  - *Sample processing:* Specimens are processed by adding the sample reagent at 2:1 ratio to the sputum sample, mixing and incubation for 15 minutes at room temperature. The sputum sample gets liquefied after the processing step.
  - *Loading the sample into cartridge:* Liquefied sample is added to the cartridge using a transfer pipette.
  - *Setting up the machine to run the test:* After switching on the system, "create test" is clicked in the GeneXpert Dx system window, test details are added, the barcode label of the cartridge is scanned and the "Start Test" is clicked to initiate testing.
  - *Loading the cartridge:* The instrument module door which displays the blinking green light is opened to load the cartridge. The door of module is closed firmly (the audible click sound should be heard). The green light stops blinking when the test starts.
  - *Obtaining the results:* When the test is completed, the green light turns off. It takes around 1 hour 55 minutes to complete test run. On completion of test run, the result is generated automatically on the monitor.
  - *Ending the test run:* When then system releases the door lock at the end of run, the module door is opened to remove the cartridge. The used cartridge is discarded.
- CBNAAT can be performed on both respiratory and nonrespiratory specimens like gastric aspirate, BAL, induced sputum, pleural fluid, CSF, lymph node aspirate etc. It cannot be on stool, urine or blood samples.
- The sensitivity and specificity of CBNAAT,
  - 98% and 99% for smear positive patient
  - 72% for smear negative culture positive patients
  - On gastric aspirate 68% and 99% respectively
  - Good with CSF and lymph node biopsy
  - Lower with pleural fluid, ascitic fluid, pericardial fluid and synovial fluids

Specimen	*Sensitivity in culture positive specimens*
Tissue biopsies	75%
Fine needle aspirates	88.3%
Gastric aspirates	78.7%
Pus samples	87.3%
CSF	85.7%
Pleural fluid	44.4%
Body fluids (peritoneal, pericardial, synovial)	50%

- Negative CBNAAT does not rule out TB.
- CBNAAT should be performed in samples collected from presumptive TB cases
- CBNAAT provides additional information about rifampicin resistance in mycobacterium tuberculosis detected cases.
- A new pediatric TB case, diagnosed by up front CBNAAT without any risk faster for drug resistant TB is currently retested with a fresh specimen. If the repeat sample is also showing rifampicin resistance, then the case is classified as MDR TB. If the repeat test is showing rifampicin sensitive, the treat the patient with first line drugs, pending confirmation by liquid culture.

Q-21. What is GeneXpert ultra test?

- GeneXpert ultra is newer generation test, PCR cartridge used in the same equipment
- Ultra has lower detection limit (16 bacilli per mL sputum) as compared to 131 per mL for GeneXpert.
- Especially useful for paucibacillary disease in children and HIV-TB coinfection.

Q-22. What is the importance of True Nat test in diagnosis of TB?

- True Nat is developed by the Indian firm Molbio Diagnostic Pvt Ltd Goa.
- It is molecular PCR-based test for diagnosis of TB and rifampicin resistance.
- *Major advantage:* It is battery operated
- Disadvantage: Not fully automated, needs centrifugation of samples like gastric aspirate.
- *Requires two steps process:* DNA extraction and then addition to the DNA chip.

Q-23. What is Line Probe Assay (LPA) test for diagnosis of TB?

- Can be used on smear positive specimen or culture isolates for Genotypic drug sensitivity test
- Rapid test for detection of additional resistance in MDR-TB patients as well as XDR TB.
- It detects,
  - TB
  - Resistance to R and H (First-line LPA)
  - Resistance to class FQ and class SLI (second-line LPA)
- LPA produces results in just 24–48 hours.

Q-24. What is Pyrosequencing (PSQ) in molecular diagnosis of TB?

- It is real time NAAT testing method.
- There is rapid sequencing of small segments of genomic DNA
- Can detect mutations associated with first and second-line ATT

Q-25. What is the role of culture in diagnosis of TB?

- Gold standard for sensitivity and specificity
- Cultures should be sent in all children who are CBNAAT negative and all presumptive DR TB
- Use of culture increases the number of TB cases found by 30–50% over smear alone.
- Approximately 10 viable bacilli/mL of sputum needed for culture compared to at least 5000 bacilli/mL of sputum for microscopy.
- Culture used for species identification, drug susceptibility testing (DST) and genotyping
- Culture also used to monitor patient response to treatment
- Two major categories of media,
  - *Solid:* Egg and agar based
  - *Liquid:* Also often referred to as broth media
- *Solid media:* Lowenstein-Jensen (LJ) media, not in use now a days.
- *Liquid media:* Mycobacterium Growth Indicator Tube (MGIT) produces results faster (2–8 weeks) than conventional LJ media.

Q-26. What is the relationship between type of disease and positivity of different microbiological tests?

	Smear	***Culture***	***Over all yield***
Primary complex	6%	22%	23%
Progressive primary	18%	46%	47%
Pleural effusion	5%	28%	32%

Q-27. What are the differentiating imaging features of tuberculoma and neurocysticercosis (NCC)?

	Parameters	*Tuberculoma*	*NCC*
CECT	Appearance	>2 cm, irregular, thick outline, marked perilesional edema	≤2 cm, thin, rounded outline with variable edema
	Location	Infratentorial or supra tentorial	Predominantly supratentorial
	Middle shift	More likely	Less likely
Contrast MRI	Appearance	T_2–usually hypointense core	Usually T_2 hyperintense core eccentric dot, scolex
	T_2 relaxation time	Shorter (83–290 ms)	Longer (305–1365 ms)
	MRS	Lipid peak present	Lipid peak absent

Q-28. What are forms of abdominal TB?

- Intestinal (39–66%) (large bowel/small bowel) (ulcerative, ulcerohyperplastic and hyperplastic).
- Nodal (4–42%)
- Peritoneal (27–40%) (Dry type, ascitic form)
- Visceral (hepatosplenic, Pancreas, Disseminated).
- One third patients has >1 site involved.

Q-29. What imaging studies are useful in diagnosis of abdominal TB?

- Plain X-ray (not diagnostic)
  - Enterolithiasis
  - Perforation
  - Features of intestinal obstruction
- USG study
  - Lymph adenopathy
  - Peritoneal thickening
  - Omental thickening and bowel wall thickening

    Ascites
- CECT
  - Abdominal LN with central necrosis, conglomerate, peripheral enhancement
  - Mesenteric thickening
  - Caked omentum, multiple SOL liver, spleen
  - Loculated ascites
- CT enterography
  - Ileocecal commonest
  - Uniform and concentric bowel thickening
  - Contracted, pulled up caecum
  - Ileocecal angle is distorted and often obtuse
  - Strictures short (usually <3 cm)

Q-30. What are CECT head findings are favoring neurotuberculosis?

- Basal meningeal enhancement
- Hydrocephalus
- Tuberculoma
- Infarcts at different areas, especially the basal ganglia.
- Precontrast basal hyper density.

Q-31. What conditions have similar radiological findings seen as in TB?

- Cryptococcal meningitis
- CMV encephalitis
- Toxoplasmosis
- Sarcoidosis
- Meningeal metastases
- Lymphoma

Q-32. What is the basis of pharmacotherapy of TB?

- Choice of anti-TB drugs is base on,
  - Bacillary load
  - Bacillary and metabolic subpopulation
  - Lag period of bacterial population
  - Pharmacokinetic profile and pathological factors
  - Drug resistant strains
- Different types of bacillary population are there in every case of TB and hence drugs are selected in a combination to attack entire (extracellular and intracellular, slow and rapidly multiplying) bacillary population for successful chemotherapy.
  - Isoniazid (INH) and Rifampicin (RMP) kill the fast-growing bacilli.
  - Pyrazinamide (PZA) acts against intracellular organisms in acidic medium.
  - RMP kills extracellular slowly growing bacilli
- Every case needs basic 4 drugs

Q-33. What is biphasic treatment of TB?

Generally, the duration of TB therapy is 6 months. It is divided into intensive phase (IP) for initial 2 months and continuous phase (CP) for later 4 months.

Intensive Phase (IP)

- The chances of naturally occurring mutants are high if the bacillary loads are more and therefore, such cases need more drugs in initial stage of disease.
- IP is for early and rapidly killing of mycobacterium tuberculosis (MTB), prevents deterioration and death, reduced infectivity and sputum conversion is achieved by 80–90%
- Addition of PZA reduces duration to 6 months due to its sterilizing effect
- Ethambutol (EMB) is useful if initial drug resistance to INH is high

Continuous phase (CP)

- CP eliminates most residual bacilli, reduces failures and relapses.
- Small number of bacilli left and so, fewer drugs are required in CP. But, in the presence of background resistance to the companion drugs, more drugs needed to prevent amplification of drug resistance.

Q-34. What is the rationale for single dose of each drug in a day?

- As dividing time of TB bacilli is about 21 hours, all the drugs are administered in such a way that they achieve peak concentration all at one time so as to hit bacilli hard.
- The drug concentration is poor in caseum and sequestrated tissues, so they should be removed by surgical method whenever it is feasible.

Q-35. What are recent case definitions in TB management?

IAP NTEP guidelines 2020 cases definitions and categories of treatment

Type of patient	*Regimens*
New microbiologically confirmed pulmonary TB	2 HRZE + 4 HRE
New clinically diagnosed pulmonary TB	
New microbiologically confirmed extrapulmonary TB	
New clinically diagnosed extrapulmonary TB	
Previously treated TB with no rifampicin resistance (recurrence, treatment after loss to follow-up, treatment after failure)	

- Molecular testing shall be done in all new cases in children with suspected TB at diagnosis
- In case of neuro or skeletal TB continuous phase is extended to 8 months

Q-36. What are the dosage of common antituberculous drugs in children as per recent NTEP guidelines?

		Range mg/kg/day	*Average mg/kg/day*	*Maximum dose (mg)*
Rifampicin	R	10–20	15	600
Isoniazid	H	7–15	10	300
Pyrazinamide	Z	30–40	35	2000
Ethambutol	E	15–25	20	1500
Streptomycin	S	15–20	20	1000

Q-37. Which Fixed Drug Combinations (FDCs) are available under RNTCP, their doses as per body weight of the patient?

- 3 Drugs FDC DT (H 50 + R 75 + Z 150) (10:15:30) for children, + non-DT Ethambutol (ETB) 100
- 4 drugs FDC adult (H 75 + R 150 + Z 400 + E 275)

Recommended drug dosage and FDC pill combinations from 0 to 18 years

Weight band (kg)	*Dose*
4-7	IP + IE
8-11	ZP + ZE
12-15	3P + 3E
16-24	4P + 4E
25-29	3P + 3E+ 1A
30-39	2P + 2E+ 2A

Q-38. What are the indications of steroids in TB?

- Definite indications
  - TBM
  - Pericarditis
  - Addison's disease
  - Military TB with alveolocapillary block
  - TB uveitis
- May be used
  - Endobronchial TB
  - Bronchial compression
  - Mediastinal compression syndrome
  - Pleurisy compression syndrome
  - Pleurisy with severe distress
  - Laryngeal TB
  - TB immune reconstitution inflammatory syndrome (IRIS)

Q-39. What is the dosage and duration of steroids in TB?

- Prednisolone 1–2 mg/kg/day or Dexamethasone 0.6 mg/kg/day
- 4 weeks and tapered over next 4 weeks

Q-40. What is the dose of pyridoxine supplementation in TB? what is the justification for its use?

- 10 mg/day is recommended to all those receiving INH therapy including neonates on INH chemoprophylaxis
  Justification for pyridoxine supplementation in ATT
- Dose of INH is increased
- High prevalence of malnutrition
- Difficult to recognize or diagnose peripheral neuropathy in children

Q-41. How should monitoring and follow-up be done in patients on antituberculous therapy?

There are two components of follow-up, clinical follow-up and laboratory follow-up.

Clinical follow-up

- An initial visit within 2 weeks of starting therapy to recheck that patient is on correct dose and combination and is tolerating all drug dose and combination and is tolerating all drugs.
- Then, every month during the treatment
- Every 6 months for 2 years after completion of treatment. Most of the treatment failures and relapses occur in first 2 years after completion of ATT, therefore follow up for 2 years is recommended.
- On each follow up visit child should be assessed for following:
  - Improvement in clinical symptoms including fever, cough, appetite, increasing weight and other clinical symptoms. It will be assessed as no improvement, partial improvement or improved after asking the parents. Most patients will show improvement in symptoms by the end of 4 weeks of therapy.
  - *Physical examination:* It includes temperature, pulse rate, respiratory rate, oxygen saturation and blood pressure, if needed. Chest indrawing, size of lymph nodes, anemia, distention of abdomen, organomegaly, etc. Chest should be examined for breath sounds, crepitations, evidence of pleural effusion. CVS and CNS should be checked in patients with involvement of these systems. Record of weight nearest to 0.1 kg (100 G) by using appropriate weighing scale on each visit is important.
- Causes of poor weight gain
  - Poor appetite
  - Vomiting

- Side effects of medicines
- Wrong diagnosis
- Comorbid conditions like SAM, HIV
- Concomitant infections such as pneumonia, diarrhea

- If the child is losing weight on assessed to be unresponsive to treatment, the patient should be reevaluated for TB or drug-resistant TB or alternative diagnosis by seeking expert advice
- Monitoring for side effects of drugs like vomiting, rashes, pain in abdomen, etc. jaundice, visual acuity and color vision are other side effects to be kept in mind.
- Treatment of co morbid conditions like HIV, SAM, Diabetes mellitus, seizures in CNS TB, complications like pneumothorax, collapse of lung, intestinal obstruction should be assessed.
- Revisit adherence to therapy at each visit. Use pill count, social support and treatment supervision, etc. should be done.

Monitoring by Laboratory Investigations

- Microbiological at the end of intensive phase and end of treatment
- MGIT culture, if no response after 4 weeks of therapy
- Liver function tests are not indicated routinely
- Follow up chest X-ray at the end of therapy or earlier, if clinically no response or development of any complication
- USG abdomen, CT/MRI scan, Echocardiograph on complication of therapy or no response or deterioration while on treatment.

Q-42. What are the guidelines for a patient who has received interrupted ATT?

- Interruption up to 4 weeks is managed by resuming the therapy
- If the drugs are interrupted for more than 4 weeks, the patient is investigated for acquisition of DRTB. If on testing RMP resistance is not detected, retreat with first line 4 drugs, and check for INH resistance then treat appropriately as drug sensitive or INH mono/poly-resistance case.
- If RMP resistance is detected, treat as MDR-TB

Q-43. What are adverse effects of anti-TB drugs?

Adverse effects of anti TB drugs

Drug	*Main adverse effects*	*Rare adverse effects*
Isoniazid	• Peripheral neuropathy • Skin rash • Hepatitis • Sleepiness/lethargy	• Convulsions • Psychosis • Arthralgia • Anemia
Rifampicin	• Abdominal pain • Vomiting • Hepatitis • Cutaneous reactions • Thrombocytopenia	• Osteomalacia • Pseudomembranous colitis • Hemolytic anemia • Acute renal failure
Pyrazinamide	• Hepatitis • Arthralgia	• Cutaneous reactions • Sideroblastic anemia
Ethambutol	• Retrobulbar neuritis	• Cutaneous reactions • Peripheral neuropathy • Arthralgia

Q-44. What are the adverse effects of second-line anti-TB drugs?

Drug	*Side effects*
Injection Kanamycin/Capreomycin	• Ototoxicity • Nephrotoxicity • Vertigo • Electrolyte imbalance
Quinolones ofloxacin, Levofloxacin, Moxifloxacin	• Arthralgia • Tendinopathy, tendinitis • Skin rash • Cardiotoxicity–QT prolongation • Convulsions • Abdominal pain, vomiting
Ethionamide	• Anorexia, metallic taste, nausea, vomiting • Excessive salivation • Hypothyroidism • Gynecomastia • Menstrual disturbances – Impotence – Acne – Hepatitis • Peripheral neuropathy
Cycloserine	• Slurred speech, convulsions, tremor, insomnia • Depression, suicidal tendency, confusion, altered behavior • Hypersensitivity reactions

Q-45. What are criteria for anti-TB drug-induced liver injury? How should it be managed?

- Risk factors for liver injury with ATT are malnutrition, associated HIV, hepatitis B, hepatitis C, hypoalbuminemia, extensive TB disease
- Defined criteria,
  - More than 5 times rise in hepatic enzyme levels even without symptoms
  - More than 3 times rise in hepatic enzyme levels with symptoms like nausea, vomiting and serum bilirubin >1.5 mg/dL
- Management of AT drug-induced hepatic injury
  - Stop INH, RMP and PZA
  - Treat with SM + EMB + Levofloxacin
  - Look for other causes of hepatitis
  - Reintroduce primary drugs once symptoms subside and liver enzymes less than twice upper limit of normal (2–6 weeks). Start with full dose of RMP. The drugs (in full dose) are to be added every 3 days, with regular LFT monitoring. A new drug is re instituted only if the ALT is less than twice the upper limit of normal.

Q-46. What are the causes for clinical or radiological deterioration during follow- up?

- Incorrect diagnosis (particularly if clinically diagnosed as TB)
- Lack of adherence to therapy
- Incorrect drugs or doses
- Not retaining drugs—may vomit out drugs due to bad taste or forceful medication
- Comorbid conditions like HIV, SAM
- Drug resistance
- Paradoxical upgrading reactions
- Need surgical intervention in abscess, sequestrated necrotic tissue

Q-47. What is paradoxical upgrading reactions or Immune Reconstitution Inflammatory Syndrome (IRIS)? What are types of paradoxical reactions? What are the differential diagnosis? What is the treatment of paradoxical upgrading reactions?

Paradoxical upgrading reactions

- It refers to enlargement of old lesions or development of unexpected new lesions during appropriate ATT
- Usually, occurs 3 to 12 weeks after beginning of ATT, most frequently seen after 6–7 weeks of starting treatment and lasts for approximately 2 months.
- Generally, it is self-limiting, resolves without serious sequelae and regresses by same ATT. It may occur post-treatment, as late as 2 years in case of TB lymphadenopathy.

Mechanism of paradoxical upgrading reactions

Acute TB can result in depression of immunity, may be aggravated by HIV and SAM.

After successful ATT and improvement in comorbid conditions, focal immune response improves

With improvement in focal immune response, there is accumulation of inflammatory exudates at previously invisible, microscopic tuberculous foci elsewhere, appearing as new lesions. Reversible radiological progression in initial treatment of TB may be noted more common, if frequent monitoring by chest X-ray is performed. It is for this reason, routine monitoring by radiographs is not recommended.

Types of paradoxical reactions

- Increase in size of mediastinal lymph nodes or areas of pulmonary infiltration in pediatric patients with primary TB
- Appearance of new lung infiltrates in patients with extrapulmonary TB
- Development of TB pleural effusion
- Increase in size of pleural effusion or appearance of effusion on the opposite side
- Appearance of new lymph nodes or enlargement of original nodes
- Increase in size or number of tuberculomas or infarctions or hydrocephalus on treatment.

Differentiation of paradoxical upgrading reactions and drug-resistant TB

- Absence of systemic symptoms is usually seen in paradoxical reactions. In paradoxical reactions, patient has no fever, cough is decreasing, appetite is improving and weight gain started, although paradoxical reactions are present
- Paradoxical reactions are the condition, diagnosed by exclusion. Coinfections should be excluded with appropriate investigations, if required.

Treatment

- Most of patients respond to continuation of same antituberculous drugs
- In severe inflammatory reaction causing compression over airways or raised intracranial pressure or intestinal obstruction, steroids are indicated
- Rarely, alternative immunosuppressive agents may be required
- Large mass, enlarged lymph nodes, abscess or pleural effusion causing respiratory embarrassment may require surgical intervention. Rapidly progressive hydrocephalus or other CNS lesion may require surgical procedure.

Q-48. What is the definition of drug-resistant TB and MDR TB?

MDR TB is defined as *Mycobacterium tuberculosis* resistant to INH and RMP with or without resistance to other drugs.

Q-49. What is presumptive case of MDR TB in children?

- Children who have contacts of adults with MDR-TB
- Who are lost to follow-up after initiating treatment
- Those who present with recurrence of disease after previous treatment
- Those who do not respond to therapy with first line drugs
- Those living with HIV patients.

Q-50. What are points indicating probable MDR–TB among children?

Criteria for diagnosis of 'probable MDR–TB' include children with signs and symptoms of active TB disease who in addition have the following risk factors.

- Close contact with a known case of MDR–TB
- Close contact with a person who died whilst on TB treatment
- Close contact with a person who failed TB treatment
- Non response or failure of a first line regimen, recognizing that both bacteriological and clinical definitions of failure should be used
- Previous treatment with second-line medications.

Q-51. What is an approach for diagnosis of DR–TB in children?

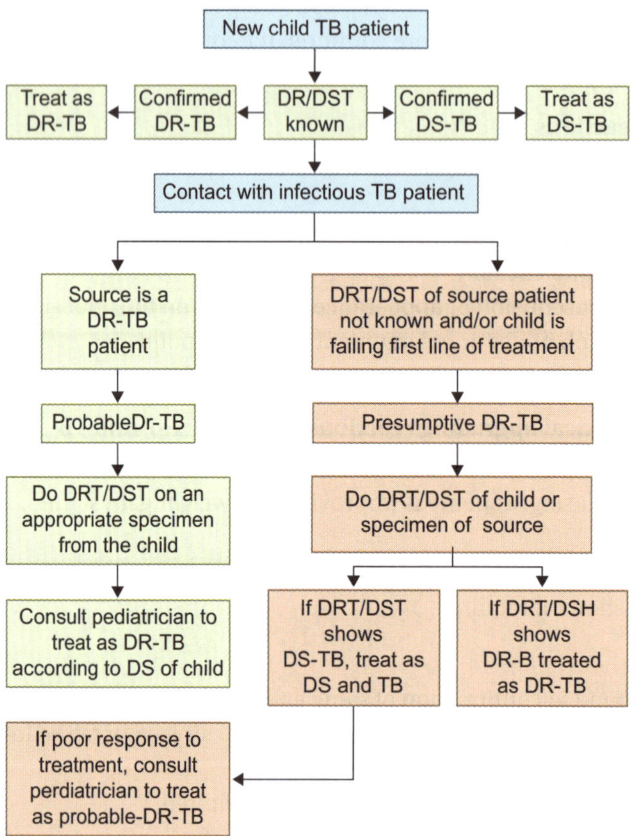

Q-52. What are the definitions of DR–TB?

- *Mono resistance TB:* Resistance to any first line anti–TB drug other than R (HE)
- MDR–TB: Resistance to at least H and R Rifampicin resistance (RR) also managed as MDR–TB
- *Poly drug-resistance TB:* Resistant to more than one first-line anti–TB drugs, other than both H and R.
- *XDR TB (extensive drug resistance):* MDR-TB + Fluroquinolones (ofx, Lfx, Mfx) and SLI (Km, Am, Cm)
- R Resistance is quite rare without H resistance. R resistance is considered as MDR– TB.

Q-53. What is the approach to diagnosis of MDR-TB in children?

- Careful history
  - History of contact with MDR-TB case
  - Failing first line TB treatment despite adherence
- Clinical examination
- HIV testing
- Microbiological confirmation and drug susceptibility testing is paramount and should always be attempted.
- Diagnosis of DR-TB in the absence of microbiological diagnosis must be thoroughly reviewed as it may often be untenable.
- Sometimes, if there is high DR TB suspicion, microbiologically negative clinically diagnosed MDR-TB can be considered provided all other alternative causes for symptoms have been rule out in the absence of negative culture or culture is not feasible due to lack of a specimen.

Q-54. What drugs are recommended for use in longer MDR-TB regimen?

Groups and steps	*Medicine*
Group A Include all three medicines	• Levofloxacin o Moxifloxacine Lfx, Mfx • Bedaquiline Bdq • Linezolid Lzd
Group B Add one or both medicines	• Clofazimine Cf2 • Cycloserine or Terizidone CS Trd
Group C Add to complete the regimen and when medicines from Groups A and B cannot be used	• Ethambutol E • Delamanid Dim • Pyrazinamide 2 • Imipenem - Cialastatin or Ipm – Clu Meropenem Mpm • Amikacin Am (S) or (streptomycin) • Ethionamide or Prothionamide Eto Pto • Para amino salicylic acid PAS

Q-55. What are implications of TB-HIV co-infection?

- Need to screen all HIV patients for TB
- Need to screen all TB patients for HIV

Q-56. What evaluation of the neonate for presence of disease should be performed in a neonate exposed to mother with TB?

- Clinical examination
  - *Vitals:* HR, RR, signs of increased work of breathing
  - Chest examination
  - Abdomen for hepatosplenomegaly
  - CNS
- X-ray chest
- USG abdomen
- Gastric aspirate

Q-57. What preventive therapy to neonate is recommended for a neonate to mother with TB?

- Recommended for whom
  - If mother has any form of active TB detected in pregnancy or often birth
  - If exposed to ay infections case of TB after birth
- Rule out active disease in neonate
- INH 10 mg/kg/day and Pyridoxine 10 mg/day for 6 months
- Close observation and no prophylaxis in case of MDR-TB in mother

Q-58. What are recommendations for isolation and breastfeeding for a neonate to mother with TB?

- No isolation
- If the baby is on IPT separation is not required
- Consideration needs for sick mother's health, nutrition and rest
- Mother's cough hygiene and etiquette are important
- Required when,
  - Mother not adhering to treatment
  - Infections XDR/MDR TB
  - Expressed breast milk can be used in such situations
- Breast feeding is safe and should be continued

Q-59. What are recommendations for preventive therapy?

- Indications
  - All symptomatic contacts (up to 5 years of age) of a smear positive case, after birth ruling out active disease and irrespective their BCG or nutritional status
  - All HIV-infected children who either has a known exposure to an infectious TB case or are TST positive but have no active TB disease
  - All TST-positive children who are receiving immunosuppressive therapy, e.g. children with nephrotic syndrome, acute leukemia, etc.
  - A child born to mother who was diagnosed to have TB in pregnancy, INH prophylaxis for 6 months, provided congenital TB is ruled out
- INH 10 mg/kg/day for 6 months

Q-60. What is perinatal tuberculosis?

Congenital TB is acquired during intrauterine life or before complete passage through birth canal. Perinatal TB is preferred term which encompasses true congenital and neonatal forms of disease. Distinction between true congenital cases and those acquired postnatally is purely of epidemiological significance and modes of presentation, treatment and immediate prognosis do not differ between two groups and may be difficult to differentiate at times.

There are two main infectious routes for congenital TB. Transplacental route, forming a primary complex in liver of an infant with secondary hematogenous spread and by aspiration or ingestion of infected amniotic fluid, leading to primary focus in lungs or GIT.

Q-61. What are diagnostic criteria for congenital TB?

Cantwell described presence of proven TB disease with at least one of the following:

- Lesions in newborn baby during the first week of life.
- A primary hepatic complex or caseating hepatic granuloma
- TB infections of placenta or maternal genital tract
- Exclusion of possibility of postnatal transmission by investigation of contacts, including hospital staff.

Q-62. What are limitations of Cantwell criteria?

- Primary may be late, after 2–3 weeks of birth.
- Difficulty in demonstration of AFB in neonates, if gastric aspirate is negative.
- Inadequate opportunities and facilities for examination of placenta or endometrium
- Percutaneous liver biopsies are also difficult to perform, especially in sick neonates with multiple comorbid factors.
- Incomplete evaluation of mother, especially if symptoms of TB are not florid and inadequate evaluation of contacts, including hospital attendants compounds the problem.

CHAPTER

46 Cerebral Palsy

QUESTIONS AND ANSWERS

Q-1. What is the definition of cerebral palsy (CP)?

In 2007, an international committee defined CP as,

- A group of permanent disorders of muscle tone, posture and movement.
- Causing limitation of activity.
- Attributable to nonprogressive disturbance that occurred in the developing fetal or infant brain. Developing brain is considered up to age of 5 years.
- CP is often accompanied by disturbances of sensation, perception, cognition, communication, behavior, epilepsy and secondary musculoskeletal problems.

Q-2. What is the epidemiology of cerebral palsy?

- Globally, population-based studies report prevalence of CP ranging from 1.5 to more than 4 per 1000 live births or children of a defined age range.
- The wide variability is due to differences in inclusion criteria and age cut offs.
- Minor increases are due to increased survival of very premature babies.
- CP is more common and severe in boys. Male neurons in culture are more sensitive to death from exposure to NMDA and nitric oxide radicals and more vulnerable to autophagy than female neurons.

Q-3. What is the pathogenesis of cerebral palsy?

- The basic pathophysiology is harmful cascade pathways triggered off by a hypoxic, ischemic, infectious or inflammatory insult resulting from heterogenous causes. The most common causes are hypoxic ischemic encephalopathy, intracranial hemorrhage, infections like bacterial meningitis, encephalitis, TBM and toxins like bilirubin encephalopathy (kernicterus), vascular causes like stroke, trauma etc.
- The excito oxidative cascade results in secondary mitochondrial energy failure.
- Impaired perfusion provokes protective redistribution of blood to vital organs including the brain.
- When reperfusion occurs, there is a massive influx of free oxygen radicals and calcium ions in the affected area due to damaged ion channels.
- This ionic imbalance causes neuronal membrane depolarization and glutamate transporter failure in the presynaptic cleft. The later is responsible for removal of glutamate from the synaptic cleft. Excess synaptic glutamate stimulates excitatory glutamate N-Methyl-D-Aspartate (NMDA) receptors causing further release of free radicles and worsening of the oxidative stress.
- Lactic acid accumulation disrupts the mitochondrial respiratory chain.
- Enzyme mediated cellular damage and release of preaptonic cytochrome C and apoptosis inducing factors lead to neuronal apoptosis and eventually necrosis of the brain cells, glia being more susceptible than neurons. Hence reversible injury processes to irreversible.
- The premature brain (<34 weeks gestation) is more prone to injury and oxidative stress. This has been established by the characteristic MRI findings like "White matter damage of immaturity" and autopsy findings such as subependymal, intraventricular and leptomeningeal hemorrhage seen in preterm babies.
- In contrast, brain structures rich in excitatory synapses like deep basal ganglia, perirolandic cortex and posterior putamen are more vulnerable in term babies.

Q-4. What is the etiology of cerebral palsy?

- A common misconception still persists that perinatal asphyxia is the most common cause of CP. However, it has been well established that it attributes to less than 10% cases of CP.
- In developed countries, most cases of CP are attributable to antenatal causes and pre term survivors. In developing countries although antenatal causes are maximal, the proportion of acquired causes is greater than in the developed countries.
- The task force report on neonatal encephalopathy and neurological outcomes (2014) has outlined four essential criteria defining an acute hypoxic event severe enough to cause CP. This includes,
  - Metabolic acidosis (pH < 7.2 and base deficit ≥12 mmol/L) in cord arterial blood at delivery.
  - Early onset of moderate or severe neonatal encephalopathy (≥34 weeks gestation).
  - Spastic quadriplegia or dyskinetic CP.
  - Exclusion of identifiable causes of CP such as trauma, coagulation disorders, infectious conditions, genetic disorders etc.
- These are five additional nonspecific criteria which suggest an insult at delivery, if collectively met,
  - Events severe enough to cause acute hypoxia in a healthy fetus like prolapsed cord, uterine rupture.
  - Sustained fetal bradycardia.
  - Apgar score <4 at 5 minutes.
  - Neonatal multisystem failure.
  - Edema and intraventricular hemorrhage on neuroimaging within 5 days.
- With the availability of newer generation genetic studies like sequencing of the whole genome, it is being increasingly recognized that genetic mutations can directly cause or indirectly result in increased susceptibility to CP.
- It is hypothesized that males are more genetically predisposed to develop mutations and get damaged by free radicals based on differences observed in cultured neurons experiments.
- Functional polymorphism in interleukin-6 gene is associated with CP in term babies.
- A large number of cases previously labeled as CP have been found to be due to genetic or metabolic disorders.

Q-5. What factors are associated with cerebral palsy?

- **Preconceptional**
  - Fertility treatment
  - Lower socioeconomic strata
- **Antenatal**
  - Multiple pregnancies
  - Maternal preeclampsia
  - Intrauterine infections
  - Chorioamnionitis
  - Neonatal stroke due to factor V Leiden
- **Natal**
  - Maternal hypotension.
  - Premature separation of membrane.
  - Low placental weight.
  - Low Apgar scores.

- **Postnatal**
  - NICU admission.
  - Ventilatory support for >7 days.
  - Neonatal sepsis.
  - Respiratory distress.
- **Factors associated with lower prevalence of CP**
  - Administration of magnesium sulphate and corticosteroids antenatally.
  - Administration of caffeine in neonates.

Q-6. What is topographic, physiologic and Modified Swedish Classification of CP?

Topographic classification (Fig. 1)	*Physiological classification*	*Modified Swedish classification*
• Quadriplegia • Hemiplegia • Diplegia • Monoplegia • Triplegia	• Spastic – Quadriplegia – Hemiplegia – Diplegia • Extrapyramidal • Mixed	• Spastic. • Tetraplegic • Hemiplegic • Diplegic • Ataxic • Dyskinetic – Choreoathetosis – Dystonia

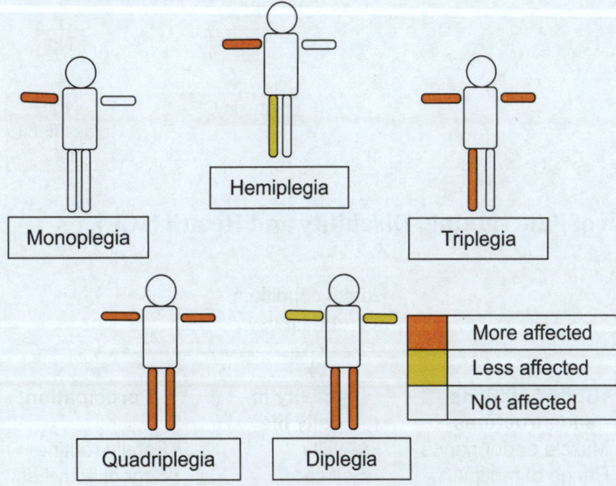

Fig. 1: Topographical classification of CP.

Surveillance of Cerebral Palsy in Europe (SCPE)

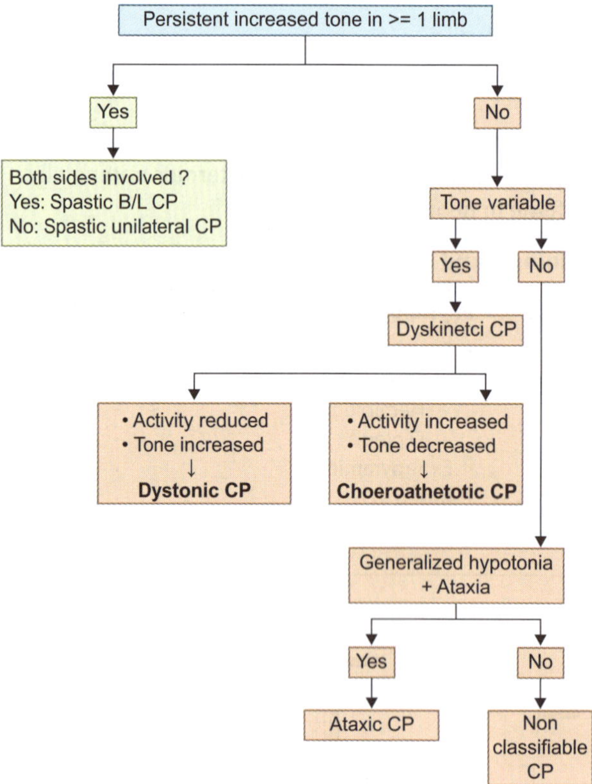

The International Classification of Functioning, Disability and Health (ICF)

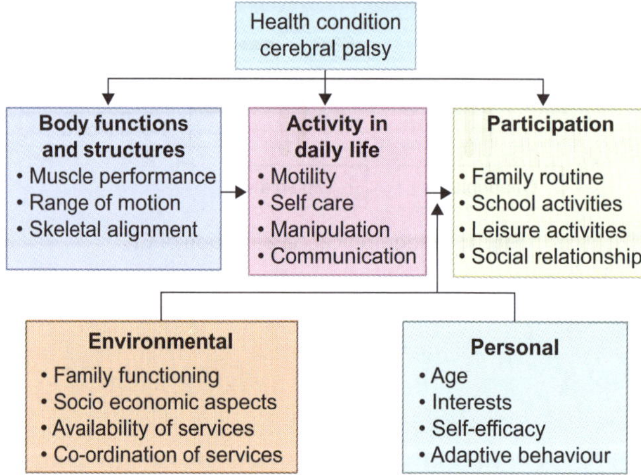

- Accurate and uniform description of nature, severity and healthcare needs, enables monitoring of change in status of individuals and comparison of data from different centers.
- Topographic classification is based on distribution pattern of limb involvement.
- Physiological classification is based on type of motor abnormality.
- Swedish and SCPE classification systems are combination of both topographic and physiological classification.
- In developed countries, spastic CP is seen in 85% with diplegia 35%, quadriplegia 20% and hemiplegia 25%, extrapyramidal 5%.

- The PGIMER Chandigarh data reports, 73% spastic with quadriplegia 51.5%, diplegia 31.5%, hemiplegia 13.8%, 7% dyskinetic, 11.2% hypotonic/ataxic and 8.8% mixed.
- The international classification of Functioning, Disability and Health (ICF) describes CP as impairment of body function and/or structures, limitation of activity, restriction of participation and environmental factors.

GMFCS: Revised and Expanded

GMFCS: REVISED and EXPANDED

	Age band				
Level	**Before 2 years**	**Between 2 and 4 years**	**Between 4 and 6 years**	**Between 6 and 12 years**	**Between 12 and 18 years**
I	Sits unsupported, gets up to stand, crawls, cruises and walks by 18-24 months without help	Walking preferred. Does not require assistance	Can walk and climb stairs. has started to run and jump	Walks in all settings. Climbs stairs without help. Can run and jump but speed, balance and coordination limited. May engage in sports	Walks in all settings. Climbs stairs without help. Can run and jump but speed, balance and coordination limited. May engage in sports
II	Sits with support of hands, can crawl, can pull to stand, and cruise few steps	Has problem in sitting if hands not free, walks with assistance	Can sit and stand but may need to pull or push against a surface. Walks short distance without help. Climbs stairs with railing. Cannot run or jump	Walks in most settings except long distance or run even terrain (hand held device). Climbs stairs with railing. Limited running and jumping. Requires adaptations to engage in sports	Walks in most settings except long distance or uneven terrain (hand-held or wheeled device). Climbs stairs with railing. Requires adaptation o engage in sports
III	Maintains trunk with minimal support of lower back, can creep on stomach	Needs assistance to assume sitting, and W-sitting. Crawling preferred though can pull to stand	Sits with trunk support. Needs help to stand, walk short distances and stairs. Long distance needs transport	Sits with seat-belt. Needs help to stand. Climbs stairs with help. Walks with hand – held device for short distance and wheeled for long distance. May engage in adapted sports	Sits with seat-belt. Needs help to stand. Climbs stairs with help. Walks with hand-held device for short distance and wheeled for long distance. May engage in adapted sports
IV	Head control present. Can roll. Trunk support required for sitting	Can sit if placed and then with support of hands. Self-mobility by rolling, creeping on abdomen or crawling	Sits in adapter chair. Needs walker for short distance and wheeled transport or longer distances	Mobility requires help. Only adaptive sitting. At home floor mobility, assisted walking or mobility device. Help needed for transfers. Outside wheeled device. Engage in adapted sports	Mobility requires help. Only adaptive sitting. At home-assisted walking or mobility device. Help needed for transfers. Outside wheeled device. Engages in adapted sport
V	Physical problems limit voluntary movements. Unable to maintain antigravity head and trunk posture in prone	May not maintain antigravity head and trunk postures. Limited sitting and standing even with equipment. No independent movement, requires physical assistance or wheelchair	May not able to maintain antigravity head and trunk postures, limitations in sitting and standing. Needs transport at all times	Needs assisted sitting. May not be able to support head and trunk. Transported in wheelchair in all settings. Transfers need complete help. Self-mobility with powered devices	Needs assisted sitting. May not be able to support head and trunk. Transported in wheelchair in all settings. Transfers need complete help. Self-mobility with powered devices

- The gross motor function classification scale revised and expanded (GMFC – R and E) rates dysfunction in self-initiated movement according to five levels that vary by age. Emphasis is on usual performance in sitting, transfers and mobility in various (home and community).

Manual Ability Classification System

Level	*Description of manual ability*
I	*Handles objects easily and successfully:* Limitations in manual tasks that require speed and accuracy (i.e., handling objects that are very small, fragile or very heavy or performing new tasks). Maintains independence in activities of daily living
II	*Handles most objects but with somewhat reduced quality and/or speed of achievement:* Certain tasks may be performed with difficulty, avoided or done using alternative methods, but usually no restriction in independence in activities of daily living
III	Handles objects with difficulty; needs help to prepare and/or modify activities: Additional support (preparation or adjustments in the environment and extra time) is required to achieve the same performance as in level II. The extent of independence depends upon the quality and quantity of support provided
IV	Handles a limited selection of easily managed objects in adapted situations: Performs parts of activities with a lot of effort and limited success with continuous support and the use of adaptive equipment.
V	*Does not handle objects and has severely limited ability to perform even simple actions:* Requires complete assistance. May at best perform extremely easy activities like pushing a button or holding something transiently

Mini-manual Ability Classification System for 1–4 years

Level	*Description of manual ability*
I	*Handles objects easily and successfully:* There is slight limitation in performing actions that require precision and coordination and may require more adult help compared to children of the same age without disabilities
II	*Handles most objects but with somewhat reduced quality and/or speed of achievement:* Some actions can be performed with difficulty, but more problems will be encountered, it will take longer and they will require more practice. The child will require help from adults more frequently compared to peers
III	*Handles objects with difficulty:* Performance is slow with limited variation and quality, and adult help is required more frequently. However, easily managed objects can be handled independently for short periods, but take much longer
IV	*Handles a limited selection of easily managed objects in simple actions:* The actions are performed slowly and with exertion. Constant adult support and help is required. Like being offered objects in adapted positions
V	*Does not handle objects and has severely limited ability to perform even simple actions:* At best they can perform simple movements (push, touch, press, and hold for a few seconds) in special situations with constant interaction with an adult who is helping him/her

- The manual ability classification scale (MACS) rates upper limb function in children above 4 years. The mini-MACS is an adaptation of MACS that is used for children between 1 and 4 years. It classifies the best overall ability to handle objects, such as toys or other objects in various settings, as well as the extent of additional support that required.

Q-7. What are clinical manifestations of CP?

Cerebral palsy has a wide variability in clinical phenotype, depending upon whether the disorder is established or still evolving, the multiple types, varying degree of motor impairment and associated comorbid conditions.

Early Signs of CP

- Persistent fisting beyond 2 months.
- Persistent primitive reflexes beyond the age at which they should disappear.
- Toe walking.
- Cortical thumb.
- Scissoring of legs—mother may complaint of finding difficulty in changing diaper and clothes.
- Hand preference before the age of 1 year.
- Lethargy.
- Irritability.
- Feeding difficulty.
- Absence of rooting and sucking reflexes.
- Seizures during neonatal period.

Common Presenting Complaints

- Delayed motor milestones.
- Locomotor difficulties.
- Abnormal movements.
- Seizures.
- Delayed speech.
- Behavioral problems.
- PGIMER, Chandigarh study reported the presenting complaints,
  - Developmental delay (88%).
  - Seizures (34.7%).
  - Gait and posture problems (22.8%).
  - Delayed speech (9.5%).
  - Behavioral problems (5.9%).

Motor Manifestations of Established CP

It is easy to make diagnosis of CP by 18–24 months when decreased motor power is associated with easily recognizable signs.

- **Abnormal tone**
  - Increased tone (Spastic, rigidity).
  - Decreased muscle tone (ataxic).
  - Variable muscle tone (dyskinetic).
- **Abnormal gait**
  - Crouched - Hip flexion, knee flexion and ankle dorsiflexion.
  - Circumductive.
- **Abnormal limb positioning**
  - Characteristic upper limb postures are elbow flexion with pronation of forearm, flexion of wrist and fingers and thumb in palm **(Figs. 2A to C)**

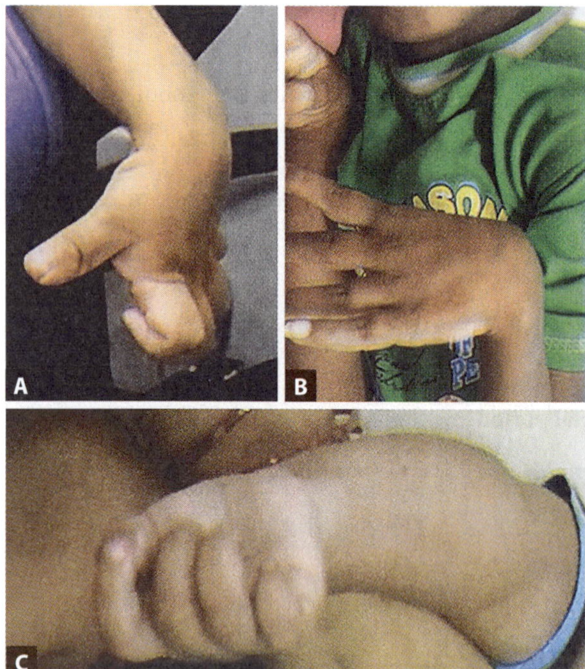

Fig. 2: Upper limb position seen in CP. (A) Flexion of wrist with slight splaying of fingers; (B) Flexion of fingers; (C) Pronation of forearm.

- Lower limb exhibit equinovalgus, equinovarus and pesvalgus, flexion of the knees and hip subluxation characterized by pelvic obliquity.
- Scissoring of lower limbs (due to excessive adductor spasms).

- **Abnormal Movements**
  - Choreoathetosis.
  - Dystonia.
  - Choreoathetosis and dystonia, both.
- **Abnormal Reflexes**
  - Deep tendon reflexes are exaggerated.
  - Persistent primitive reflexes.
  - Persistent extensor planters.
  - Failure of appearance of postural reflexes.

Manifestations of Evolving CP

- Delayed motor milestones.
- Slightly more than normal tightness or limpness.
- Difficulty while diapering or dressing the infant.
- Difficulties in breast feeding.
- Repetitive tongue movements.
- Impaired hearing or vision.
- Non paralytic squint.
- Recurrent regurgitation.
- High degree of suspicion on follow-up examination of high-risk babies, NICU graduates.

Signs indicative of early CP while performing developmental maneuvers

Developmental maneuver	*Significant finding*
Supine	• Head persistently in midline • Persistent fisting • Reduced and/or asymmetric spontaneous movements • Not tracking till 180° by 12 weeks • Not turning head to sound
Prone	• Head to side, not in midline by 12 weeks • Chin not raised off plane of surface by 6 weeks • Face not at 45-90° and no weight bearing on forearms by 12 weeks • Pelvis still not flat by 12 weeks • Knees drawn under abdomen without extension of legs by >6 weeks
Pull to sit	• Pronounced head leg • Spasms of hamstring felt in popliteal space and feeling of resistance with flexion and knees • Entire body rising spontaneously to feet
Held sitting	• Inability to lift chin up intermittently • Rounding of back pronounced.
Held standing	• Unable to lift chin up momentarily beyond 8 weeks • Unable to bear weight at all • Abnormal degree of planter flexion.
Ventral suspension	• Excessive head leg with limbs, hanging limply • Advanced head control–head above level of plant with increased extension of LL
Axillary suspension	• Abnormal/asymmetrical extension of LL • Abnormal adduction/scissoring of LL • Feeling of sensation of slipping

Changing Manifestations of CP

- Though the insult is one time (nonprogressive), the manifestations of CP are known to change. This is due to several reasons like ongoing CNS maturation, recognition of symptoms at appropriate age, influence of interventions, development of complications like deformities and contracture, etc.
- Hypotonia evolving into spasticity due to ongoing myelination.
- Speech delay or impairment of cognition becomes appreciable when the child is older.
- Influence of interventions like physiotherapy, speech therapy, sensory stimulations etc. may show improvement.
- Development of complications like seizures, intercurrent illnesses, deformities, contractures etc. may manifest with loss of some achieved functions.
- Nutritional problems like PEM, obesity, rickets also may show changing manifestations of the disease.

Q-8. What is pseudoregression in CP? What factors are responsible for it?

Some milestones which the child had already achieved, are lost and it may be interpreted as regression of milestones, creating dilemmas of degenerative disorders to the treating person. Actually, it is not regression of milestones, but transient loss of some milestones due to development of some complications and they are regained on correction of the situation. The conditions causing pseudo regression are as follows:

- Poorly controlled seizures.
- Overmedication with anticonvulsants.
- Intercurrent systemic illnesses.

- Nutritional deficiencies causing secondary neurological problems. Nutritional deficiencies known in these patients are iron deficiency anemia, deficiencies of vitamin B_{12}, folic acid, vitamin D, zinc, etc.
- Infantile tremor syndrome.
- Development of joint deformities and contractures.
- Movement disorders.
- Progressive hydrocephalus.
- Hypothyroidism.
- Depression and emotional problems.
- Behavioral problems.

Q-9. What are comorbid conditions in Children with CP?

- Cognitive impairment.
- Speech and language problems
- Hearing impairment
- Sensory impairment
  - Cortical blindness
  - Hearing impairment
  - Periconceptional deficit
  - Oromotor hypersensitivity
- Epilepsy
- **Ocular manifestations**
  - Strabismus
  - Refractory errors
  - Optic atrophy
  - Nystagmus
  - Visual impairment
- Behavioral problems
- **Gastrointestinal problems**
  - Feeding problem
  - Poor dental hygiene
  - GI motility disorders
  - GERD
  - Constipation
- Macro and micronutritional deficiencies
- Excessive irritability and crying due to pain. It may be due to muscle spasms, orthopedic problems, GERD, constipation, etc.
- Sleep disorders.
- Orthopedic problems
  - Rickets
  - Joint deformities and contractures.
  - Fractures

Q-10. What are clinical manifestations specific to type of CP?

Spastic quadriplegic (Figs. 2A to C)

- Most severely affected CP in term babies
- Intellectual disability
- Epilepsy.
- Squint/visual impairment.

- Pseudobulbar palsy.
- Speech abnormalities.
- Deformities.

Spastic Diplegic CP

- Most commonly seen in preterm babies (85%).
- Lower limb and trunk are more involved.
- Difficulties in changing diaper and clothes due to scissoring of legs.
- Commando crawl (self-propulsion by use of arms).
- Intellectual disability and epilepsy are less common.
- Learning disability and sensory problems may be present.

Hemiplegic CP (Fig. 3)

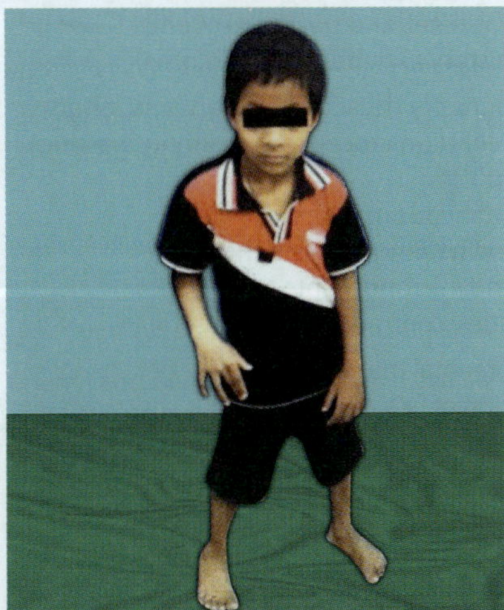

Fig. 3: Spastic hemiplegic CP. Right upper limb with flexion at elbow joint and slight flexion and splaying of fingers. Standing with legs wide apart.

- Common in term babies.
- Involvement of arms is more than legs.
- Early indicators are persistent fisting and cortical thumb.
- Hand preference in infancy.
- Asymmetry of position of upper limb with flexion at elbow joint and slight flexion and splaying of fingers. Standing with legs wide apart.
- Circumduction gait.
- Epilepsy and intellectual disability is relatively common.

Dyskinetic CP

- Initial hypotonia, gradually evolves into dystonia, rigidity and abnormal postures.
- Intellectual disability and epilepsy less common.
- Speech difficulties, tongue thrust and drooling are common.
- Dystonia, truncal twisting and facial grimacing.
- Choreoathetosis with choriform movements.

Ataxic CP

- Caused by cerebellar injury.
- Hypotonia.

- Difficulty in balance and motor coordination.
- Tremors.

Mixed CP

- Combination of both spastic and extra pyramidal CP.

Evaluation of a child with CP

Component	*Salient aspects to be evaluated*
History	Presenting complaints.
	• Feeding and diet in details • Developmental history • Motor manifestations • Comorbid conditions • Bladder and bowel habits • Antenatal, natal, and postnatal events • Family history (3 generation pedigree)
General physical examination	• Anthropometry (Head size, weight and length or height) • Growth chart (microcephaly, stunting, wasting) • Dysmorphism • Neurocutaneous markers • Vision and hearing assessment • Macro and micronutrients deficiencies • Deformities, contractures
Development	• Developmental maneuvers • Calculation of DQ • Dissociation and deviation of milestones • Pseudo regression • Behavioral problems
Neurological examination	• Posture • Alertness • Interest in surrounding • Cranial nerves • *Observe movements:* Abnormality, symmetry, range • Posture, gait • *Muscle tone:* Inspection, feel muscles, shake limbs, resistance to passive movements • Reflexes
Assessment of oromotor functions	• Primitive reflexes • Feeding • Tongue thrust, movements • Jaw thrust • Sucking and swallowing • Gag reflex (hyperactive) • Neck–hyperextension

Q-11. What investigations would you perform in a case of CP?

CP is clinical diagnosis, still investigations are required to exclude CNS malformations, neurometabolic disorders and to assess presence and comorbidities. It will help for deciding present status and planning of further management.

Neuroimaging

- The pattern, extent and severity of lesions may determine etiology and timing of insult. MRI is preferable over CT scan as detection of neuroanatomic abnormalities is higher, except where cranial calcification is anticipated.

- If development malformations are found genetic testing can be considered.
- If there is evidence of stroke, workup for coagulopathy can be done.
- Normal neuroanatomy may be found in 10–20% cases and up to 25% of children with periventricular leukomalacia do not have significant impairment.
- The sensitivity of an abnormal MRI at term to predict risk of CP in infancy is 90%
- When MRI is normal, but there is clinical suspicion of metabolic disorder as per history (positive family history, episodes of deterioration or metabolic decompensation) or examination (spastic diplegia or choroathetoid CP without definite etiology), metabolic and genetic testing may be considered.

Topographic and Radio Imaging Correlation

Topographic classification	*MRI findings*	*Suggested etiology*
Diplegic CP	• *White matter damage of immaturity (WMDI):* Periventricular • Leukomalacia posterior >anterior • Periventricular cyst/ scars in WM • Enlargement of ventricles • Squared posterior ventricles	• Prematurity • Ischemia • Infection • Metabolic
Quadriplegic CP	• Cortical and subcortical lesions • Extensive WMDI • Multi cystic encephalopathy • Cortical malformations	• Ischemic injury • Infection • Metabolic • Genetical • Developmental
Hemiplegic CP	• Asymmetrical WMDI • Stroke (in utero/neonatal). • Focal infarct (cortical/subcortical) • Cortical malformation	• Thromboembolic disorder • Infection • Genetic • Developmental • PV hemorrhagic infarctions
Dyskinetic CP	• Basal ganglia lesions • Scars in putamen and thalamus	• Severe birth asphyxia • Kernicterus • Mitochondrial • Genetic
	• Scars in globus pallidus, hippocampus • Scars in putamen, caudate and brain stem	Metabolic disorder

For Assessment of Gait

- Video Gait Analysis is an optoelectronic computer-based system that objectively analyses gait and documents joint movements in multiple planes and levels.
- It is particularly helpful in preoperatively to determine cause of crouch gait like equines, hamstring tightness, lever arm dysfunction etc. in toeing to see femur or tibial torsion.

For assessment of comorbidities

- Assessment of behavioral issues.
- Visual assessment.
- Hearing assessment.
- Dietary intake.
- Micronutrient deficiencies.
- Orodental hygiene.
- Radiographs for hip joints and spine for scoliosis.

How would you describe the final diagnosis of CP?

Following components should be included:

- Physiological.
- Topographic.
- ICF/functional.
- Neuroradiological classification.
- Etiology.
- Timing of insult.
- Comorbid conditions.
- Complications.
- Nutritional status.

It helps in planning holistic management, counselling, monitoring progress and prognostication.

Q-12. What is the treatment of CP?

- Intervention should be started once CP is diagnosed or suspected.
- Rehabilitation in CP is not proper terminology. It is used in adults. There is disability in adults following CNS insults and it is tried to reestablished through some interventions. In children, it is early intervention for habilitation.
- Without intervention the natural course is rapid deterioration of gait and motor functions.
- Goals are enhancing acquisition of new skills, treating comorbid conditions and decreasing complications. It should be done by a team of multi specialists in a single center.
- The team members comprise of a pediatrician, neurologist, developmental pediatrician, physiotherapist, occupational therapist, ophthalmologist, audiologist, speech and language therapist, orthopedic surgeon, dental surgeon, clinical psychologist, genetic specialist and special educator. The pediatrician should be key person to coordinate with others.
- **Physiotherapy**
  - It involves repetitive exercise directed at a specific muscle group with a joint. It also includes the equipment required to develop the strength and motor skills required in sitting, standing, walking balancing etc. and control of movement.
  - The basic principle is encouraging movement that is as normal as possible maintaining correct posture in daily activities.
  - Physiotherapy may not have long term benefits for children with severe disease or beyond 5 to 7 years of age.
- **Occupational therapy**
  - It includes use of technique and adaptive equipment to develop skills required for activities of daily living.
  - The aim is increasing functional skill and independence.
- **Speech therapy**
  - Parents are educated how to provide a stimulating environment, help in exercises for improving muscle tone and tongue and throat to decrease drooling and to deal with feeding problems.
  - Communication can be augmented with devices like specialized keyboards, talking typewriters and electronic speech generating devices.
- **Management of spasticity**
  - Physical therapy with use of splints and orthopedic devices.
  - Commonly used drugs are Botulinum A toxin, Diazepam, Tizanidine, Baclofen, Dantrolene, etc.
  - Surgery may be indicated with development of contractures and deformities.
- **Drugs for dystonia**
  - Levodopa (0.5 to 2 mg/kg/day).
  - Trihexyphenidyl (0.25 mg/day BD).
  - Carbamazepine.

- Oral glycopyrrolate for drooling.
- Drugs for constipation and GERD.
- Visual and Hearing rehabilitation.
- Dietary advice.
  - Sufficient fluids.
  - Micronutrient supplementation.
  - Calories should be restricted to avoid obesity.
- Management of sleep disorders, Management of pain, spasticity, GERD, Sleep hygiene etc. Melatonin can be prescribed.
- Oral hygiene and dental care.

Q-13. What preventive measures can be taken for CP?

- **Primary prevention**
  - Antenatal care.
  - Conducting delivery at place with basic facility.
  - Administration of antenatal steroids and magnesium sulfate in indicated cases. Monitoring high risk newborns.
  - Exclusive breast feeding.
  - Discouraging pre lacteal feeds.
  - Teaching danger signs and early referral.
  - Caffeine in indicated babies.
  - Prevention of neonatal hypothermia.
- **Secondary prevention**
  - Developmental surveillance.
  - Frequent screening in high-risk babies.
  - Early detection and timely intervention.

Parental Counseling

- Establish rapport. Greet the parents. Introduce yourself
- I collected the information in details regarding illness of your child, examined him/her thoroughly and checked the reports of all investigations performed.
- From analysis of all these informations, I came to conclusion that your child is suffering from cerebral palsy
- Cerebral palsy is the condition which occurs due to various insults to the developing brain, usually under the age of 5 years. In many cases, the cause may not be obvious and may not be able to locate. The common risk factors in a case of cerebral palsy are prematurity, birth asphyxia, brain hemorrhage, meningitis, neonatal jaundice, congenital malformations etc.
- Unfortunately, your baby was premature (30 weeks), there was delayed cry, baby required NICU admission for several weeks, had seizures, needed ventilatory support and several medicines
- Following all these issues, it has resulted in brain damage which is one time damage what we say cerebral palsy. It is static, nonprogressive condition
- All these handicaps to the child are features of the disease, cerebral palsy
- The brain of an infant or young child is growing. Fortunately, in such conditions, growing parts of brain take up the functions of damaged brain what we say neuroplasticity. It is the good hope for us. Therefore, neuro development in your child may be late and slow, but the progress will be evident in due course of time
- Normal children develop by their own at appropriate age. We have to make special efforts to achieve good development of such children
- Medical team and family have to work together to achieve the goal. The medical team is consisting of myself as a pediatrician, pediatric neurologist, physiotherapist, orthopedic surgeon, dental surgeon, ENT and

ophthalmic surgeons and dedicated nursing staff. Not only parents, but whole family should join the hands for the cause.

- I will prescribe necessary medicines and explain you in details for various problems like GERD, constipation, muscle stiffness etc. Early stimulation and appropriate interventions are quite helpful. Good nutrition and tender nursing care are essential components of management. Immunization schedule should be followed up as per advice.
- Regular follow-up is necessary
- Well organized team work, regular follow up, our enthusiasm and constant efforts are required to achieve the goal of making the child independent and training him professionally according to his ability
- You are free for any question, query or clarification
- I will provide you my contact number. Please, contact me at any time, if you need any help.

CHAPTER

47

Nephrotic Syndrome

QUESTIONS AND ANSWERS

Q-1. What is the definition of nephrotic syndrome (NS)?

Nephrotic syndrome is characterized by

- Nephrotic rang of proteinuria
  - > 40 mg/m^2/hour or
  - 1000 mg/m^2/day or
  - Spot urinary protein / urinary creatinine ≥2 or
  - 3 + to 4 + by dipstick
- Hypoalbuminemia (serum albumin <3 g/dL)
- Edema

Q-2. What is steroid sensitive nephrotic syndrome (SSNS)?

NS having complete remission within 6 weeks of treatment with prednisolone at a dose of 60 mg/m^2/day or 2 mg/kg/day or maximum 60 mg/day.

Q-3. What is initial (primary) steroid resistant NS?

Failure to achieve complete remission after 6 weeks initial therapy with prednisolone 60 mg/m^2/day or 2 mg/kg/day or maximum 60 mg/day.

Q-4. What is late (secondary) steroid resistant NS?

Initially steroid sensitive NS which becomes steroid resistant in a subsequent relapse.

Q-5. What is complete remission of NS?

Complete remission of NS is defined as,

- Urinary protein nil or trace dipstick or
- Urinary protein/urinary creatinine <0.2 or
- 24 hours urinary protein <100 mg/m^2/day for 3 consecutive early morning specimens.

Q-6. What is partial remission of NS?

Partial remission of NS is defined as,

- Urinary protein 1+/2+ dipstick or
- Urinary protein/urinary creatinine 0.2 to 2 or
- 24 hours urinary protein 100-1000 mg/m^2/day and
- Serum albumin >3 g/dL and
- Absence of edema

Q-7. What is relapse of NS?

Criteria for relapse of NS are,
- Urine albumin 3+/4+ by dipstick or
- Urine protein/urine creatinine ≥2 or
- 24 hour urine protein >1000 mg/m^2/day for 3 consecutive early morning specimens.

Q-8. What is definition of frequent relapses?

Two or more relapses in the first 6 months after stopping initial therapy or 3 relapses in any 6 months or ≥4 relapses in one year.

Q-9. What is definition of steroid dependence?

Two consecutive relapses when an alternate day steroids or within 14 days of discontinuation of steroids.

Q-10. What is stable remission of NS?

Sustained remission or infrequent relapses during immunosuppressive therapy.

Q-11. What is complicated relapse of NS?

Relapse associated with life-threatening complications like hypovolemia requiring inpatient care, severe infections like peritonitis, cellulitis, meningitis or thrombosis.

Q-12. What is significant steroid toxicity?

- Hyperglycemia (Fasting glucose >100 mg/dL, post prandial glucose >140 mg/dL or HbA1C > 5.7)
- Obesity (BMI ≥ 27 kg/m^2)
- Short stature (height < –2SD for age) with height velocity < –3SD for age)
- Raised intraocular pressure
- Cataract
- Myopathy
- Osteonecrosis
- Psychosis

Q-13. What is difficult to treat steroid sensitive NS?

Both of the following:
- Frequent relapses
- Significant steroid toxicity with infrequent relapses
- Failure of ≥2 steroid sparing agents (including levamisole, cyclophosphamide, mycophenolate mofetil)

Q-14. What investigations should be performed in patients with SSNS?

- Essential at onset
  - Urinalysis
  - Complete blood counts
  - Blood urea, creatinine, electrolytes, total protein, albumin, total cholesterol
  - Tuberculin test
- Additional evaluation, at onset or relapse
  - *Chest radiograph:* Positive tuberculin test or history of contact, suspected LRTI
  - *Renal ultrasonography:* Planned for kidney biopsy, presence of gross hematuria, suspected renal vein thrombosis
  - *Complete blood counts:* Suspected systemic infection or hypovolemia
  - Blood urea, creatinine, albumin, electrolytes; severe edema, hypovolemia/dehydration, oliguria/anuria, prolonged (>72 hour) diuretic therapy

- *Complement C3, C4, antinuclear antibody, antistreptolysin O:* Gross, persistent microscopic hematuria, sustained hypertension, suspected secondary cause (SLE, IgA vasculitis, C3 glomerulopathy)
- *Serum transaminases:* Hepatitis B surface antigen, antibody against hepatitis C virus, history of jaundice or liver disease

- Periodic monitoring if relapsing illness serum creatinine, electrolytes and albumin.

Q-15. What are the indications of kidney biopsy in NS?

- Persistent microscopic hematuria, gross hematuria, or acute kidney injury not attributed to hypovolemia.
- *Systemic features:* Fever, rash, arthralgia, low C3.
- Initial or late corticosteroid resistance
- Prolonged (>30-36 months) therapy with calcineurin inhibitors CCND or reduced kidney function during their use.

Q-16. What are differentiating features of nephrotic syndrome and poststreptococcal glomerulonephritis (PSGN)?

Features	*Nephrotic syndrome*	*PSGN*
Age	Most common 2–6 years	Most common 5–12 years
Preceding history	Often mild viral URTI	• Pyoderma, 3–6 weeks preceding • Throat infection 1–2 weeks preceding
Past history of similar episodes	Relapses are common	Usually no recurrent episode
Clinical features		
Edema	• Starts with mild edema and becomes generalized massive edema • Ascites and hydrocele in males • Pitting edema	Usually puffiness of face and mild edema
Hematuria	Gross hematuria does not occur, may be microscopic heaturia in some patients	Cola colored urine is common, may be presenting feature
Hypertension	Not common, occasionally, may be transient	Very common, may present with hypertensive encephalopathy
Oliguria	Not common	Very common and important feature
Loin pain	Uncommon	Common
Hypervolemia	Does not occur intravascular volume may be low	Very common. Acute LVF may be life threatening complication
Complications	• Infectious • Peritonitis • Deep vein thrombosis	• Acute LVF • Hypertensive encephalopathy • Pulmonary edema • Metabolic acidosis • Hyperkalemia • Acute renal failure

Q-17. What are the causes of NS in children?

- Idiopathic (90%)
  - Minimal change NS (MCNS) —most common (85% of idiopathic)
  - Focal segmental glomerulosclerosis (FSGN) (10%)
  - Mesangio-proliferative glomerulonephritis (MPGN) (5%)
- Other primary NS (most common in adults)
  - Membranous glomerulonephritis (MGN)
  - Membranoproliferative glomerulonephritis (MPGN)
- Secondary NS (10% of cases)

- SLE, HSP, PAN
- Sickle cell disease
- *Infections:* Hepatitis B, C, Malaria
- NS associated with lymphoma, leukemia
- *Drug-induced:* D-penicillamine, Gold salts, NSAIDs, mercury, phenyotin
- Endocarditis

- Congenital NS
  - *Finnish type:* Autosomal recessive
  - Secondary to congenital syphilis, CMV, toxoplasmosis, HIV, hepatitis B

Q-18. What is adequate biopsy specimen in renal biopsy?

- Should include cortico-medullary junction
- Should contain approximately 20 glomeruli

Q-19. What is the treatment of first episode of NS?

Prednisolone at a dose of 60 mg/m^2/day (2 mg/kg/day, maximm 60 mg/day) in 1-2 divided doses for 6 weeks, followed by 40 mg/m^2 (1.5 mg/kg, maximum 40 mg) as single morning dose on alternate day for next 6 weeks and then discontinued.

Q-20. What is the treatment of relapses of NS?

Prednisolone at 60 mg/m^2/day <2 mg/kg/day, maximum 60 mg) in single or divided doses until remission (urine protein nil/trace for 3 consecutive days), followed by 40 mg/m^2/day (1.5 mg/kg/day, maximum 40 mg/day) on alternate days for 4 weeks.

Q-21. What is the management of frequent relapses and steroid dependence NS?

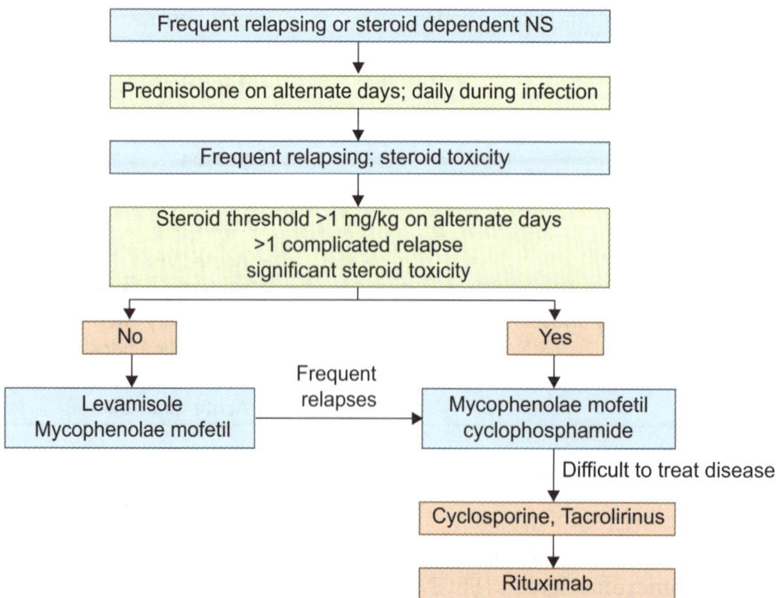

- The initial strategy is to administer prednisolone at a dose of 0.5-0.7 mg/kg on alternate days. In patients with stable remission (sustained remission or infrequent relapses), therapy may be tapered to 0.2-0.3 mg/kg on alternate days for 6-12 months. Daily therapy at the same doses for 5-7 days during minor infections, prevents infection associated relapses.

- Patients who relapse at steroid threshold >0.7 mg/kg or show steroid toxicity require therapy with steroid sparing medications. The choice of agents is based on disease severity, adverse effects, patient age, cost of therapy and parental preference. Levamisole and mycophenolate mofetil (MMF) are preferred medications for mild disease. Patients with high steroid threshold (>1 mg/kg on alternate days), complicated relapses and those with significant steroid toxicity may be treated with MMF at higher doses (1000-1200 mg/m^2/day) or cyclophosphamide. The use of cyclophosphamide is avoided in children <5-7 years old and in peri-pubertal boys due to reduced efficacy and risk of gonadal toxicity, respectively.
- Patients who relapse despite therapy with two or more steroid sparing agents (difficult to treat steroid sensitive disease) are considered for therapy with calcineurin inhibitors and failing that, rituximab. The use of rituximab is avoided in young children due to risk of hypogammaglobulinemia.

Immunosuppressive medications for frequent relapses

Medication	*Dose*	*Duration*	*Adverse effects*	*Recommended monitoring*
Prednisolone	0.5-0.7 mg/kg on alternate days	6-12 months	• Cushingoid features • Short statute • Hypertension • Raised intraocular pressure • Glucose intolerance • Cataract • Elevated transaminase	Screen for side effects • Anthropometry at 3-6 months • Eye evaluation at 6-12 months • Blood sugar and transaminases at 3-6 months
Levamisole	2-2.5 mg/kg on alternate day	2-3 years	• Leukopenia • ANCA positive vasculitis • High transaminases • Seizures	• Blood count at 2-3 months • Transaminases at 4-6 months
Cyclophosphamide	2-2.5 mg/kg on alternate day	8-12 weeks	• Leukopenia • Alopecia • Infections • Discolored nails • Hemorrhagic cystitis • Gonadal toxicity • Malignancies	• Blood counts at 2 weeks • Maintain hydration • Discontinue during significant infection • Co-administer with prednisolone 1 mg/kg on alternate days
Mycophenolate mofetil	600-1200 mg/m^2/day in divided doses AUC > 45 mg	2-3 years	• Abdominal pain • Diarrhea • Nausea • Weight loss • Viral warts • Leukopenia • Elevated transaminases	• Screen for adverse effects • Blood count and transaminases 3-6 months
Cyclosporine	4-5 mg/kg/day in divided doses, trough 80-120 ng/mL	2-3 years	• Nephrotoxicity • Hyperkalemia • Hepatoxicity • Gingival hyperplasia • Hypertrichosis • Hypertension	Screen for cosmetic side effects, tremors, diarrhea, hypertension, creatinine, potassium
Tocrolimus	0.1-0.2 mg/kg in divided doses, trough 4-8 ng/mL	2-3 years	• Dyslipidemia • Tremors • Seizures • Headache • Diarrhea • Glucose tolerance • Hypomagnesemia	• At 4 weeks LFT, glucose, uric acid, magnesium • Lipids at 3-6 months

Contd...

Contd...

Medication	*Dose*	*Duration*	*Adverse effects*	*Recommended monitoring*
Rituximab	375 mg/m^2 slow IV infusion	2 doses, 1 week a part	• Chills, fever • Serum sickness • Bronchospasms • Acute lung injury • Neutrophenia • *P. jirovecii pneumonia* • Reactivation of hepatitis B-K • Hypogamma-globulinemia	• Predose—CBC, transaminases hepatitis and HIV serology IgG level • Post-therapy CD19 counts, CBC, IgG

Q-22. How to treat difficult to treat steroid sensitive NS?

- Calcineurin inhibitors (CNI), either cyclosporine or tacrolimus
- Rituximab in patients who have either failed CNI or have received these agents for a prolonged duration.
- Rituximab should be administered during disease remission after ruling out acute and chronic infections and should target B-cell depletion.

Q-23. What are the features of hypovolemia during relapse?

- Clinical features
  - Abdominal pain, vomiting, lethargy
  - Prolonged capillary refill time, cold extremities
  - Tachycardia, low volume pulses
  - Low blood pressure, postural hypotension
- Biochemical indices
  - Elevated hematocrit
  - Blood urea (mg/dL) to creatinine (mg/dL) ratio >100
  - Fractional excretion of sodium <0.5%.
  - Urinary potassium index [(urine potassium/urine $N^+ + K^+$) >0.6]
  - *Ultrasonography:* Decreased inferior vena cava diameter, increased coallapsibility index.

$$\text{Fractional excretion of sodium} = \frac{\text{Urine Na+} \times \text{serum creatinine}}{\text{Serum Na+} \times \text{urine creatinine}} \times 100$$

Q-24. What is the management of edema in NS?

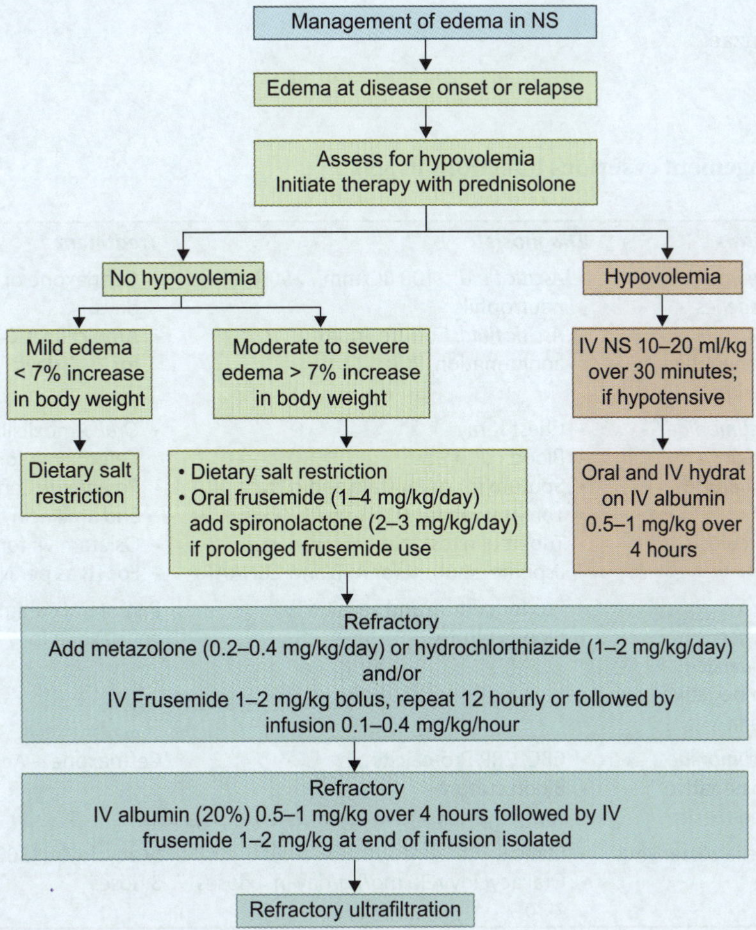

Q-25. What factors are responsible for infections in NS?

- Immunosuppressive drugs
- Anasarca
- Urinary losses of IgG and complement factors

Q-26. What are common infections in NS?

- Peritonitis
- Pneumonia
- Cellulitis
- Sepsis
- Varicella

Q-27. What are common organism responsible for infections in NS?

- Bacterial
  - Pneumococci
  - *H. influenzae*
  - *Staphylococcal aureus*
- Viral
  - Varicella
  - Rhinovirus

- Adenovirus
- Influenza
- Para influenzae
- RSV
- EBV

Q-28. What is the management of serious infections in NS?

Infection	*Organisms*	*Diagnosis*	*Treatment*
Peritonitis	• *S. pneumoniae* • *S. pyogenes* • *E. coli* • Gram negative bacteria	• *Ascitic fluid:* >100 BC/mm^3, >50% neutrophils • *Ascitic fluid:* Culture, index agglutination, PCR	• Ceftriaxone or ceftaxine for 7-10 days • Ampicillin + Gentamicin / Amikacin for 7-10 days
Pneumonia	• *S. pneumoniae* • *S. aureus* • *H. influenzae* • H1N1 • Tuberculosis	• Chest X-ray • Blood culture • Sputum for gram stain and culture • Throat swab for H1N1 by PCR • Tuberculin test, pleural tap, gastric aspirate, sputum for AFB and CBNAAT	• *Oral:* Amoxicillin, Coamoxiclar, Cefuroxime for 10-14 days • *Parenteral:* Ceftriaxone or ampicillin and amikacin for 7-10 days • Osletamivir for 5 days • For TB as per NTEP
Cellulitis	• *S. aureus* • *S. pyogenes* • *H. influenzae* • Gram-negative bacteria	• Pus for culture and sensitivity • Blood culture	Parenteral co-amoxiclav, cloxacillin + ceftriaxone for 7-10 days
Sepsis	• *S. pneumoniae* • Gram negative bacteria	• CBC, CRP, Pro-calcitonin • Blood culture	Ceftriaxone + Amikacin for 10-14 days
Varicella	• Varicella zoster virus	• Clinical • Oral acyclovir 30 mg/kg/day in 4 doses 7-10	IV acyclovir (1500 mg/m^2/day) in 3 doses

Q-29. What are the principles of immunization with live vaccines in patients with nephrotic syndrome?

Immunosuppression	*Advice*
Receiving high dose prednisolone (>2 mg/kg/day, >20 mg/day if >10 kg for <14 days	Vaccinate immediately after discontinuing treatment
Receiving high dose prednisolone >2 mg/kg/day >20 mg/day if >10 kg) for >14 days	Vaccinate one month after discontinuing corticosteroids
Receiving low-moderate dose prednisolone <2 mg/kg/day or <20 mg/kg)	No live vaccine until discontinuation of steroid therapy
Low dose alternate day prednisolone and pressing need for vaccine	Live vaccine may be administered
Patients receiving cyclophosphamide	Avoid live vaccines until off therapy for 3 months
Patients receiving calcineurin inhibitors, levamisole or mycophenolate mofetil	Avoid live vaccines until off therapy for 1 month
Therapy with rituximab	Avoid live vaccines until after β-cell recovery (6-9 months)
Immunocompetent siblings and household contacts	Do not administer OPV, may receive MMR, rotavirus and varicella vaccines
Household contacts older than 1 year	Administer influenza vaccine annually

Q-30. What specific vaccines are recommended for patients of NS?

Vaccine	Age	Previously received	Vaccine	Schedule
Pneumococcal: Conjugate (PCV 13 preferred to 10 valent)	6-72 months	Completely immunized (3 doses at 6,10,14 weeks and booster at 12-15 months)	PCV 13/10 PPSV 23	One dose >2 years old. One dose >2 years old and 8 weeks after last PCV 13/10
Polysaccharide (PPSV 23)		No or incompletely immunized	PCV 13/10, PPSV 23	2 doses > 8 weeks apart. One dose > 2 years old and 8 weeks after last PCV 13/10
	> 72 months	Completely immunized	PPSV 23	1 dose
		No or incompletely immunized	PCV 13/10 PPSV 23	1 dose. One dose >8 weeks after PCV 13/10
Varicella	>15 months	No evidence of immunity	Live attenuated	Two doses at 4-8 weeks apart
Influenza	>6 months	-	Inactivated	Annually
Hepatitis B	Any	No or anti HBSC 10 m/kg/ml	Subunit (10 ug/0.5 mL)	3 doses at 0, 1, 6 months or in accelerated schedule with >4 weeks gap between doses 1 and 2, >8 weeks between 2 and 3 and >16 weeks between doses 1 and 3

Q-31. What is the postexposure management of unimmunized patients with NS exposed to varicella?

Contraindication to live vaccine	Strategy	Timing after exposure
No	Administer varicella vaccine	As soon as possible <5 days
Yes	Options (in order of preference) • Varicella zoster immununoglobulin (VARIZIA) • 125 IU/kg body weight • Maximum 625 IU • Intramuscular	<10 days, preferably <4 days
	• Oral acyclovir • 80 mg/kg in 4 divided doses • Maximum 3.2 G • Daily for 7 days OR Oral valvacyclovir (>3 months old) 60 mg/kg (maximum 3 G) daily in 3 divided doses for 7 days	Begin 6-10 days after exposure
	Intravenous immunoglobulins 400 mg/kg	< 10 days

CHAPTER 48

Vaccines

QUESTIONS

HEPATITIS B VACCINE

Q-1. What is the importance of Birth dose of hepatitis B vaccine (HBV)?

Vertical transmission is responsible for more than 50% of all childhood hepatitis B infection. The risk of development of chronic HBV infection is inversely related to the age of acquiring infection. Newborns usually do not develop acute symptoms but have a high risk of developing chronic carrier state. Approximately 90% of newborns infected at birth become chronic carriers and 25% of these will develop chronic liver disease including cirrhosis or hepatocellular carcinoma later in life. Therefore, it is necessary to give hepatitis B vaccine within 24 hours of birth for prevention of vertical transmission of infection.

Q-2. What is recommended schedule for hepatitis B vaccination?

- Standard pediatric dose contains 10 µg of the antigen.
- Immunocompromised and special groups require double dose.
- The pediatric formulation is recommended till 12 years of age.
- It is given as three dose schedule 0-1-6 months for adults and older children as catch-up schedule. For infants, 0, 4–6 weeks and 14–24 weeks schedule can be used.
- For programmatic reasons, four doses may be given. Here, birth dose is followed by 3 doses in a combination vaccine at 6,10 and 14 weeks. The additional dose is not harmful.
- In immunocompromised and those with chronic renal failure, 0, 1, 2 and 12 months (4 doses) schedule is recommended with double doses.

Q-3. What are the recommendations for immunizing a neonate born to a hepatitis B surface antigen (HbsAg) positive mother?

- In infants born to HbsAg positive mothers, the first dose of HBV should be given at birth, within 12 hours, along with hepatitis B immunoglobulin (HBIG) in the dose of 0.5 mL. Both vaccine and HBIG should be given at same time, on separate thighs by intramuscular route. Three more doses of HBV should be administered at 6-10-14 weeks as part of combination vaccines.
- The HBIG may be given up to 7 days of birth but the efficacy of HBIG after 48 hours is not known.
- If HBIG is not available or unaffordable, Hepatitis B vaccine may be given at 0,1 and 2 months with an additional dose between 9 months and 12 months.
- All infants born to HbsAg positive mothers should be tested for HbsAg and anti-HbsAg antibodies at the age of 9-15 months to identify carrier or nonresponders.

Q-4. Is it safe for the HbsAg positive mother to breastfeed?

Yes, breastfeeding can be given along with HBIG and vaccine to the baby as per recommendations.

Q-5. What is the dose of HBIG?

The dose of HBIG in neonates is 0.5 mL and adults 0.06 mL/kg.

Q-6. Can hepatitis B vaccine be given to preterm babies and babies less than 2 kg?

Preterm infants and low birth weight infants with birth weight <2000 g have a decreased response to hepatitis B vaccine administered before the age of 1 month. However, by the chronological age of 1-month, preterm babies irrespective of their birth weight and gestational age are likely to respond as adequately as full term infants.

ROTAVIRUS VACCINES

Q-7. Which are the different rotavirus (RV) vaccines available in India?

Monovalent Rotavirus Vaccines

- Rotarix: It is produced by GSK. Rotarix is a live attenuated monovalent vaccine, containing human strain 89–12 [type GIPIA (8)].
- Indian Neonatal Rotavirus live vaccine: The strain is 116E. It is developed by Bharat Biotech of India. It is live vaccine, containing naturally attenuated monovalent, bovine-human reassortant strain, G9P [II], with the VP4 of bovine rotavirus origin and all other segments of human rotavirus origin. It is marked as Rotavac by Bharat Biotech of India and Rotasure by Abbott Vaccines.

Polyvalent Rotavirus Vaccines

- **Rotateq:** It is pentavalent bovine—human, reassortant vaccine, produced by Merck and Company. It contains five reassortant rotaviruses developed from human and bovine parent rotavirus strains that express human rotavirus outer capsular proteins of five common circulating strains, [G1, G2, G3, G4 and P8 (subgroup PIA)].
- **Bovine rotavirus Pentavalent Vaccine (BRV-PV) (Rotasil):** It is a pentavalent rotavirus vaccine developed from bovine (UK) human rotavirus reassortant strains (seortypes G1, G2, G3, G4 and G9) by Serum Institute of India.

Q-8. What is the Advisory Committee on Vaccines and Immunization Practices (ACVIP) schedule for RV vaccines?

- Minimum age 6 weeks for all available RV vaccines.
- Only two doses of RV-1 (Rotarix) are recommended.
- **Rotavirus (RV) 5, RV-116E, RV-BRV-PV:** 3 doses at 4 weeks interval, beginning at 6 weeks (not less than 15 weeks) to be completed by 32 weeks.
- **Rotavirus 1 (Rotarix):** Two doses beginning at 6 weeks (not less than 15 weeks) with 4 weeks interval between two doses to be completed by 32 weeks.
- If any doses in series were missed or if vaccine product is unknown for any dose in series, a total of three doses of RV vaccine should be completed.

Catch-up Vaccination

- The maximum age for the first dose is 14 weeks and 6 days.
- Vaccine should not be initiated for infants aged 15 weeks, 0 days or older.
- The maximum age for the final dose is 32 weeks.

Q-9. What is the risk of intussusception following RV vaccination?

The currently available RV vaccines are quite safe and the risk of intussusception is very small in comparison to previous vaccine, Rotashield. Rotashield was voluntarily withdrawn by the manufacturer in 1999 due to an increased frequency of intussusception in the first 2 weeks after vaccination.

Q-10. What is the schedule for RV vaccine in Universal Immunization Program of India?

The RV vaccine is administered in three doses at 6, 10 and 14 weeks along with pentavalent vaccines. The maximum upper age limit for giving first dose is 1 year. If the child has received first dose of RV vaccine by 12 months of age, two more doses of the vaccine should be given with an interval of 4 weeks between two doses to complete the course in the second year. In private practice, the schedule should be followed up as per IAP recommendations.

PNEUMOCOCCAL VACCINES

Q-11. What different pneumococcal vaccines are available in India?

Pneumococcal Conjugate Vaccines

Serotype → *Vaccine →*	*1*	*3*	*4*	*5*	*6A*	*6B*	*7F*	*9V*	*14*	*18C*	*19A*	*19F*	*23F*	*22F*	*33F*
PCV-10 (GSK)	√		√	√		√	√	√	√	√		√	√		
PCV-10 (SII)	√			√	√	√	√	√	√		√	√	√		
PCV-13 (Pfizer)	√	√	√	√	√	√	√	√	√	√	√	√	√		
PCV-14	√	√	√	√	√		√	√	√	√	√	√	√	√	√

Pneumococcal Polysaccharide Vaccine 23 Valent (PPSV-23)

Q-12. What is the advantage of conjugate pneumococcal vaccines over PPSV?

Pneumococcal conjugate vaccine is T-cell-dependent vaccine. It is efficacious in a child less than 2 years of age. It is more immunogenic, boostable, provides hard effect, reduced nasopharyngeal carriage and helps to curtain antibiotic resistance.

Q-13. What is the dose and schedule of PCV10 and PCV13 as recommended by ACVIP?

- The dose is 0.5 mL, given by IM route on anterolateral aspect of thigh.
- 6 weeks to 6 months. (PCV10 and PCV13):
  - *Primary doses:* 6-10-14 weeks.
  - *Booster dose:* Between 12 and 15 months. The booster dose can be administered 6 months after the third primary dose.
- *7 to 12 months:* Previous unvaccinated infants should receive two primary doses at a minimum interval of 4 weeks, followed by a booster dose in the second year of life.
- *12 to 24 months:* Two doses at interval of 8 weeks.
- *2 to 5 years*: (PCV 13) single dose
  PCV10: Two doses at interval of 8 weeks.
- 12 months to 5 years (PCV10) —unvaccinated children should receive two doses with an interval of 8 weeks.

Q-14. What are the recommendations for pneumococcal vaccines in high-risk individuals?

Age	*Previous doses of any pneumococcal vaccines*	*Recommendations*
<23 months	Nil	Usual recommendations
24–71 months	4 doses of PCV 13	• One dose of PPSV-23 after 8 weeks of last dose of PCV-13 • One repeat dose of PPSV-23 after 5 years
24–71 months	<3 doses of PCV 13	• 2 doses of PCV13 at least 8 weeks apart • One dose of PPSV-23 after 8 weeks of last dose of PCV-13 • One repeat dose of PPSV-23 after 5 years
24–71 months	One dose of PPSV-23	• Two doses of PCV-13 at interval of 8 weeks and at least 8 weeks after PPSV-23. • One dose of PPSV-23 5 years after first dose of PPSV-23 and 8 weeks after PCV-13
6–18 years with medical conditions	Nil	• One dose of PCV-13. • One dose of PPSV-23 after 8 weeks of PCV-13 • Second dose of PPSV-23 after 5 years of first dose
	One dose of PCV-13	• One dose of PPSV-23. • Second dose of PPSV-23 after 5 years.
	>1 dose of PPSV-23	• One dose of PCV 13 after 8 weeks of PPSV-23 • Second dose of PPSV-23 after 5 years

Q-15. What is the schedule of pneumococcal vaccine in NIP of India?

- 6 weeks, 14 weeks and 9 months of age.
- 0.5 mL, IM.
- Anterolateral aspect of right thigh.

INFLUENZA VACCINES

Q-16. Which are types of influenza vaccines?

- Two types, Injectable inactivated influenza vaccines (IIV) and cold adapted live attenuated intranasal vaccines (LAIV).
- They can be trivalent or quadrivalent.
- IIV can be split viron or subunit vaccines. There is not much difference in efficacy between these two types of vaccines and can be used any of them.

Q-17. What are the Northern (NH) and Southern (SH) influenza vaccines and which one should be used in India?

Influenza vaccines come in market twice a year that is the northern and southern vaccines. WHO collects nasopharyngeal swab samples from patients suspected influenza like illness periodically from various parts of the world throughout the year and collects the data from time to time. Based on the data, it meets twice a year and recommends representative strains that will best match the circulating strains in the last 6 months all over the world to be included in NH and the SH vaccines.

Each year in the months of February to March, it meets and provides strain for the northern hemisphere vaccines which come in the market in the month of September of that year for use before the subsequent winter season as influenza season peaks in winter in the northern zone countries.

It also meets in the month of August and September each year to suggest strains to be included in southern vaccines that then come out in the market in March the next year to be used before monsoon as influenza peaks during monsoon in the southern zone countries.

So, one should use appropriate vaccine based on whether the peak of influenza is in winter (use northern vaccine) or monsoon (use southern vaccine).

Influenza peaks are in monsoon months and hence behaves like a southern zone country and hence we should use southern vaccine in the month of April to August to cover the monsoon peak, except in Jammu and Kashmir where the influenza peaks during winter and hence we should use northern vaccine there. In the northern parts of India, there is equal peak during winter and during monsoon and hence, one can use either of the vaccines.

Q-18. What about the schedule and route of administration of inactivated influenza vaccines?

- Dose of inactivated influenza virus vaccines (IIV) is 0.25 mL for 6 to 36 months old subjects and 0.5 mL for >36 months old subjects. However, 0.5 mL dose is found to be safe and more immunogenic than 0.25 mL in 6-36 months old subjects and hence, is preferred dose even at that age.
- *6 months to 9 years:* Two doses for the first time and subsequently one dose every year.
- For >9 years of age, only one dose for the first time and thereafter every year.
- IM on anterolateral aspect of thigh in infants and deltoid region in older children.

Q-19. An unimmunized child has just recovered from influenza illness. Does he need a flu shot and when?

Yes, he needs flu vaccine to protect him from the other strains in the vaccine. He can receive vaccine after clinical recovery.

MEASLES, MUMPS AND RUBELLA VACCINES (MR AND MMR)

Q-20. What is the composition of measles—rubella (MR) and Measles, Mumps and Rubella (MMR) vaccines?

- Measles vaccine is derived from live-attenuated strains of Edmonston- Zagreb (Tresivac) or Schwarz (Priorix) strains of measles virus.

- Rubella vaccine is derived from liver-attenuated strains of RA—27/3 rubella virus in both MR and MMR vaccines.
- Mumps vaccine is derived from different formulations having different strains of the virus which include Leningrad-Zagreb (Tresivac), Lemingrad-3, Urabe- AM 9, Jeryl-Lynn strains.
- Measles, Mumps and Rubella vaccines are available in lyophilized forms. It can be stored at 2-8°C, should be protected from light and the reconstituted vaccine should be used within 6 hours.
- The dose is 0.5 mL and should be administered by sub cutaneous route. The vaccine should be reconstituted by diluent provided with the vaccine.
- Measles containing vaccines, especially multidose vials can be get contaminated as it does not contain preservatives.

Staphylococcal is the most common organism which can cause toxic shock syndrome which may be fatal.

Q-21. What are the adverse effects of MR/MMR vaccine?

- Quite safe and effective.
- Mild fever, tenderness at injection site can occur in few cases.
- Post vaccination rash may appear, for lasting for 2 to 3 days.
- Mild measles like illness may develop between 7 and 12 days postvaccination.
- Thrombocytopenia may develop, but it is rare.
- Mild reduced cell-mediated immunity for transient period.
- Encephalitis is very rare.
- Febrile seizures are known to occur.
- Subacute sclerosis pan encephalomyelitis (SSPE) is very rare to develop after 7-8 years of vaccination due to measles component.
- Transient parotitis may occur.
- Mild aseptic meningitis.
- Anaphylaxis is rare due to measles component.
- Arthralgia and lymphadenopathy may develop due to rubella component.

Q-22. What are contraindications for MR and MMR vaccines?

- Being a live viral vaccine, measles contains vaccines (MCV) is contraindicated in severely immunocompromised subjects.
- Should not be given to a pregnant lady
- HIV is contraindication, but can be given as early as 6 months where in CD_4 counts are well preserved.
- History allergy to constituents of vaccines.
- Malnutrition, low grade fever, mild URTI and diarrhea like minor illnesses are not contraindications.

Q-23. What are the recommendations for MR and MMR vaccines by IAP and NIP?

- Recommendations by IAP
  - First dose of Measles containing vaccines (MCV) as MR/MMR at 9 months.
  - Second dose as MMR at age of 15 months.
  - Third dose of MMR between 4 and 5 years of age.
- As per National Immunization Program
  - MR between 9 and 12 months of age on right deltoid region.
  - MR between 16 and 24 months of age on right deltoid region.

Q-24. What are recommendations for catch-up vaccination of MMR vaccine?

All the school-aged children above 5 years of age, if not vaccinated earlier should be at least vaccinated with 2 doses of MMR vaccine with minimum interval of 4 weeks between the two doses.

Q-25. What about postexposure prophylaxis?

- If MMR vaccine is administered within 72 hours of exposure, it may provide some protection or modify the course of disease.
- Immunoglobulin IgG is another option, which can be administered by IM route, within 72 hours of exposure.
- IV IgG can be used in immunocompromised persons.

Q-26. Why is IAP recommending MMR vaccine, while Government of India MR vaccine?

- IAP recommends MMR vaccine at 9 months of age, 16–24 months of age and 4–5 years of age, while Government of India considers mumps as mild disease without significant morbidity and mortality. Besides, cost of vaccine can be brought down by MR vaccine instead of MMR especially in mass use for public.
- However, IAP considers mumps morbidity significant as much as rubella. Mumps complications are known like aseptic meningitis, encephalitis, pancreatitis, orchitis, transverse myelitis etc. Mumps can also cause fetal aqueductal stenosis leading to congenital hydrocephalus when pregnant woman develop mumps.

Q-27. If there is an outbreak, can we vaccinated children younger than 9 months?

- During outbreak of measles in the community, MMR vaccine can be given at 6 months of age. Still, this dose should not be counted in regular schedule of 3 doses of MMR vaccine.

Q-28. What is MR vaccination campaign? What is its role?

- According to the global measles and rubella strategic plan 2012, all the six WHO regions have committed to measles elimination and rubella control.
- Government of India is a signatory in this mission of measles elimination and rubella control by 2020. However, with two dose routine immunization, it was a challenging task to cover almost all children with uncertain information and nonavailability of vaccination records. Based on the huge success of polio vaccination campaign in elimination of polio from our country, MR campaign was designed as one dose campaign irrespective of previous vaccination or disease status in the age group between 9 months and 15 years.
- The MR vaccine received during campaign will not be counted and will be an extra dose on an above two doses of MR vaccines.
- An additional dose of MR vaccine, does not harm.
- Government of India completed the campaign with vaccinating 31 crores of children between 9 months and 15 years.
- A follow-up MR campaign will be required as a periodic event every 3–5 years guided by country specific surveillance data. The periodicity will depend on RI coverage, existence of pockets of unprotected children and vaccine efficacy.
- This follow-up campaign will target only those children, born after last campaign aged 9 months, to achieve and sustain high level of population immunity.

Q-29. Why so much hype about rubella control?

Rubella is basically mild exanthematous viral illness. It was first understood as a significant health problem when a pandemic of congenital rubella syndrome (CRS) occurred in 1964–65. If rubella develops to pregnant lady in first trimester, it can lead to CRS with disastrous consequences in fetus/newborn such as still birth, mental retardation, congenital heart disease (PDA), cataracts, deafness, blindness, etc. In view of this, all the regions of WHO have made declarations for elimination of measles and rubella control.

TYPHOID VACCINES

Q-30. What are different typhoid conjugate vaccines?

There are different typhoid conjugate vaccines made from polysaccharide derived from *S. typhi* or *Citrobacter freundii* conjugated with a carrier protein which is either *Pseudomonas aeuroginosa* Exo protein A (rEPA), tetanus toxoid (TT), diphtheria toxoid (DT) or cross-reactive material (CRM 197), a nontoxic mutant of diphtheria toxin.

Q-31. What are the characteristics of typhoid conjugate vaccines?

- Contains 25 μg Vi polysaccharide antigen linked to tetanus toxoid protein.
- Liquid preparation, 0.5 mL.
- Administration by intramuscular route.
- 6 months onwards, up to 45 years of age.
- *Storage:* 2 to 8°C.
- *Schedule:* Single dose at 6 months of age.

Q-32. Do you need to given the typhoid vaccine after the child has had a culture proven typhoid?

Yes, typhoid vaccine should be given even after culture proven typhoid disease. It can be given after complete recovery from the illness, usually 4–6 weeks after recovery. Typhoid disease does not confer complete or long-lasting immunity.

HEPATITIS A VACCINES

Q-33. What are different vaccines against Hepatitis A?

Both inactivated and live-attenuated hepatitis A vaccines are available. The inactivated vaccines are derived from HM 175/GBM strains grown on MRC-5 human diploid cell lines. The live attenuated vaccine is derived from H2 strain of hepatitis A virus after serial passage in human diploid cell line.

Q-34. What are currently available inactivated hepatitis A vaccines?

- *Harvix 720:* Each 0.5 mL pediatric dose of vaccine contains 720 ELU of viral antigen, adsorbed onto 0.25 mg of aluminum as aluminum hydroxide.
- *Harvix 1440:* Each 1 mL adult dose of vaccine contains 1440 ELU of viral antigen, adsorbed on 0.5 mg of aluminum as aluminum hydroxide.
- Havrix is free from any preservative.
- It should be stored at 2-8°C.
- Harvix 1440 is not available in India at present.
- It should be given by IM route on anterolateral aspect of thigh in younger children and on deltoid in older children and adults.
- Avaxim (Sanofi)
  - Marketed in two formulations, 80 u to 160 u.
  - The 80 u formulation is recommended from 12 months to 15 years of age. It contains 80 u antigen in 0.5 mL with 0.15 mg of aluminum hydroxide per dose.
  - The 160 u formulation is recommended in more than 15 years of age. It contains 160 u in 0.5 mL with 0.3 mg of aluminum hydroxide per dose.

Q-35. What is the schedule for inactivated hepatitis A vaccine?

Minimum age for administration of inactivated hepatitis A vaccine is 12 months of age. Two doses schedule is there at interval of 6 months. It is given by IM route.

Q-36. What is the currently available live attenuated hepatitis A vaccine?

- Live-attenuated hepatitis A vaccine is manufactured in China and available in other countries including India.
- The vaccine is derived from H2 strain or *Lactobacillus* acidophilus (LA)-1 strain of hepatitis A virus.
- Live-attenuated hepatitis A vaccine is well studied in India. There are published evidences on long term follow-up in Indian subjects with live attenuated vaccine. 10 years follow-up study from India showed long-term immunity after single dose. No significant safety concern was reported in the study.

Q-37. What is the catch-up schedule for hepatitis A vaccine?

Two doses, at least 6 months apart of inactivated hepatitis A vaccine or a single dose of live vaccine. For inactivated vaccine, pediatric formulation is recommended till 18 years of age and adult formulation thereafter.

Q-38. Is there any role of hepatitis A vaccine for postexposure prophylaxis?

Hepatitis A vaccine may be given for postexposure prophylaxis to the household contacts of hepatitis A case, those with immune deficiency and chronic liver disease. It should be given as early as possible preferably within 14 days.

Q-39. What is the role of hepatitis A vaccine in hepatitis B carriers and those suffering from chronic liver disease?

Patients with chronic liver disease and hepatitis B carriers are at increased risk of complications when they are infected with hepatitis A. Hence, they should be protected by giving hepatitis A vaccine.

VARICELLA VACCINES

Q-40. Which are the varicella vaccines available?

- Variped (MSD)
- Varilrix (GSK)
- Biovac-V (Wockhardt)
- Varivax (Life Science)
- Nexipox (Novo)
- Zuvicella (Zuventus)

Q-41. What is IAP schedule for varicella vaccination?

- First dose at 15–18 months and second dose is recommended preferably 3 months after the first dose or at age of 4–6 years.
- For catch up vaccination in children 12 months to 12 years, two doses should be given 12 weeks apart. For catch-up vaccination in children 13 years and above, two doses should be given 4–12 weeks apart. It is given by subcutaneous route.

Q-42. What is breakthrough varicella?

Varicella which occurs in children vaccinated more than 6 weeks after vaccination is called breakthrough varicella. It is usually milder and may present with short lasting maculopapular rashes and may not progress to the vesicular stage. Break through varicella has mild fever, less number of lesions and shorter duration of illness. However, it is infective, can result in transmission to susceptible contacts and rarely may result in severe complications and death.

Q-43. What are the contraindications of varicella vaccination?

- History of hypersensitivity to one or more components of the vaccine.
- Primary immunodeficiency.
- HIV.
- High dose systemic steroid therapy. (≥2 mg/kg/day for >14 weeks).
- Patients with malignancy on chemotherapy.
- Pregnant woman.

Q-44. How useful is varicella vaccination in post exposure prophylaxis?

Among children, protective efficacy was reported as more than 90% when vaccination occurred within 3 days of exposure.

HUMAN PAPILLOMA VIRUS (HPV) VACCINES

Q-45. What are the vaccines available to prevent HPV infection?

Three HPV vaccines are now being marketed, a bivalent, a quadrivalent and a monovalent vaccine. All the HPV vaccines are produced by recombinant technology and contain virus like particles (VLPs) of the dominant L1 capsid protein.

- Gardasil is a quadrivalent vaccine containing L1 VLPs of types 16, 18, 6 and 11 with aluminum as adjuvant.
- Cervavac is a quadrivalent vaccine, containing L1 VLPs of types 16,18,6 and 11 with aluminum as adjuvant.
- Gavdasil 9 is a nine valent vaccine containing types 6,11,16,18,31,33,45,52 and 58.

Q-46. What are ACVIP recommendations on HPV vaccine schedule?

- *Girls 9–14 years:* Two doses of any vaccine at interval of 6 months (0-6 months).
- *Girls 15 years and older:* Three doses in the schedule of 0-1-6 months for bivalent HPV and 0-2-6 months for quadrivalent HPV vaccines.
- Gardasil 9 is approved for boys between 9 and 14 years of age.
- HPV4 by SII is recommended for females and males between 9 and 26 years of age.
- IM is route of administration.

ANTIRABIES VACCINES (ARVS)

Q-47. Which animals can transmit the rabies?

- Potentially, all mammals can develop rabies and transmit it to humans.
- About 95% of human rabies cases are caused by dog bites and 2% by cat bites.
- Human rabies has also been reported due to bites by monkeys, mongooses, jackals, foxes, wolves and other carnivorous animals. Horses, donkeys, cattle and buffaloes can also transmit rabies.
- Squirrel, rabbit and domestic rats do not transmit rabies and do not warrant consideration for postexposure prophylaxis.
- Human to human transmission of rabies may occur following corneal or other transplantation.

Q-48. Why are children more susceptible to rabies?

Approximately 40% of cases occur in children less than 15 years of age. Children are more often affected as their inquisitive nature make them more susceptible to bites. Smaller stature of the child makes them more vulnerable to be bitten on face or neck. They may not inform the parents and small bites or licks may go unnoticed.

Q-49. What is the incubation period of rabies?

The incubation period is generally 20–60 days, shortest may be 5–6 days. It has been reported very long time also as long as 7 years.

Q-50. What is the immediate preventive measure to be taken?

The wound should be cleaned with soap and running water for 15 minutes, immediately. Application of viricidal agent such as povidone–iodine is useful. Suturing of the wound should be avoided.

Q-51. What are the various ARVs available?

- Human Diploid cell vaccine (HDCV).
- Purified Chick Embryo Cell Vaccine (PCEVC).
- Purified Vero Cell Vaccine (PVCV).
- Purified Duck Embryo Vaccine (PDEV).

All these modern tissue culture vaccines are equally effective.

Q-52. What are different classes of bites and preventive measures to be taken?

- *Category I:* Touching or feeding animals. Licks on intact skin. Contact of intact skin with secretion or excretion of a rabid animal or human case.
- *Category II:* Nibbing of uncovered skin. Minor scratches or abrasions without bleeding. It needs wound hygiene + vaccine.
- *Category III:* Single or multiple transdermal bites or scratches. Licks on broken skin. Contamination of mucous membrane with saliva, exposure to bats.

  This category needs wound hygiene + rabies immunoglobulin (RIG)/monoclonal antibodies (Mabs) + Vaccines.

  All category III bites, all wild animal bites and category II bites in immunocompromised should be given RIG or Mabs. RIG/Mabs is not indicated if patient has received a complete course of post exposure prophylaxis (PEP) or pre- exposure prophylaxis (PrEP) previously.

Q-53. What are the latest WHO guidelines on PrEP, PEP and re-exposure prophylaxis?

- For re-exposure, vaccination is not recommended, if complete PrEP/PEP already received within less than 3 months previously.
- *If received more than 3 months previously:* 1 site IM on day 0 and 3, or 1 site ID on day 0 and 3, or 4 sites ID on day 0.

  It should be remembered that Drug Controller General of India (DCGI) has not approved the revised schedule in India due to lack of data from India. Government institutions still follow the older schedule.

Q-54. What are recommendations for use of RIGs/Mabs?

- All class III bites by a suspected rabid animal.
- Class II bites in immunocompromised persons.

Q-55. What is the schedule to administer RIGs/Mabs?

- Immediately within 24 hours of animal bite along with first dose of vaccine.
- If vaccine alone was started, then till 7 days after starting the first dose of vaccine, it can be given.
- It can be administered even a week or more later if the person has not received any vaccine.
- Human Rabies Immunoglobulins (HRIG) is available in 2 mL vials with a strength of 150 iu/mL. The dose of HRIG is 20 units/kg body weight to a maximum of 1500 iu.
- Equine Rabies Immunoglobulins (ERIG) is available in 5 mL vials with a strength of 300 iu/mL and the dose is 40 iu/kg to a maximum of 3000 iu.
- As per latest recommendations from the WHO, skin testing prior to ERIG administration is not required.
- As much as possible should be infiltrated around the wound and below it. There is no recommendation for intramuscular administration of remaining RIG.
- If volume is less, it can be diluted with normal saline to the desired volume.
- The calculated dose should not be exceeded.
- Suturing should be avoided, but if there is large gap it can be done after infiltration of wound with RIGs/Mabs. The suture should be kept loose and minimum in numbers. It should not interfere with free bleeding and drainage. Secondary suturing should be preferred whenever feasible.

Q-56. What are guidelines for PrEP?

Pre-exposure prophylaxis is recommended for persons at risk of occupational or vocational exposure to rabies. These include diagnosticians, laboratory and vaccine workers, veterinarians, postmen, etc. IAP recommends that all children at high risk of being bitten by dogs and children with pets at home should be vaccinated. The schedule of PrEP is 0 and 7 days (2 doses) by IM route.

The main advantages are that it simplifies post exposure management. There is no need of RIG/MAbs following subsequent class III exposures.

Q-57. What are the guidelines for intradermal (ID) rabies vaccination?

In Government setup ID vaccines are given routinely for cost and dose sparing. For ID route, one dose is 0.1 mL. The vaccine in one vial can therefore fractionated to provide multiple doses.

A systemic review of vaccine potency has shown that current vaccines, when administered by ID route for either PEP or PrEP have efficacy equivalent to or higher than that of same vaccine administered by IM route.

JAPANESE ENCEPHALITIS VACCINES

Q-58. Who should be vaccinated with Japanese Encephalitis (JE) vaccines?

This vaccine is not an outbreak response vaccine. It is recommended for universal vaccination in endemic areas. All children from 1 to 18 years should be vaccinated in endemic area. As JE encephalitis does not induce herd immunity, high vaccination coverage should be achieved and sustained in population at risk of disease.

Q-59. What are recommendations on JE vaccination for travelers?

JE vaccine is recommended for persons moving to a JE endemic country to live long term, one month or longer and frequent travelers to JE endemic areas. JE vaccination should also be considered for short term, less than 1-Chinese hamster month travelers with an increased risk of JE based on planned travel duration, season, location, activities and accommodations. The schedule should be completed at least one week before travel.

Q-60. What are the JE vaccines are available?

- Inactivated mouse brain derived
  - Uncertain protection
  - Multiple doses
  - Unacceptable neurological adverse events
  - Productions ceased
- *Live attenuated JE vaccine:* **SA-14-14-2.**
- *Killed JE vaccines:* **JEEV and JENVAC.**
- *Live-attenuated recombinant:* SA 14-14-2 chimeric vaccine.

Q-61. What is regarding live-attenuated SA-14-14-2 vaccine?

This was the first vaccine used in campaign mode in India in 2006. It is given as two dose schedule, 9 months and 18 months. This vaccine is not available in private market for office use.

Q-62. What are IAP recommendations for JE vaccine use?

- Recommended only for individuals living endemic districts, both rural and urban.
- *Minimum age:* 8 months.
- *Two dose schedule:* 9 months along with measles and MR vaccine and second at 18 months with DPT booster.
- Not available in private market for office use.
- Storage at 2–8°C.
- Administered by IM or SC route.

Inactivated Vero cell culture derived Kolar strain 821564XY JE vaccine by Bharat Biotech.

- *Minimum age:* 1 year.
- *Primary immunization:* Two dose of 0.5 mL, by IM route at 4 weeks interval.
- Need for booster still undetermined.

Catch-up vaccination:

All susceptible children up to 15 years of age should be administered during disease outbreak.

YELLOW FEVER VACCINE

Q-63. Who should receive Yellow Fever Vaccine?

This vaccine is not meant for routine vaccination in India. The vaccine is indicated in the following persons:

- All travelers of age more than 9 months and traveling to/from yellow fever endemic zones.
- All children 9–12 months of age and above in yellow fever endemic countries.
- In the event of outbreak in these countries, all unvaccinated infants of age 6–8 months are also vaccinated.
- WHO recommends that all endemic countries should introduce yellow fever vaccine into their routine immunization programs.

Q-64. How is yellow fever vaccine is stored and administered?

- Single dose of 0.5 mL SC or IM.
- Freeze-dried vaccine is available in single and multi dose vials.
- Storage at 2–8°C along with sterile water as diluent.

Q-65. What is the procedure for validation of vaccination for travelers to endemic countries for yellow fever?

- An International Certificate of Vaccination or Prophylaxis (ICVP) duly dated, stamped and signed by the center administering the vaccine, is issued to each vaccinee as per International Health Regulations.
- All travelers visit the embassy of their destination country (endemic for yellow fever) and submit the ICVP before departure.
- Validity of the ICVP has changed from 10 years to duration of the life of the person vaccinated.
- From 11 July, 2016 the ICVP against yellow fever is valid for life of the person vaccinated. This life time validity applies automatically to all existing and new certificates, beginning 10 days after the date of vaccination.
- If the procedure for validation of the certificate is not followed, the traveler may be quarantined, denied entry or can be revaccinated in their destination country at the point of entry (airport/sea port).
- If due to medical contraindication, the physician at vaccination center can issue a waiver by filling out and signing the Medical Contraindication to Vaccination section of ICVP. However, the traveler must be advised that issued waiver may not be acceptable to the destination country leading to their quarantine, refusal of entry or even vaccination at their airport.
- Under International Health Regulation (IHR), any changes, deletions, erasures or additions may cause an ICVP to be rendered invalid.
- Further specific guidelines in relation to yellow fever international travelers are available on WHO website.

Q-66. What are the guidelines for travelers entering India from endemic countries for yellow fever?

Any traveler with exception of less than 9 months arriving by air or sea to India without a certificate is quarantined (detained in isolation) for up to 6 days if that person

- Arrives within 6 days of departure from a residential area in a country with risk of yellow fever virus transmission.
- Has actually visited that area while in transit (except those passengers and members of flight crew who while in transit through an airport in a country with risk of yellow fever virus transmission, remained in the airport during their entire stay and the health officer agrees to such an exception).
- Arrives on a ship that started from or touched at any port in a country with risk of yellow fever virus transmission up to 30 days before its arrival in India, unless such a ship has been disinfected in accordance with the procedure recommended by WHO.
- Arrives on an aircraft that has been a country with risk of yellow fever virus transmission and has not been disinfected in accordance with the India Aircraft Public Health Rules, 1954 or as recommended by WHO.

Q-67. What are contraindications and precautions observed in relation with yellow fever vaccination?

Contraindications	*Precautions*
Allergy to vaccine component	Age 6–8 months
Age <6 months	Age ≥60 years
Symptomatic HIV or CD4 T lymphocytes count <200/mm^3(or <15% of the total in <6 years child)	Asymptomatic HIV and CD4 T lymphocytes count 200–499/mm^3 or between 15 and 24% child <6 years old
Thymus disorders associated with abnormal immune cell dysfunction	Pregnancy
Primary immunodeficiency	Breastfeeding
Malignant neoplasm	
Transplantation	
Immunosuppressive therapy	

Q-68. Where can one get vaccinated for yellow fever in India?

As of March 2017, there are total 41 yellow fever vaccination centers in India. Out of these, 17 are in west zone, 9 each are in north and south zones and 3 each in central and east zone. The vaccination charges are approved by the Ministry of Health and Family Welfare, Government of India is INR 300 per dose.

Q-69. Where is the yellow fever vaccines produced in India?

By Central Research Institute (CRI), Kasauli and supplied to various recognized centers.

ZOSTER VACCINES

Q-70. What are the vaccines available against zoster?

- Live zoster vaccine (Merck) (Zostavax)
- Recombinant zoster vaccine (Shingrix) by GSK.

Q-71. What are characteristics of Recombinant Zoster Vaccine (RZV) (Shingrix)?

- The active antigen, which is recombinant surface glycoprotein E (gE) antigen, is supplied in a freeze-dried form. It has to be reconstituted at the time of use with accompanying vial of AS01B adjuvant suspension component. The gE antigen is obtained by culturing genetically engineered Chinese hamster ovary cells, which carry a gE antigen.
- 0.5 mL by IM route.

Q-72. What is the schedule of RZV?

- 0.5 mL each dose, 0 and 2 to 6 months.
- By IM route.

Q-.73. What are the recommendations regarding use of zoster vaccines?

- More than 50 years, irrespective or prior receipt of varicella vaccine, does not require screening for history of chickenpox.
- Adults with chronic medical conditions.

Q-74. Catch-up Immunization in Adolescents

Vaccine	*Schedule*
MMR	Two doses at 4–8 weeks interval
Hepatitis B	Three doses, 0, 1 and 6 months
Hepatitis A	Two doses at 0 and 6 months
Typhoid TCV	Single dose
Varicella	Two does at 3 months apart
Tdap	Single dose
Influenza	One dose every year

Q-75. What are suggested vaccinations for all healthy adults in India?

- Td/Tdap every 10 years.
- Annual influenza vaccination.
- Zoster (Shingles) over 50 years of age.
- One dose of PCV-13 followed by PPSV-23 after 6- 2 months.

VACCINATION FOR TRAVELERS

Q-76. What are the vaccines that residents of India need before traveling to other countries?

General Recommendations

The travelers should have completed all age specific immunization for their own protection. In addition, one must also be immunized against diseases endemic in the area or country to which one is travelling or steps out international zone (transit area) in transit, if not immunized earlier as per age. The traveler should go through the travel advisory of the own country, places in transit and countries visiting.

- *Yellow fever vaccine:* It is mandatory to visit certain countries where yellow fever is endemic.
- *Meningococcal meningitis vaccine:* It is mandatory to travelers for Hajj. Study in USA, UK and other specified countries.
- *Polio vaccine:* It is mandatory for Hajj Pilgrims and travelers from Pakistan, Afghanistan and other notified areas or countries which are still endemic to wild polio virus or are experiencing polio outbreaks. As per the Government of India regulation, people traveling from India to wild polio virus endemic countries like Pakistan, Afghanistan, Nigeria and those travelling in countries where polio virus is in circulation following importation (Ethiopia, Kenya, Somalia and Syria) will require to take a dose of bivalent OPV at least 4 weeks before the travel date irrespective of age/The bOPV vaccination certificate will be issued after the additional dose and it will remain valid for a year.
- *Measles containing vaccine (MCV):* Many countries which had eradicated or eliminated measles are facing serious outbreaks and deaths due to measles. Two doses of MMR given after the age of 12 months at least 4 weeks apart are essential before entry into certain countries. Documentary proof is needed else the point of entry may quarantine the traveler pending antibody titers or vaccination as per their requirement.
  Evidence of immunity to measles and rubella for international travelers include:
- Written documentation of having received the measles and rubella vaccines.
- Laboratory evidence of rubella and measles immunity, positive serological test for measles and rubella specific IgG antibodies.

Q-77. What are the vaccines travelers to India need before entering India as per immigration requirement?

- *Yellow fever vaccination:* For those traveling from or stay in transit in countries endemic for yellow fever.
- *Polio vaccines:* Any person of any age residing in any of countries endemic for polio, traveling to India, is supposed to take a single dose of bOPV 4 weeks before the travel date.

Q-78. What are the vaccines that Indian travelers need for domestic travel inside India?

- **Cholera**
  Endemic in West Bengal and adjacent states, during large religious gatherings as Kumbh melas.
- *Japanese encephalitis:* Eastern and North eastern states of India. JE vaccines are not recommended for routine use, but only for individual living in endemic areas. Government of India has identified around 231 districts to be endemic for JE. JE vaccine is also recommended to travelers to JE endemic districts.

ADVERSE EVENTS FOLLOWING IMMUNIZATION (AEFI)

Q-79. What is AEFI?

AEFI is defined as any untoward medical occurrence which follows immunization and which does not necessarily have a casual relationship with the usage of the vaccine. The adverse event may be any unfavorable or unintended sign, abnormal laboratory finding, symptom or disease. It might have not been caused by vaccine components or process of vaccination but have a temporal relationship with administration of vaccine.

Q-80. What are different types of AEFI?

- *Vaccine product-related reaction:* An AEFI is caused or precipitated by a vaccine due to one or more of the inherent properties of the vaccine product, e.g. extensive limb swelling following DPT vaccination.
- *Vaccine quality defect-related reaction:* An AEFI that is caused or precipitated by a vaccine that is due to one ore more quality defects of the vaccine product including administration device as provided by the manufacturer, e.g. failure by the manufacturer to completely inactivate a lot of IPV leads to cases of paralytic polio. Syringe and needle defects are included in this category.
- *Immunization error-related reaction:* An AEFI that is caused by inappropriate vaccine handling, prescribing or administration and thus by its nature is preventable, e.g. transmission of infection by contaminated multidose vial. Toxic Shock Syndrome following administration of contaminated multi dose vial of measles vaccine is example of this category.
- *Immunization anxiety-related reaction:* An AEFI arising from anxiety about the immunization, e.g. vasovagal syncope in an adolescent following vaccination.
- *Coincidental event:* An AEFI that is caused by something other than the vaccine product, immunization error or immunization anxiety, e.g. fever after vaccination and malarial parasites isolated from blood. It is temporal association.

Q-81. What are possible causes of immunization errors?

- Nonsterile injection.
- Reconstitution/administration errors, e.g. reconstitution with wrong diluent.
- Injection at incorrect site, e.g. BCG by subcutaneous route, vaccination on buttocks.
- Improper maintenance of cold chain
- Contraindication ignored.

Q-82. What are the grades of AEFI?

- *Minor AEFI:* Local swelling, pain and redness at injection site.
- *Severe AEFI:* High grade fever following DPT, Inconsolable crying for more than 3 hours following DPT. Does not require hospitalization and no sequelae.
- *Serious:* Resulting in disability, death, occurs in clusters, results in congenital anomaly or birth defect.

Q-83. What is the timeline for AEFI investigations?

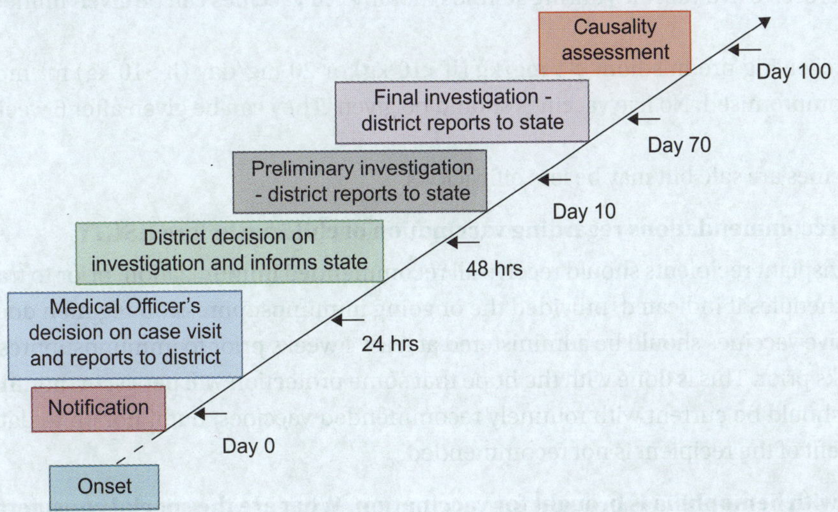

VACCINATION IN SPECIAL SITUATION

Q-84. What are the general principles in vaccinating immunocompromised?

- In severe immunodeficiency, all live vaccines are generally contraindicated.
- All inactivated vaccines may be given, but immunogenicity and efficacy may be low.
- Higher dose, more number of doses may be required, e.g. hepatitis B.
- Antibody titers should be checked postimmunization.
- Regular booster may be required.

Q-85. What are the recommendations regarding vaccination of children with primary immunodeficiency disorders?

- *B-lymphocyte (humoral) deficiency disorders:*
  - In severe disorders like X-linked agammaglobulinemia and common variable immunodeficiency, all live vaccines are contraindicated, inactivated vaccines may not elicit adequate response, but can be given. Administration of IVIG may interfere with immune response to vaccines.
  - In milder disorders like selective IgA deficiency and IgG subclass deficiency, BCG, OPV and yellow fever vaccines are contraindicated. Other live vaccines appear to be safe. All vaccines are likely to be effective, but immune response may not be adequate.
- *T-lymphocyte (cellular) deficiency disorders:*
  - In severe disorders like SCID, complete DiGeorge syndrome, all live vaccines are contraindicated. Inactivated vaccines are safe and may be effective.
  - In partial defects like Wiskott-Aldrich syndrome and Ataxia telangiectasia, all live vaccines are contraindicated, while inactivated vaccines may be effective.
- *Complement deficiency:* All vaccines can be given and are effective.
- *Phagocytic function disorders:* In chronic granulomatous disease (CGD), leukocyte adhesion defect (LAD) and myeloid peroxidase deficiency, all live bacterial vaccines are contraindicated. Live viral vaccines and all inactivated vaccines are safe and effective.

Q-86. What are recommendations regarding vaccination of children on steroids?

- Children on alternate day steroid therapy, inhaled corticosteroid formulations, intraarticular steroids and topical steroids are not immune compromised and vaccines can be given.

- Children receiving prednisolone >2 mg/kg/day (if <10 kg) or <20 mg/day (if >10 kg) for less than 2 weeks should not receive live vaccines during steroids therapy. All vaccines can be given immediately after stopping steroids.
- Children receiving prednisolone >2 mg/kg (if <10 kg) or 20 mg/day (if >10 kg) for more than 2 weeks are immunocompromised. No live vaccines should be given. They can be given after 6 weeks of discontinuation of steroids.
- Killed vaccines are safe but may be less efficacious.

Q-87. What are the recommendations regarding vaccination of children before HSCT?

In general, transplant recipients should receive all recommended immunization, prior to transplantation and on accelerated schedules if indicated, provided the ongoing immunosuppression regimen does not contraindicate vaccination. Live vaccines should be administered at least 4 weeks prior to immunosuppression and inactivated vaccine 2 weeks prior. This is done with the hope that some protection will persist in months after transplant.

The donor should be current with routinely recommended vaccines, but if not up to date, vaccination of the donor for benefit of the recipient is not recommended.

Q-88. A 5-year-boy with hemophilia is brought for vaccination. What are the special considerations?

- Children with bleeding disorders may be more prone to hematoma formation following intramuscular (IM) injections. When an IM route of administration is essential, it is preferable to schedule it after administration of replacement therapy.
- A 23 G or smaller gauze needle is to be used, firm pressure should be applied at injection site and it should not be rubbed.
- It can be given by subcutaneous route, if IM route is not advisable.
- Children with mild to moderate thrombocytopenia and platelet functional defects, can be safely vaccinated with precautious mentioned.

Q-89. What are the vaccine recommendations for children schedules for a cochlear implant?

Children with cochlear implants are more prone to bacterial meningitis. They may have other anatomic factors that may increase the risk for meningitis. *Streptococcus pneumoniae* is the most common etiological agent for bacterial meningitis. They should receive all age-appropriate vaccinations, including, pneumococcal, Hib and influenza vaccines. Children 2 years old and older and adults should receive a dose of PPSV 23, 8 weeks after the last dose of Conjugate Pneumococcal Vaccine. The schedule should be completed at least 2 weeks prior to implant.

Q-90. A 6-week preterm infant is still in the NICU for ongoing care. Can the infant receive all vaccines due at 6 weeks?

In medically stable infants, all inactivated vaccines required at 6 weeks of age can be administered simultaneously to pre term or low birth weight infants, except for oral rotavirus vaccine, as this a transmissible vaccine and can pose a risk to other sick newborns in the NICU. While rotavirus vaccine is to be deferred till discharge, IPV should be preferred over OPV.

Q-91. What are the recommendations for individuals who have recently received antibody containing products?

- Inactivated vaccines can be given safely.
- Live vaccines including MMR and varicella should be avoided for 3 months.
- Antibody containing products should be avoided for 2 weeks after these vaccinations.
- OPV and yellow fever vaccine may be given at any time.
- Rotavirus vaccine should be avoided for 6 weeks,
- Following IVIG therapy, measles and varicella containing vaccine should be given after 8–10 months.

Q-92. A 10-month-old child presented with high-grade fever, cough, coryza and conjunctivitis of 5 days duration. He developed these skin rashes on 4th day of fever.

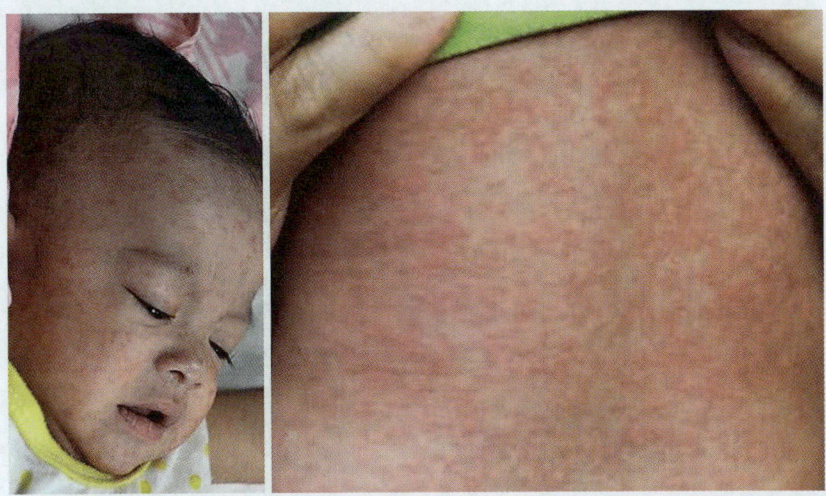

A. What is probable diagnosis?
B. What is the pathognomonic sign of this condition? What is its morphology?
C. What is the late CNS complication of this disease? What are the characteristics of this CNS complication?
D. Which strain of the organism are used for vaccine preparation?
E. What is the National Immunization Schedule in India for prevention of this disease?

Q-93. A 7-year-old boy had fever for a day, developed these skin lesions on next day, first on trunk and face then spread to extremities associated with itching.

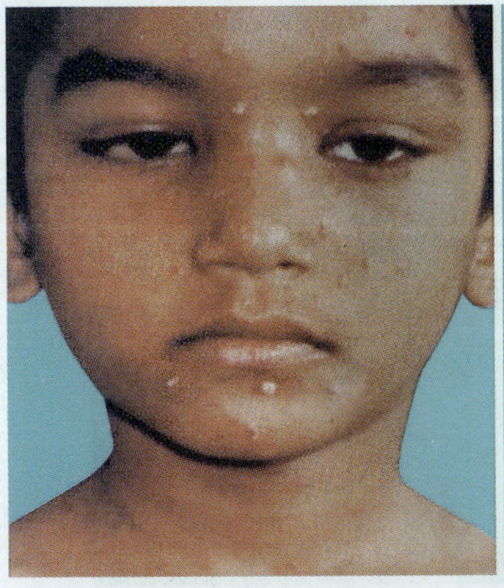

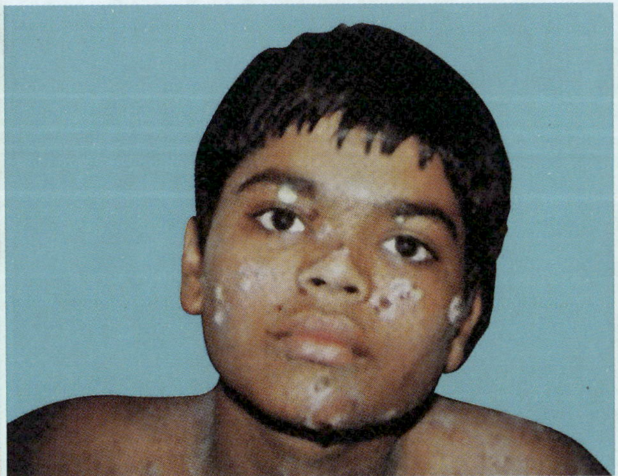

A. What is the probable diagnosis?
B. What are the morphological characteristics of the skin lesions?
C. What bacterial complications are known to occur in this disease? Name the common bacteria.
D. This child developed the CNS complication involving gait and speech problems. Name the disorder.

Q-94. Mother had fever and vesicular skin lesions at 10 weeks of pregnancy. It was diagnosed as some viral infection. Her baby was born with multiple anomalies of skin, limbs, eyes and brain.

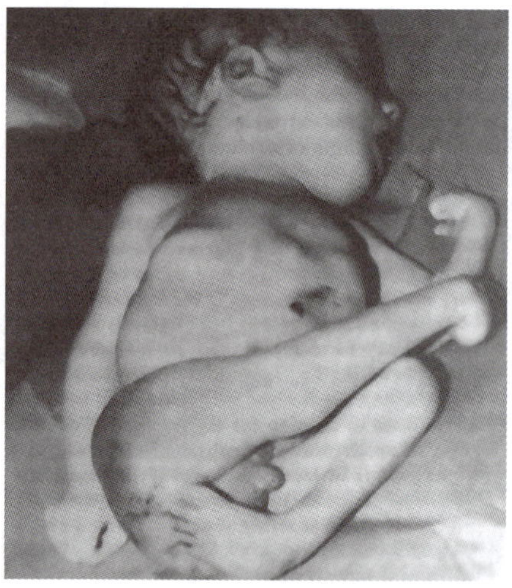

A. What is probable diagnosis?
B. What are characteristic skin lesions in this disorder?
C. What anomalies of eyes are known to occur in this condition?
D. What skeletal anomalies can develop in this disease?
E. What CNS anomalies are seen in this condition?

Q-95. Mother had fever and vesicular skin lesion 2 days prior to delivery. The baby developed these skin lesion on 8th day of life. Unfortunately, the baby died.

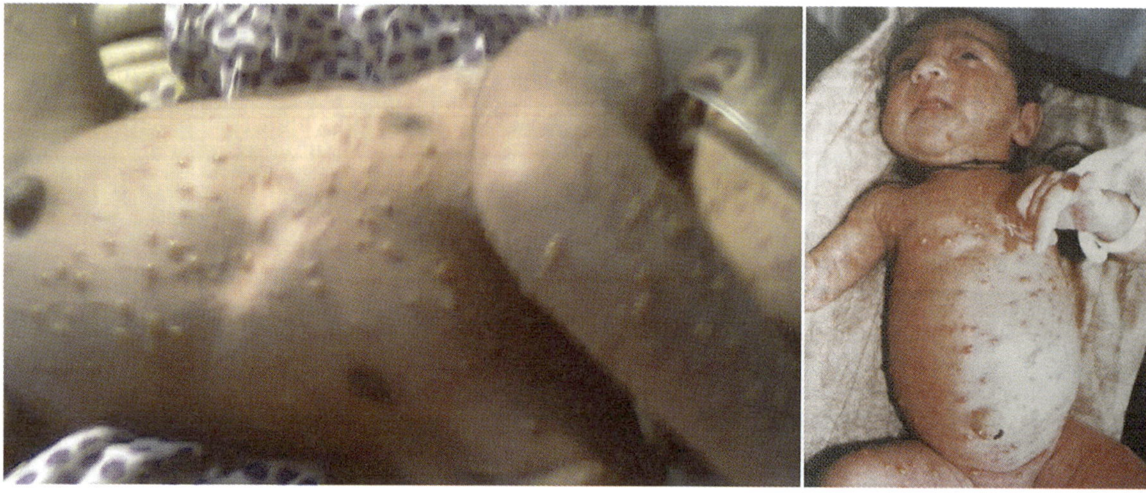

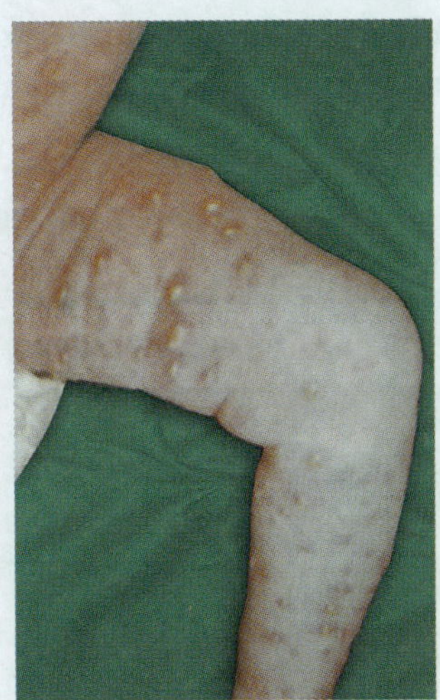

A. What is probable diagnosis?
B. What is high risk period to develop this disease to mother during pregnancy which may result in fatal neonatal infection?
C. What drug for passive immunity should be given to the newborn as soon as possible to prevent this infection? What is alternative, if previous one is not available?
D. What is the treatment of this neonatal infection?

Q-96. An adolescent had severe pain over trunk and then developed these skin lesions over the same area. The skin lesions were more pruritic and painful.

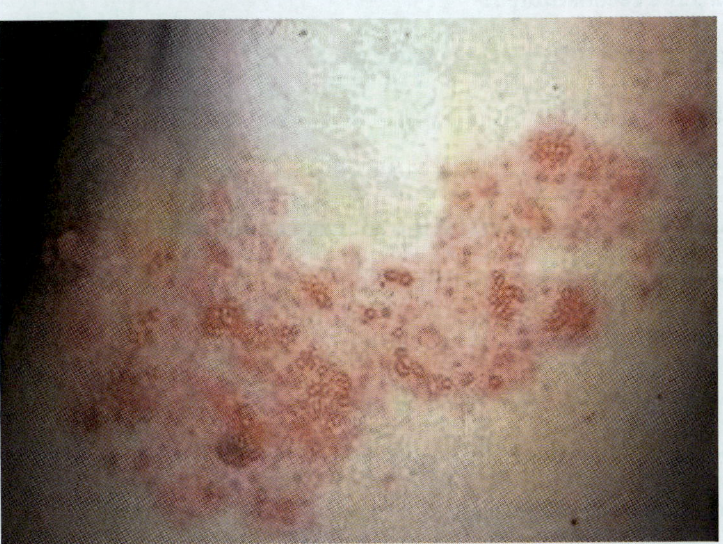

A. What is the probable diagnosis?
B. What is the genesis of this condition?
C. In which individuals it is more common?
D. Any preventive measure for this disease is available? Mention details of the measure

Q-97. The newborn presented with eye problem as shown in the picture. The baby was having intrauterine growth restriction, hepatosplenomegaly, cardiac murmur and thrombocytopenia. Mother had fever and skin rashes at 10 weeks of pregnancy.

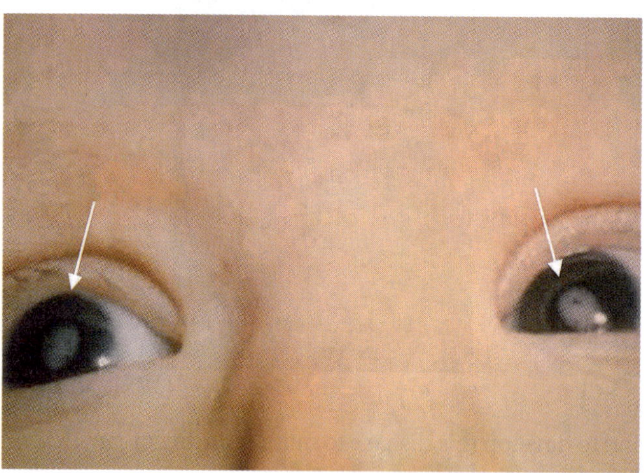

A. What is probable diagnosis?
B. What cardiac anomalies are common in this disorder?
C. What is the triad for clinical diagnosis of this condition?
D. An adolescent girl is not vaccinated for this infection. What will be your advice to prevent this congenital infection to her offspring?

Q-98. How is the BCG vaccine reconstituted?

Q-99. For what time reconstituted BCG vaccine can be used?

Q-100. What is the dosage of BCG vaccine?

Q-101. What is the route of administration of BCG vaccine?

Q-102. What are the criteria suggesting successful intradermal administration?

Q-103. What are severe complications of BCG vaccination?

Q-104. What are the contraindications of BCG vaccination?

Q-105. Why is the reactivation of BCG scar in Kawasaki disease?

Q-106. What are the various available vaccines for diphtheria, pertussis and tetanus together?

Q-107. What is the role of adjuvant in DPT vaccine?

Q-108. What are the absolute contraindications for DPT vaccines?

Q-109. What are the precautions for administering DPT vaccines?

Q-110. What is the recommended schedule for DTwP/DTaP in India?

Q-111. Is it necessary to immunize individual who developed the disease diphtheria, tetanus or pertussis?

Q-112. Why is the concentration of diphtheria and pertussis antigens reduced in Tdap, while tetanus remains same?

Q-113. Can Tdap be given as second booster at 5 years of age?

Q-114. What are the recommendations for tetanus prophylaxis following an injury?

Q-115. What is the reactogenicity of repeated doses of tetanus toxoid?

Q-116. What are the recommendations for vaccination of pregnant women with Tdap/Td?

Q-117. What is cocooning?

Q-118. If the mother did not receive Tdap in pregnancy, can she receive it after the delivery?

Q-119. When was last case of wild polio reported in India? Where?

Q-120. When India was certified as polio free?

Q-121. What are the characteristics of OPV? What are the different types of OPV?

Q-122. What is bivalent OPV (bOPV)?

Q-123. What is monovalent OPV (mOPV)?

Q-124. What are drawback of OPV?

Q-125. What was tOPV replaced by bOPV?

Q-126. What is the importance of birth dose of OPV (OPV-O)?

Q-127. What is fractional IPV (fIPV)?

Q-128. What is the IAP recommended IPV schedule?

ANSWERS

A-92. A. Measles

B. Kolpik spots is the pathognomonic sign of measles

Koplik spots appear on the buccal mucosa at the level of premolars. The resemble grains of white sand surrounded by red base. They appear 1-2 days before the onset of rash.

C. Subacute Sclerosing Panencephalitis (SSPE)

Behavioral and intellectual deterioration followed by myoclonic epilepsy are characteristics of SSPE

D.

- Edmonston-Zagreb
- Schwarz-Moraten

E. MR vaccine at 9 months of 16-24 months of age

A-93. A. Varicella (Chickenpox)

B. Pleomorphic skin lesions

Simultaneous presence of skin lesions in various stages (multi morphological skin lesions at a time).

C.

- Impetigo
- Cellulitis
- Lymphadenitis
- Necrotizing fasciitis
- Abscess

D. Postchickenpox cerebellitis

A-94.

A. Congenital varicella syndrome
B. Cicatrix, a zigzag scarring in a dermatomal distribution
C.
- Chorioretinitis
- Microphthalmia
- Cataract

D. Limb hypoplasia and digital defects
E. Cortical atrophy
Extensive aplasia of brain

A-95.

A. Neonatal varicella
B. From 5 days prior to delivery to 2 days afterwards
C.
- Varicella Zoster Immunoglobulin (VZIG) 125 IU/kg, minimum 62.5 IU in a neonate
- Intravenous Immunoglobulin 400 mg/kg single dose

D. Acyclovir intravenous 10 mg/kg/dose 3 times a day, 14 days for skin/eye involvement, 21 days for disseminated or CNS disease.

A-96.

A. Herpes zoster
B. This condition represents reactivation of a latent varicella zoster viral infection and occurs several years after primary infection with varicella zoster virus.
C. It is common in immunocompromised individuals like HIV
D. Yes, vaccines are available against herpes zoster.
It is recommended for people 50 years of age or older, irrespective of prior history of herpes zoster. It is also indicated for 18 years and older who are immunocompromised.

A-97.

A. Congenital Rubella syndrome
B.
- Patent ductus arteriosus
- Congenital cataract
- Sensorineural deafness

C. One dose of MMR vaccine

A-98.

- The BCG vaccine is supplied as lyophilized (freeze-dried) preparation in vacuum sealed, dark colored, multidose vital with normal saline as diluent.

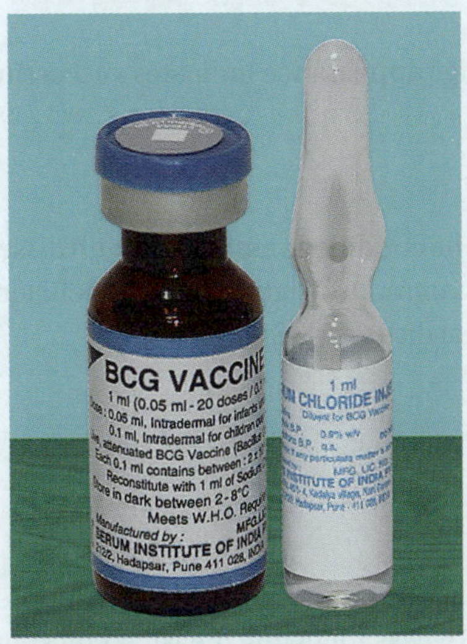

- The ampoules of freeze-dried BCG vaccine are dark colored, long and sealed under vacuum.

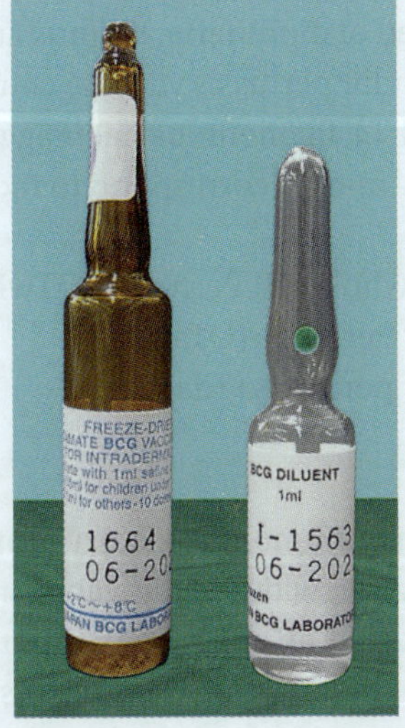

- They have to be opened carefully gradually filling at the junction of neck and the body of the ampoule so that air does not rush causing spillage.
- The vaccine is reconstituted by dissolving it in normal saline and not distilled water which is quite an irritant.
- The diluent should always be kept with the vaccine in the main compartment of the refrigerator to maintain its temperature at the time of reconstitution.

A-99. Reconstituted BCG vaccine should be used within 6 hours. It should be stored at 2–8°C and protected from light. It should be discarded within 6 hours of reconstitution. As the vaccine does not contain preservatives or antibiotics, bacterial contamination may lead to toxic shock syndrome, if it is kept for long time after reconstitution.

A-100.

- The standard dose of BCG vaccine is 0.1 mL volume. Dosage does not depend upon the age or weight of the baby.
- Some experts recommend a dose of 0.05 mL to newborns aged less than 4 weeks as they consider a higher incidence of regional lymphadenitis on full dose administration.

A-101. Intradermal.

A-102. A wheel of 5 mm with Peau-di-orange appearance indicates successful intradermal administration of the vaccine.

A-103.

- Osteitis and osteomyelitis
- Disseminated BCG disease. The conditions associated with disseminated BCG disease are severe combined immunodeficiency (SCID), common variable immunodeficiency (CVID), HIV infection and Mendelian susceptibility to mycobacterial disease (MSMD).

A-104.

- Primary immunodeficiency
- HIV
- Leukemia
- Lymphoma
- BCG should be withheld in children who are on immunosuppressive or radiation therapy
- It is best to avoid BCG for 4–6 weeks following measles, chickenpox or hepatitis B like infections

A-105. It is possibly due to cross reactivity between Mycobacterial and Human Homologue Heat Shock Protein. It occurs in 30 to 50% cases of Kawasaki disease.

A-106. The combination vaccines are composed of diphtheria, tetanus and pertussis in the form of whole-cell inactivated component (WP) or as acellular pertussis vaccine containing variable amount of inactivated bacterial components, pertussis toxin (PT), filamentous haemagglutinin (FHA), pertactin (PRN) and fimbrial haemagglutinin. The small alphabets 'd' and 'P' correspond to reduced amounts of diphtheria and acellular pertussis components respectively.

- Diphtheria, Tetanus toxoids and whole cell Pertussis (DTwP).
- Diphtheria Tetanus and acellular Pertussis (DTaP).
- Tetanus, diphtheria and acellular pertussis (Tdap).
- Tetanus and diphtheria (Td).
- Diphtheria and Tetanus (DT).

A-107. Adjuvants are chemical substances with immunomodulatory properties which enhance host antigen specific immune responses compared to those given without adjuvants. Inactivated whole cell pertussis bacilli absorbed on insoluble aluminum salts act as an adjuvant in diphtheria, pertussis and tetanus (DPT) vaccines. Adjuvants help antigen to elicit high and long-lasting immune response with lesser concentration of antigens. Aluminum salts, aluminum phosphate and aluminum hydroxide are commonly used adjuvants.

A-108.

- Severe allergic reaction to vaccine component following a prior dose.
- Progressive neurological disease.
- Encephalopathy not due to another identifiable cause occurring within 7 days of vaccination. Neurological side effects are attributed to pertussis component and occurrence of encephalopathy warrants further immunization with DT component.

A-109.

- Fever 105°F (40.5°C) or higher within 48 hours of vaccination and no other cause is identified for fever.
- Collapse or shock like state called as Hypotonic Hyporesponsive Episode (HHE) within 48 hours.
- Persistent inconsolable crying lasting for 3 hours or more, occurring within 48 hours.
- Convulsions with or without fever occurring within 3 days.

A-110.

- *Primary doses:* 6, 10 and 14 weeks.
- *Booster doses:* 18 months and 5 years.
- *Catch-up schedule:* 0, 1 and 6 months. This can be given up to 7 years of age.

- *Beyond 7 years and adults:* Tdap or Td, 0, 1 and 6 months. The first two doses at least at interval of 4 weeks and third dose 6 months after the second dose, first dose should be preferably Tdap. Booster dose of Td should be given every 10 years. Persons those who have never received Tdap should be given one dose of Tdap as one of these boosters.

A-111. Yes, because the disease does not confer adequate protection.

A-112. The reactogenicity of diphtheria and pertussis antigen is related to the dose of antigen, while that of tetanus is related to number of doses.

A-113. Although Tdap is licensed for use above 4 years of age, it is avoided as a second booster. Full dose of DTwP or DTaP should be performed. If Tdap has been given, there is no need to repeat the dose, but ensure that the child gets the 10 years Tdap booster.

A-114. The recommended dose for TIG is 250 IU IM, gives as soon as possible after the injury. If more than 24 hours have elapsed, 500 IU should be given. TIG should be given slowly using 23-gauge needle, because of its viscosity.

	Clean minor wounds		***Other wounds***	
	TT/Td/Tdap	TIG	TT/Td/Tdap	TIG
≥3 doses	Yes if >10 years since last booster	No	Yes if >5 years since last booster	No
<3 doses or uncertain or unimmunized	Yes	No	Yes	Yes

A-115. Repeated doses of tetanus toxoid result in very high antitoxin levels. In this situation, an additional dose may result in antigen—antibody complex formation, which gets deposited in the skin, glomeruli etc. This is known as "Arthus reaction." It also causes fever and local pain.

A-116. One dose of Tdap is recommended for pregnant women between 28 and 37 weeks to protect the new born and infants from pertussis. The second dose, if required for tetanus, is given as Td after 4 weeks and at least 2 weeks prior to delivery.

A-117. The term "cocooning" means vaccinating the contacts of an infant or immune compromised individuals. It is the practice of immunizing household people and healthcare professionals to prevent transmission to newborns. It is practice for protection of newborns against pertussis. All individuals who would come in contact with newborn is administered a booster of Tdap including antenatal one dose of Tdap to mother.

A-118. Yes, the mother and close care givers of the new born should be given a Tdap dose.

A-119. The last reported case of wild polio in India was on January 13, 2011 in Howrah, West Bengal.

A-120. March 27, 2014

A-121.

- OPV is a live-attenuated vaccine.
- The licensed formulations of OPV are:
  - Monovalent OPVs against type 1 ($mOPV_1$), type 2 ($mOPV_2$) and type 3 ($mOPV_3$).
  - Bivalent OPV (bOPV) containing type 1 and 3.
  - Trivalent OPV is no longer in use since April, 2016.
  - The type 2 strain of OPV is immunodominant and in formulating tOPV, the amount of type 2 virus is reduced compared with other viruses. This feature of the vaccine has led to the disappearance of WPV in 1999.
- OPV is administered orally as 2 drops (0.1 mL) dose. OPV is a highly heat sensitive vaccine and has Vaccine Vial Monitor (VVM).
- In high income countries, seroconversion rates in children following administration of 3 doses of tOPV approach 100% for all 3 polioviruses. However, in developing countries, it is 73, 90 and 70% to types 1, 2 and 3 respectively after 3 tOPV doses.
- OPV induces intestinal immunity, thus preventing virus shedding and transmission, resulting in population protection.

A-122. bOPV contains serotypes 1 and 3. bOPV elicits a better immune response against poliovirus type 1 and 3 than tOPV, but not give immunity against type 2.

Since April 2016, globally, tOPV is replaced with bOPV in routine immunization.

A-123. mOPV confer immunity to one of the three serotypes of OPV. mOPV elicits a superior immune response to the serotype which it contains than tOPV. There is no any response to remaining two strains.

mOPVs for type 1 (mOPV1) and type 3 (mOPV3) poliovirus were relicensed in 2005. Monovalent OPV type 2 (mOPV2) has been stockpiled in the event of a CVDPV2 out break.

A-124. Two major drawbacks of OPV are Vaccine Associated Paralytic Polio (VAPP) and Vaccine Derived Poliovirus (VDPV).

VAPP: OPV is associated with VAPP in approximately 1 in 2.7 million doses of OPV. VAPP is caused by a strain of polio virus that has mutated from the original attenuated vaccine strain contained in OPV. It can occur in the recipient of OPV or can occur in a close unvaccinated or nonimmune contact of the vaccine recipient who is excreting the mutated virus.

The risk of VAPP varies by dose and by setting. In developed countries, the risk is greatest with the first dose. In developing countries, the risk of VAPP is higher from subsequent doses than following the first dose.

As the virus causing VAPP is not transmissible, there are no outbreaks associated with VAPP. Thus, VAPP is a risk to an individual and not to the community.

VDPV: It is a strain of polio virus which has mutated from the original strain contained in OPV. This strain may regain neurovirulence and transmissibility. The latter is known as a circulating VDPV (CVDPV) is associated with sustained person to person transmission and circulating in the environment.

There are three types of VDPV:

1. cVDPV (Circulating Vaccine Derived Polio Virus)
2. iVDPV (Immunodeficiency related Vaccine derived polio virus), reported in immunodeficient patients.
3. aVDPV (Ambiguous Vaccine derived polio virus) currently have unclassified source.

A-125. The last case of type 2, wild polio virus was reported in 1999. Since 2009, 97% of CVDPV cases of 40% of VAPP are due to type 2. Hence, type 2 was dropped from tOPV with the purpose of reducing risks of VAPP and cVDPV associated with type 2 in the OPV.

A-126. Since 1985, WHO has recommended administration of one dose of OPV at birth in countries at risk for polio, where the serological response to 3 doses of OPV, in the primary immunization schedule, was found to be suboptimal.

The birth dose should be administered at birth or as soon as possible after birth within the first 15 days. Although data on birth dose seroconversion rates show great variability, low rates in India, this OPV-O increases the seroconversion rates of subsequent doses and induces mucosal protection before enteric pathogens may interfere with the immune response. OPV-O is advised even with IPV schedule in India.

A-127. With switch from tOPV to bOPV, it was recommended to include IPV in NIP in all OPV using countries, but bulk production of IPV was the challenge, led to severe global shortage of IPV.

Meanwhile, there is conclusive evidence that two fractional doses administered via intradermal (ID) route offer higher immunogenicity compared to one full intramuscular (IM) dose of IPV. As a result, a two dose fIPV schedule has been strongly recommended by the WHO.

A fractional dose is one-fifth (1/5) of a full dose (0.1 mL) of IPV, injected via intradermal (ID) route. It is given on right arm at the insertion of deltoid muscle.

A-128.

- bOPV at birth.
- IPV by IM injection in full dose at 6-10-14 weeks.
- Booster at 15–18 months and 4–6 years.

CHAPTER 49

Electrocardiogram

The contraction of heart generates electrical currents which are distributed throughout the body to the skin. Application of two electrodes to any two parts of the body leads the cardiac current to a recording galvanometer. This graphic representation of electrical currents of the heart is called electrocardiogram (ECG).

CONDUCTION SYSTEM OF HEART

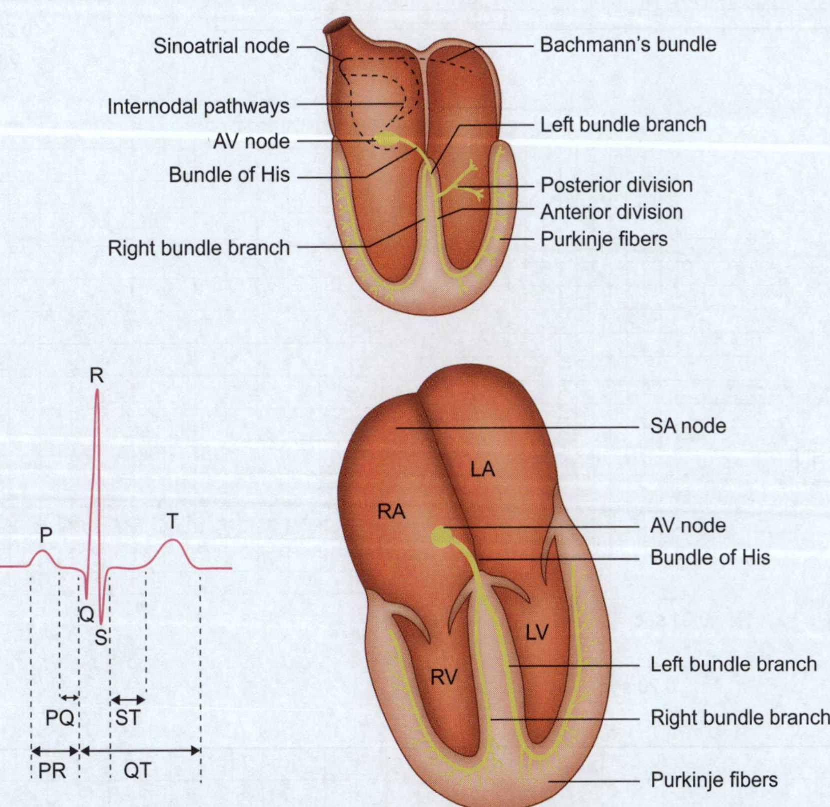

Functioning of Conduction System

- The sinoatrial node (SA node), a clump of specialized tissues in the right atrium is the pace maker, generates an electrical stimulus.
- The electrical impulse spreads through the atria, stimulating them to contract.
- The impulse travels to the atrioventricular node (AV node), where it slows down briefly.
- The impulse continues down the bundle of His, which divides into the right and left bundle branches.
- The impulse travels through the bundle branches to the right and left ventricles, stimulating them to contract.

ECG Paper

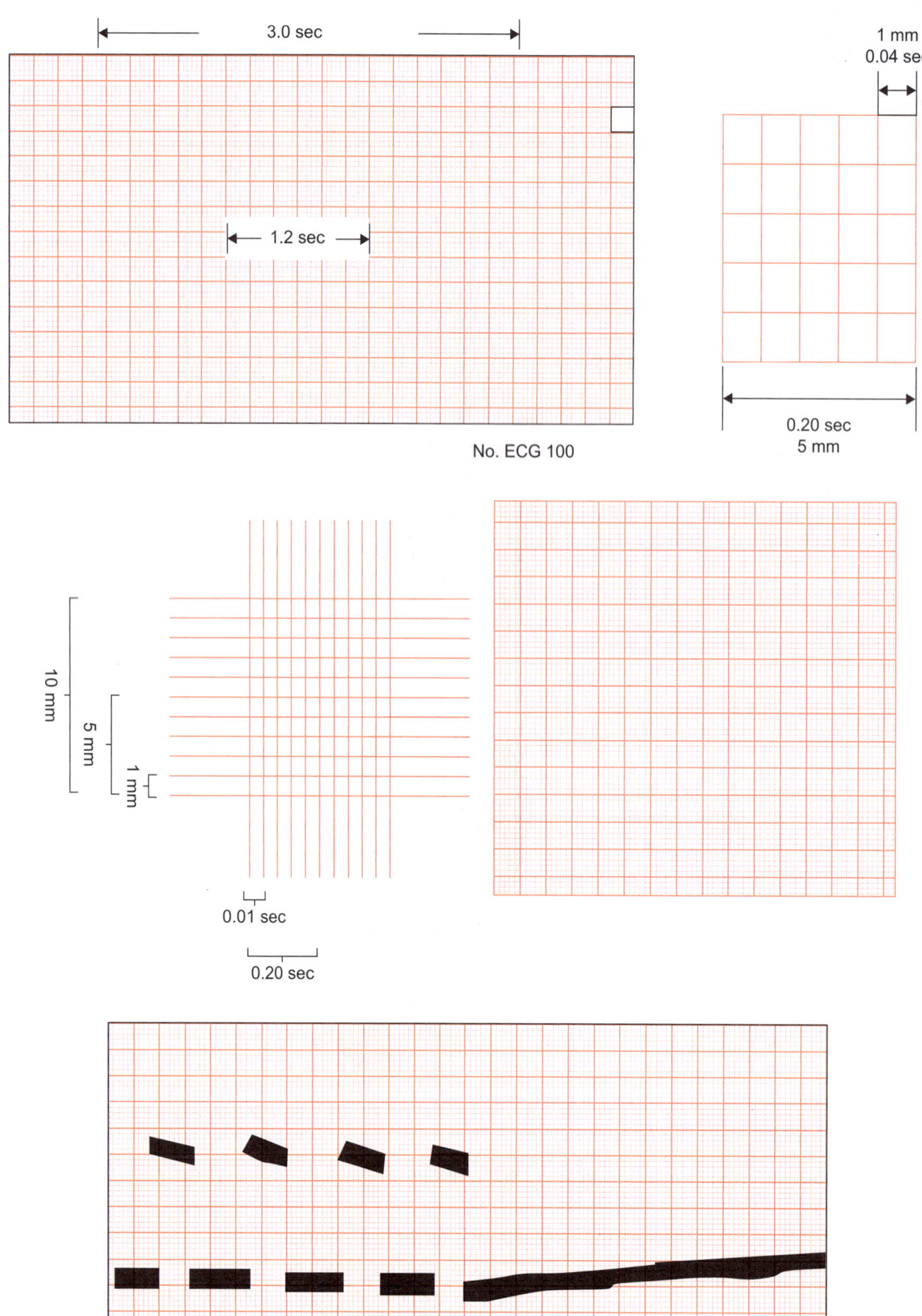

3.0 sec
1.2 sec
No. ECG 100
1 mm
0.04 sec
0.20 sec
5 mm
10 mm
5 mm
1 mm
0.01 sec
0.20 sec

- ECG paper has small and large squares. The small square are 1 mm squares and large squares are 5 mm squares.
- The standard speed of ECG paper is 25 mm/sec. Time is measured on the horizontal axis and voltage on the vertical axis.
- One second is divided into 25 small divisions of 1 mm each. The distance between two thick lines being 0.2 seconds and distance between two thin lines is 40 msec (0.04 sec). Five thick squares constitute 1 second.
  Horizontal one small square = 0.04 sec. One large square = 0.04 × 5 = 0.2 sec.
- Vertically, 1 mm = 0.1 mv.

Calibration

The ECG machine is generally calibrated in such a way that 1 millivolt produces a deflection of 10 mm in ECG record. Usually, the calibration mark will be there at the beginning.

Timelines, Voltage Lines and Correct Standardization in an Electrocardiogram

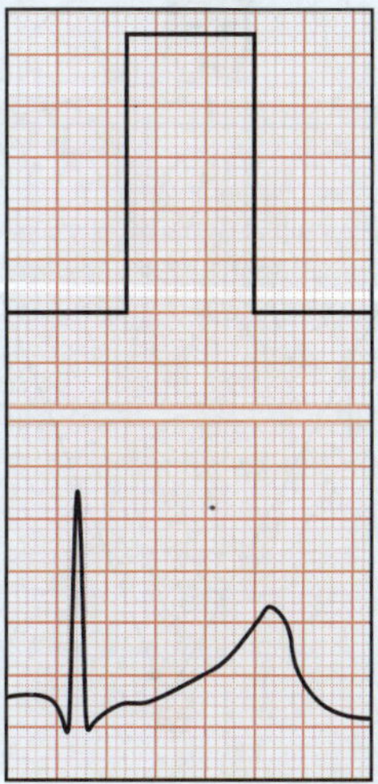

Good standardization (10 mm square wave pattern)

Calculation of Heart Rate

- 1500 ÷ number of small divisions between two R – R waves.
- Since the ECG paper moves at the speed of 25 mm/sec. it moves 25 × 60 = 1500 mm = 1500 small divisions in 1 min.
- Time taken between two R-R waves means one beat. Therefore, beats per minutes means 1500 ÷ small division between R- R waves

Leads of ECG

- An electrode placed on the body is called a lead. Lead is also used as a term for actual tracing obtained.
- Bipolar limb leads (Standard Leads) (In reality, it is combination of two tracings)
  - Lead I: Rt. Arm - left arm
  - Lead II: Rt. Arm - left leg
  - Lead III: Left arm - left leg
  - Lead II = Lead I + Lead III
- Unipolar Leads
- Designated as V (Voltage leads)
- One electrode (exploring electrode) in close proximity to the heart, while other (in different electrode) is far removed from it so that its potential is more or less reduced to zero.

Unipolar leads

Unipolar limb leads	**Unipolar chest leads**
(Augmentation 50%) • aVR (Rt. arm lead) atrial and ventricular cavities • aVL (left arm lead) left lat. cardiac wall • aVF (left leg lead) diaphragmatic or inferior surface of the heart	• V1 to V6 • Ve, VSC, • V3R, V4R (Rt. ant. chest corresponding to V 3–4) ↓ Important in children not to miss RVH and atrial hypertrophy

13 Leads ECG is Recommended in Pediatric Patients, Including either V_3R or V_4R

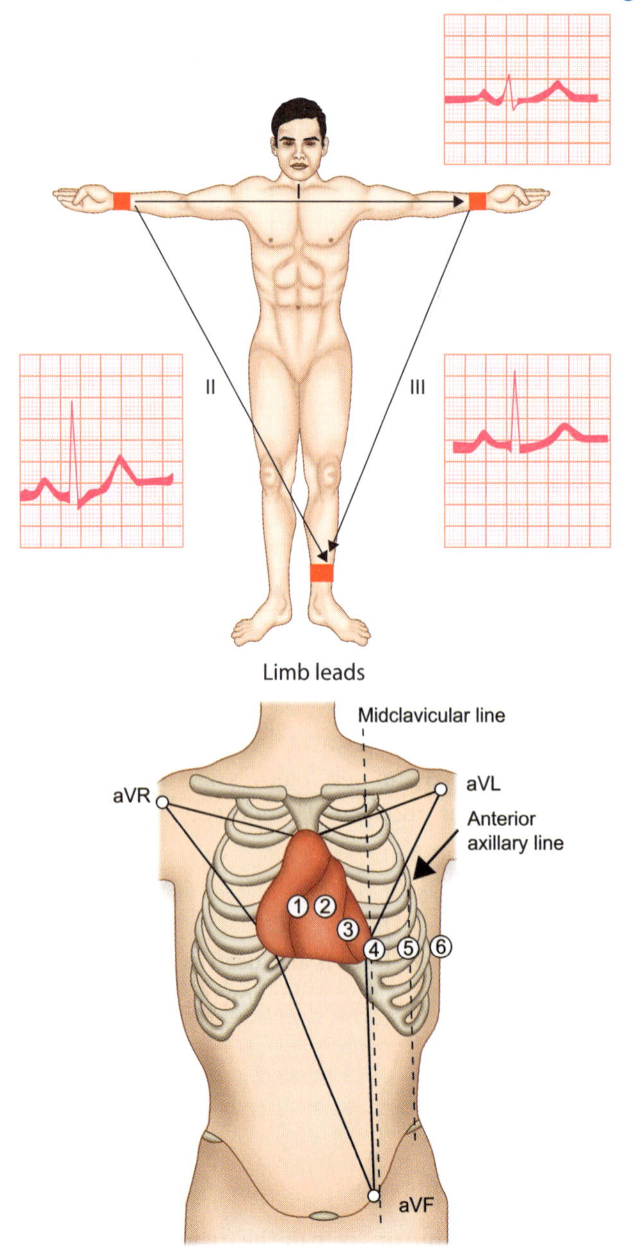

Limb leads

Augmented limb leads, and precordial leads

NORMAL ECG COMPLEXES

Nomenclature

- *Cardiac cycle time:* 0.8 sec. (with heart rate 75/min)
- *Atrial systole:* 0.1 sec.
- *Atrial diastole:* 0.7 sec.
- *Ventricular systole:* 0.3 sec.
- *Ventricular diastole:* 0.5 sec.
- P wave, QRS complex, T wave
- *Two important intervals:* PR interval, QT Interval
- *Two important segments:* PQ segment, ST segment
- *P wave:* SA node through both the atria to the AV node
- *PR segment:* Time taken by AV node (slowest conducting tissue) to conduct the impulse
- *QRS complex:* Q Wave → activity in IVS
- RandS waves → ventricular activity
- *ST segment:* Time gap between depolarization and repolarization
- *T wave:* Ventricular repolarization
- *U wave:* (20 to 30%) late ventricular repolarization
- Repolarization of atria
- *Isoelectric line:* The point at which ST segment joins the QRS complex → Junction 'J'

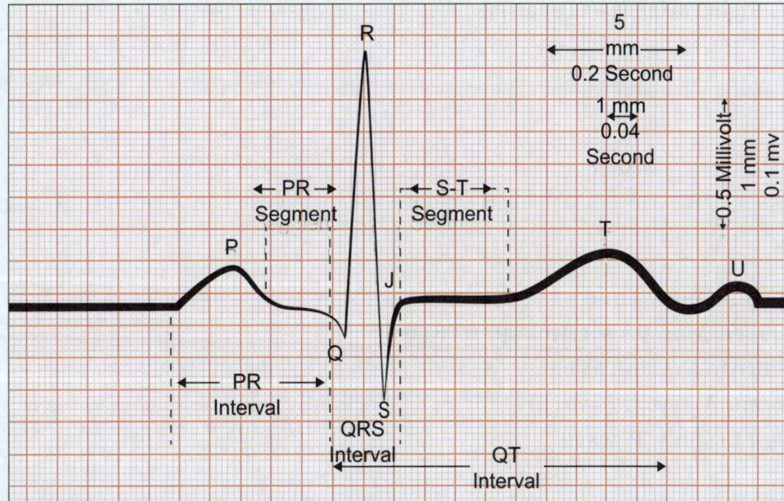

Waves, Intervals and Segments

Waves, segments and intervals	*Normal values*
P wage (best seen in leads II and V_1)	Height not more than 2.5 mm width not more than 2.5 mm (i.e. 0.1 seconds)
PR interval (best seen in Leads II and V_1)	3 to 5 mm (i.e., 0.12 to 0.20 seconds)
Q wave	Depth not more than ¼ the size of the R wave in the same lead width not more than 1 mm (i.e., <0.04 seconds)
R and S wave (best seen in precordial leads)	R in V_{1-2} < S in V_{1-2} S in V_{1-2} < 20 mm R in V_{5-6} < 25 mm S in V_{5-6} < 5 mm
QRS complex	At least of 10 mm height in precordial leads and 5 mm in limb leads (less than this is known as "Low Voltage complex")

Normal Values of Waves, Intervals and Segments

QRS axis	Older people -30° to +90° Younger people 0° to +110°
ST segment	No specific duration. Must be in the same level as the PR segment
T wave	At least 10% of the R wave in the same lead. No upper limit
QT interval (measured in mid-precordial leads)	As this varies with heart rate, it is usually corrected to read QT_c = [QT / RR interval] which must be <0.42 seconds for males and <0.44 seconds for females

- Upward deflections: +ve
- Downward deflections: -ve
- QandS wave → Never +ve
- R wave → Never -ve
- Q wave → always infront of R
- Monophasic → +ve or -ve deflection
- Biphasic/Diphasic → +ve and -ve
- Intervals in ECG → contain some waves
- Segments in ECG → No waves

P Wave

- *Two components:* I → Right Atrial, II → Let atrial

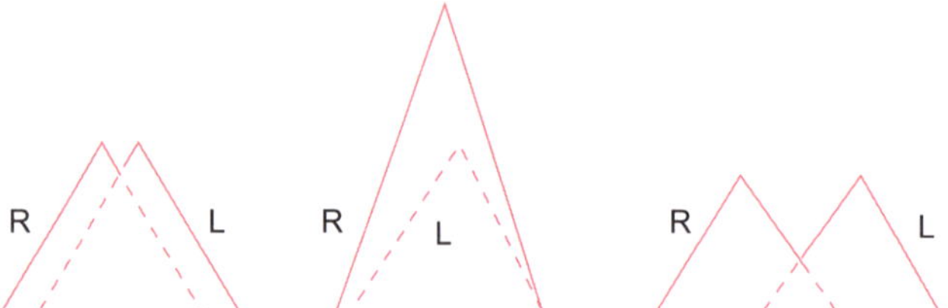

- *Normal amplitude:* 1.5 min max. 3 min
- *Normal duration:* 0.06 sec. Max. 0.1 sec. (infants 0.08 sec)
- Negative in aVR, positive in aVL and aVF
- May be biphasic in V_1 and V_2 +ve (R) -ve (L)
- Leads V_1 and II are best to study 'P' wave

Q Wave

- Due to depolarization of interventricular septum (IVS)
- Commonly present in leads I, II, III, aVR and almost always in V_5 and V_6. Absent in V_4R and V_1
- Absent Q waves in V_6 with,
  - Corrected TGA
  - Single ventricle
  - Mirror image dextrocardia
  - Left bundle branch block (LBBB)
- Present Q waves in V_1 with,
  - Severe RVH
  - Corrected TGA
  - Single ventricle
  - May be normally in newborn

- Deep Q waves (but not wide)
    - LVH of volume overload type, e.g. in VSD
    - Occasionally RVH
    - Combined VH (VSD + PHT)
    - Cardiomyopathy
- Deep and wide Q waves
    - Myocardial infarction
    - Myocardial fibrosis
    - Idiopathic hypertrophic, subaortic stenosis
- Normal duration not >0.04
  Depth not >2 mm (Max. ¼ of R)
- Deep Q in III → may be due to high diaphragm
  (Decrease or absent on deep inspiration)

PR Interval

(As Q wave is not seen many times)

- PR Interval → P duration + PQ segment
  (Atrial depolarization) (Physiological delay at AV node)
- <3 years → 0.08 sec
- 3 to 16 years → 0.1 sec
- >16 years → 0.12 sec
- Prolonged PR interval (I° block) (abnormal delay at AV node)
    - *Myocarditis:* Rheumatic fever, Enteric fever
    - *CHD:* Endocardial cushion defects, ASD, Ebstein's anomaly)
- *Toxicity:* Quinine
- Hyperkalemia
- Ischemia/profound hypoxia
- Normal heart
- Short PR Interval:
    - Wolff-Parkinson-White (WPW) syndrome
    - Lown-Ganong-Levine syndrome
    - Glycogen storage disease
- Variable PR Interval:
    - Wandering atrial pacemaker
    - Wenckebach phenomenon

QRS Complex

- Duration not >0.1 sec.
- Amplitude: *Standard leads:* 5 mm
  lead II occasionally 20 to 30 mm
  Precordial: 25 to 30 mm
- Widening:
    - Ventricular premature beats (VPB)
    - Bundle branch block (BBB)
    - Hyperkalemia
    - Aberrant conduction
- *High voltage:* LVH, Thin chest wall

- **Low voltage**
  - Pericardial effusion
  - Constrictive pericarditis
  - Myxedema
  - Cardiac failure
  - Wide spread myocardial damage
  - Obesity, emphysema, thick chest wall, edema

ST Segment

- Isoelectric and horizontal
  - In limb leads → ↑/↓ 1 mm → Normal
  - In V_5-V_6 → shift up to 2 mm → Normal
- **Depressed**
  - Digitals
  - Coronary insufficiency
  - LVS
  - Subendocardial injury
  - RVS
- **Elevated**
  - Pericarditis
  - Myocardial infarction

T Wave

- **In V_5** → <1 year → 11 mm
  >1 year → 14 mm
- **In V_6** → <1 year → 7 mm
  >1 year → 9 mm
- Tall T wave
  - Normal
  - Hyperkalemia
  - Volume overload
  - Myocardial ischemia (without infarction)
  - Diaphragmatic infarction (Tall T Wave in V_1 and V_2)
  - CVA
  - Post myocardial infarction
- Low/Flat T wave
  - Normal in newborn
  - Pericarditis
  - Hypothyroidism
  - Myocarditis
  - Hypokalemia
  - Myocardial ischemia
  - Hyperglycemia
  - Digitalis effect
  - Hypoglycemia

Common Morphologies of the P Wave: T Wave and ST Segment

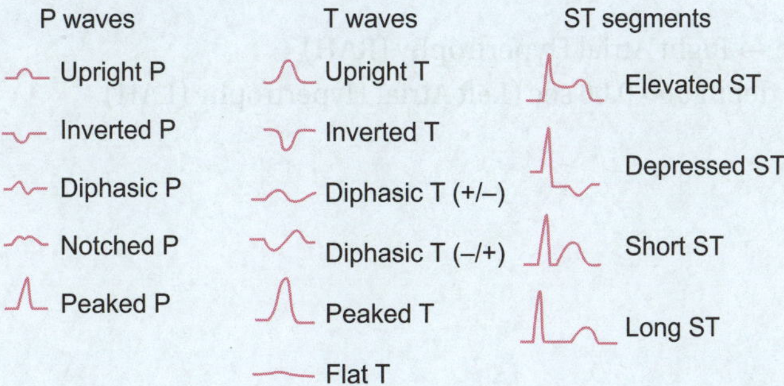

U Wave

- A small wave of low voltage is sometimes seen following the T wave, in the same direction as T
- Often best seen in V_3
- Prominent in hypokalemia (usually in V_3-V_5)

J Wave

- The junction of QRS complex and ST segment

J Segment

- In hypothermia, J wave appears as a hump like wave, usually superimposed on distal limb of QRS complex

Q-T Interval

- Ventricular depolarization (QRS) + Ventricular repolarization (to end of T Wave)
- Varies with her rate and not with age
- Corrected QT Interval QTc (Bazett's formula) not > 0.44 s ec. $\frac{\text{QT measured}}{\sqrt{\text{RR interval}}}$ (0.49 sec. my be normal for 5 to 6 months of age)
- *Prolonged:*
  - Hypocalcemia
  - Myocarditis
  - Long QT syndrome
  - Head injury
  - Cerebrovascular accident (stroke)
  - Diffuse myocardial damage
  - Quinidine
  - Procainamide
- *Shortened:*
  - Hypercalcemia
  - Hyperkalemia
  - Digitalis

CHAMBER ENLARGEMENTS

- Most common abnormality seen in pediatric ECGs
- Atrial enlargement
  - 'P' wave is studied in leads II, V_1 and V_2
  - Increased in amplitude of P wave

- Increased in duration of P wave
- Biphasic P wave in V_1-V_2
  +ve phase of P > 1.5 mm → Right Atrial Hypertrophy (RAH)
  –ve phase of P >1.5 mm depth or > 0.06 sec (Left Atrial Hypertrophy (LAH)

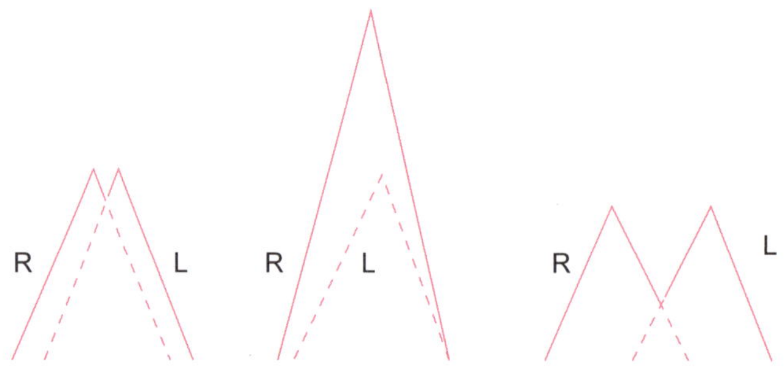

Normal 'p' wave 'P' Pulmonale 'P' Mitralae

'P' Pulmonale

(Right Atrial Enlargement)

- Frequently associated with Cor pulmonale
- Also called as P congenital as associated with RA strain in pulmonary hypertension (PH) or cyanotic CHD
- Tall, peaked P wave in V_1 as right atrial force is directed towards this lead
- Changes are also best seen in lead II since both atrial forces run parallel to this lead

'P' Mitralae

(Left Atrial Enlargement)

- Frequent association with mitral valve disease so called as P Mitrale
- Second or left atrial component of P wave in lead II is delayed giving wide and notched P wave
- In V_1, P wave is biphasic with prominent or mainly negative component as left atrium is directed away from V_1 lead
- In infants, P wave duration > 0.08 sec. (0.1 sec or more in any lead)

Combined Atrial Enlargement

- Increase in both amplitude and duration of P wave
- Lead II → P wave is tall
- V_1 → +ve deflection is taller
  –ve deflection is broader

Ventricular Hypertrophy

Abnormalities are seen in:

- QRS voltage
- R/S ratio
- Strain pattern
- QRS duration
- QRS axis
- Nonspecific changes

Criteria for RVH

- R wave in V_1 or V_4R greater than normal (7-8 mm)
- R>S in V_1
- S wave > normal for age in V_6
(15 mm in first week, 10 mm in 1 to 24 weeks,
7 mm in 6-12 months and 5 mm >1 year)
- Greater R wave in V_1 and prolongation of QRS duration
- Upright T waves in V_4R and V_1 with R>S in V_1
- Right axis deviation
- Q wave in V_1 (qR and qRS), may be normal in 10% neonates.
(May be normal in 10% neonates)

Criteria for LVH

- R in I + S in III > 25 mm
- R in aVL >12 mm
- S > 25 mm in V_1
- R > 25 mm in V_5
- R in V_5 + S in V_1 >35 mm (>30 mm in infant)
- Left axis deviation
- R/S ratio in V_1 and V_2 < lower limit for age (0.5)
- Q waves in V_5 and V_6 >5 mm + tall asymmetrical T waves
- Flat or inverted T Waves in I or aVR

Criteria for BVH

- At times the potentials from two hypertrophied ventricles cancel each other and so ECG may appear normal
- It may be diagnosed if,
  - Precordial leads show RVH in V_1 and V_2 and LVH in V_5 and V_6
  - RVH + left axis deviation
  - Deep Q waves in V_5 and V_6
  - LVH + Rt. Axis deviation

Causes of RVH

- Pulmonary stenosis
- Pulmonary hypertension
- Fallot's tetrad
- TGA

Causes of LVH

- Aortic stenosis
- Aortic regurgitation
- Coarctation of aorta
- Moderate sized VSD
- PDA
- MR
- Systemic hypertension
- Congestive and obstructive cardiomyopathy

Right Bundle Branch Block (RBBB)

Criteria

- rSR pattern in aVR, V_1 and V_2
- QRS duration > for age
  > 0.12 sec. for complete RBBB
  0.1 to 0.12 sec. for incomplete RBBB
- Wide and slurred S in I, V_5 and V_6
- *Causes:*
  - RV conduction delay
  - Ebstein's anomaly
  - RVHCoarctation of aorta
  - RV volume over load
  - ASD
- After open heart surgery (VSD, TOF)

Left Bundle Branch Block (LBBB)

Criteria

- RSR' pattern in V_5-V_6
- QRS duration > for age
- Loss of Q waves in I, V_5 and V_6
- Slurred and wide 'R' waves in I, aVL, V_5 and V_6
- Wide 'S' waves inV_1-V_2
- ST depreciation and T inversion common in adults in association with ischemic and hypertensive heart diseases.

HYPERKALEMIA

- Best seen in II, III and left chest leads
- Tall-slender-peaked-tented T waves ($S.K^+$ 6.7 mEq/L)
- PR interval prolonged, P waves broader and flattened ($S.K^+$ 7 mEq/L)
- Wider QRS → S. K^+ 8.8 mEq/L
- Absent P wave → S. K^+ 9 mEq/L
- Ventricular fibrillation, ventricular standstill ($S.K^+$ 12-14 mEq/L)
- *Causes:*
  - Chronic renal failure
  - Acidosis
  - Or acute renal failure
  - Hyperadrenogenital crisis
  - Iatrogenic
  - Shock

HYPOKALEMIA

- Sagging of ST segment
- Diminished T wave
- Fusion of appearance of U wave and T waves
- Arrhythmias → Heart block, ventricular tachycardia, ventricular fibrillation

- *Causes:*
  - Malnutrition
  - Diuretics
  - Vomiting

ECG Findings of Hypokalemia and Hyperkalemia

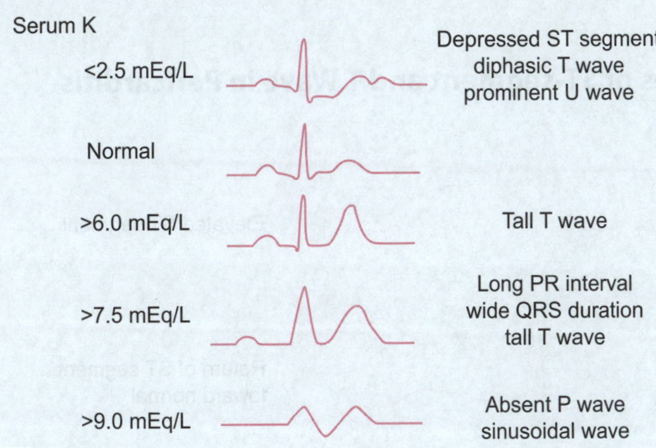

HYPOCALCEMIA

- ST-segment prolonged
- QTc interval prolonged
- *Causes:*
  - Rickets
  - Respiration/Metabolic alkalosis
  - RTA
  - Pseudohypoparathyroidism
  - CRF

HYPERCALCEMIA

- QTC shortened
- ST segment shortened

ECG Findings of Hypercalcemia and Hypocalcemia

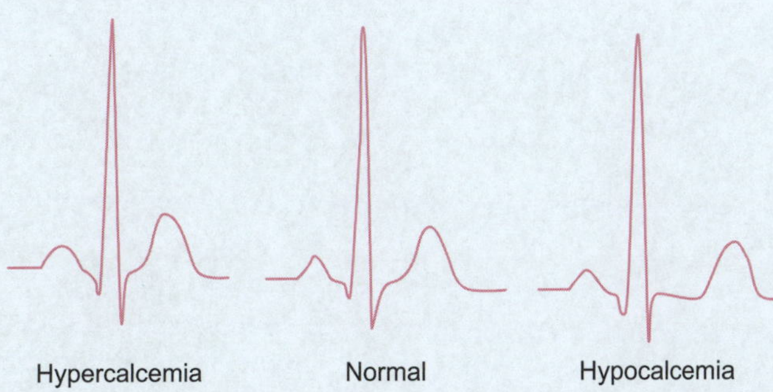

PERICARDITIS

- Pericardial effusion may produce low QRS voltages (QRS voltages <5 mm)
- Sub pericardial myocardial damage produces time dependent changes in the ST segment and T wave
- ST-segment elevation occurs in the leads representing the LV (Pardee's sign)
- The ST-segment shift returns to normal within 2 to 3 days. The T wave is small but still up right
- After 2-3 weeks of onset, T wave becomes sharply inverted and there is isoelectric ST segment. It may persist for 2-3 months

Time-dependent Changes of ST-segment and T Wave in Pericarditis

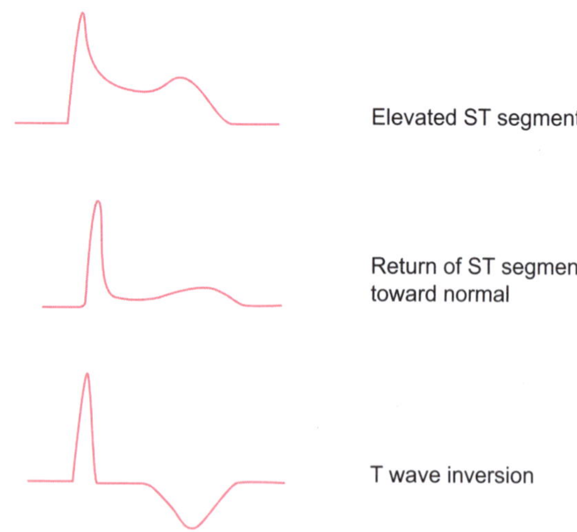

MYOCARDITIS

- Nonspecific changes, may include in all phases of cardiac cycle.
- Disturbances of AV conduction (I° and II° AV block)
- Low QRS voltages (<5 mm in all LL)
- Diminished amplitude of T wave
- Prolonged QTc interval
- Arrhythmias
- Ectopic beats

MYOCARDIAL INFARCTION

- Rare in infants and children
- *Causes:*
  - ALCAPA
  - Hypertension
  - Kawasaki disease
  - Diabetes mellitus
  - Infective endocarditis
  - Atherosclerosis
  - SLE
  - Syphilis
  - Polyarteritis nodosa
  - Coronary artery embolization

DISTURBANCES OF AV CONDUCTION

AV Blocks: Disturbances in Conduction between Normal Sinus Impulse and Eventual Ventricular Response

- I degree AV block: Prolongation of PR Interval
- II degree AV block
- III degree AV block (complete heart block)

I-degree AV Block

- Prolonged PR interval beyond upper limit for age
- *Causes:*
  - Rheumatic fever
  - Cardiomyopathies
  - CHDs, (ASD, Ebstein's anomaly)
  - Cardiac surgery
  - Digitalis toxicity

  Continued disturbances of AV conduction can lead to

II-degree AV Block

- Some, but not all, P waves are followed by QRS complexes (dropped beats)
- Mobitz Type I (Wenckebach Phenomenon)
- Mobitz Type II
- Two-to-one (or higher) AV block

Mobitz Type I

- *Causes:*
  - Myocarditis
  - Cardiomyopathy
  - Myocardial infarction
  - CHD
  - Cardiac surgery
  - Digitalis toxicity

Mobitz Type II

- AV conduction is 'all or none'

  AV conduction is either normal or completely blocked
- Block is at level of bundle of His. It is more serious than type I, may progress to complete heart block
- Treat the cause
- Prophylactic pace maker therapy

Higher AV Block

QRS complex follows every second, third or fourth P wave → 2:1, 3:1, 4:1 block

III-degree AV Block

(Complete Heart Block)

- Atrial and ventricular activities are entirely independent
- P waves are regular (Regular P-P interval)

- QRS complexes are also regular (Regular R-R interval) much slower rate than P rate
- Congenital complete heart block
  - Duration of QRS complex is normal as pace maker for ventricular complex is at a level higher than the bifurcation of bundle of His
  - Ventricular rate is faster (50-80/min) than that in the acquired type

III-degree AV Block

Causes

- Congenital
- Isolated anomaly
- Maternal SLE
- Sjögren Syndrome
- Structural heart disease (L-TGA)
- *Acquired:*
  - Cardiac surgery
  - Diphtheria
  - Severe myocarditis
  - Cardiomyopathies
  - Acute renal failure
  - Tumors
  - Mumps

  No treatment in asymptomatic

Symptomatic:
- *Atropine, isoproterenol*
- *Ventricular pace maker*

WOLFF-PARKINSON-WHITE SYNDROME

- A form of pre-excitation
- Results from an anomalous conduction pathway (bundle of Kent) between atrium and ventricle, by passing normal delay of conduction in AV node
- *Criteria:*
  - Short PR interval
  - Delta wave (initial slurring of QRS complex)
  - Wide QRS duration
  - Supraventricular paroxysmal atrial tachycardia, often intractable, causing death.

SECTION 4

Common Procedures

Common Procedures in Pediatric Practice

INTRODUCTION

It is very essential for every medical student and practicing pediatrician to learn performing common pediatric procedures. The procedures are best learnt by observation, performing the procedure under supervision and repetitive performances. It should be practical, methodological, and safe for both patients as well as for the individual who performs the procedure.

GENERAL CONSIDERATIONS

Healthcare Counseling

Healthcare counseling (HCC) is a relatively new concept that amalgamates human biology, human psychology, and medical sociology principles, and applies the same in real-time clinical situations. HCC is especially important for the child population as the pediatricians need to partner the parenting responsibilities in different illness care settings covering the period from newborn to adolescence.

Explain to the parents in detail regarding the procedure including its indications, technique of the procedure, possible complications, etc. If the child is older and able to understand, talk to him also in simple language. By this, cooperation is available from parents as well as the child. It decreases the anxiety of all and the procedure can be performed smoothly. An informed consent is a must for all the procedures. In certain procedures such as lumbar puncture, pleural and pericardial tapping, liver biopsy, renal biopsy, exchange transfusion, bone marrow aspiration, and biopsy, it is prudent to get signed consent along with HCC to avoid medicolegal problems.

Procedure Room and Lighting

Separate procedure room is desirable. It should have good daylight and should be well-illuminated and well-equipped. All the equipment and drugs to perform the procedure as well as to manage any emergency if it arises should be made available.

Containers

It is very important to confirm that proper containers are available for collection and transferring the specimens.

Identification of the Patient

It should be a routine to identify the child before performing the procedure. It should be confirmed with hospital staff as well as the parents that you are dealing with the correct child.

Sedation

Children are afraid of procedures and their reactions in the form of crying and struggling and frightened appearance increases the parental anxiety. It affects the performance of the person who is performing the procedure. It results in increased rate of failure and complications related to procedure. In this situation, sedation to the child may help. Promethazine 1 mg/kg/dose or triclofos sodium 20 mg/kg/dose by oral route will suffice in most of the cases. Diazepam, ketamine, and general anesthesia are other options as per indications.

Restraint

Physical restraint of the frightened child may be essential for the successful outcome of any practical procedure. The child may be wrapped with a blanket taking care to prevent aspiration or airway obstruction. The help of the person who is assisting is very crucial in deciding the outcome of the procedure.

Anesthesia

Local anesthesia may be achieved by infiltrating tissues around the site with 0.5–2% lignocaine. The maximum dosage of 1% lignocaine that can be infiltrated is 0.3 mL/kg. An alternative is to apply lignocaine cream to small area of the skin 60 minutes prior to performing the procedure, protected by adhesive dressing. Sedation or general anesthesia may be needed in certain cases.

Asepsis

The physician should scrub hands and forearm using an effective cleaning agent like 4% chlorhexidine or hexachlorophene before undertaking any procedure. Wearing of sterile gloves by the doctor is very important both for his and the patient's safety. The site of the patient's skin is then cleaned with 70% isopropyl alcohol and the surface is allowed to dry, the surface is then again washed three times with 10% povidone-iodine or 0.5% chlorhexidine gluconate in 70% isopropyl alcohol. It should be cleaned in a circular fashion from the center outward.

INTRAMUSCULAR INJECTION

Common Sites

Muscles commonly used for intramuscular (IM) injection are vastus lateralis, deltoid, and gluteus medius. Children do not have well-developed gluteus medius and therefore, it is not the site of preference for IM injections. It has been documented that some vaccines such as hepatitis B and antirabies vaccines administered at gluteal region produce very poor antibody response.

The vastus lateralis (anterolateral aspect of thigh) is the preferred site in infants. The site in vastus lateralis is the middle-third of the area between the greater trochanter and lateral femoral condyle **(Figs. 1A and B)**.

In case of deltoid, the site for injection is midway between acromion process and deltoid insertion, which is 3–5 cm below the acromion process. This site may be used in children above 5 years and adults. The quantity of drug should be <5 mL. Only watery injections with less viscosity should be injected at deltoid region.

Technique (WHO Technique)

- The site of injection should be exposed well.
- For anterolateral aspect of thigh, the child may be laid supine or be held in mother's lap. For deltoid, child may be held in mother's lap or may sit.
- The muscle selected for injection should be relaxed.
- The skin over injection site should be cleaned with spirit. A circular motion of swab is used, proceeding from puncture site and extending outward for 5 cm. Let the spirit evaporate and skin become dry otherwise spirit entering into tissues is painful.
- The syringe is filled with the medicine.
- In children, usually 23 G needle with 25-mm length are used for IM injections.
- Stretch the skin flat and push the needle down at 90° **(Fig. 2)**.
- Aspiration before injecting the vaccine is not required.
- Inject the vaccine at the rate of 1 mL per 10 seconds.
- The needle is withdrawn and injection site is pressed for few seconds. Do not rub the injection site.
- Needle should be withdrawn smoothly with steady movement.
- Discard the needle and syringe as per standard guidelines.

Alternative to WHO technique, Advisory Committee on Immunization Practices (ACIP) technique may be used. It is also called *bunching technique*. In this technique, bunch the muscle and direct needle inferiorly along long axis of leg at an angle of 45°. It stabilizes leg and increases the muscle mass.

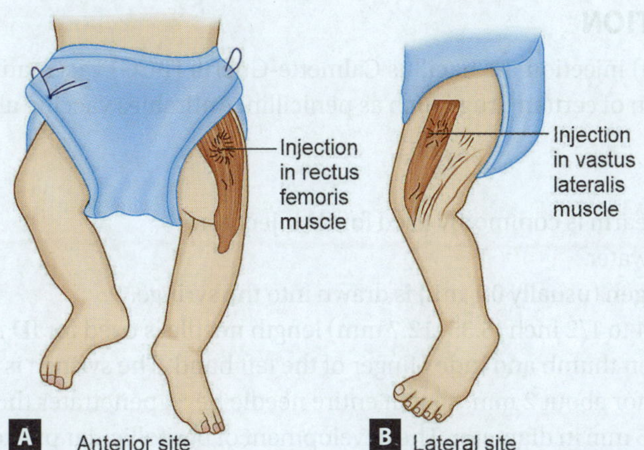

Figs. 1A and B: Site for intramuscular injections (IM) in an infant.
Source: Prajapati BS. Essential Procedures in Pediatrics, 1st edition. New Delhi: Jaypee Brothers Medical Publishers; 2003.

SUBCUTANEOUS INJECTION

Drugs or vaccines are injected subcutaneously when slow absorption and long duration of action are desired. Another indication of subcutaneous (SC) injection route is a coagulopathy, which makes IM injection hazardous, for fear of development of IM hematoma. Insulin and heparin such as drugs as well as measles, mumps, and rubella (MMR), varicella vaccines are given by SC route.

Technique

- Common sites are arm, anterior abdominal wall and thigh. Atrophic and infected areas are avoided.

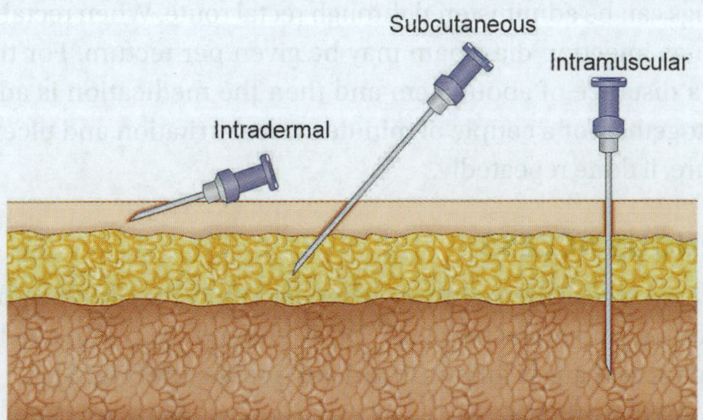

Fig. 2: The position of the needle during different ways of administering injections.
Source: Wechter EH, Philips J, Holaday B. Nursing Care of Children, 10th edition. Philadelphia: JB Lippincott Co; 1985.

- The skin is cleaned and disinfected with spirit.
- 26 G needle with 13-mm length is commonly used for SC injection.
- The skin is raised into a fold with thumb and index finger of the left hand.

- The midpoint of the fold is pierced with the needle held at 45° with its surface. The tip of the needle is advanced into the SC tissue **(Fig. 2)**.
- Aspiration is not required.
- Drugs or vaccine is injected, needle is withdrawn and site is pressed for few minutes.

INTRADERMAL INJECTION

Indications for intradermal (ID) injection are bacillus Calmette-Guérin (BCG) vaccination, Mantoux test, skin tests for allergy, and test for sensitization of certain drugs such as penicillin. Antirabies vaccine also can be given by ID route.

Technique

- Ventral (volar) aspect of forearm is commonly used for ID injection.
- Skin is cleaned with sterile water.
- A measured amount of antigen (usually 0.1 mL) is drawn into the syringe.
- 26 G or 27 G needle with 1/4 to 1/2 inch (6.35–12.7 mm) length needle is used for ID injection.
- The skin is held taut between thumb and index finger of the left hand. The syringe is held at an angle of 10–15° with the skin. Needle is inserted for about 2 mm, so that entire needle bevel penetrates the skin and the injected solution raises a small bleb of about 5 mm in diameter. The development of perifollicular puckering (Peau d'orange) indicates successful ID injection **(Fig. 2)**.
- The needle is withdrawn.
- The site is circled and it is recorded in patient's chart.
- The reaction is observed in defined time.

RECTAL ADMINISTRATION OF DRUGS

It is a safe and easy way of administering drugs. The human rectum represents a body cavity in which drugs can be easily introduced and retained. The absorption of the drugs is well through this route. Rectal administration of drugs is indicated in patients who are not able to take orally due to nausea and vomiting, having convulsions, uncooperative children, before surgery, etc. If the child can understand, it should be explained to him. The child should be relaxed. He is kept in lateral position with knees flexed toward abdomen or in supine position with legs taken upward toward abdomen and the drug is inserted into the rectum through anal orifice, and buttocks are held firmly to prevent expulsion of the drug. Paracetamol, diazepam, midazolam, paraldehyde, glycerine, bisacodyl, diclofenac sodium, steroids, neomycin, artesunate, and many more drugs can be administered through rectal route. When rectal preparations are not available, some liquid preparations such as injection diazepam may be given per rectum. For this purpose, a lubricated tube is inserted into the rectum to a distance of about 5 cm and then the medication is administered through it using a syringe. The buttocks are held together for a couple of minutes. Local irritation and ulcerations in rectum may develop as complication of this procedure, if done repeatedly.

PERIPHERAL INTRAVENOUS ACCESS

Peripheral intravenous (IV) access is one of the mainstays of modern medicine. It allows blood sampling, administration of medicines, fluids, nutrients, blood, and blood products. Intracaths and scalp vein needles are commonly used for this purpose. Various sites for venous access are as follows in order to preference **(Fig. 3)**:

- Veins on dorsum of hand
- Superficial radial vein on radial aspect of wrist
- Superficial veins over volar aspect of forearm
- Basilic vein and median cubital vein over antecubital fossa
- Superficial veins over dorsum of foot and long saphenous vein on medial aspect of leg above the ankle
- Veins of scalp in newborns and infants
- External jugular vein

Straight, large, and easily accessible peripheral veins in healthy SC tissues are ideal for venous access. Veins of the upper extremities are preferred because there are many potential sites and more comfortable to the patient. The distal and superficial veins are preferred as complications are more, following extravasation and thrombophlebitis in proximal and deep veins. When the veins are not visible, they can be palpated at common sites and can be accessed.

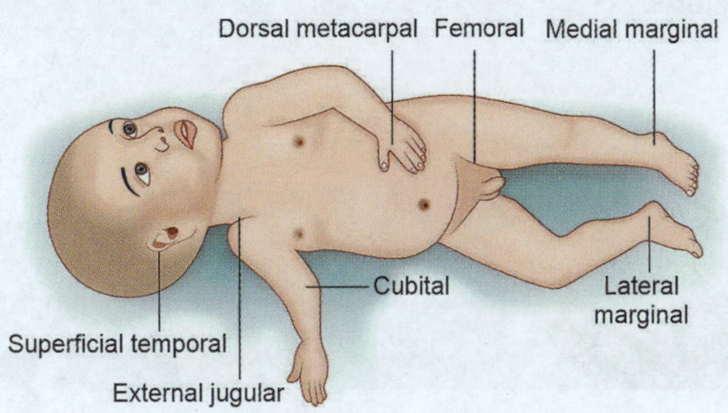

Fig. 3: Common sites for venipuncture.
Source: Prajapati BS. Essential Procedures in Pediatrics, 1st edition. New Delhi: Jaypee Brothers Medical Publishers; 2003.

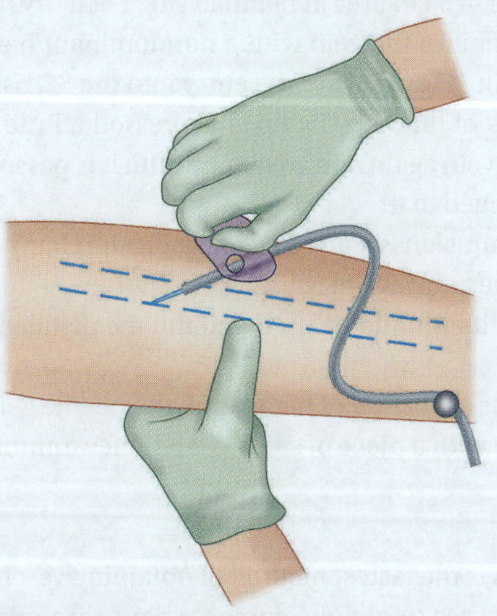

Fig. 4: Technique of venipuncture with scalp vein needle.
Source: Prajapati BS. Essential Procedures in Pediatrics, 1st edition. New Delhi: Jaypee Brothers Medical Publishers; 2003.

Scalp vein needle is a hollow needle with butterfly plastic handle, and a plastic tube, at the other end of which, a syringe or infusion set can be attached. It is useful for venous sampling of blood and short-term use of IV route **(Fig. 4)**. Vein is counter punctured very easily on movement of the limb.

Intracaths are plastic catheters over a hollow metallic needle. The metallic needle just projects beyond the tip of plastic catheter. The metallic needle is to provide stiffness during insertion into the vein, after which it is withdrawn. The plastic catheter is then advanced further gently so that vein is not counter punctured. The plastic catheter is well tolerated. Intracaths and scalp vein needles are available in various sizes from 26 G to 16 G. In children commonly, we use 26 G–21 G depending on age of the child and requirement.

Technique

- A tourniquet is placed over the limb, 3–4 cm proximal to the site selected for venipuncture, taking care not to pinch the skin of the child. The pressure should be such that it occludes venous flow but allows arterial blood flow.

- Tapping sharply over the vein causes mechanical reflex dilatation of the vascular walls. It should be light otherwise pain will cause vasoconstriction.
- Active or passive pumping of extremity enhances blood flow and distends veins.
- A warm moist towel may be applied to the site for several minutes. It causes venous dilatation.
- Aseptic precautions are mandatory.

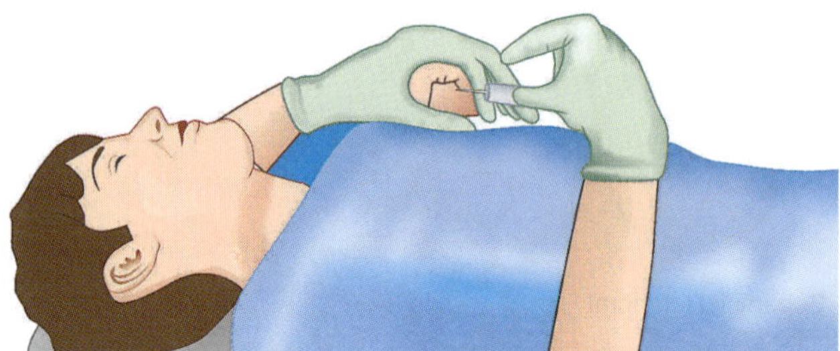

Fig. 5: For inserting the intravenous (IV) cannula on the dorsum of the hand.
The hand may be held flexed at the wrist to occlude venous return and make the veins prominent.

- The methylated spirit is applied over 4–5 cm area at planned site. Let it dry.
- The skin is pulled taut distally to stabilize the vein with a nondominant hand. It is punctured by the needle bevel. up at 15–30° angle parallel to the vein **(Fig. 5)**. After the entry into the SC tissue, the needle is aligned parallel to the skin surface and along the long axis of the vein. Its tip is depressed a little and is advanced until it penetrates the vein. Then, it is made parallel to the vein again and advanced until it is passed fully into the vein. Blood is collected if indicated and then the IV set is attached to it.
- The tourniquet is removed and the infusion is started by releasing the clamp on the tubing. A hub of the cannula and IV set are secured to the skin with the adhesive plaster.
- For flushing the cannula, normal saline should be used and not the distilled water. Distilled water causes pain at IV site and it also causes hemolysis.
- If venipuncture is performed only for collection of blood, pull the needle gently after collecting the required sample and apply steady pressure at the site with a piece of spirit swab for few minutes.

INTRAOSSEOUS INFUSION

Peripheral percutaneous venous access is the fastest method of obtaining vascular access in children. However, during life-threatening emergencies, rapid access to venous compartment through peripheral or central venous route is occasionally difficult or an impossible procedure for a pediatrician to perform. Small peripheral vessels in children often collapse during shock and efforts at setting up an IV line in a peripheral vein may fail. When IV access cannot be established within three attempts or 90 seconds time, intraosseous route should be used as per the recommendations.

Common Sites

- Anteromedial surface of the proximal tibia, one- or two-finger breadths distal to tibial tuberosity to avoid damage to epiphyseal growth plate
- 2–3 cm above the lateral condyle of the femur in the midline
- Medial surface of the distal tibia proximal to the medial malleolus

Technique (Fig. 6)

- Specially designed needles, Jamshidi type available for intraosseous infusion should be used, if available. Hypodermic needle can also be used. 20–16 FG needle can be used for children below 18 months of age, and 16–12 FG for older children.

- Identify the site of placement.
- Patient's leg should be restrained, a small sandbag is placed behind the knee.
- The use of local anesthesia is optional, but usually recommended as it may be more painful once the child is resuscitated.
- Aseptic precautions are must.
- Insert the needle perpendicular to the skin and advance to the periosteum and then with a screwing motion penetrate into the marrow. A distinct "give way" sensation indicates that your needle is in marrow. Confirm that the needle is firmly embedded in the bone.
- Insertion of needle to a depth of 1 cm is usually adequate as the distance from skin through the cortex is rarely >1 cm in infants and children.
- The needle should maintain erect posture without support.
- Trocar is removed and correct position is verified by aspiration of marrow and easy flushing with 5–10 mL of normal saline without signs of extravasation.

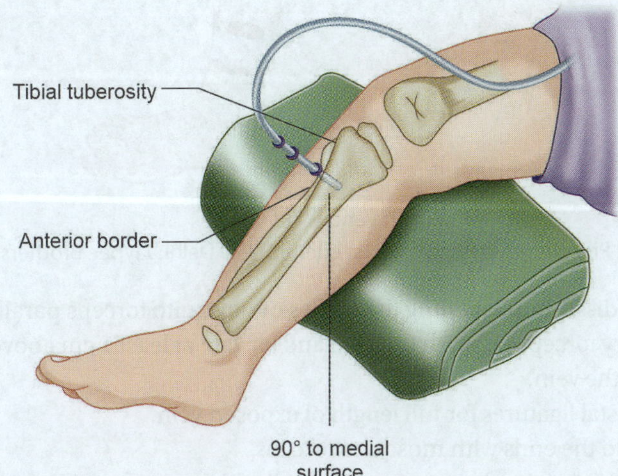

Fig. 6: Intraosseous cannulation technique.
Source: Chameides L. Textbook of Pediatrics Advanced Life Support. Dallas: American Heart Association—American Academy of Pediatrics; 1988.

- The needle should be secured and apply sterile dressing over the site.
- It should be watched for local complications such as extravasation and infection.
- As soon as the peripheral IV route is established, intraosseous needle should be removed.
- Emergency drugs and fluids can be administered via intraosseous route, essentially the same dosage and rates as given by IV route.

VENOUS CUTDOWN (VENESECTION)

Venous cutdown is now rarely resorted to in the present scenario of cannulas and intraosseous access. It is mainly useful when routine IV access has failed in conditions such as shock or when large amounts of fluids have to be given for a long time as in total parenteral nutrition.

Sites

- *Lower limb:* Most preferred site is saphenous vein near ankle.
- *Upper limb:* Median cubital or basilic vein in front of elbow
- Cephalic vein at the wrist at anatomical snuff box
- External jugular vein in the neck

Technique (Fig. 7)

- Get all the instruments ready.
- Prepare the part aseptically. Then it is draped with sterile towels.
- 0.5% Xylocaine is infiltrated subcutaneously at the site of incision. In emergency, local anesthesia can be skipped.
- A 1–2 cm long transverse incision is made 1.5 cm above and in front of medial malleolus over the saphenous vein.

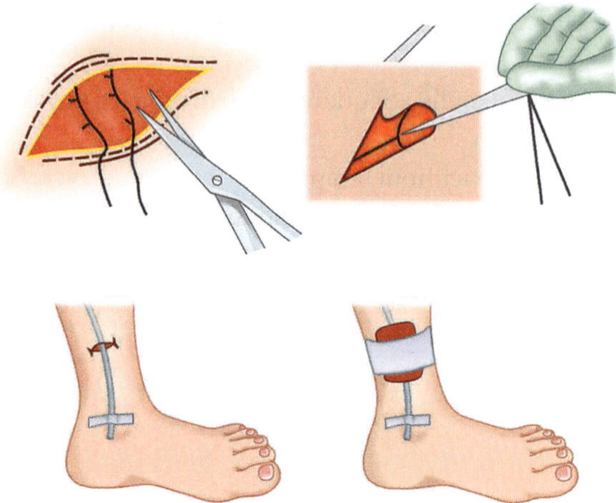

Fig. 7: Venous cut down.

Source: Prajapati BS. Essential Procedures in Pediatrics, 1st edition. New Delhi: Jaypee Brothers Medical Publishers; 2003.

- The vein is exposed by blunt dissection, opening the blades of mosquito forceps parallel to the vein.
- Pass the tip of mosquito artery forceps beneath the vein and elevate at least 1 cm above the vein.
- Pass two silk ligatures under the vein.
- Separate the proximal and distal ligatures for full length of exposed vein.
- Tie the distal ligature and hold the ends with mosquito forceps.
- With venesection scissors put "v"-shaped cut on anterior wall of the vein at middle of the exposed part.
- Introduce polyethylene tube of suitable size proximally through the cut in the vein till the free flow of blood is obtained.
- Cannula is fixed by tying proximal ligature on the vein with cannula in vein.
- Ends of proximal and distal ligatures are trimmed.
- Wound is sutured by silk sutures in a way so that cannula or tube does not get kinked or obstructed.
- Dressing is applied and remaining part of the tube is properly fixed with dressing.
- IV drip is connected to the venesection needle.

Complications

- Wound infections
- Thrombophlebitis
- Deep vein thrombosis
- Air embolism
- Injury to adjacent nerves and vessels.

  As alternate route is possible, earliest venesection tube should be removed.

EXTERNAL JUGULAR VEIN PUNCTURE

The external jugular vein is formed below the ear and behind the angle of mandible, passes downward and obliquely backward across the surface of sternocleidomastoid muscle and ends in subclavian vein lateral to anterior scalene muscle.

Technique (Figs. 8 and 9)

- Place the patient in supine. Both the shoulders should touch the table and head is rotated fully to one side and extended partly over the end of the table so as to extend the vein. Making the child cry makes the vein prominent.
- Restraining the child properly is very important.
- Clean the overlying skin.
- Use proper size of the cannula. Keep the cannula in the direction of the vein with the point aimed toward the same shoulder.
- Make the venipuncture midway between the angle of mandible and midclavicular line.

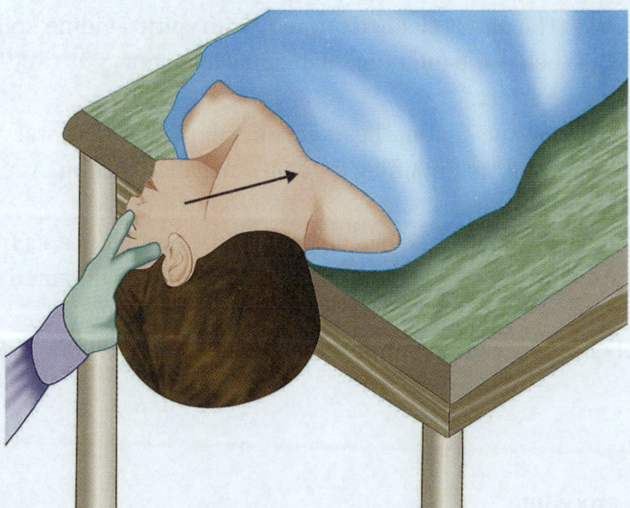

Fig. 8: Position for jugular vein (both internal and external) puncture. The arrow shows the direction of insertion of the needle for external jugular vein puncture.
Source: Silver HK, Kempe CH, Bruyn HB. Handbook of Pediatrics, 13th edition. Singapore: Lange-Maruzen Asia Publications; 1980.

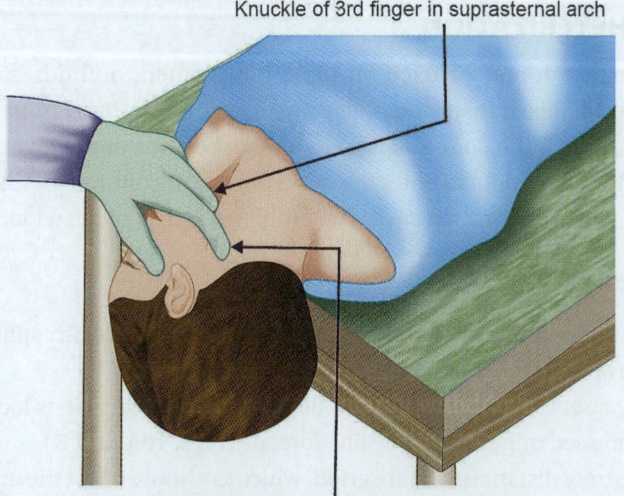

Fig. 9: Internal jugular vein puncture technique.
Source: Silver HK, Kempe CH, Bruyn HB. Handbook of Pediatrics, 13th edition. Singapore: Lange-Maruzen Asia Publications; 1980.

- Proceed as described for veins of extremities.
- After removing the needle, apply constant pressure at puncture site for 5 minutes while the child is sitting.

FEMORAL VEIN PUNCTURE

In view of the risks of femoral venipuncture, it should be used as a last resort for collection of blood samples in neonates and infants.

Technique

- Restraining the infant in frog leg position.
- Clean the inguinal area properly. The part is cleaned properly with spirit—iodine-spirit.
- The femoral artery is located just below the midpoint of inguinal ligament.
- The femoral vein lies medial to the artery.
- Skin is pierced about 1–2 cm as below the inguinal ligament directly over the femoral vein and the needle is advanced at an angle of 30–45° with the skin while maintaining the gentle negative suction. As the vein is punctured, the blood is withdrawn in the syringe.
- If no blood is obtained while needle is inserted, suction should be maintained as the needle is slowly withdrawn. Sometimes needle passes through both the walls of the vein and blood is obtained only when the needle is being withdrawn.
- On removal of needle, apply firm pressure over the site of puncture for at least 3–5 minutes to avoid oozing and hematoma formation.

Precautions

- As far as possible avoid this procedure.
- Strict asepsis is a must as there is potential risk of septic arthritis and osteomyelitis.
- Be careful regarding piercing the femoral artery, which can be identified by bright red color of blood as jet flow of it. If artery is pierced inadvertently, remove the needle and apply pressure for a long time and check the limb periodically for pulsations, color, and warmth.

UMBILICAL VEIN CATHETERIZATION

It is used for exchange transfusion. It may be used for rapid replacement of fluids and blood especially in extreme preterm neonates. Nowadays, exchange transfusion is also preferred by peripheral route.

The umbilical vein spirals through the cord and is at 12 o'clock position at the level of the abdominal wall. Here, it turns cephalad and runs slightly toward right to enter the porta hepatis. It continues with left portal vein, communicates with left hepatic vein and then with inferior vena cava. The umbilical vein is much wider than umbilical arteries.

Technique

- The child should be in supine position with gentle restraining. A padded crucifix splint is used to restrain the baby.
- Sterilize and drape the skin around the umbilical stump.
- The cord is then cut cleanly about 2 cm above the umbilicus and umbilical vein is located at 12 o'clock position. The blood clot in the vein is expressed or pulled out by fine forceps **(Figs. 10A and B)**.
- Mark the catheter for the correct distance to be inserted, which is about 20% of the crown heel length.

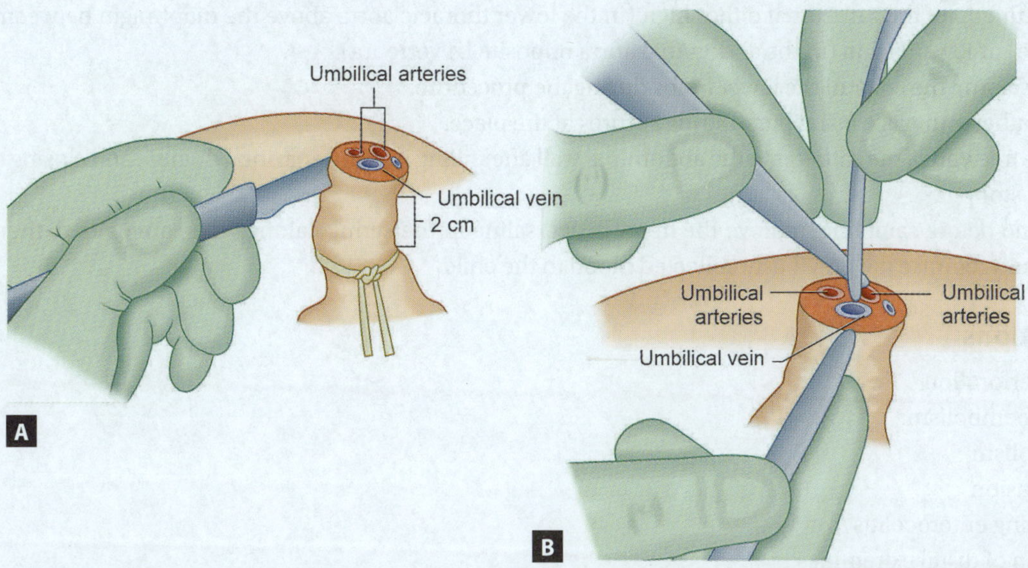

Figs. 10A and B: (A) Cutting the umbilical cord for vessel catheterization; (B) Insertion of umbilical catheter in umbilical vein.
Source: Prajapati BS. Essential Procedures in Pediatrics, 1st edition. New Delhi: Jaypee Brothers Medical Publishers; 2003.

- The catheter is passed into the vein slowly and gently, giving caudal traction on the cord stump till free flow of blood is obtained.
- Flush the catheter with heparinized saline.
- The free end of the catheter should be strapped to the abdominal wall.

Special Points

- If the cord is dried up, it can be excised flush with the umbilicus, which can expose the orifice of the umbilical vein at 12 o'clock position. This can be gently dilated with Hagar's dilator and then catheterized.
- If both these methods fail, supraumbilical cut down will become necessary.
- Remove the umbilical vein catheter within 24–48 hours.
- The catheter tip should be advanced up to thoracic portion of the inferior vena cava.
- While passing the catheter, the resistance is felt at the ductus venosus. The catheter should be passed 1–2 cm beyond this point.

Complications

- Infection
- Vessel perforation
- Thrombosis of portal vein and portal hypertension in the future
- Liver infarction
- Liver abscess
- Necrotizing enterocolitis
- Cardiac arrhythmias

UMBILICAL ARTERY CATHETERIZATION

It is used for periodic monitoring of arterial blood gases and for constant monitoring of blood pressure in a neonate. There are two umbilical arteries and the lumen appears patent.

Technique

- Prepare the umbilical stump as for venous catheterization.
- Identify the artery and insert the catheter gently in the caudal direction, pulling the umbilical stump superiorly.

- Position the tip of the catheter at either high (in the lower thoracic aorta above the diaphragm between T4 and T11 vertebrae) or low position (in the abdominal aorta opposite L4 vertebra).
- Keep observing the color of the lower limbs during the procedure.
- Fix the catheter in place using purse string sutures at the place.
- Strap the free end of the catheter to the abdominal wall after filling it with heparinized saline and closing the end with a rubber stopper.
- Every time before sampling, remove the heparinized saline in the syringe along with same blood, then collect the sample and reinfuse the previously collected blood to the child.

Complications

- Vessel perforation
- Thromboembolism
- Air embolism
- Hypertension
- Necrotizing enterocolitis
- Infarction of distal extremities
- Renal infarction.

RADIAL ARTERY CATHETERIZATION

It is very useful and frequently used for repeated sampling of arterial blood and for continuous arterial pressure monitoring. The radial artery is easily accessible at the wrist in the groove between the tendon of the flexor carpi radialis medially and the distal radius laterally.

Before puncturing the radial artery, carry out the Allen test to assess the ulnar collateral circulation.

Allen Test (Figs. 11A to D)

- Make the patient's hands warm to make pulsations easily demonstrable.
- Have the patient open and close the handheld out in front and then clinch the first tightly closed.
- Occlude both radial and ulnar arteries for 30 seconds. Have the patient open the hand. Hand becomes pale due to occlusion of radial and ulnar arteries.
- Release the pressure over the ulnar artery and observe the open hand for return of normal pink color. Return of normal color within 6 seconds indicates patency of the ulnar artery and an intact arch with good collateral circulation.

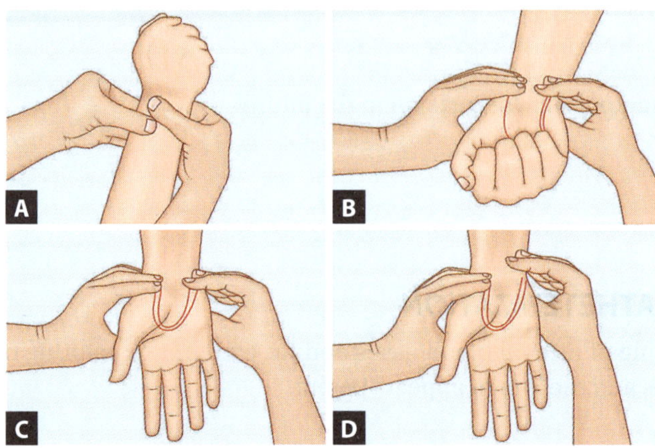

Figs. 11A to D: Allen test.

Source: Prajapati BS. Essential Procedures in Pediatrics, 1st edition. New Delhi: Jaypee Brothers Medical Publishers; 2003.

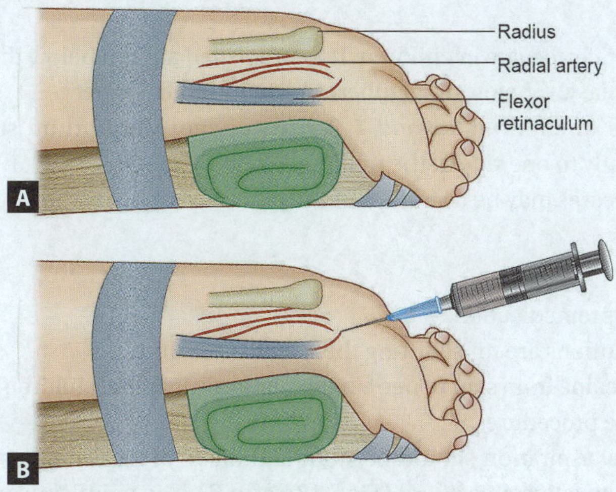

Figs. 12A and B: Radial artery—(A) Anatomy; (B) Catheterization technique.

- Delay of appearance of normal color from 10 seconds to 15 seconds indicates slow filling of the ulnar artery and collaterals.
- Persistent blanching for >15 seconds indicates an incomplete arch or poor collaterals.
- Same test can be performed to check patency of radial artery.
- If ulnar collateral circulation is good, radial artery puncture can be performed.

Technique (Figs. 12A and B)

Patient's hand should be supported and dorsiflexed at the wrist approximately 60° with both hands and lower forearm secured to a board. A roll of gauze behind the wrist will maintain dorsiflexion.

- Locate the radial artery just proximal to head of radius.
- Clean the area and observe the absolutely aseptic precautions.
- Infiltrate the skin with local anesthetic agent.
- Insert the catheter needle at about 30° angle to the surface of the skin and advance the catheter and needle stylet into the artery until blood appears in hub of the needle.
- Remove the needle and attach the hub of the catheter to the connecting tubing.
- Secure the catheter at the place with silk sutures.
- Fix the wrist in a neutral position to the board. It is essential as flexion at wrist can disturb the arterial line.
- Cover the insertion site with sterile dressing.

Special Points

- Do not perform the procedure, if Allen's test is delayed.
- Observe the color of palm periodically after cannulation.
- Before sampling blood, flush the line with 2% normal saline.
- Do not infuse medications and blood products through the arterial line except flushing fluid.

BONE MARROW ASPIRATION

This is a very common ward procedure indicated in children with blood dyscrasias, malignancies and undiagnosed fevers. Needle aspiration, trephine biopsy, and surgical biopsy are three methods available for bone marrow examination. Needle aspiration is commonly practiced in most of the cases in children. It should be done with caution when a defect in clotting mechanism is suspected.

Common Sites

- *Iliac crest:* This is the most preferred site in children. It is performed at 1 cm below the posterior iliac crest.
- *Tibia:* At the upper end of tibia, just below tibial tuberosity on its medial aspect.
- *Sternum:* It should be used in children beyond 7–8 years of age. Manubrium sterni can be used 1 cm above sternomanubrial angle, slightly to one side of the midline.
- Rarely, lumbar spinous processes may be used.

Technique

- Atropine should be given as premedication.
- Aseptic and antiseptic precautions are must during the whole procedure.
- Local infiltration of 1% lignocaine from skin to periosteum. In some irritable children, general anesthesia is desirable for successful outcome of the procedure.
- The needle for bone marrow aspiration should be stout and made of hard stainless steel. It is about 7–8 cm long with a well-fitting stylet and an adjustable guard **(Figs. 13A and B)**. The point of needle and edge of bevel should be sharp. The Sahan and Klima needles are most commonly used needles. Some people prefer to use stout hypodermic needles so that these can be disposed after use and complications of reuse of the needle can be avoided.
- The needle with the guard adjusted 0.5–1 cm from the tip of the needle is introduced into the iliac crest or sternum with screwing or boring movements keeping the needle vertical. The force required varies but needs to be considerable. Sudden giving in of resistance indicates entry of the needle into the bone marrow. Leave the needle and if it remains steady, it indicates that the needle is in the bone marrow.

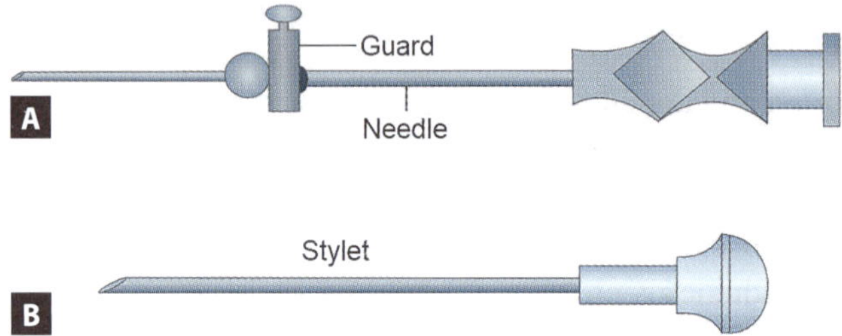

Figs. 13A and B: Bone marrow aspiration needle.

Source: Prajapati BS. Essential Procedures in Pediatrics, 1st edition. New Delhi: Jaypee Brothers Medical Publishers; 2003.

- The stylet is withdrawn and marrow is aspirated with the syringe. About 0.2 mL of marrow is aspirated. This procedure is performed swiftly to obtain only bone marrow particles as slow sluggish aspiration causes dilution of marrow with blood.
- To prevent dilution of marrow with blood, aspirate material only till it appears beyond nozzle of syringe. It is sufficient material for examination. Aspiration beyond it increases the chances of marrow dilution.
- The needle is withdrawn and smear is prepared with marrow. With good material and well-prepared smear marrow, particles can be seen by naked eyes.
- Press the site for 5 minutes. Apply tincture of benzoin seal at puncture site.
- Along with smears of bone marrow, smears from peripheral blood should be prepared and sent for examination.

Complications

- Local pain and hematoma
- Injury to mediastinal structures in case of aspiration at sternum
- Infection
- Dry tap

LUMBAR PUNCTURE

This procedure is performed to obtain cerebrospinal fluid (CSF) sample for analysis in diagnosing infections and other disorders of central nervous system. It is also used for monitoring CSF pressure, intrathecal drug administration, and removing CSF in some cases of hydrocephalus.

Contraindications

- Marked raised intracranial pressure (ICP) with closed fontanel because of the risk of herniation of brain substance through foramen magnum. Papilledema is a marker of raised ICP.

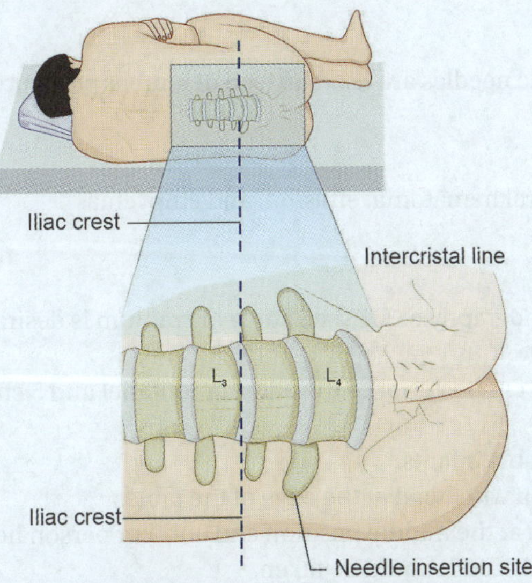

Fig. 14: Position for lumbar puncture.
Source: Prajapati BS. Essential Procedures in Pediatrics, 1st edition. New Delhi: Jaypee Brothers Medical Publishers; 2003.

- Local infection
- Cardiovascular and respiratory instability

Technique

- Informed written consent is must.
- The patient is placed on his side at the edge of the table or bed with the knee drawn up toward abdomen and the head flexed to get maximum flexion of the spine **(Fig. 14)**. If the child is newborn or child has respiratory problem, child should be firmly fixed at shoulders and buttocks only without flexing neck and drawing up knees. In infants, sitting position allows easier identification of the midline. An experienced assistant has a vital role in positioning, restraining, and comforting the patient.
- Aseptic and antiseptic precautions are must.
- Routinely, local anesthesia is not used. But in older children those are irritable; local anesthesia may be useful for performing the procedure smoothly.
- Site of puncture is defined by palpating the iliac crest, which corresponds to L3–L4. Hold the needle between index and middle fingers. In children, instead of lumbar puncture needle with stylet, simple hypodermic needle is commonly used. This should be avoided.
- Gently introduce the needle in midline at above mentioned space, needle being directed toward umbilicus. Entry into the subarachnoid space is indicated by giving the way sensation and free flow of CSF.
- Collect the CSF 0.5 cc in ethylenediaminetetraacetic acid (EDTA) bulb for cell count and 1 cc in plain bulb for biochemistry. It should also be collected in sterile bulb for culture.

- CSF for cell count should be examined at the earliest, usually within 30 minutes.
- Remove the needle and apply firm pressure for few minutes.
- Apply tincture benzoin seal at puncture site.
- In a case of raised ICP, head should be kept little down to prevent herniation of brain through foramen magnum.
- Monitor the patient for some time after the procedure for pulse and respiration.

Complications

- Infection
- Coning
- Headache
- Injury to local structures
- Epidermoid tumor (if hypodermic needles are used instead of lumbar puncture needles)

SUBDURAL TAP

It is indicated for diagnosis of subdural hematoma, effusion, and empyema.

Technique

- Before subdural tapping, ultrasonography or CT scan study of cranium is desirable.
- Informed written consent is must.
- Scalp should be shaved, at least 5 cm posterior to the anterior fontanel and 5 cm lateral to midline and anteriorly up to forehead.
- Sedation may be required in irritable infants.
- Child should be in supine position with head at the edge of the table.
- One person should hold the head at the middle position and another person hold the shoulders **(Fig. 15)**.
- Strict aseptic and antiseptic precautions should be taken.
- Sterilize the area.
- Lateral margins of anterior fontanel are palpated along the coronal sutures and the site is chosen either far lateral as possible or at the area of maximum transillumination.
- It should be at least 2–3 cm from the midline to prevent injury to the underlying sagittal sinus.
- A zig-zag puncture is used to prevent later leakage of subdural fluid.
- A disposable no. 20 G needle is used. The skin is first pulled to one side and then needle is passed perpendicular to the scalp through the suture line and into the subdural space to a depth of approximately 0.3–0.6 cm. A definite pop giving the way is felt on entering the subdural space. The flow of fluid will be there on entering the subdural space. If flow of fluid is not there, slight adjustment or rotation of the needle may be necessary.

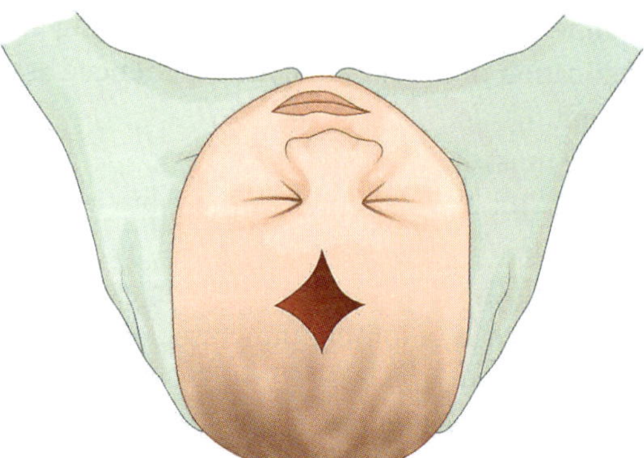

Fig. 15: Position of head for performing subdural tap.
Source: Prajapati BS. Essential Procedures in Pediatrics, 1st edition. New Delhi: Jaypee Brothers Medical Publishers; 2003.

- The subdural fluid is allowed to drain spontaneously. The fluid should not be aspirated for fear of drawing pial vessels into the point of needle.
- The subdural fluid is collected in EDTA and plain tubes for examination. Smear for Gram stain should be prepared. It should also be collected for culture.
- The subdural tap must be performed on both the sides. Samples from both the sides should be kept separate and labeled properly indicating right and left side.
- Maximum 10 mL of fluid should be tapped from each side.
- Subdural fluid will be either blood stained or xanthochromic but not clear. If it is clear, it is most likely CSF through ventricular tapping.
- Remove the needle and sterile benzoin seal is done. Dressing should be done tightly with sterile gauze and adhesive tape.

Complications

- Trauma to blood vessels and hematoma formation
- Infection leading to subdural empyema

VENTRICULAR TAP

This procedure is useful in newborns for diagnosis of ventriculitis and intraventricular hemorrhage. It is also performed to relieve the acute rise of ICP in noncommunicating hydrocephalus. In some conditions, it may be done to administer intraventricular drugs.

Technique

- Before ventricular tapping, ultrasonography or computed axial tomography (CAT) scan study of cranium should be done.
- Informed written consent should be taken.
- Scalp should be shaved.
- Sedation, if necessary
- Aseptic and antiseptic precautions
- Child should be in supine position with head at middle edge of the table.
- One person should hold the head at middle position and another person should hold the shoulders.
- The ventricle is entered by passing no. 23 FG needle in neonates and no. 22 FG in infants, 4–5 cm long disposable needle through lateral margin of anterior fontanel and keeping the direction of needle slightly inward toward inner canthus of opposite eye or nasion **(Fig. 16)**.
- Depending on the degree of ventricular dilatation and size of the patient, the ventricle is reached at the depth of about 2.5 cm.
- Entering the ventricle, gives the way.
- No syringe suction should be applied.
- CSF should be collected in EDTA and plain tubes for examination. Smear should be prepared for Gram stain.
- After removing the needle, press at puncture site for some time.
- Sterile benzoin seal is done. Dressing should be done with sterile gauze and adhesive tape.
- In a case of hydrocephalus, CSF can be drained in large quantity.
- For administering drugs in ventricles, drug should be taken in the syringe and after ventricular puncture, it should be attached with the needle. Let the CSF come in syringe, get the medicine diluted in CSF and then inject back into the ventricle. Drug should not be diluted in any solution.

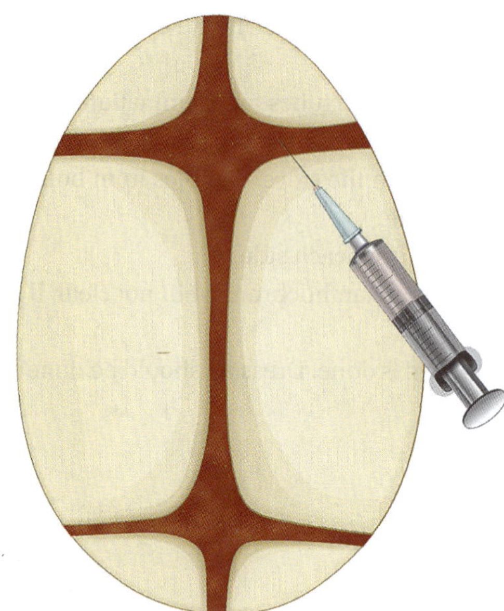

Fig. 16: Ventricular tapping—the needle should be directed forward and inward toward nasion.
Source: Prajapati BS. Essential Procedures in Pediatrics, 1st edition. New Delhi: Jaypee Brothers Medical Publishers (P) Ltd; 2003.

Complications

- Ventriculitis
- Injury to brain tissues
- Intraventricular hemorrhage

NASOGASTRIC TUBE INSERTION

Nasogastric tube is passed for either aspiration of gastric contents or administration of feeds or therapeutic substances. Nowadays, silastic and polyethylene tubes are being used because they have less tissue reactions.

Indications

Diagnostic

- Gastric aspirate test for diagnosis of neonatal septicemia
- Shake test for lung maturity in preterm babies
- Examination of gastric contents for *Mycobacterium tuberculosis*
- Assessment of upper gastrointestinal (GI) tract bleeding
- Measurement of gastric volume

Therapeutic

- Paralytic ileus
- Intestinal obstruction
- Enteral feeding
- Administration of therapeutic substances

Contraindications

- Esophageal stricture
- Ingestion of alkali—may cause esophageal perforation

- Head and neck injury preventing passage of tube
- Nasal fracture

Technique

- The head is raised in semiupright position.
- The distance from nose to earlobe and from ear lobe to xiphoid process is determined to measure the length of the tube to be passed. The point is marked on the tube **(Figs. 17A and B)**.
- The more patent nostril is selected for passing the tube.
- The terminal part of the tube is lubricated with a lubricant. It is avoided in newborns to prevent aspiration of an oily substance. In that case, it is wet with water.
- The tube is passed into the nostril, its curve directs downward as it passes along the floor of the nose. In case of difficulty, it is tried in another nostril. Resistance is felt when it reaches the nasopharynx. Getting the patient to sip a little water helps to overcome it.

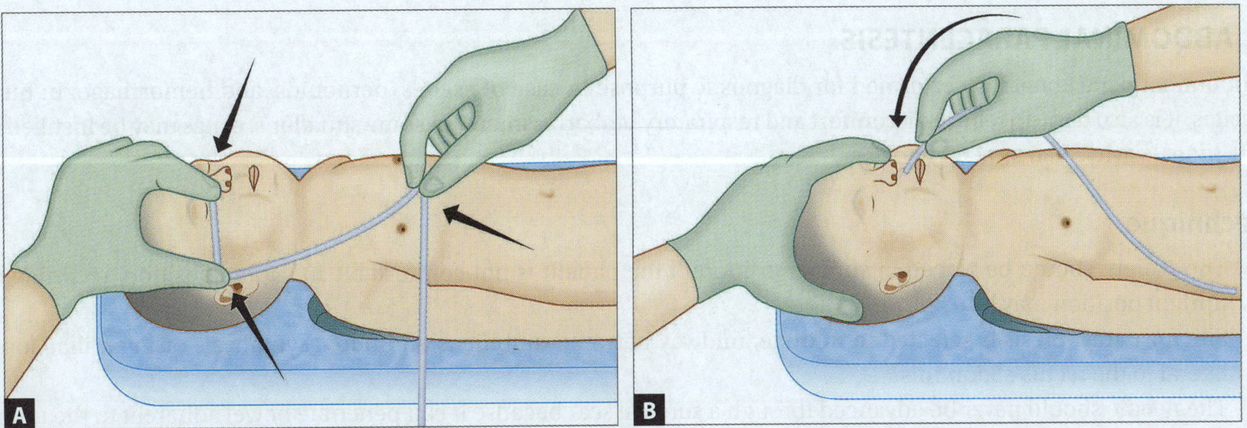

Figs. 17A and B: Method of inserting a nasogastric tube in a child.
Source: World Health Organization. Management of the child with a serious infection or severe malnutrition: guidelines for care at the first-referral level in Developing Countries Department of Child and Adolescent Health and Development. Geneva: World Health Organization; 2000.

- With swallowing of the saliva or water by the patients, the tube is advanced into the esophagus.
- If the patient gags or the tube coils up in the mouth, the tube is withdrawn partly and again it is passed.
- The tube is passed up to the mark as measured length of the tube to be passed.
- Confirmation of proper placement is done by the following tests:
  - Aspiration of stomach contents on applying suction at the outer end of the tube with a syringe indicates that the tube lies in the stomach.
  - Air is injected into the tube while epigastric area is auscultated. A sound is heard if the tube is in the stomach.
  - Placing a tube in a glass of water and escape of air bubbles in the water indicate that the tube lies in the trachea.
  - Placement of a radiopaque tube can be assessed by radiography.
- The tube is fixed with a tape in a butterfly fashion around the tube or with vertical tapping over the nose and the tube. The tapping is done in such a way that the tube rests in the middle of the nasal lumen and not directly in contact with mucosa. It is not taped over the forehead as it may cause pressure necrosis of the nose.
- The feed or drug should be allowed to go in the tube by gravity method. It should not be pushed by piston. The tube should be flushed with water periodically.
- While removing the tube, pinch the tube end to prevent spilling of the contents into the trachea.

Complications

- Pulmonary aspiration
- Esophageal perforation
- Gastric perforation
- Nasal necrosis
- Esophageal stricture

  Instead of nasogastric tubing, nowadays orogastric tubing is preferred to avoid certain complications.

GASTRIC LAVAGE

It is useful in removing the poisonous substance from the stomach. In corrosives and hydrocarbons ingestion, gastric lavage is contraindicated. In corrosives, passing the tube may cause perforation. Since passing the gastric tube is likely to induce vomiting, it increases the risk of aspiration of hydrocarbons into the trachea and lungs, which causes pneumonia.

After passing the tube in the stomach as described in nasogastric tube insertion, lavage of the stomach using aliquots of normal saline is done in cases of poisoning. It is continued till the color of the lavage is normal.

ABDOMINAL PARACENTESIS

Abdominal paracentesis is performed for diagnostic purpose in case of ascites, peritonitis, and hemorrhage. In huge ascites, it is also done to relieve discomfort and respiratory embarrassment. In some situations, drugs may be instilled in peritoneal cavity such as malignancies.

Technique

- The patient should be placed in supine position. If the patient is not comfortable in supine position, reclining or upright position may be used.
- Site for paracentesis is selected in midline, midway between umbilicus and pubic symphysis or in an iliac fossa lateral to the rectus abdominis.
- The needle should never be advanced through a surgical scar because it can penetrate bowel adherent to the under surface of the scar, or lacerate an omental or mesenteric vessel.
- Informed written consent should be taken.
- Aseptic and antiseptic measures must be taken.
- Injection atropine as premedication
- One percent lignocaine is infiltrated under skin and into the deeper structures at the site selected for paracentesis. Wait for few minutes for full effect of anesthetic agent.
- The hypodermic needle 20 FG is attached to 20 mL syringe. It is passed into the peritoneal cavity perpendicular to the skin. As the needle enters the peritoneal cavity, it gives the way and ascitic fluid starts to drain through the needle.
- In a case of tense ascites, needle should be passed obliquely or skin should be retracted caudally before insertion of the needle to produce a Z-track effect on withdrawing the needle so that needle tract after paracentesis gets sealed properly and persistent drainage can be prevented after removal of the needle.
- After removal of fluid, 10–15 mL for diagnostic purpose, the needle is withdrawn and a seal of tincture benzoin is applied locally.
- If the paracentesis is for therapeutic purpose, the needle should be connected with IV set and regulator of IV set is adjusted in such a way that ascitic fluid is drained slowly. One liter of fluid may be drained over a period of 2–3 hours.
- The patient should be watched following the procedure.

COMPLICATIONS

- Intestinal perforation or laceration
- Peritonitis

- Postparacentesis shock
- Electrolyte imbalance
- Hypoproteinemia
- Perforation of urinary bladder
- Pneumoperitoneum

LIVER BIOPSY

Nowadays, liver biopsy is done under the ultrasound (USG) guidance rather than blind biopsy.

Indications

- Chronic hepatitis
- Undiagnosed hepatomegaly
- Neonatal hepatitis
- Cirrhosis of liver
- Fever of unknown origin

Contraindications

- Bleeding tendency
- Massive and tense ascites
- Severe portal hypertension

Prerequisites

- Bleeding time, clotting time, platelet count, and prothrombin time
- Ultrasound study of liver
- *Premedication:* Atropine 0.01 mg/kg IM 30 minutes before the procedure.

Technique

- Vim-Silverman needle, Menghini's needle, and Tru-cut needles are used for liver biopsy. Tru-cut needle is disposable, easy to operate, and has more success rate, so it is common in use.
- Informed written consent is a must.
- Patient is kept in supine position, near the edge of the bed or table with the right arm under the head and left arm by the side.
- Preparation of the local area
- Aseptic and antiseptic precautions are must.
- 1% lignocaine is infiltrated in the skin, intercostal muscles, and Glisson's capsule. Wait for some time for good effect of the anesthetic agent. Some children may require sedation or general anesthesia.
- The Tru-cut needle is introduced under USG guidance into the liver substance with the inner needle retracted. The latter is then advanced, holding the outer cutting sheath steady. The outer sheath is then advanced to cut the liver in the biopsy notch. The whole apparatus is then withdrawn together quickly. The entire sequence should take only few seconds.
- The Vim-Silverman needle has trocar and bifid needle to cut the liver tissue. In Menghini's needle, the cut piece of liver is sucked into the syringe applied with negative pressure.
- On removal of the needle, the puncture site is sealed with tincture of benzoin.

THORACOCENTESIS (INTERCOSTAL DRAINAGE)

Thoracocentesis refers to temporary insertion of a needle or a catheter into the pleural space for removal of fluid or air from the pleural cavity. The fluid is collected for diagnostic purpose and in some situations, it is done for therapeutic purpose to remove fluid or air, which is in large quantity and causes respiratory embarrassment. Drugs can also be instilled in the pleural cavity by this procedure, if it is indicated, such as in a case of malignancy.

Technique

- Written consent is must.
- *Injection:* Atropine as premedication
- Site of insertion of needle can be decided by chest X-ray, dull note on percussion, and USG study of thorax. Best way to perform the procedure is under USG guidance.
- It should be performed in sitting position of the patient. Patient can lean forward on the table of suitable height with head resting on his forearms **(Fig. 18)**.
- Strict aseptic and antiseptic measures should be taken.
- 1% lignocaine is infiltrated at the upper border of the rib below the space chosen. Anesthetizing wide area and generous infiltration of local anesthetic agent for good anesthesia help to get good cooperation of the patient, performing the whole procedure comfortably leading to successful performance with minimal chances of complications. Wait for some time for good effect of anesthetic agent.
- A wide-bore needle is connected on one side of the three-way stopcock and opposite to it a syringe is attached. Three-way stopcock is arranged in such a way that there is a single track between the needle, stopcock, and syringe.
- The needle is inserted into the chest in the same manner as for the anesthetic needle, finding the intercostal space and stepping over the lower rib with care, thereby preventing damage to underlying structures **(Fig. 19)**. Slight suction is applied to the syringe so that the fluid is aspirated in the syringe immediately as the needle enters the pleural space.

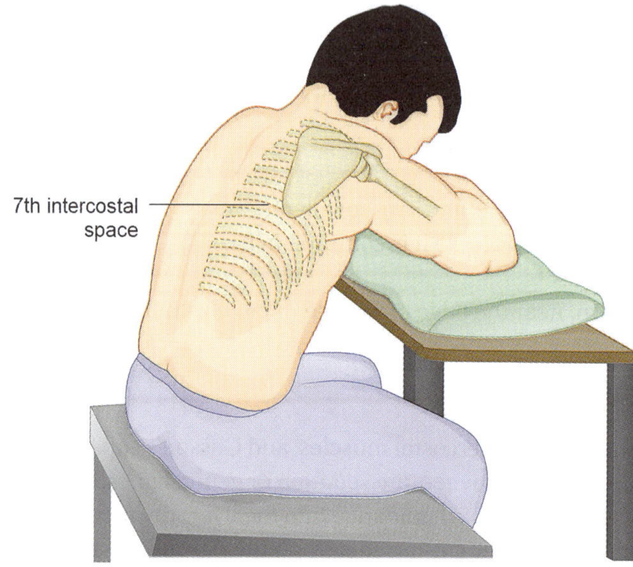

Fig. 18: Another position for doing thoracocentesis.
Source: Johnson KB. The Harriet Lane Handbook—a manual for pediatric house officers, 13th edition. New Delhi: Jaypee Brothers Medical Publishers; 1993.

- Fluid should be withdrawn slowly and steadily.
- A forceps should be attached to the needle at the skin level, which helps to prevent excessively deep insertion of the needle into the thorax.
- The fluid is aspirated in the syringe and then three-way stopcock is turned to connect the syringe with the outlet, which is attached to IV set.

- Collect the fluid in EDTA and plain tubes. It is also collected for culture. Smear should be prepared for Gram's stain and Ziehl-Neelsen stain.
- The three-way tap is now turned again to connect the syringe with the needle and the pleural space, a further aspiration is carried out. It is expelled into the drainage bag by turning the three-way tap. The drainage bag or bottle should be placed well below the level of the patient's chest.
- As fluid is removed, the lung expands and this often makes the patient to cough.
- The needle is withdrawn and puncture site is covered with a benzoin seal. A sterile gauze is put over it and adhesive tape is applied.

Complications

- Pneumothorax
- Hemothorax
- Infection
- Unilateral pulmonary edema
- Hypoproteinemia

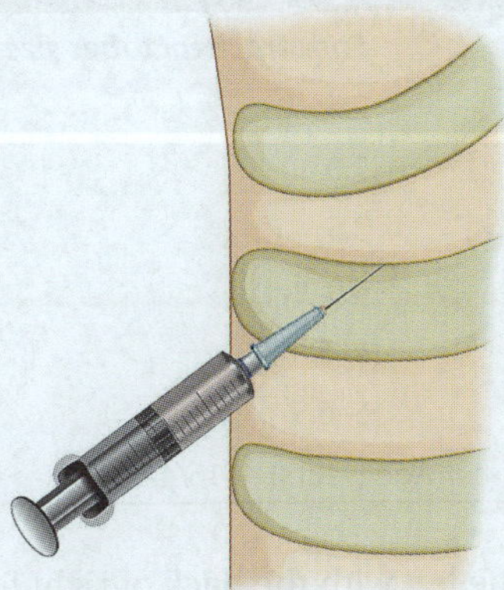

Fig. 19: Site of needle for pleural fluid aspiration.

Source: Prajapati BS. Essential Procedures in Pediatrics, 1st edition. New Delhi: Jaypee Brothers Medical Publishers; 2003.

ENDOTRACHEAL INTUBATION

Endotracheal intubation is a procedure, which every pediatrician and one working in intensive care units must be well conversant with. The critically ill patient often requires endotracheal intubation. It secures patent airway. It is a prerequisite for mechanical ventilation. Endotracheal suction can most efficiently be done through an endotracheal tube (ET). It is indicated when bag and mask resuscitation fails in a case of an asphyxiated newborn.

Indications

- *In neonatal asphyxia:*
  - Bag and mask resuscitation fails.
  - Apparently, stillborn baby after adequate suctioning of upper airways
  - Infants with diaphragmatic hernia
  - Meconium aspiration
- Cardiorespiratory arrest due to any cause
- Central nervous system depression in a case of head injury or comatose child

- Diseases of peripheral nervous system, poliomyelitis, Guillain-Barré syndrome, tetanus, organophosphorus poisoning, etc.
- Administration of general anesthesia

Equipment

- Laryngoscope—with straight blade for neonates
- Endotracheal tubes for various sizes with stylet **(Table 1)**

Technique

- The patient is placed in a supine position. The operator stands beyond the patient's head. Patient's neck is slightly extended with the head in midline.
- Clear the oropharynx with gentle suctioning.
- Empty the stomach.
- Hold the handle of laryngoscope in left hand with thumb and first three fingers; stabilize the hand with fifth finger resting on patient's cheek. The blade should be pointing away from oneself.

TABLE 1: Endotracheal tube size according to weight of child.

Weight/age	*Endotracheal tubes size (ID in mm)*
<1,000 g	2.5
1,000–2,000 g	3.0
2,000–3,000 g	3.5
>3,000 g	4.0
1–5 years	4–5
5–12 years	5–6.5
Approximately size of ET, internal diameter (ID) in mm = Age (years) + 16/4.	

- Open the baby's mouth and push the tongue left with the back of right forefinger and steady the head with the rest of right hand.
- While visualizing insert the blade, midline until the tip is between base of tongue and epiglottis within the vallecula **(Figs. 20A and B)**.
- If the infant is making respiratory effort, free flow of oxygen with an oxygen tubing held close to the infant's mouth and nose is to be provided during intubation.
- Open the mouth further by pulling on laryngoscope handle, simultaneously tilt the blade tip upward slightly to elevate epiglottis and visualize the glottis. Use base of the tongue as pivot rather than maxilla.
- Suction is needed.
- Have the assistant to palpate suprasternal notch with index finger, applying gentle pressure, if desired.
- Hold the tube with concave curve anterior and pass it down to right side of the mouth, outside the blade, along with maintaining visualization.
- As the patient inspires, pass the tube through cords 2 cm into trachea or until immediately after tip passes under assistant's finger in suprasternal notch.
- The tube is then held firmly at the lips with the right hand, and the laryngoscope and stylet are carefully removed.
- Initially, confirmation of the tube placement is accomplished by attaching a resuscitation bag with the connector and ventilating the infant. With correctly placed tube, the air entry is heard on both sides of the chest, breath sounds are of equal intensity and air is not heard entering the stomach. While listening to the breath sounds, the stethoscope is to be placed at approximately the nipple line.
- Note the centimeter marks on the tube at the level of upper lips and then secure the tube to the infant's face.

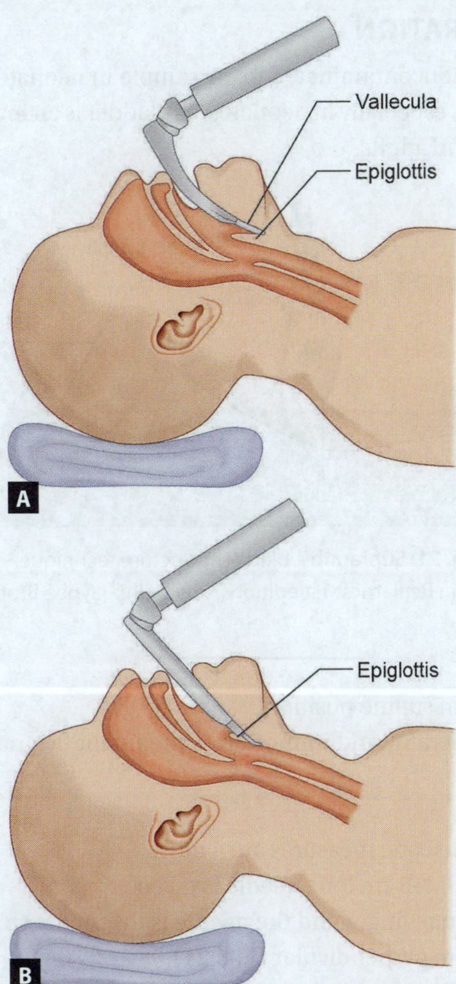

Figs. 20A and B: Position of laryngoscope blade when using (A) Curved blade, it is in the vallecula; (B) Straight blade, it is over the epiglottis.

Source: Prajapati BS. Essential Procedures in Pediatrics, 1st edition. New Delhi: Jaypee Brothers Medical Publishers; 2003.

- Final confirmation of placement of the tube can be obtained by chest film, if it is needed.
- Attempts to intubate should not exceed 30 seconds. If you are unable to intubate within 30 seconds, abort and continue with bag and mask and then try again after a few minutes. Repeated attempts may cause serious glottic edema and bleeding.
- Intubation is not a matter of prestige. If you are unable to do so, please ask for help.
- ET route is also used for administration of some drugs such as epinephrine, atropine, and naloxone.

Complications

- Hypoxia
- Bradycardia
- Apnea
- Pneumothorax
- Injury and lacerations to tongue, gums, pharynx, epiglottis, trachea, vocal cords, etc.
- Infections
- Postextubation stridor can be managed by nebulized epinephrine or steroids.

Some physicians prefer nasotracheal intubation when long-term ventilation is required.

SUPRAPUBIC BLADDER ASPIRATION

This procedure is performed to collect noncontaminated urine sample in neonates and infants. It is a safe and reliable way of collecting urine samples. It is easy, especially in neonates, as bladder is an intra-abdominal organ in these patients unlike a pelvic organ in older children and adults.

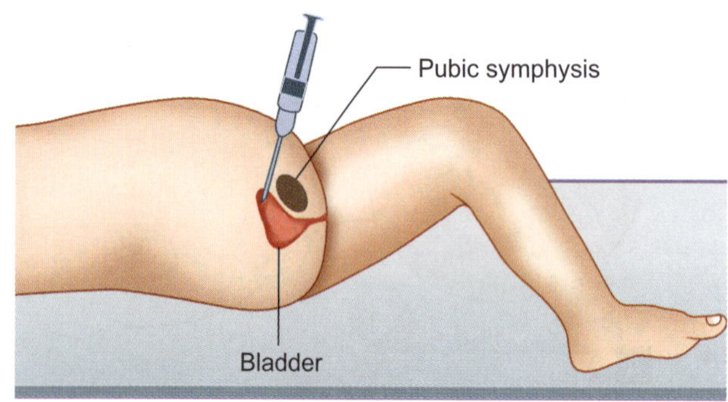

Fig. 21: Suprapubic bladder puncture technique.
Source: Prajapati BS. Essential Procedures in Pediatrics, 1st edition. New Delhi: Jaypee Brothers Medical Publishers (P) Ltd; 2003.

Technique

- The infant is placed on a flat surface in supine position.
- The assistant stands opposite the operator and immobilizes the infant by grasping the thorax with one hand and thighs and hips with the other.
- Make sure that the bladder is full.
- Local part is cleaned. Aseptic and antiseptic measures are a must.
- A 10-cc disposable syringe with 22 FG, 4–5 cm long needle is taken.
- The pubic symphysis is located with one finger and the needle is inserted 2 cm above the symphysis in the midline with syringe held at 10–20° angles from perpendicular **(Fig. 21)**.
- With a single steady motion, the needle is inserted until a perceptive change in resistance is felt as the needle enters the bladder.
- Light aspiration is applied to aspirate the urine specimen.
- After removal of needle, a seal of tincture benzoin is applied at puncture site.

PERITONEAL DIALYSIS

Dialysis involves the use of semipermeable membranes that permit the simultaneous passage of smaller molecular weight solutes and water while retarding or inhibiting the movement of large-sized particles. The basic principle controlling the transmembrane movement of solute and water are similar whether the membrane is artificial (hemodialysis) or natural (peritoneal dialysis).

Indications

- Blood urea >300 mg/dL
- Serum hyperkalemia—K^+ >6.5 mEq/L not responding to medical line of treatment
- Severe acidosis
- Pulmonary edema
- Acute left ventricular failure
- Drug intoxications such as barbiturates and salicylates
- Life-threatening electrolyte imbalance

Contraindications

- Peritonitis.
- Abdominal adhesions
- Laparotomy done
- Pleuroperitoneal communication

Technique (Fig. 22)

- Informed written consent
- Aseptic and antiseptic measures are must.
- Injection atropine 0.01 mg/kg IM 30 minutes before the procedure as the premedication
- Sedation, if required
- Proper restraining
- Bladder is emptied by its own or catheterization, if it is necessary
- Abdominal wall is prepared, painting spirit—betadine spirit. Towel draping
- The catheter is usually placed in the midline few centimeters below the umbilicus.
  If midline insertion is not possible, the catheter can be inserted in the flank area, outside the line of inferior epigastric artery.
- The site is anesthetized by injecting 1% lignocaine up to peritoneum.

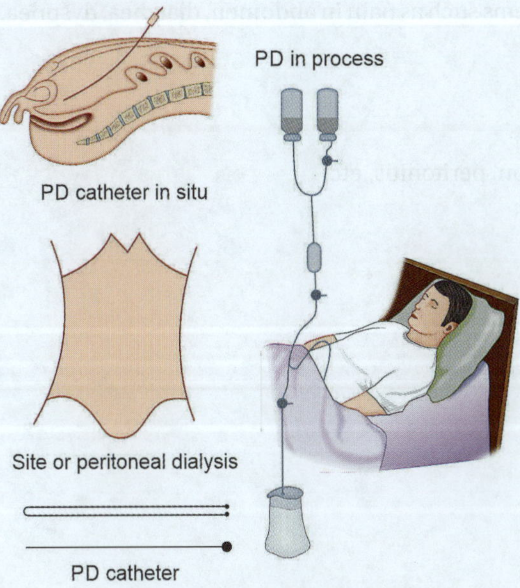

Fig. 22: Peritoneal dialysis (PD).
Source: Prajapati BS. Essential Procedures in Pediatrics, 1st edition. New Delhi: Jaypee Brothers Medical Publishers (P) Ltd; 2003.

- If there is no ascites, distend the abdomen with 10 mL/kg dialysate solution using 17–20 FG angiocath or needle.
- Needle is withdrawn and a knife blade is used to enlarge the puncture wound in the skin.
- If ascites is present, a very small penetrating incision is made in the skin and the trocar with catheter is stabilized with the fingers of one hand on the skin while the other hand introduces the trocar through the abdominal wall with an alternating drilling motion.
- Penetration up to peritoneum is detected by a definite sensation of giving the way and also by the appearance of fluid in the catheter when trocar is removed.
- On reaching the peritoneal cavity and before removing the trocar, the catheter is gradually advanced in the peritoneal cavity in right or left paracolic gutter and trocar is gradually withdrawn.

- When the catheter is sufficiently introduced in the peritoneal cavity, trocar is removed totally. All the fenestrations on the catheter must be within the peritoneal cavity to avoid SC fluid infiltration in the abdominal wall. In neonates and infants, IV catheters or simple feeding tube can be used.
- The catheter should be stabilized with adhesive plaster.
- The catheter is connected with the administration tubing through small connector, and dialysis fluid is flown.
- Because hyperkalemia is often present, potassium-free fluid is used for the first three–six cycles.
- Time of input of dialysis fluid will be about 10–15 minutes. The fluid is kept in the peritoneal cavity for about 30 minutes. Time for output of dialysis fluid will be about 15–20 minutes. Each cycle will take about an hour. First few cycles should be of half an hour (rapid cycles).
- Record the weight of the patient prior to the procedure and every 12 hours.
- Total duration of dialysis is about 40 hours depending on the clinical and biochemical parameters.
- Warm the dialysate to body temperature.
- Infuse it by gravity flow.
- Each cycle should be of 30–50 mL/kg.
- Blood sugar, blood urea, serum creatinine, serum electrolytes and serum proteins should be checked 12 hourly.
- In the presence of fluid overload, use hypertonic dialysate.
- Tip of the catheter should be sent for culture.
- Close the site of dialysis by sterile bandage
- Peritoneal dialysis-related problems such as pain in abdomen, diarrhea, dyspnea, bleeding, and fluid delivery should be sorted out appropriately.

Complications

- Pain may be due to over distention, peritonitis, etc.
- Bleeding
- Dialysate leak
- Outflow obstruction
- Peritonitis
- Metabolic complications
- Thrombosis
- Pulmonary complications

RENAL BIOPSY

Indications

- Steroid-resistant nephrotic syndrome
- Asymptomatic proteinuria
- Glomerulonephritis associated with conditions such as systemic lupus erythematosus, Henoch–Schönlein purpura, etc.
- Rapidly progressive glomerulonephritis.

Contraindications

- Bleeding diathesis
- Solitary functioning kidney
- Ectopic/horseshoe-shaped kidney
- Severe uncontrolled hypertension

Prerequisites

- Bleeding time, clotting time, partial thromboplastin time (PTT) or activated partial thromboplastin time (APTT), and platelets count
- Blood grouping and cross-matching
- Hypertension and uremia should be controlled.
- Informed written consent is a must.

Technique

- Atropine 0.01 mg/kg IM before 30 minutes of the procedure.
- The patient is placed in the prone position on a firm bed. A pillow is placed under patient's abdomen. This compresses and fixes the kidneys to the posterior abdominal wall, bringing the kidneys closer to the skin and limiting possible ballottement of the kidney by the biopsy needle.
- Ultrasonography is commonly used to mark the location of kidneys and point of entry of the needle into the kidney perpendicular to the skin surface and to obtain depth of tissue from skin surface. Usually, lower pole of left kidney is selected for biopsy.
- The area is prepared and local anesthesia is given. Irritable children may need general anesthesia.
- A 23-gauge exploring lumbar puncture needle is passed downward and obliquely toward the lower pole of the kidney. A needle can be felt going through different structures and renal capsule. Experienced person feels "give-in" feeling up on penetration of capsule of kidney.
- The patient is asked to take slow deep breathings. If the needle is in the kidney, a characteristic pendular movement is seen with respiration, the hub of needle swings through a wide arch, moving toward head during inspiration, and toward buttock during expiration. If the needle is not in the kidney tissue, it is slightly advanced until it penetrates kidneys and moves characteristically on breathing. The depth of the kidney below the skin is measured on the stem of the needle.
- A small nick is made over anesthetized area with a scalpel.
- Franklin modified Vim–Silverman needle and Tru-cut needle are commonly used in the practice. Tru-cut needle is easy to use and having less failure rate. Therefore, Tru-cut needle is preferred nowadays.
- Tru-cut needle is one-piece apparatus with a length of 11.4 cm or 15 cm. The needle with cannula covering the obturator is advanced in the kidney to desired length in a direction perpendicular to skin surface.
- The patient is asked to hold the breath in deep inspiration.
- The obturator is advanced by firm tap on the handle. The specimen is cut by downward movement of cannula over obturator.
- Entire assembly is removed.
- The patient is asked to breathe normally.
- Firm pressure is applied over biopsy site for few minutes and the site is sealed with tincture benzoin. Two good cores of tissue (8–10 mm long) are needed for adequate histological examination. One is immediately fixed in buffered formalin and other in saline (for immunofluorescence study).

Postprocedure Management

- The patient is asked to remain in prone position for 2 hours and in bed for 24 hours.
- Monitoring temperature, pulse, respiratory rate (RR), and blood pressure (BP) 1 hourly for 6 hours and then 4 hourly for 24 hours.
- Urine should be collected in separate bottles during each voiding and should be checked for hematuria.
- Patient is asked to take ample liquids orally.
- Diuretics may be given in case of oliguria to flush any clot in the passage.
- If no frank hematuria and vitals are normal, patient can be discharged after 24 hours with instructions not to do exertion for a week.

Complications

- Hematuria
- Perinephric hematoma
- Arteriovenous (AV) fistula

PERICARDIOCENTESIS

Pericardiocentesis is a procedure for removal of fluid from pericardial cavity for diagnostic purpose or to relieve cardiac tamponade. It is occasionally a life-saving procedure. It is a risky procedure. It should be performed only by skilled person under continuous cardiac monitoring. Echocardiographic diagnosis is must before performing the procedure. It gives idea regarding amount of fluid and also helps to determine the anatomical approach.

Prerequisites

- Echocardiographic diagnosis
- Coagulation profile
- Resuscitation kit including defibrillator
- Cardiac monitor
- IV line
- Premedication with injection atropine 0.01 mg/kg IM 30 minutes before the procedure

Technique

- Informed written consent should be taken.
- Sedation may be required in some patients. If possible, it should be avoided.
- Child should be seated leaning backward at approximately 60° and carefully restrained.
- The best site is xiphocostal angle. The other sites are fourth, fifth, or sixth intercostal spaces 1–2 cm medial to the border of cardiac dullness on percussion.
- Aseptic and antiseptic precautions are must.
- 1% xylocaine is infiltrated in the skin at left xiphocostal angle, 3–4 cm below left costal margin. The needle is advanced initially perpendicular to the skin surface and after traversing the soft tissue under the rib cage, its tip is pointed to the left shoulder. While advancing the needle in the deeper structures, if it reaches to pericardial cavity, the pericardial fluid is withdrawn in the syringe. Local anesthetic agent should not be injected in the pericardial cavity.
- The pericardiocentesis needle is passed along the same path until the fluid is obtained. The distance from skin to the pericardium is <5 cm in a child. A distinct "give" or "pop" is felt when the pericardium is punctured. Pericardial fluid can then be aspirated.
- Getting the fluid confirms the position of needle into the pericardial cavity. Normal saline can be injected under two-dimensional (2D) echo monitoring, which shows bubbles of saline.
- If the blood or bloody fluid is withdrawn, it is vital to determine if cardiac chamber or coronary artery has been punctured. Still uremia and malignant diseases can give rise to hemorrhagic pericardial effusion. Blood obtained from heart or coronary vessel clots immediately.
- Fluid is sent for appropriate examinations.
- The needle is withdrawn and benzoin seal is done at puncture site.
- Postprocedure monitoring of heart rate, RR, and BP should be done. 2D echo may be performed to study postpericardiocentesis condition.

Complications

- Hemopericardium
- Arrhythmias

- Vasovagal reactions
- Infection
- Pneumothorax
- Air embolism
- Perforation of an abdominal viscus, commonly stomach
- Cardiac arrest and death

FINE-NEEDLE ASPIRATION BIOPSY

Fine-needle aspiration biopsy (FNAB) is very useful for cytological and bacteriological evaluation of a mass or a lymph node. It is minimally invasive and requires no sedation. It aids in tissue diagnosis and in determining the course of management.

Requirements

- 1^2 1.5^2 20–25 FG needles. 22 FG 1^2 long is the most commonly used size of needle.
- 10–20 mL plastic disposable syringes
- Clean glass slides
- About 70–90% ethanol for routine wet fixation
- Containers for culture media whenever needed

Technique

- Sterilize the area.
- Anesthesia is usually not required, local anesthetic agent may be used in uncooperative and irritable children.
- Immobilize the lump to be biopsied between your thumb and finger with one hand.
- Hold the syringe in the other hand and insert needle into the assigned area, perpendicular to the skin surface and position the needle within the target tissue.
- Pull the syringe plunger to apply negative pressure.
- While maintaining suction, make several passes through the mass or node.
- Release the negative pressure while needle remains in the target tissue.
- Withdraw the needle.
- Detach the needle, draw 2–3 mL air into the syringe, reattach the needle, and blow the aspirates on to the slide.
- Apply the pressure over the puncture site with cotton swab for 5 minutes.
- Deep biopsies can be done with assistance of radiological imaging techniques such as USG.
- The following situations can give unsatisfactory yield during FNAB:
  - When needle misses the lesion tangentially.
  - When central area is cystic, necrotic, or hemorrhagic and devoid of diagnostic material.
  - When there is a small malignant lesion close to a dominant benign mass.
  - When the target tissue is fibrosclerotic and poor in cells.

CHAPTER 51

Miscellaneous

AUDIOGRAM

QUESTIONS

Q-1. What is an audiogram?

An audiogram is a graph that shows the softest sounds a person can hear at different pitches or frequencies. The closer the marks are to the top of the graph, the softer sounds that person can here. Where the patient's results fall on the audiogram indicate the different degrees of hearing loss. The audiogram shown below indicates the different degrees of hearing loss.

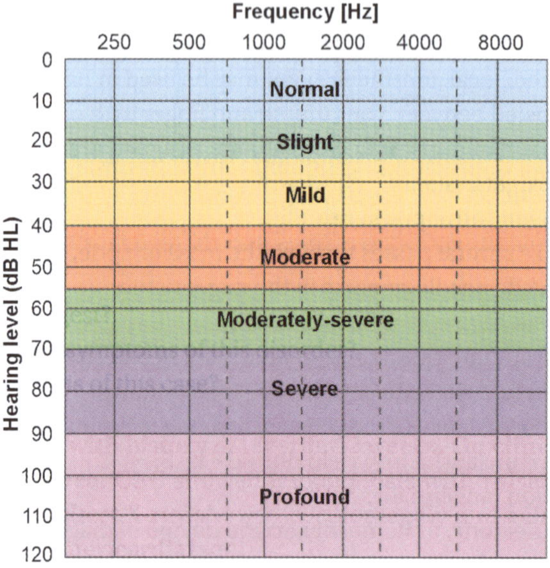

Q-2. What does an audiogram show?

- *Frequency:* The horizontal line on the graph shows the pitch of the sound measured in hertz (Hz).
- *Loudness:* The vertical line on the graph shows the intensity of sound measured in decibel (dB).
- *Symbols:*
  - An 'O' is used to represent responses on the right ear.
  - An 'X' is used to represent responses to the left ear.

Q-3. What the numbers mean?

- Across the top of the graph, there are numbers from 250 to 8000. These numbers (measured in Hz) represent the frequencies (pitches) of the sound.
- On the left side of the graph, there are numbers from -10 to 110. These numbers (measured in dB) represent the intensity (loudness) of the sound presented.

Common Sounds and their Intensity (dB)

- *Near total silence:* 0 dB
- *Whispering:* 15 dB
- *Refrigerator Hum:* 40 dB
- *Normal conversation:* 60 dB
- *Vacuum cleaner:* 70 dB
- *Lawnmower:* 90 dB
- *Car Horn:* 110 dB
- *Fire work:* 140 dB
- *Jet Take off:* 150 dB

Audiometric Testing

- Evoked otoacoustic emission (EOAE) test function of outer hair cells, often used as a newborn hearing screen.
- Audiometry brainstem response (ABR) use electrodes to monitor brain activity response to sound stimulus, can be done at any age, but will often need to be sedated after age of 6 months.
- *Behavioral observation audiometry (BOA) (0–5 months):* Observes child response to sound stimulus. Does not assess laterally.
- *Visual reinforcement audiometry (VRA) (6 months to 2 years):* Child turns to visual cue in response to sound stimulus.
- *Conditioned play audiometry (CPA) (2–5 years):* Child interacts with toy or object in response to sound stimulus. Can assess laterally.
- *Conventional pure-tone audiometry (>5 years):* Raising hand in response to sound stimulus.

Degrees of Hearing Loss

Degree of hearing loss	*Thresholds (dB)*	*Description*
Normal	0–25 adult, 0–15 infant	Normal hearing
Mild	20–40	Unable to hear soft sounds. Can hear conversations in a quiet setting but may have difficulty in noisy environments
Moderate	41–55	Has difficulty in hearing some quieter conversations
Moderate severe	56–70	Has difficulty in hearing a normal conversation. May lip read or use hearing aids to assist with communication
Severe	71–90	Can understand speech only if the speaker is in close proximity
Profound	>90	Generally, cannot understand speech. Unable to hear 'loud' stimuli such as lawn mowers or passing cars

Types of Hearing Loss

- Conductive
- Sensorineural
- Mixed

Conductive Hearing Loss

- A conductive hearing loss occurs when sound from the environment is unable to be conducted to the structures of the inner ear.
- *Causes:*
  - Cerumen impaction
  - Tympanic membrane perforation
  - Middle ear fluid collection
  - Otosclerosis
- Conduction hearing loss can be assessed with Rinne and Weber tests.

Sensorium Hearing Loss

- *Causes:*
  - *Infections:* Meningitis, encephalitis, mumps, syphilis, etc.
  - *Medicines:* Aminoglycosides, furosemide, quinine, chloroquine
  - Familial
  - Temporal bone fractures
  - Congenital malformations
  - Acoustic neuroma, meningioma, etc.

Interpretation of Audiogram

A.

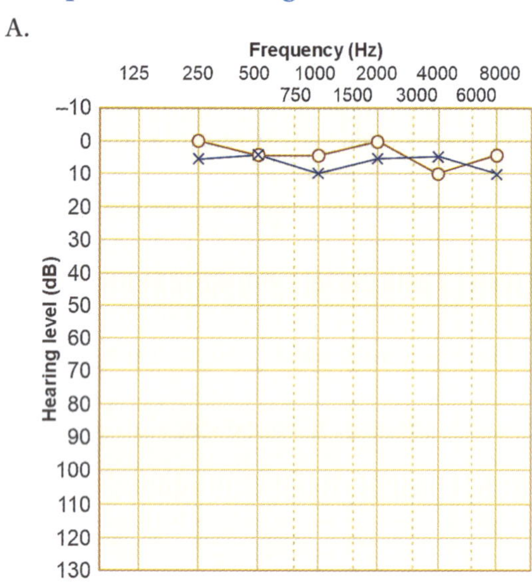

B.

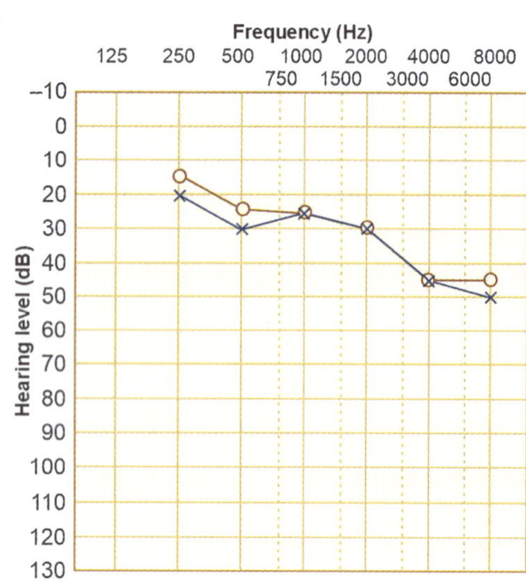

C.

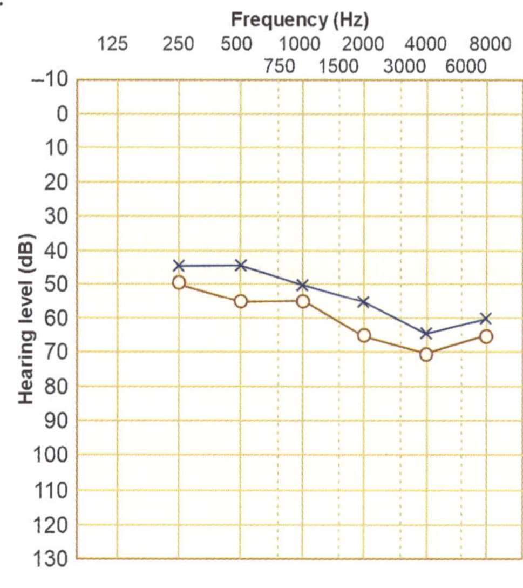

D.

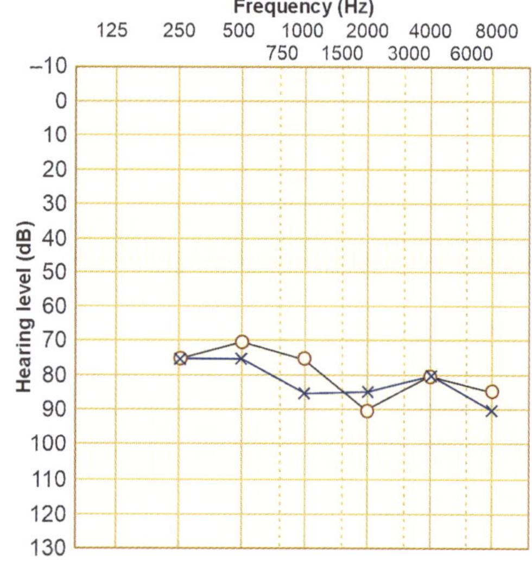

ANSWERS

A. Normal hearing
B. Mild hearing loss
C. Moderate hearing loss
D. Severe Hearing loss

SPIROGRAM

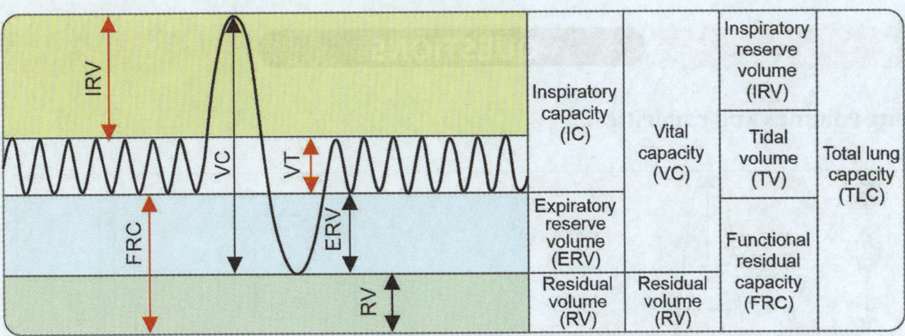

Spirometry

Spirometry is a method used to measure lung capacities and lung volumes. The instrument used for this purpose is called a spirometer. The subject usually breathes into the mouthpiece of this instrument and the further process is recorded in the form of graph. The graphical record that is used for inference is termed a spirogram.

Spirogram

Spirogram is the graphical record of lung capacities and lung volumes using a spirometer. In the above diagram, the upward deflection depicts inspiration and the downward deflection depicts expiration.

A typical spirogram comprises the following details of lung capacities and lung volumes:

- *Tidal volume (TV):* It is the volume of air respired in and out in a normal single respiration. It signifies the depth of breathing. Normal TV is 500 mL (0.5 L).
- Inspiratory reserve volume (IRV) is the volume of additional air that could be inhaled forcefully after a normal end inspiration. Normal value of IRV is 3300 mL (3.3 L).
- Expiratory reserve volume (ERV) is the volume of additional air that could be expired forcefully after a normal end expiration. Normal ERV is 1000 mL (1 L).
- *Residual volume (RV):* It is the volume of air that remains in the lungs even after forceful expiration. Normally, lungs cannot be completely emptied even after forceful expiration. Some amount of air always remains in the lungs even after the forced expiration. The normal RV is 1200 mL (1.2 L).

Static lung capacities are the mixture of 2 or more lung volumes. They are four types IC, VC, FRC and TLC.

- *Inspiratory capacity (IC)* is the maximum volume of the air that is inspired after normal expiration, it is the sum of TV and IRV (3800 mL).
- *Vital capacity (VC):* It is the maximum volume of air can be expelled out of the lungs forcefully after a deep inspiration. It is the sum of IRV, ERV, TV (4800 mL).
- *Forced vital capacity (FVC)* is the volume of air that could be exhaled rapidly and forcefully after a deep inspiration. It is usually equal to VC unless there is a pulmonary disease.
- *Functional residual capacity (FRD):* It is the volume of air in the lungs after a passive expiration. It is usually measured with the help of plethysmography, nitrogen wash out or helium dilution methods and not spirometry. It is the sum of RV and ERV (2200 mL).
- *Total lung capacity (TLC):* It is the volume of air present in the lungs after a maximal inspiration. It includes the sum of all the volumes (6000 mL).

PULMONARY FUNCTION TESTS

QUESTIONS

Q-1. Mark the lung volumes and capacities.

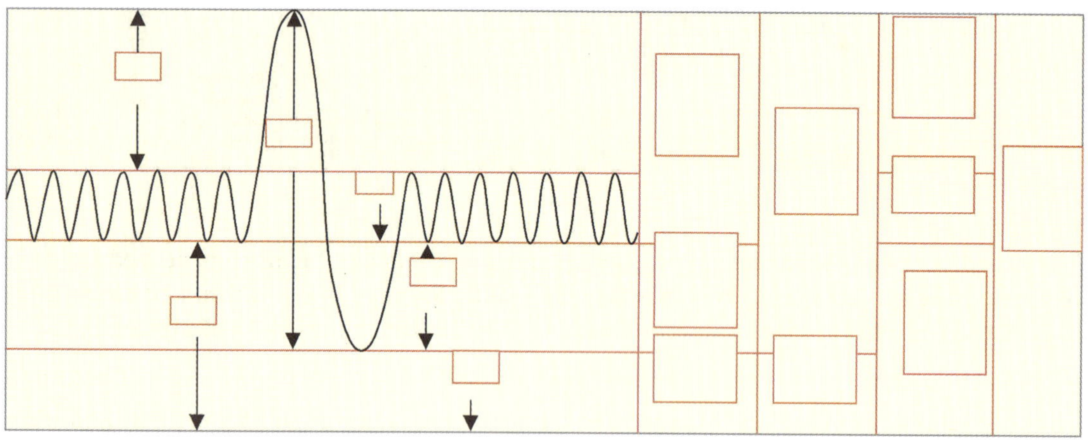

Q-2.

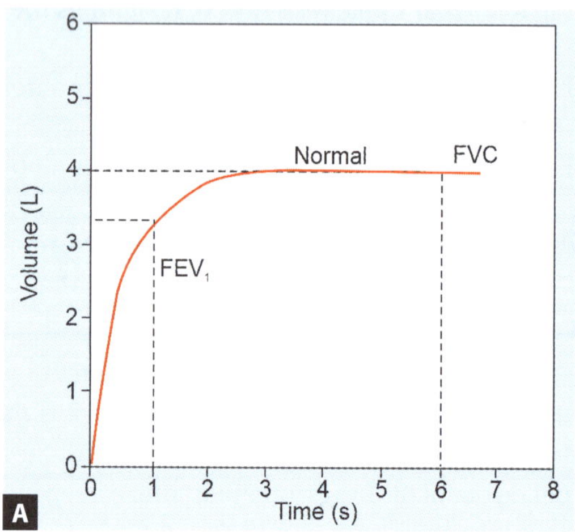

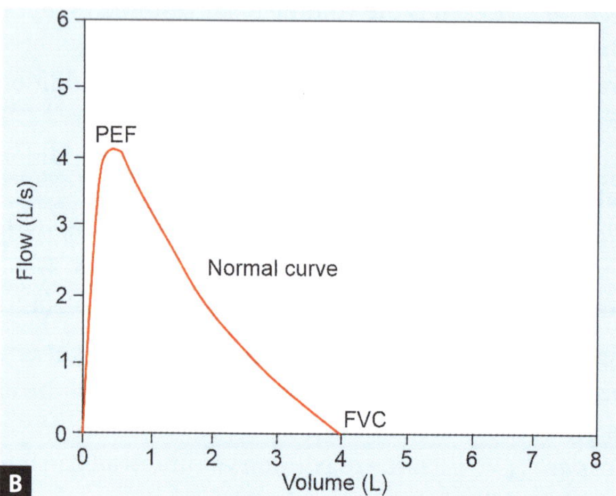

A. What is called curve 'A'?

B. What is called curve 'B'?

C. What is the interpretation of curve A?

D. What is the interpretation of curve B?

Q-3. Mention your interpretations of curves A, B and C.

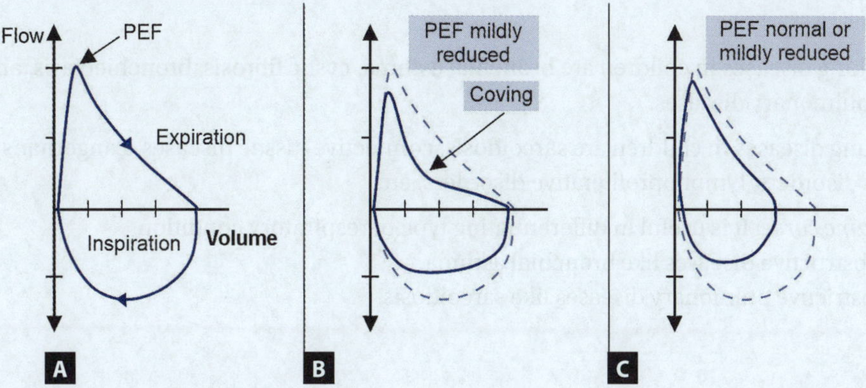

Q-4. Name obstructive lung diseases in children

Q-5. What are restrictive lung disease in children?

Q-6.

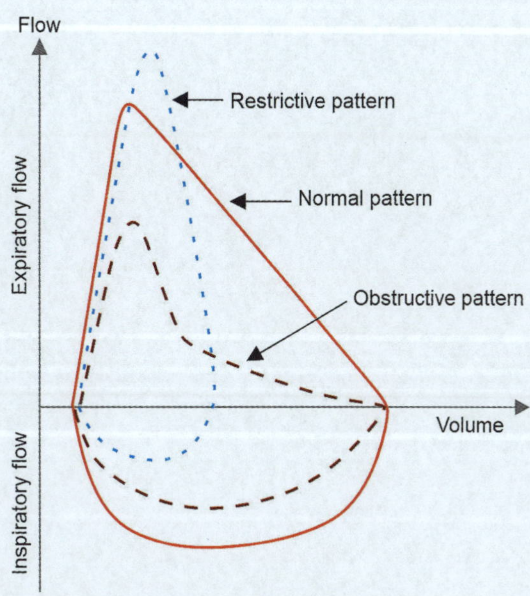

A. Identify the graphic picture and gives its use in clinical practice.
B. Give one example of green and black flow.

ANSWERS

A-1. Spirogram diagram

A-2. A. Volume time curve.
B. Flow volume curve.
C. Curve 'A' shows a 'Plateau' was reached well before the 6 second forced expiratory time (FET) was reached.
D. Curve 'B' shows a good start with a high peak flow. The flow gradually falls as volume falls.

A-3. *A:* Normal
B: Obstructive
C: Restrictive

A-4. Obstructive lung diseases in children are bronchial asthma, cystic fibrosis, bronchiectasis, and chronic obstructive pulmonary diseases.

A-5. Restrictive lung diseases in children are sarcoidosis, connective-tissue diseases, Langerhans cells histiocytosis, eosinophilic disorders, lymphoproliferative disorders, etc.

A-6. A. *Flow volume curve:* It is useful in differentiating type of respiratory condition.
B. *Green:* Obstructive diseases like bronchial asthma.
C. *Black:* Restrictive pulmonary diseases like sarcoidosis.

TYMPANOGRAM

Tympanogram is a test of middle ear functioning. It looks at the flexibility (compliance) of the eardrum to changing air pressure, indicating how effectively sound is transmitted into the middle ear. This objective test also allows us to view the functioning of the Eustachian Tube, the upper auditory pathways and the reflex contraction from the middle ear muscles. Impedance testing is crucial in distinguishing a conductive loss from a sensorineural hearing loss. A typical tympanometry result indicates the ear canal volume (cm^3), the max pressure (daPa) and the peak compliance (mL).

Interpretation of Tympanogram

A tympanogram provides information regarding the compliance of the middle ear system (how well sound passes through the eardrum to the middle ear system), ear canal volume and middle ear pressure. Compliance is plotted vertically on the tympanogram, and is measures in mL or mmho. Maximum compliance of middle ear system occurs when the pressure in the middle ear cavity is equal to the pressure in external auditory canal. This compliance (Static acoustic admittance) is represented by the highest peak of the curve on the graph. Pressure is indicated on the horizontal axis of the graph, and is measured in decaPascals (**Figure:** Type A Tympanogram).

Type A Tympanogram

It looks like a teepee and indicates a normal middle ear system, free of fluid or physiological anomalies which would prevent the admittance of sound from the middle ear into the cochlea.

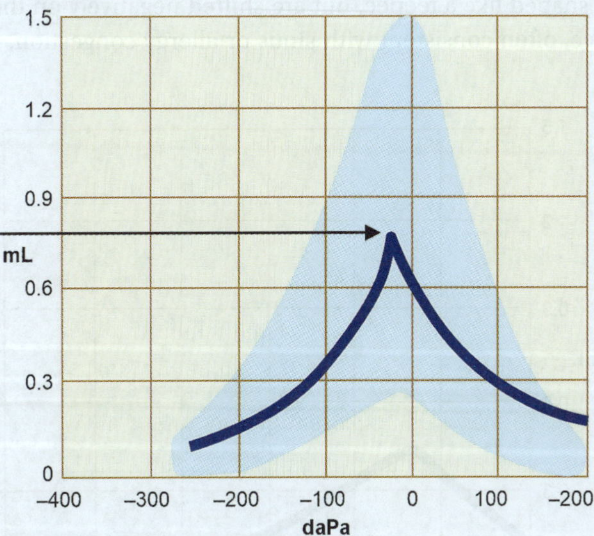

Type B Tympanogram

Type B tympanograms are a flat line, which is consistent with middle ear pathology, such as fluid or infection behind the eardrum. In some cases, these tympanograms are seen when there is a hole in the eardrum, the difference lies in the ear canal volume, the larger ear canal volume indicates a perforation in the eardrum.

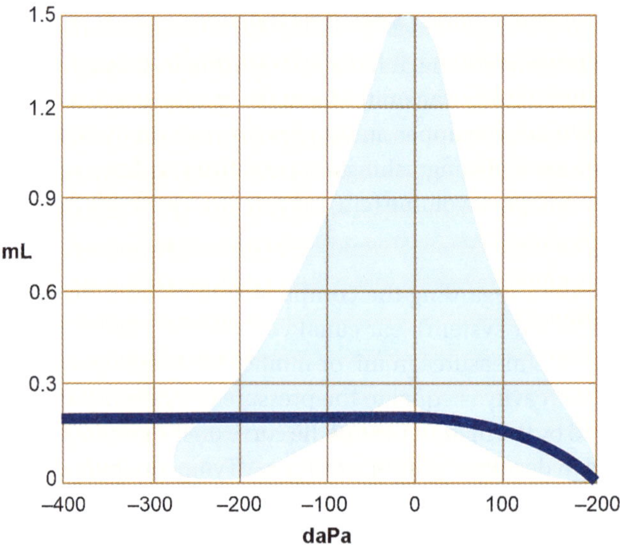

Type C Tympanogram

Type C tympanograms are still shaped like a teepee, but are shifted negatively on the graph. This indicates negative pressure in the middle ear space, often consistent with sinus or allergy congestion, or an end stage of a cold or ear infection.

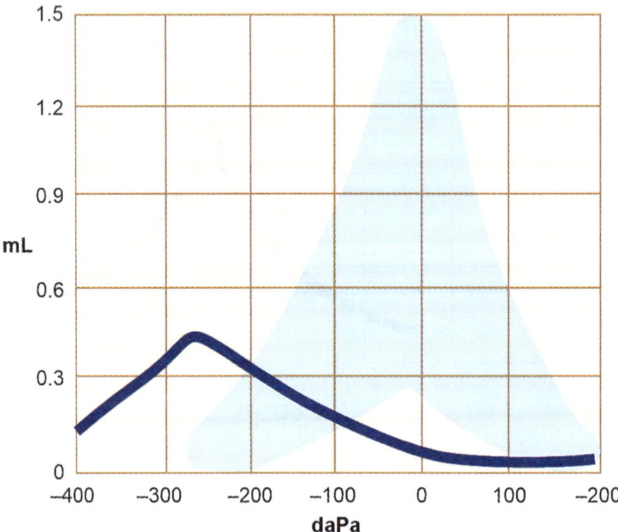

QUESTIONS

Q-1. Identify the types of tympanograms with once example for each one.

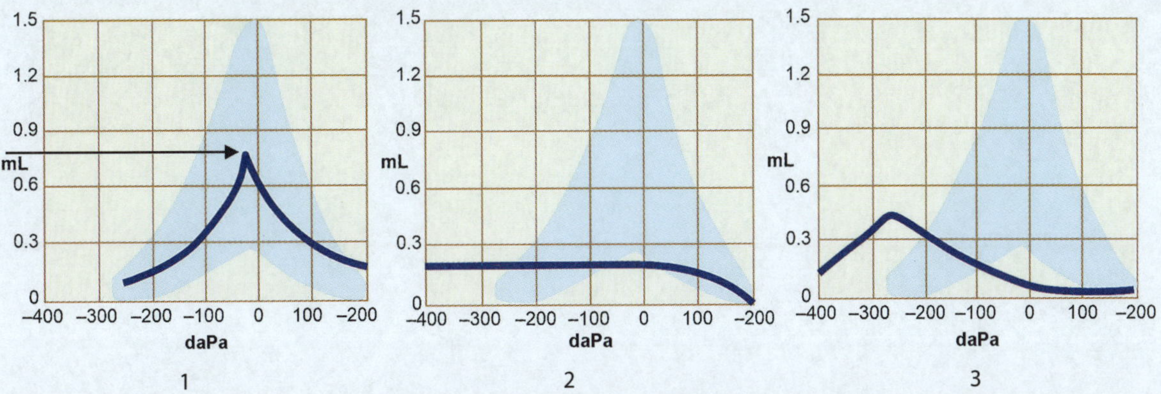

ANSWERS

A-1. 1. *Type A Tympanogram:* Normal middle ear

2. *Type B Tympanogram:* Perforation of eardrum
3. *Type C Tympanogram:* Sinus or allergy congestion

Index

Page numbers followed by *f* refer to figure.

D

E

F

G

H

I

Q

R

S

T